Blackwell's Five-Minute
Veterinary Consult

Clinical Companion

Small Animal
Toxicology

Blackwell's Five-Minute
Veterinary Consult

Clinical Companion

Small Animal
Toxicology

Gary D. Osweiler, DVM, MS, PhD, DABVT
Lynn R. Hovda, RPH, DVM, MS, DACVIM
Ahna G. Brutlag, DVM
Justine A. Lee, DVM, DACVECC

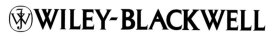

A John Wiley & Sons, Inc., Publication

Blackwell Publishing was acquired by John Wiley & Sons in February 2007. Blackwell's publishing program
has been merged with Wiley's global Scientific, Technical, and Medical business to form Wiley-Blackwell.

Editorial Office
2121 State Avenue, Ames, Iowa 50014-8300, USA

For details of our global editorial offices, for customer services, and for information about how to apply
for permission to reuse the copyright material in this book, please see our Website at www.wiley.com/
wiley-blackwell.

Library of Congress Cataloging-in-Publication Data

Blackwell's five-minute veterinary consult clinical companion. Small animal toxicology / Gary D. Osweiler
... [et al.].
    p. ; cm. – (Blackwell's five-minute veterinary consult series)
    Other title: Small animal toxicology
    Other title: Five-minute veterinary consult clinical companion
    Includes bibliographical references and index.
    ISBN 978-0-8138-1985-3 (pbk. : alk. paper)
    1. Veterinary toxicology–Handbooks, manuals, etc.   I. Osweiler, Gary D.   II. Title: Small animal
toxicology.   III. Title: Five-minute veterinary consult clinical companion.   IV. Series: Five minute
veterinary consult.
    [DNLM: 1. Poisoning–veterinary–Handbooks.   2. Veterinary Drugs–toxicity–
Handbooks.   3. Animals, Domestic–Handbooks.   SF 757.5 B632 2010]
    SF757.5.B63 2010
    636.089'59–dc22
                                    2010016558

9780813819853

A catalog record for this book is available from the U.S. Library of Congress.

Set in 10.5 on 13 pt Berkeley by Toppan Best-set Premedia Limited
Printed in Singapore by Markono Print Media Pte Ltd

1 2011

Dedication

This Clinical Companion book in small animal toxicology is a specialty extension of *The 5-Minute Veterinary Consult: Canine and Feline* by Drs. Larry Tilley and Frank Smith. We are grateful for their vision and innovation which fostered this clinical specialty series. The book owes its completion to our many excellent authors and to the associated editors whose breadth, depth and perseverance supported a timely completion.

Thanks also to thoughtful veterinary colleagues who have shared their questions, experiences and wisdom over the years to provide us a daily education in toxicology as a clinical specialty. On a personal note, I thank Sue and our children and grandchildren whose enthusiastic interest in animals is a continuing reminder of the world we share with the animals around us.
— Gary Osweiler

To old friends, many gone but never forgotten, and to Bob and Tyne, the anchors in my life.
— Lynn R. Hovda

I would like to dedicate this book to my colleagues at Pet Poison Helpline. My interest in toxicology has been sparked, nurtured, and sustained by their mentorship, knowledge and enthusiasm. I am deeply grateful for their continued support and friendship. In addition, I would like to thank my partner Nathan for his patience and love (and for cooking me dinner every night).
— Ahna G. Brutlag

To my parents, Ting and Anna, for their wisdom and faith, and to Dan and JP, for being the calm to my craziness.
— Justine A. Lee

Contents

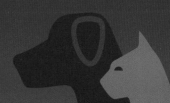

section **3**	**Reference Information**

See the supporting companion website for this book: www.wiley.com/go/osweiler

Preface

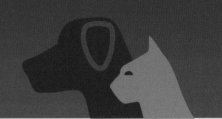

This new publication, *Blackwell's Five-Minute Veterinary Consult Clinical Companion: Small Animal Toxicology*, follows the lead of the successful *Five-Minute Veterinary Consult: Canine and Feline* 5th edition. The Five-Minute concept of providing essential and relevant information in an organized and easy to access format for veterinary clinicians continues in the Clinical Companion series. In addition, the focused and relevant information in this text provides an excellent support for teaching veterinary toxicology in professional curricula. Certainly, other very detailed texts are available to take the interested clinician and student into additional depth and breadth. These include other toxicology texts as well as detailed volumes in pharmacology, pathology, and chemistry that support concepts and tools of toxicology.

Blackwell's Five-Minute Veterinary Consult Clinical Companion: Small Animal Toxicology provides greatly expanded, in-depth coverage of toxicology. It is a logical, consistent, and sufficiently detailed resource designed to guide appropriate clinical decision making while accessing specific information quickly and efficiently. The coverage is organized by traditional categories of overview, etiology/pathophysiology (including mechanism of action, pharmacokinetics, toxicology, and systems affected), signalment/history, clinical features, key differential diagnoses, diagnostics, and therapeutics. Incorporated is information essential to toxicology evaluation such as dosage, absorption, distribution, metabolism, excretion, toxic doses, prevention, and public health issues. In addition, information discussing prompt detoxification and supportive therapy, as well as specific antidotes and drug therapies, is reviewed.

ORGANIZATION AND FORMAT

The first section of this book, Clinical Toxicology, provides organized and detailed information on the determination of dosage, effective detoxification, and effective life support measures that are often responsible for saving animals' lives even before a diagnosis can be confirmed. The Clinical Toxicology section offers information on the use of diagnostics to suggest or confirm specific poisonings and provide the basis for both therapy and prognosis.

The second section of this book, Specific Toxicants, is organized around well-recognized, broad categories of toxicants generally familiar to clients and the veterinarian alike. This section details 100 individual topics that present current problems in small animal toxicology. The selection of these topics is based on evidence from published literature, animal poison control centers, and veterinary colleges in North America. The multiple-author format and use of four editors provides a broad range of experiences by those whose professional careers are in the clinical specialties of toxicology, internal medicine, and emergency and critical care. Their professional experience increases the relevance of the topics chosen and presented.

Finally, the third section of this book, Reference Information, provides useful references including conversion tables, diagnostic values for toxicants, regulatory resources, and important resources for toxicology.

KEY FEATURES

Within each major category of specific toxicants, the individual chapters are arranged alphabetically to provide orderly access to the topics. Specific headings within each chapter are consistent and include the following categories: Definition/Overview, Etiology/Pathophysiology, Signalment/History, Clinical Features, Differential Diagnosis, Diagnostics, Therapeutics, and Comments (including client education, patient monitoring, and expected course and prognosis). Additionally, each chapter includes up to six pertinent and clinically relevant references to provide additional direction to the clinician or student.

APPENDICES

The reference information provided in the final section of this text contains comprehensive tables listing metallic toxicants, toxic plants, and topical products as well as the names of more toxicology publications, including major online resources from professional and governmental organizations.

Gary D. Osweiler, Lynn R. Hovda,
Ahna G. Brutlag, Justine A. Lee

Contributor List

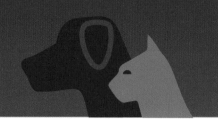

Catherine M. Adams, DVM
Pet Poison Helpline and SafetyCall
    International, PLLC
Minneapolis, Minnesota

Catherine Angle, DVM, MPH
Pet Poison Helpline and SafetyCall
    International, PLLC
Minneapolis, Minnesota

Danielle M. Babski, DVM
Resident, Emergency and Critical Care
Veterinary Teaching Hospital
University of Georgia
Athens, Georgia

Karyn Bischoff, DVM, MS, DABVT
Assistant Professor, Department of
    Population Medicine and Diagnostic
    Sciences
Cornell University
and
Diagnostic Toxicologist
New York State Animal Health
    Diagnostic Center
Ithaca, New York

Benjamin M. Brainard, VMD, DACVA,
    DACVECC
Assistant Professor
College of Veterinary Medicine
University of Georgia
Athens, Georgia

Ahna G. Brutlag, DVM
Assistant Director of Veterinary
    Services
Pet Poison Helpline and SafetyCall
    International, PLLC
Minneapolis, Minnesota

Erica Cargill, CVT
Pet Poison Helpline and SafetyCall
    International, PLLC
Minneapolis, Minnesota

Dana L. Clarke, VMD
Resident, Emergency and Critical
    Care
Matthew J. Ryan Veterinary Hospital at
    the University of Pennsylvania
Philadelphia, Pennsylvania

Seth L. Cohen, DVM
Associate Veterinarian
Kenwood Pet Clinic
Minneapolis, Minnesota

Elise M. Craft, DVM
Resident, Emergency and Critical
    Care
College of Veterinary Medicine
University of Minnesota
Saint Paul, Minnesota

Kenneth J. Drobatz, DVM, MSCE,
  DACVIM, DACVECC
Director, Emergency Services
Professor of Critical Care
Mathew J. Ryan Veterinary Hospital at
  the University of Pennsylvania
Philadelphia, Pennsylvania

Teresa K. Drotar, DVM
Veterinary Medical Officer
Training Specialist
Professional Development Staff
Veterinary Services
APHIS/USDA
Ames, Iowa

Kristin M. Engebretsen, PharmD,
  DABAT
Clinical Toxicologist
Emergency Medicine Department
Regions Hospital
Saint Paul, Minnesota
and
Clinical Associate Professor
Department of Experimental and
  Clinical Pharmacology
College of Pharmacy, University of
  Minnesota
Minneapolis, Minnesota

Dean Filandrinos, PharmD, MS
Senior Clinical Toxicologist
Vice President, Operations
Pet Poison Helpline and SafetyCall
  International, PLLC
and
Clinical Assistant Professor
Department of Experimental and
  Clinical Pharmacology
College of Pharmacy, University of
  Minnesota
Minneapolis, Minnesota

Sarah L. Gray, DVM
Resident, Emergency and Critical
  Care
College of Veterinary Medicine
University of Minnesota
Saint Paul, Minnesota

Nancy M. Gruber, DVM
Pet Poison Helpline and SafetyCall
  International, PLLC
Minneapolis, Minnesota

John Gualtieri, PharmD, MT (ASCP)
Senior Clinical Toxicologist
Vice President, Drug Safety and
  Pharmacovigilance
Pet Poison Helpline and SafetyCall
  International, PLLC
and
Clinical Assistant Professor
Department of Experimental and
  Clinical Pharmacology
College of Pharmacy, University of
  Minnesota
Minneapolis, Minnesota

Lauren E. Haak, PharmD
Pet Poison Helpline and SafetyCall
  International, PLLC
Minneapolis, Minnesota

Jeffery O. Hall, DVM, PhD, DABVT
Professor and Head, Diagnostic
  Toxicology
Utah Veterinary Diagnostic
  Laboratory
Department of Animal, Dairy, and
  Veterinary Sciences
Utah State University
Logan, Utah

Stephen B. Hooser, DVM, PhD,
    DABVT
Director, Animal Disease Diagnostic
    Laboratory
Purdue University
West Lafayette, Indiana

Lynn R. Hovda, RPH, DVM, MS,
    DACVIM
Director of Veterinary Services
Pet Poison Helpline and SafetyCall
    International, PLLC
Minneapolis, Minnesota
and
Adjunct Professor, Veterinary
    Population Medicine Department
College of Veterinary Medicine,
    University of Minnesota
Saint Paul, Minnesota

Tyne K. Hovda
Research Assistant
Pet Poison Helpline and SafetyCall
    International, PLLC
Minneapolis, Minnesota

Hwan Goo Kang, DVM, PhD
Senior Researcher
Veterinary Bioscience Division
National Veterinary Research and
    Quarantine Service
Anyang, Kyunggido
Republic of Korea

Megan I. Kaplan, DVM
Resident, Emergency and Critical Care
Allegheny Veterinary Emergency
    Trauma and Specialty
Monroeville, Pennsylvania

Daniel E. Keyler, PharmD
Codirector, Toxicology Research
Department of Pharmacology and
    Toxicology Research
Minneapolis Medical Research
    Foundation
Minneapolis, Minnesota
and
Clinical Professor
Department of Experimental and
    Clinical Pharmacology
College of Pharmacy, University of
    Minnesota
Minneapolis, Minnesota

Christy A. Klatt, DVM
Commission Veterinarian
Minnesota Racing Commission
Shakopee, Minnesota

Amie Koenig, DVM, DACVIM,
    DACVECC
Assistant Professor
College of Veterinary Medicine
University of Georgia
Athens, Georgia

Anita M. Kore, DVM, PhD, DABVT
3M Medical Department
Corporate Toxicology and Regulatory
    Services
Saint Paul, Minnesota

Justine A. Lee, DVM, DACVECC
Associate Director of Veterinary
    Services
Pet Poison Helpline and SafetyCall
    International, PLLC
Minneapolis, Minnesota

Stephen H. LeMaster, PharmD, MPH
Senior Clinical Toxicologist
Pet Poison Helpline and SafetyCall
    International, PLLC
Minneapolis, Minnesota
and
Clinical Assistant Professor
Department of Experimental and
    Clinical Pharmacology
College of Pharmacy, University of
    Minnesota
Minneapolis, Minnesota

Ta-Ying Debra Liu, DVM
Resident, Emergency and Critical Care
Matthew J. Ryan Veterinary Hospital at
    the University of Pennsylvania
Philadelphia, Pennsylvania

Josephine L. Marshall, CVT
Pet Poison Helpline and SafetyCall
    International, PLLC
Minneapolis, Minnesota

Krishona L. Martinson, PhD
Equine Extension Specialist and
    Assistant Professor
Department of Animal Science
University of Minnesota
Saint Paul, Minnesota

Charlotte Means, DVM, MLIS, DABVT,
    DABT
Senior Toxicologist
ASPCA Animal Poison Control Center
Urbana, Illinois

Michael Murphy, DVM, PhD, DABVT,
    DABT, JD
Veterinary Medical Officer
Food and Drug Administration, Center
    for Veterinary Medicine
Rockville, Maryland

Gary D. Osweiler, DVM, PhD, DABVT
Professor
Veterinary Diagnostic and Production
    Animal Medicine
College of Veterinary Medicine
Iowa State University
Ames, Iowa

Garret E. Pachtinger, VMD
Resident, Emergency and Critical Care
Mathew J. Ryan Veterinary Hospital of
    the University of Pennsylvania
Philadelphia, Pennsylvania

Katherine L. Peterson, DVM
Pet Poison Helpline and SafetyCall
    International, PLLC
Minneapolis, Minnesota

Michael E. Peterson, DVM, MS
Reid Veterinary Hospital
Albany, Oregon
and
Oregon State University
College of Veterinary Medicine
Corvallis, Oregon

Konnie H. Plumlee, DVM, MS,
    DABVT, DACVIM
Laboratory Director
Veterinary Diagnostic Laboratory
Arkansas Livestock and Poultry
    Commission
Little Rock, Arkansas

Robert H. Poppenga, DVM, PhD,
    DABVT
Professor of Veterinary Clinical and
    Diagnostic Toxicology
California Animal Health and Food
    Safety Laboratory
School of Veterinary Medicine
University of California
Davis, California

Lisa L. Powell, DVM, DACVECC
Associate Clinical Professor
College of Veterinary Medicine
University of Minnesota
Saint Paul, Minnesota

Birgit Puschner DVM, PhD, DABVT
Professor
Department of Molecular Biosciences
School of Veterinary Medicine
University of California
Davis, California

Jane Quandt, DVM, MS, DACVA,
    DACVECC
Associate Clinical Professor
College of Veterinary Medicine
University of Minnesota
Saint Paul, Minnesota

Carey L. Renken, MD
College of Veterinary Medicine
Iowa State University
Ames, Iowa

Mark Rishniw, BVSc, MS, PhD,
    DACVIM (cardiology and internal
    medicine)
Director of Clinical Research
Veterinary Information Network
Davis, California
and
Postdoctoral Associate
College of Veterinary Medicine
Cornell University
Ithaca, New York

Amber Roegner, BS
Graduate Student in Pharmacology/
    Toxicology
Department of Molecular Biosciences
School of Veterinary Medicine
University of California
Davis, California

Kelly M. Sioris, PharmD
Senior Clinical Toxicologist
Pet Poison Helpline and SafetyCall
    International, PLLC
Minneapolis, Minnesota
and
Clinical Assistant Professor
Department of Experimental and
    Clinical Pharmacology
College of Pharmacy, University of
    Minnesota
Minneapolis, Minnesota

Leo J. Sioris, PharmD
Senior Clinical Toxicologist
Chief Executive Officer
Pet Poison Helpline and SafetyCall
    International, PLLC
Minneapolis, Minnesota
and
Professor
Department of Experimental and
    Clinical Pharmacology
College of Pharmacy, University of
    Minnesota
Minneapolis, Minnesota

Sean Smarick, VMD, DACVECC
Staff Intensivist and Hospital Director
Allegheny Veterinary Emergency
    Trauma and Specialty (AVETS)
Monroeville, Pennsylvania

Rebecca S. Syring, DVM, DACVECC
Staff Veterinarian, Section of Critical
    Care
Matthew J. Ryan Veterinary Hospital of
    the University of Pennsylvania
Philadelphia, Pennsylvania

Patricia A. Talcott, DVM, PhD, DABVT
College of Veterinary Medicine
Washington State University
Pullman, Washington

Mary Anna Thrall, DVM, MS, DACVP
Professor
School of Veterinary Medicine
Ross University
Basseterre, St. Kitts
West Indies

Tina Wismer, DVM, DABVT, DABT
Senior Director of Veterinary Outreach
  and Education
ASPCA Animal Poison Control Center
Urbana, Illinois

Blackwell's Five-Minute
Veterinary Consult
Clinical Companion

Small Animal Toxicology

Clinical Toxicology

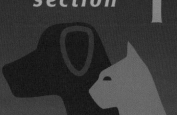

Decontamination and Detoxification of the Poisoned Patient

 DEFINITION/OVERVIEW

- In veterinary medicine, the primary treatment for toxicant exposure should be decontamination and detoxification of the patient.
- The goal of decontamination is to inhibit or minimize further toxicant absorption and to promote excretion or elimination of the toxicant from the body.
- Knowledge of the underlying mechanism of action, the pharmacokinetics (including absorption, distribution, metabolism, and excretion), and the toxic dose of the toxicant are imperative in determining appropriate decontamination and therapy for the patient.
- Decontamination can only be performed within a narrow window of time for most substances; therefore, it is important to obtain a thorough history and time since exposure.
- Decontamination categories may include ocular, dermal, inhalation, injection, GI, forced diuresis, and surgical removal to prevent absorption or enhance elimination of the toxicant.

Ocular Decontamination

- If ocular exposure has occurred, thorough evaluation and appropriate medical care of the eye may be necessary.
- Proper decontamination is often difficult for the pet owner, as it requires restraint of the animal.
- If the product is corrosive, owners should flush the eye at home with physiological saline (e.g., contact lens solution *without* any cleaners, soaps, etc.) or tepid water for 15–20 minutes prior to transportation to a veterinarian. This will help maximize decontamination and secondary injury to the cornea. Immediate veterinary care is imperative. Owners should be advised to prevent injury or rubbing of the eye until veterinary attention is sought. An Elizabethan collar should be used, if available.
- If the product is considered a *non*corrosive irritant, owners should flush the eye at home with physiological saline (e.g., contact lens solution *without* any cleaners, soaps, etc.) or tepid water for 10–15 minutes. Ophthalmic ointments or medications should *not* be used, and the pet should be monitored carefully for

an extended period of time to prevent iatrogenic corneal abrasion or ulceration from rubbing the eyes. Owners should be advised to prevent injury or rubbing of the eye. An Elizabethan collar should be used, if available. Any change in condition (e.g., blepharospasm, pupil size change, pruritis, ocular discharge) should prompt immediate medical attention.

Dermal Decontamination

- The goal of dermal decontamination is to prevent oral reexposure from the pet grooming itself and to prevent transdermal absorption.
- Owners should be advised to prevent the pet from grooming, and cautioned to protect themselves from exposure to the toxicant while transporting the pet to the veterinary clinic.
- When decontaminating a patient, it is important that pet owners and veterinary staff be protected from the toxic agent (e.g., pyrethrin, organophosphate, corrosive or caustic chemical, etc.). Appropriate protection should be used (e.g., rubber gloves, waterproof apron, face shield, etc.).
- Oil-based toxicities (e.g., pyrethrins) should be bathed off in tepid water and a liquid dish degreasing detergent (e.g., Dawn, Joy, etc.). The patient should be bathed and rinsed multiple times as soon after exposure as possible. Pet shampoos are typically insufficient to remove the oil-based product, and clinical signs may continue despite medical treatment due to continued absorption. Avoid the use of shampoos containing insecticides, coal tar, antibiotics, or antifungals.
- In fractious, tremoring cats exposed to pyrethrins, relaxation first with methocarbamol (see chap. 83, "Pyrethrins and Pyrethroids") may be beneficial. Once calmed, appropriate dermal decontamination can take place more easily.
- Gentle clipping of the hair may also help remove the toxin, particularly in long-haired pets or patients that cannot be bathed.
- If caustic, acidic, or alkaline exposure has occurred to the skin, careful, gentle decontamination must occur. The skin should be thoroughly flushed with copious amounts of tepid water for 15–20 minutes, making sure not to traumatize the area with abrasive scrubbing or high-pressure water sprays.
- Avoid the use of "neutralizing" agents on the skin (e.g., an acid for an alkaline exposure), as this may result in a chemical reaction that results in more serious dermal injury.
- Monitor temperature appropriately. Due to cooling from the bathing process, patients may become hypothermic and should be treated with heat support if necessary.

Inhalant Decontamination

- The patient should be removed from the source of exposure and evaluated. Often, simple removal is all that is necessary.

- Further treatment may include administration of a humidified oxygen source, monitoring of oxygenation and ventilation (e.g., via arterial blood gas analysis, pulse oximetry, co-oximetry, etc.) and rarely, mechanical ventilation. Please see chapters 103–104 on toxic gases for more information.
- The nares and upper airway help filter particulate matter, helping prevent lower airway exposure. The use of bronchoscopy is typically unnecessary.
- The area where the inhalant exposure occurred should be adequately ventilated to prevent reexposure by persistent toxic fumes.

Injection Decontamination

- Injection decontamination typically applies to embedded stingers or venom sacs in the animal's skin. The stinger and venom sac should be removed with gentle manipulation (e.g., tweezers) after careful examination of the affected area.
- Snake bites should not be decontaminated via incision and "sucking" of the venom from the bite wound, nor should hot or cold compressions or tourniquet application be used. Please see chapters 45–51 for more information on envenomations.

Gastrointestinal Decontamination

- The medical recommendation to decontaminate a pet at home must be thoroughly evaluated by the veterinarian or veterinary staff.
- A thorough history should be obtained from the pet owner prior to emesis induction (for home emesis or veterinary emesis induction).
- It is important to understand the contraindications for emesis induction to prevent secondary complications such as aspiration pneumonia, protracted emesis, hematemesis, or caustic or corrosive injury to the esophagus, oropharynx, and GIT.
- Important factors when considering emesis induction:
  - Time frame—A thorough history and time frame since ingestion must be obtained prior to recommendations for emesis induction. If several hours have passed, toxic contents may have moved out of the stomach. Emesis induction is indicated for most toxins ingested within 1 hour. Certain toxins like salicylates, opioids, anticholinergics, and TCA antidepressants can delay gastric emptying; with these specific toxins, one can induce emesis up to 4 hours postingestion, provided the patient is asymptomatic.
  - Underlying medical problems—Certain breeds with known brachycephalic syndrome (e.g., stenotic nares, everted saccules, hypoplastic trachea, and elongated soft palate) may be at higher risk for aspiration, and emesis induction at a veterinary facility may be safer. Dogs with a prior history of laryngeal paralysis, megaesophagus, aspiration pneumonia, upper airway disease, etc., should not have emesis induction performed due to the high risk of aspiration pneumonia.

- Symptomatic patients—Patients that are already symptomatic should not undergo emesis induction. Symptomatic patients that are excessively sedate may have a decreased gag reflex or a lowered seizure threshold and may be unable to protect their airway, resulting in aspiration pneumonia.
- Corrosive or caustic agent—Emesis induction may cause additional damage to the esophagus, oropharynx, and GIT when these agents are expelled.
- Hydrocarbons—Low-viscosity liquids can be easily aspirated into the respiratory system, resulting in severe aspiration pneumonia. Examples include gasoline, kerosene, motor oil, transmission fluid, tiki torch oil, citronella, etc. See chapter 9 on hydrocarbons for more information.

Effectiveness of Emesis Induction:

- The effectiveness of emesis induction is based on several factors, including:
  - Emetic agent used
  - Time elapsed since ingestion
  - Physical characteristics of the toxin ingested
  - Toxicant's effect on gastric emptying
  - Presence of gastric contents (see chap. 101 on phosphides)
- The more rapidly emesis is induced postingestion, the greater yield of recovery of gastric contents. Studies have shown that gastric recovery within 1 hour after toxin ingestion was approximately 17%–62%. When emesis was induced within an even shorter time span (within 30 minutes), mean recovery of gastric contents was approximately 49% (range 9%–75%).
- While delayed emesis after 1 hour may still be successful, the amount of gastric recovery significantly decreases as time passes.
- Emesis induction performed after 4 hours is likely of no benefit, with the exception of large bezoars or concretions of toxic agents (if still present in the stomach). Examples include:
  - Large wads of xylitol gum
  - Large amounts of chocolate
  - Grapes and raisins
  - Iron tablets which may form a concretion or bezoar
  - Blood or bone meal
  - Foreign material (see chap. 63 on foreign bodies)
  - Drugs that delay gastric emptying (e.g., opioids, anticholinergics, salicylates, TCA antidepressants)

RECOMMENDATIONS FOR HOME EMESIS

- The decision to recommend emesis induction at home is based on the clinical judgment of the veterinary facility.

- Numerous "antidotes" and "emetics" exist on the Internet, and pet owners may find and use inappropriate information. Rumors of grease, clay, dirt, vegetable oil, milk, bread, etc. all have been reportedly used by pet owners as antidotes or emetics.
- In addition, pet owners may use an inappropriate dose based on an estimated weight of the patient, resulting in an ineffective dose or side effects (e.g., protracted vomiting, hematemesis). Appropriate counseling by the veterinary staff is imperative (on which emetic to use, how much to use, if home emesis induction is warranted, etc.).
- As time is of the essence with emesis induction, it is often more effective to seek veterinary attention immediately rather than attempt emesis induction at home. This depends on the comfort and ability of the pet owner and availability of appropriate emetics at home. Rather than send a pet owner to a local store to purchase hydrogen peroxide and wait 10 minutes for the effect of the emetic (which may or may not be productive), it may be more efficient to seek veterinary care for prompt emesis induction.
- Certain human medications have a rapid onset of action, and clinical signs can be seen as early as 15–30 minutes. In these situations, emesis induction is not recommended at home and is best done under the supervision of a veterinarian. Examples include selective serotonin reuptake inhibitors, baclofen, and benzodiazepine or non-benzodiazepine agents (e.g., sleep aids like Ambien).

Emetic Agents

- Currently the only recommended oral emetic is 3% hydrogen peroxide. Others that have been previously recommended include table salt (sodium chloride, or NaCl), liquid dishwashing detergent, or 7% syrup of ipecac.
- Common veterinary emetics available at a veterinary clinic include apomorphine (tablets, capsules, or injectable) and alpha$_2$-adrenergic agonist agents like xylazine. Hydrogen peroxide is also commonly used by veterinarians as an emetic.

3% Hydrogen Peroxide
- Hydrogen peroxide is the *current* recommendation for at-home emesis induction in dogs. Only the 3% concentration should be used, as higher concentrations can result in severe gastritis.
- Hydrogen peroxide is ineffective in cats and is *not* recommended, as they froth and foam from administration, rarely vomit, and may develop a severe gastritis. Cats ingesting toxic products should be sent directly to the veterinarian for emesis induction under veterinary supervision.
- Hydrogen peroxide is thought to act as an emetic by direct gastric irritation. The product should be nonexpired (e.g., fresh, bubbly) to be most effective.
- Dose of hydrogen peroxide: 1–5 mL/kg orally, not to exceed 50 mL in dogs.

- It should be acknowledged that this dose has been exceeded by many veterinarians without ill-effect; however, persistent emesis and hematemesis may result.
- Emesis induction typically occurs within 10 minutes. If the first dose is ineffective as an emetic, a second dose can be repeated.
- Hydrogen peroxide is generally safe, but more than two doses should not be administered at home before seeking veterinary attention.
- Pet owners should be informed that they must carefully syringe hydrogen peroxide (via turkey baster, oral syringe, etc.), as most dogs will not electively drink this on their own, delaying emesis even further. Owners should be careful to prevent aspiration during administration.
- Hydrogen peroxide works best if a small amount of food is present in the stomach (e.g., the pet owner should be informed to feed a few dog treats or small amount of kibble prior to emesis induction).
- Another option is to soak a small amount of food or bread with the prescribed amount of hydrogen peroxide.

Table Salt (Sodium Chloride)
- The use of salt as an emetic is *no* longer recommended due to the risks of hypernatremia, persistent emesis, and hematemesis.
- Salt acts as an emetic by direct gastric irritation.
- Dose of salt in dogs and cats: 1 to 3 teaspoons orally.
- Emesis induction typically occurs within 10–15 minutes.
- In children treated with salt as an emetic, hypernatremia, secondary cerebral edema, and neurologic complications have been seen (see chap. 61 on salt toxicity).

Liquid Dish Detergent (e.g., Dawn, Palmolive, Joy)
- The use of liquid dish detergent is not typically recommended, although it may be considered more benign than table salt or syrup of ipecac.
- Detergents containing phosphate are most effective (thus excluding eco-friendly products).
- Liquid dish detergent acts as an emetic due to direct gastric irritation.
- Dose: 10 mL/kg of a *mixture* of 3 tablespoons of detergent to 8 ounces of water.
- Emesis induction typically occurs within 20 minutes.
- It is imperative that pet owners and veterinary staff ensure that the appropriate product is used, rather than electric dishwater soap or laundry detergents. These types of detergents should *never* be used due to their alkaline nature, which may cause severe injury to the GIT.

7% Syrup of Ipecac
- Syrup of ipecac is *no* longer recommended as an emetic in both human and veterinary medicine.
- Syrup of ipecac is derived from *Cephaelis ipecacuanha*, which is a dried root indigenous to South America.

- Syrup of ipecac acts as an emetic due to direct gastric irritation and stimulation of the CTZ. This is likely due to the active alkaloid compounds emetine and cephaeline.
- Syrup of ipecac is not to be confused with ipecac fluid extract, which is much more potent (14×).
- Dose: dogs, 1–2 mL/kg PO; cats, 3.3 mL/kg; cumulative dose in either species is not to exceed 15 mL; dose may be repeated once.
- Emesis induction typically occurs within 10–30 minutes but may take up to 1 hour.
- Potential complications from syrup of ipecac administration include:
  - Delayed effect
  - Lack of effectiveness in approximately 50% of small animals
  - Distaste (particularly to cats)
  - Protracted emesis, hematemesis, lethargy, diarrhea, depression
  - Potential cardiotoxic arrhythmogenic action

VETERINARY EMETIC AGENTS

Apomorphine (tablets, capsules, or injectable)

- Apomorphine is an effective emetic used by veterinarians.
- Apomorphine acts directly on the CTZ.
- Dose: dogs, 0.02–0.04 mg/kg IV or IM; or direct application of the tablet form into the subconjuctival sac. The injectable apomorphine can also be administered SQ; however, this is not currently the recommended route due to delayed onset of action and a prolonged duration of effect. If subconjunctival apomorphine is used, thorough flushing of the subconjunctival sac must be performed after emesis induction, or protracted vomition may occur.
- Emesis occurs within 4–6 minutes.
- If emesis does not occur, a second titrated dose (e.g., half of a tablet) can be used. If emesis does not occur after a second dose, an additional oral dose of hydrogen peroxide may be beneficial. (Clinically, some breeds like Labrador retrievers seem to require an additional peroxide dose.)
- Apomorphine is not recommended for cats, as it is an ineffective emetic and may result in CNS stimulation.
- The use of apomorphine as an emetic should be carefully considered with opioid or sedative toxicity, due to the potential for severe sedation.
- If a patient exhibits excessive CNS sedation or respiratory depression after apomorphine administration, naloxone can be used as a reversal (dose: 0.01–0.04 mg/kg, IV, IM, or SQ). However, naloxone will not reverse the emetic effect of apomorphine due to different receptor effects.
- Apomorphine tablets can be purchased through veterinary pharmaceutical companies.

Xylazine

- Xylazine is an emetic used by veterinarians for emesis induction in cats, but it may occasionally be effective in dogs.
- Xylazine is a centrally mediated alpha$_2$-adrenergic agonist.
- Dose: cats, 0.44–1 mg/kg, IM or SQ.
- Emesis induction typically occurs within 10 minutes but is not always effective.
- The use often results in profound CNS and respiratory depression, and cats should be carefully monitored for excessive side effects.
- Xylazine can be reversed with alpha$_2$-adrenergic antagonists:
  - Yohimbine: 0.1 mg/kg IM, SQ, or IV slowly
  - Atipamezole (Antisedan): 25–50 µg/kg IM, IV

Gastric Lavage (fig. 1.1)

- The goal of gastric lavage is to remove gastric contents when emesis induction is unproductive or contraindicated.
- Human studies have shown that if gastric lavage was performed within 15 to 20 minutes after toxicant ingestion, gastric lavage recoveries were minimal (38% and 29%, respectively). If lavage was performed at 60 minutes postingestion, only 8.6%–13% was recovered.
- As most poisoned patients present to the veterinary clinic after 1 hour, the clinical usefulness of gastric lavage is debated.

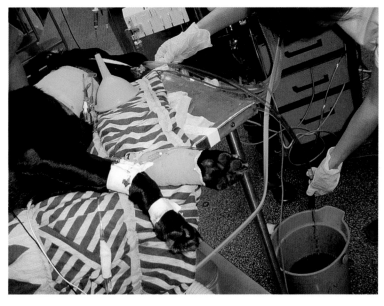

■ **Fig. 1.1.** A patient undergoing gastric lavage. Note IV catheter placement, intubation with an endotracheal tube with an inflated cuff, and gastric lavage. (Photo courtesy of Justine A. Lee)

- Despite low gastric recovery and labor intensiveness, the use of gastric lavage is indicated in certain circumstances:
  - A symptomatic patient that is already excessively sedate, unconscious, tremoring, or seizing that still needs controlled decontamination (e.g., metaldehyde, organophosphates)
  - Material that is large in size or has formed a bezoar or concretion (e.g., bone meal, iron tablets, large amounts of chocolate, etc.)
  - Large toxic ingestions of capsules or tablets approaching the LD_{50} (e.g., calcium channel blockers, beta-blockers, baclofen, organophosphorous and carbamate insecticides)
- A newer modality is to administer AC via orogastric tube prior to lavage to prevent further absorption of the toxin, and then to lavage out the charcoal-toxin complex. Following copious lavage, AC is then readministered. There is lack of data evaluating this technique, and this modality still needs to be evaluated.
- Complications of gastric lavage include:
  - Aspiration pneumonia
  - Risks of sedation
  - Hypoxemia secondary to aspiration pneumonia or hypoventilation from sedation
  - Mechanical injury to the mouth, oropharynx, esophagus, or stomach
- Contraindications for gastric lavage include:
  - A corrosive agent, where esophageal or gastric perforation can occur with orogastric tube placement
  - A hydrocarbon agent, which may be easily aspirated due to its low viscosity
  - Sharp objects ingested (e.g., sewing needles, etc.)
- Many veterinarians may not feel comfortable performing gastric lavage, but it can be easily accomplished when organized with the appropriate supplies in a team-oriented approach.
  - Begin by preparing all materials in an organized fashion:
    - ◻ White tape
    - ◻ Mouth gag
    - ◻ Sterile lubrication
    - ◻ Gauze
    - ◻ Warm lavage fluid in a bucket
    - ◻ Bilge or stomach pump
    - ◻ Funnel
    - ◻ Step stool
    - ◻ Sedatives predrawn and labeled
    - ◻ Sterile ETT with a high-volume, low-pressure cuff
    - ◻ Empty syringe to inflate the cuff
    - ◻ Material to secure and tie-in the ETT

- □ IV catheter supplies
  - □ Activated charcoal predrawn in 60-mL syringes ready for administration
  - □ Sedation reversal agents if necessary
- Place an IV catheter.
- Sedate and intubate with ETT; secure ETT in place and connect to oxygen ± inhalant anesthesia source. Inflate cuff to prevent aspiration of gastric contents or lavage fluid. Place the patient in right lateral recumbency.
- Premeasure an appropriately sized orogastric tube to the last rib and mark this line with white tape. This will be the maximum distance to pass the tube.
- Lubricate the orogastric tube, and pass the tube into the stomach using gentle, twisting motions. Blowing into the other end of the tube to inflate the esophagus with air may assist with passing of the tube into the stomach.
- Confirm orogastric tube placement by:
  - □ Palpation of the orogastric tube on abdominal palpation
  - □ Blowing into the orogastric tube and simultaneously ausculting for "bubbles" or blowing in the stomach
  - □ Palpation of the neck for two tubelike structures (trachea, esophagus with tube placement)
- Infuse tepid or warm water by gravity flow via funnel, bilge, or stomach pump. The volume of the stomach is approximately 60–90 mL/kg; therefore, copious amounts of fluid can be used to gavage. Fluid recovery (by gravity) should be emptied into an empty bucket.
- The stomach should be frequently palpated to monitor over-distension of the stomach, and massaged/agitated to help break up contents within the stomach; this will hopefully allow small material to be removed via gastric lavage.
- Several lavage cycles (>5–10) should be performed to maximize decontamination of the stomach. All of the gavage fluid, if possible, should be removed prior to AC administration.
- The gastric lavage fluid should be examined for the presence of plant material or pills, and can be saved for toxicological testing.
- Prior to removal of the orogastric tube, the appropriate amount of activated charcoal (with a cathartic for the first dose) should be instilled.
- The AC contents can then be flushed further into the orogastric tube with water or by blowing forcefully into the tube.
- Prior to removal of the orogastric tube, it is imperative that the tube be kinked off to prevent lavage fluid from being aspirated. Once kinked, the tube should be removed quickly in one sweeping movement.

- The patient should continue to be intubated until gag reflex is present. Positioning the patient in sternal recumbency with the head elevated may help prevent aspiration.

Whole Bowel Irrigation (WBI)

- The goal of WBI is to clean the GIT by removing toxins and normal intraluminal GI contents.
- This is done by enteral administration of large amounts of polyethylene glycol electrolyte solution (PEG-ES, or PEG; e.g., Golytely) until effluent (e.g., stool) is clear.
- WBI is frequently done in human medicine, but less so in veterinary medicine.
- Indications in veterinary medicine include bowel preparation for endoscopy, colonoscopy, or for emergency detoxification for specific toxicants.
- WBI should be performed with toxic levels of iron tablets, large ingestions of sustained-release medicines, or ingestion of enteric-coated tablets.
- Due to the massive amount of PEG-ES that needs to be ingested, administration must typically occur via a temporary feeding tube.
- Dose of PEG-ES: 25–40 mL/kg, followed by continuous oral infusion via naso-esophageal or nasogastric tube of 0.5 mL/kg/hour. Alternatively, 30–40 mL/kg can be gavaged every 2 hours.
- Stool typically appears within 2–4 hours, and WBI should be continued for approximately 8–12 hours until the effluent is clear.
- The use of antiemetics may be necessary. Metoclopramide (0.2–0.5 mg/kg, SQ) would be an appropriate choice due to its antiemetic and gastric emptying effects.
- Complications of WBI include nausea, vomiting, bloating, abdominal discomfort, and possible aspiration pneumonia.
- Contraindications for WBI include a foreign body obstruction, ileus, perforated bowel, shock, refractory emesis, and significant GI hemorrhage.

Activated Charcoal (AC)

- The goal of AC is to act as an adsorbent and to prevent systemic administration.
- While less commonly used in human medicine, AC still remains the primary treatment of choice for detoxification of a patient.
- AC is produced by heating wood pulp to extreme temperatures (900°C), washing it with inorganic acids, and drying it. This results in "activated" charcoal particles with a high surface area that promotes absorption. One gram of AC has approximately $1000 \, m^2$ of surface area.
- AC contains carbon moieties that adsorb compounds with varying affinity.
  - Nonpolar compounds bind to AC well.
  - Heavy metals and alcohols (e.g., ethylene glycol) typically are not absorbed by AC.

- Xylitol binds poorly to AC.
- The interaction between the bound toxin to AC could potentially undergo desorption; hence, the addition of a cathartic to help promote GIT transit time is imperative to help decrease the time for desorption to potentially occur.
  - Administration of AC with a cathartic as long as 6 hours out may still be beneficial with toxicosis, particularly if the product has delayed release (e.g., extended or sustained release) or undergoes enterohepatic recirculation.
  - The use of AC with a magnesium-containing cathartic should be used judiciously in cats.
- Dose: 1–5 g of AC per kg of body weight; in general, the higher dosage used, the more effective the adsorption.
- Certain situations or toxicities warrant multidose administration of AC. Drugs undergoing enterohepatic recirculation, or sustained, extended, or long-acting release products will require multidose administration of AC.
- Dose: for multidose charcoal (1–2 g/kg, PO q 4–6 hours for 24 hours).
  - Additional doses of AC should *not* contain a cathartic, due to increased risks for dehydration via fluid losses from the GIT.
- There are several types of AC commercially available, and the labeled directions should be followed appropriately for each specific type, as the dose is dependent on the product used and concentration. Many types also contain a cathartic already present (e.g., typically 70% sorbitol).
- AC tablets and capsules are not as effective as AC liquid slurries.
- Few animals will ingest AC voluntarily, and administration may need to occur via forced but careful syringe feeding or orogastric tube administration.
- Due to the thick viscosity of AC, it is often difficult to administer via NE or NG tube administration.
- Rarely, reports of hypernatremia have been clinically seen with AC administration. This is likely due to the sorbitol effect (see "Cathartics"). The patient should be assessed for hydration status. Appropriate fluid supplementation (SQ, IV) should be used to prevent dehydration and hypernatremia.
- Contraindications for AC include endoscopy, abdominal surgery of the GIT, gastric or intestinal obstruction, perforation of the GIT, late-stage presentation with clinical signs already present, dehydration, lack of borborgymi, ileus, hypernatremia, hypovolemic shock, a compromised airway (risk for aspiration pneumonia), caustic substance ingestion, and hydrocarbon toxicosis (due to increased risk for aspiration pneumonia).
- The use of antiemetics should be considered, due to the high prevalence of vomiting from cathartic administration (or from the emetic previously used to decontaminate the patient):
  - Maropitant 1 mg/kg, SQ q 24 hours; not labeled for cats
  - Ondansetron 0.1–0.2 mg/kg, SQ, IM, IV q 6–12 hours

- Metoclopramide 0.2–0.5 mg/kg, SQ, IM q 8–12 hours; or CRI at 1–2 mg/kg/day IV; generally less effective as an antiemetic than maropitant or ondansetron, but provides gastric emptying and a prokinetic effect.

Cathartics

- Cathartics are designed to increase the speed and transit time of the GIT, promoting fecal excretion of the toxin; more importantly, carthartics decrease the time allowed for toxin absorption through the GIT.
- Two of the most common types of cathartics used in the poisoned patient include:
  - Saccharide cathartics (e.g., sorbitol)
  - Saline cathartics (e.g., magnesium citrate, magnesium sulfate, sodium sulfate)
- Dose: sorbitol (70% solution, 1–2 mL/kg, PO, given within 60 minutes of toxin ingestion).
- Side effects of sorbitol administration: vomiting, dehydration, secondary hypernatremia, abdominal cramping or pain, and possible hypotension.
- Contraindications for cathartics are similar to those for AC listed above.
- Mineral oil is *no* longer recommended as a cathartic due to the high risks of aspiration.
- The use of cathartics alone is no longer recommended or beneficial.
- Cathartics should not be used in a dehydrated patient, due to the risks of voluminous fluid losses through the GIT and secondary hypernatremia. For patients receiving either multidoses of AC with or without cathartics, serum sodium levels and hydration status should be carefully monitored.

Fluid Therapy

- Fluid therapy is one of the cornerstone therapies of emergency management of the poisoned patient to:
  - Correct dehydration
  - Maintain perfusion at a cellular level
  - Vasodilate the renal vessels, flush the renal tubules, and diurese (particularly with nephrotoxic agents like NSAIDs, lilies, etc.)
  - Treat hypotension (particularly with drugs like beta-blockers, calcium channel blockers, ACE-inhibitors, etc.)
- Fluid therapy can also be used to aid in detoxification of the patient by increasing renal excretion of toxicants by forced diuresis, provided the toxicants undergo renal excretion.
- Dose: The dose of IV fluids to administer is dependent on the clinical state and physical examination findings of the patient.
  - In a healthy patient, fluid rates of 4–6 mL/kg/hour can be used to force renal clearance of the toxicant.

- Neonates have a higher maintenance fluid rate (80–100 mL/kg/day), and fluid rates should be adjusted accordingly.
- Patients with cardiac disease, respiratory disease, or those who have ingested toxicants that may increase the patient's risk of pulmonary edema (e.g., TCA antidepressants, phosphide rodenticides, etc.) should have judicious fluid administration.
- Careful assessment of hydration should be made based on PCV/TS, weight gain, CVP, and physical examination findings.
- The additional use of diuretics can be used in hydrated patients to increase forced diuresis:
  - Furosemide 2–4 mg/kg, IV, SQ, IM q 6–8 hours
  - Mannitol 1–2 g/kg, IV slow over 20–30 minutes q 6–8 hours
- Highly protein-bound toxins are not cleared efficiently by diuresis (e.g., NSAIDs).
- Drugs that respond well to forced diuresis include:
  - Phenobarbital
  - Amphetamines
  - Salicylate
  - Lithium
  - Bromide

Surgical Decontamination

- Surgical removal of toxic agents may occasionally need to be performed, particularly if the toxicant is caustic or corrosive (e.g., batteries), results in a bezoar that cannot be removed by gastric lavage (e.g., iron tablets, bone meal), results in foreign body obstruction (e.g., Gorilla glue), or continues to leach their toxic effect (e.g., Amitraz collars, zinc pennies, fentanyl or nicotine patches, etc.). Please see chapter 63, "Foreign Bodies," for more information.
- Prior to surgery, patients should have radiographs done to verify presence of the agent and presence of an obstructive pattern. Keep in mind that not all foreign bodies may be radiopaque. Patients should be properly volume resuscitated with IV fluid therapy and antiemetic therapy, and have their electrolyte, glucose, or acid-base imbalances corrected prior to anesthesia.

CONCLUSIONS

- Aggressive decontamination and detoxification of the poisoned patient is imperative and is still considered the mainstay therapy in veterinary medicine.
- The clinician should feel well versed in appropriate decontamination methods to treat poisoned patients.

Abbreviations

AC   = activated charcoal
ACE   = angiotensin converting enzyme

CNS	= central nervous system
CRI	= continuous rate infusion
CTZ	= chemoreceptor trigger zone
CVP	= central venous pressure
ETT	= endotracheal tube
GI	= gastrointestinal
GIT	= gastrointestinal tract
IM	= intramuscular
IV	= intravenous
NE	= nasoesophageal
NG	= nasogastric
NSAIDS	= nonsteriodal anti-inflammatory drugs
PCV	= packed cell volume
PEG-ES	= polyethylene glycol electrolyte solution
PO	= *per os* (by mouth)
q	= every
SQ	= subcutaneous
TCA	= tricyclic antidepressants
TS	= total solids
WBI	= whole bowel irrigation

Suggested Reading

Peterson ME. Toxicological decontamination. In Peterson ME, Talcott PA, eds. Small Animal Toxicology, 2nd ed. St. Louis: Elsevier Saunders, 2006, pp. 127–141.

Cope RB. A screening study of xylitol binding in vitro to activated charcoal. Vet Human Tox 2004; 46:336–337.

Plumb DC. Veterinary Drug Handbook, 6th ed. Ames: Blackwell Publishing Professional, 2008.

Author: Justine A. Lee, DVM, DACVECC
Consulting Editors: Justine A. Lee, DVM, DACVECC; Lynn R. Hovda, DVM, MS, DACVIM

chapter 2

Emergency Management of the Poisoned Patient

DEFINITION/OVERVIEW

- Management of the acutely poisoned patient includes initial telephone triage, appropriate communication and history gathering from the pet owner, thorough physical examination, and initial stabilization.
- It is imperative to understand the toxicant's mechanism of action, the pharmacokinetics (absorption, distribution, metabolism, and excretion), and the toxic dose to know how to treat the patient appropriately.
- Once this is understood, prompt decontamination and detoxification of the patient should be done. Please see chapter 1, "Decontamination and Detoxification of the Poisoned Patient," for more information.
- Initial stabilization should include the ABCDs:
  - Airway
  - Breathing
  - Circulation
  - Disability
- Appropriate diagnostic testing (e.g., CBC, chemistry, blood gas analysis, electrolytes, UA) should be performed, as this may help guide or titrate therapy. Additional diagnostics include radiographs and specific toxicant testing (e.g., ethylene glycol [EG]). Please refer to the specific toxicant's chapter for further information.
- Appropriate monitoring of the critically ill, poisoned patient should include the following:
  - Continuous ECG (cECG)
  - Blood pressure monitoring (BP)
  - Central venous pressure (CVP)
  - Urine output (UOP)
  - Pulse oximetry
  - End-tidal carbon dioxide ($ETCO_2$)
  - Blood gas analysis
- Appropriate antidote (e.g., fomepizole, 2-PAM, naloxone, etc.) therapy should be initiated promptly with any poisoning; however, the majority of toxins do not have a readily available antidote. Symptomatic and supportive care will be

discussed later in this chapter. Please see chapter 3, "Antidotes and Other Useful Drugs," for further information specific to antidotes.

ABCDs of the Poisoned Patient

Airway

- Any patient presenting comatose, unconscious, neurologically impaired (e.g., decreased or absent gag reflex), or with severe respiratory distress or dyspnea should be intubated with an endotracheal tube (ETT), connected to an oxygen source, and treated with positive pressure ventilation (PPV) or manual delivery of breaths (see "Breathing").
- Pulse oximetry and $ETCO_2$ monitoring should be used appropriately to monitor the patient; likewise, the use of arterial blood gas (ABG) analysis should be considered the gold standard for measuring oxygenation and ventilation.

Breathing

- If the patient is apneic, mechanical ventilation and PPV are indicated at 10–20 bpm, with a tidal volume of 6–15 mL/kg.
- Hypoventilation is defined as a partial pressure of carbon dioxide (PCO_2) ≥45 mm Hg. Hypoxemia is defined as an arterial partial pressure of oxygen (PaO_2) ≤80 mm Hg. In general, a "50:50 rule" (PCO_2 ≥50 mm Hg with a PaO_2 ≤50 mm Hg) is an indication for PPV and oxygen supplementation.
- First, determine why the patient is hypoventilating or hypoxemic:
  - Was it due to excessive sedation from a toxicant? If the toxicant has a reversal agent (e.g., amitraz, yohimbine; benzodiazepine, flumazenil; fentanyl patch, naloxone; respectively), prompt reversal should occur. If a reversal agent is not available, supportive PPV until the patient is able to ventilate appropriately is indicated.
  - Why is the patient hypoxemic? Is there evidence of abnormal lung sounds (on auscultation) or the presence of a fever or cough? Chest radiographs should be performed to rule out disease in the following anatomical locations: airway (upper and lower), pulmonary parenchyma, pleural space, and thoracic wall. Rule-outs including aspiration pneumonia, atelectasis, pulmonary edema, pleural effusion, or multilobular hemorrhage [secondary to long-acting anticoagulant rodenticides (LAAC)] should be considered. Other rule-outs include hypemic hypoxia, where hemoglobin is unable to carry oxygen adequately (e.g., carboxyhemoglobin, methemoglobin, etc.).
- Supportive mechanical ventilation (see fig. 2.1) is indicated until the patient meets the following criteria:
  - Able to ventilate and oxygenate without assistance
  - Spontaneous respirations
  - Resolution of severe dyspnea
  - Return of neurologic status (e.g., palpebral or gag reflex)

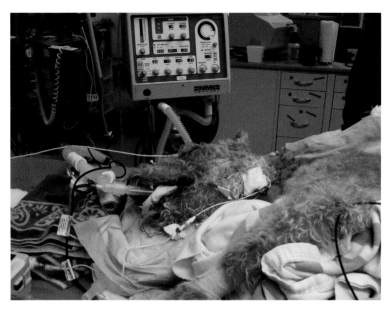

■ **Fig. 2.1.** A patient undergoing mechanical ventilation. Note the intensive monitoring and supportive care, including IV access, monitoring equipment (continuous monitoring of pulse oximetry, ECG, rectal temperature, CVP, blood pressure), and intubation with an endotracheal tube with an inflated cuff. (Photo courtesy of Justine A. Lee)

- PCO_2 ≤50 mm Hg
- PaO_2 ≥60 mm Hg (Oxygen supplementation can then be administered via less invasive modalities, such as an oxygen cage.)
■ Readers are referred to the references on mechanical ventilation for more information.

Circulation
■ The patient should be assessed for effective circulation based on the following physical examination parameters: mentation, mucous membrane color, CRT, heart rate, pulse quality and pressure, and body temperature.
■ Altered circulation may be due to various toxicants:
- Excessive sedation—benzodiazepines, baclofen, opioids, sedatives or hypnotics, others
- Agitation—SSRIs, TCAs, benzodiazepines, amphetamines, others
- Inadequate perfusion (secondary to hemorrhagic shock, hypovolemic shock, profound hypotension, etc.)—LAAC, ACE inhibitors, beta-blockers, calcium channel blockers, iron, others.
- Hypoxemia—LAAC, carbon monoxide, smoke inhalation, or secondary causes such as aspiration pneumonia, atelectasis, pulmonary edema, pleural effusion, etc.
- Hypoglycemia—volatile alcohols, xylitol, sepsis, and prolonged tremoring or seizure activity from neurotoxins

- Neurologic—5-FU, amphetamines, SSRIs, baclofen, ivermectin, bromethalin, benzodiazepines, lamotrigine, pyrethrins, organophosphates, metaldehyde, cocaine, amphetamines, mushrooms, salt, blue-green algae, others
- Appropriate therapy should be initiated promptly. This may include the following:
  - Reversal agents like naloxone or flumazenil to reverse extreme sedation or hypoventilation
  - Sedation for agitation
  - Fluid resuscitation (including crystalloids, colloids, blood products) to maintain blood pressure, perfusion, and treat dehydration
  - Oxygen therapy
  - Dextrose administration—if patient is hypoglycemic <60 mg/dL (normal 70–110 mg/dL), administer 0.5–1.5 mL/kg of 50% dextrose IV, diluted 1:3 with a crystalloid, over 1–2 minutes, followed by a CRI in IV fluids (2.5%–5% dextrose supplementation).
  - Treatment for cerebral edema, including 15°–30° head elevation, perfusion with IV fluid therapy, oxygen administration, and mannitol.
  - Please see "Treatment" for more specific information on each therapy.

Disability
- Prior to treatment, the poisoned patient should be evaluated for gross neurological disability. Initial neurologic examination should include the following:
  - Mentation
  - Pupillary light reflex (PLR) and assessment if pupils are equal and responsive to light
  - Ambulation
  - Spinal reflexes
- Assessing neurologic function prior to treatment, if possible, is imperative as patients with severe toxicosis (e.g., organophosphate, metaldehyde, bromethalin), may have suffered severe hypoxemia or even cardiopulmonary arrest. Assessing neurologic function allows better prognostic guidance to pet owners.
- For more information on treatment for neurologic disorders, please see "Neurologic Support" below.

SUPPORTIVE CARE AND TREATMENT

- As stated previously, few toxicities have antidotes, and treatment is often symptomatic and supportive, including the following:
  - Monitoring and supportive care
  - Fluid therapy
  - Cardiovascular support
  - Gastrointestinal support

- Neurologic support
- Analgesia/sedation
- Miscellaneous treatment

Monitoring

■ Monitoring of the poisoned patient may include any of the following:
  - cECG
  - BP
  - CVP
  - UOP
  - Pulse oximetry
  - ETCO$_2$
  - Blood gas analysis

Continuous ECG

■ In general, patients with underlying heart disease, cardiac dysrhythmias, myocardial hypoxia, pain/stress, splenic disease, or severe acid-base/electrolyte disturbances may be more at risk of arrhythmias and should be monitored with a cECG.

■ Likewise, poisoned patients should also be monitored with cECG when risks of arrhythmias, tachycardia, bradycardia, or severe electrolyte or acid-base abnormalities exist.
  - Specific toxins include cardiac medications (e.g., beta-blockers, calcium channel blockers, digoxin), albuterol, SSRIs, amphetamines, lamotrigine, cardiac glycoside-containing plants, *Bufo* toads, and amitraz. This list is not exclusive.
  - The ECG should be used to look for the presence of dysrhythmias, bradycardia, or tachycardia.

■ In general, the following parameters should warrant treatment if detected on an ECG:
  - Dog: HR <50 bpm or >180 bpm
  - Cat: HR <120 bpm or >240 bpm
  - Presence of severe VPCs
    □ R on T phenomenon (often predisposing to serious ventricular arrhythmias like ventricular fibrillation)
    □ VPCs >180 bpm
    □ Pulse deficits
    □ Hypotension
    □ Clinical signs of poor perfusion (e.g., prolonged CRT, dull mentation, etc.)

■ General treatment information for arrhythmias: (Readers are directed to a veterinary cardiology or critical care book for more details due to the large scope of information.)

- Bradyarrhythmias (dog: HR <50 bpm; cat: HR <120 bpm)
  - □ Atropine: 0.02–0.04 mg/kg IV, IM, SQ
  - □ Glycopyrrolate: 0.01 mg/kg IV, IM, SQ
  - □ If nonresponsive, advanced therapy including high-dose insulin, intravenous lipid emulsion, and temporary pacemaker placement may be necessary.
- Supraventricular tachyarrhythmias (SVTs) (dog: HR >180 bpm; cat: HR >240 bpm).
  - □ SVTs are differentiated from VPCs by ECG appearance. SVTs typically retain a normal-appearing QRS.
  - □ Esmolol: 250–500 µg/kg IV slow over 2 minutes, then 10–200 µg/kg/min CRI
  - □ Verapamil: 0.025–0.15 mg/kg IV q 5 minutes, up to total dose of 0.15–0.2 mg/kg
  - □ Digoxin: 0.005–0.01 mg/kg PO q12h
  - □ Diltiazem: 0.125–0.35 mg/kg IV slowly, repeat every 15 minutes to maximum dose of 0.75 mg/kg
  - □ Amiodarone: 10–25 mg/kg PO q 12 × 7 days, then wean slowly.
- Ventricular arrhythmias
  - □ SVTs are differentiated from VPCs by ECG appearance. VPCs have a QRS that is 90% abnormal, wide, and bizarre.
  - □ Lidocaine
    - ◦ Dogs: 2–4 mg/kg IV bolus, then 25–100 µg/kg/min IV CRI.
    - ◦ Cats: 0.25 mg/kg IV bolus, then 10 µg/kg/min IV CRI (Use with caution in cats due to the risk of neurotoxicity.)
  - □ Procainamide: 2 mg/kg IV bolus, repeated to maximum cumulative dosage of 20 mg/kg, then 25–50 µg/kg/min IV CRI (dogs only)
  - □ Amiodarone: 10 mg/kg PO q 12 × 7 days, then wean slowly or 1.3 mg/kg IV load once, followed by 0.03–0.1 mg/kg/min
  - □ Magnesium sulfate: 30 mg/kg (= 0.243 mEq/kg) IV slowly to effect

Blood Pressure (BP)

- Blood pressure should be measured frequently in hypotensive patients, as it is a reflection of cardiac output, blood volume, and vascular tone.
- Blood pressure can be monitored by direct arterial blood pressure, Doppler, or oscillometric (e.g., Dinamap) measurement. These are listed in order of accuracy.
  - Direct arterial blood pressure is advantageous because it is continuous and very accurate, but it is invasive, requires specialized equipment, requires a high level of skill to maintain and place an arterial line, and if disconnected (and unobserved) can lead to catastrophic bleeding.
  - Indirect blood pressure monitoring can be performed with oscillometric or Doppler monitoring and is often more economical.

- □ The HR must match on the oscillometric Dinamap or the results are not considered accurate.
- □ Appropriate cuff selection is imperative, with the cuff being approximately 40% of the limb circumference.
- Causes for hypotension include hypovolemia (low preload), peripheral vasodilation, decreased systemic vascular resistance, decreased cardiac output, and poor cardiac contractility.
- Causes for hypertension in veterinary medicine include renal disease, cardiac disease, hyperadrenocorticism, pain, fear, immune-mediated hemolytic anemia, pheochromocytoma, etc.
- In the poisoned patient, hypotension may be seen from the following toxicants:
  - Cardiac medications (e.g., beta blockers, calcium channel blockers, cardiac glycoside–containing plants, *Bufo* toads)—resulting in arrhythmias or severe bradycardia, which results in poor cardiac contractility, decreased afterload, and decreased systemic vascular resistance.
  - Beta agonists (e.g., albuterol, salmeterol, clenbuterol)—resulting in severe tachycardia, which prevents adequate ventricular filling.
  - ACE inhibitors, diuretics—resulting in volume depletion, decreased systemic vascular resistance, and potentially decreased preload.
  - Sedatives (e.g., baclofen, opioids, others)—resulting in severe sedation and CNS depression.
- The primary treatment for hypotension is IV fluid therapy, provided there is no underlying heart disease. These treatment guidelines must be modified for patients with a heart murmur, known cardiac disease (e.g., dilated or hypertrophic cardiomyopathy), etc. When treating hypotension, make sure the patient is adequately volume-resuscitated first before reaching for any vasopressors. Our ideal goal of therapy is to achieve the following endpoints of resuscitation:
  - Mean arterial pressure (MAP) ≥65 mm Hg
  - CVP ≥8–12 mm Hg
  - UOP ≥0.5 mL/kg/hour
  - Normal lactate 1–2 mmol/L
  - Normal base excess (BE) −3 to +3 mmol/L
- If the patient is hypotensive (MAP <60 mm Hg or systolic <90 mm Hg), volume resuscitate.
  - Any balanced, isotonic crystalloid (e.g., NormR, LRS): 20–30 mL/kg IV aliquots over 15–20 minutes—repeat 2–3× as needed, monitoring frequently for response to therapy.
  - If no improvement, consider colloid bolus (e.g., Hetastarch): 5 mL/kg IV aliquots over 20–30 minutes—repeat 2–3× as needed.
  - If no improvement, consider the following:
    - □ If coagulopathic (PT/PTT prolongation, as seen with LAAC): plasma 10–20 mL/kg IV over 1–4 hours

- ☐ If anemic: blood products (e.g., whole blood, etc.) 10–20 mL/kg IV to effect over 1–4 hours
- If the patient is hypertensive (MAP >160 mm Hg or systolic >200 mm Hg), several factors must be addressed, including agitation, pain, underlying metabolic disease (e.g., heart disease, renal disease, hyperadrenocorticism, immune-mediated hemolytic anemia, etc.), neoplasia (e.g., pheochromocytoma), toxicant induced (SSRIs, amphetamines), etc.
  - The use of judicious sedation/analgesia, anxiolytics, anticonvulsants, vasodilators, or ACE inhibitors is necessary.
  - If the hypertension is toxicant related and concurrent agitation is simultaneously observed, the use of aggressive sedation is recommended for patients with stable cardiovascular systems.
    - ☐ Acepromazine
      - ○ Dog: 0.05–0.2 mg/kg, IV, IM, SQ PRN to effect. Doses of up to 1 mg/kg may be necessary in severe cases, but in general no more than 3 mg total per dog is recommended.
      - ○ Cat: 0.05–0.1 mg/kg IV, IM, SQ PRN. Doses of up to 1 mg/kg may be necessary in severe cases, but it is generally not recommended to give more than 1 mg total per cat.
    - ☐ Chlorpromazine
      - ○ Dog: 0.5–1 mg/kg, IV, IM, SQ PRN to effect
      - ○ Cat: 0.5 mg/kg, IV, IM, SQ PRN to effect
    - ☐ Torbugesic 0.1–0.8 mg/kg, IV, IM, SQ PRN to effect
    - ☐ Diazepam 0.1–0.5 mg/kg, IV only, PRN to effect
      - ○ Diazepam is contraindicated with SSRI, benzodiazepine, or non-benzodiazepine toxicosis (e.g., sleep aids). See the specific chapter for further information.
  - If the patient is still hypertensive, the use of anti-hypertensives is indicated to prevent vascular injury, retinal detachment, etc.
    - ☐ In the poisoned patient, persistent hypertension typically responds well to aggressive, frequent sedation of the patient. However, if the patient is persistently hypertensive, the additional use of anti-hypertensives may be necessary:
    - ☐ Amlodipine (calcium-channel blocker):
      - ○ Dog: 0.1–0.25 mg/kg, PO q 12–24 hours PRN to effect
      - ○ Cat: 0.625 mg *total* per cat, PO q 12–24 hours PRN to effect
      - ○ Use cautiously in patients with cardiac or hepatic disease. Do not use in hypotensive patients or those with toxicants that may result in hypotension (e.g., calcium-channel blockers, beta-blockers, etc.).
    - ☐ Hydralazine (vasodilator)
      - ○ Dog: 0.5–2 mg/kg, PO q 8–12 to effect.
      - ○ Cat: 2.5 mg *total* per cat, PO q 12–24 to effect.

Central Venous Pressure (CVP)

- CVP is the hydrostatic pressure in the cranial vena cava and approximates right atrial pressure.
- CVP monitoring can be performed to estimate right ventricular end-diastolic volume and the relationship between blood volume capacity and blood volume. It indirectly correlates to intravascular volume, right heart function, and venous compliance, correlating with preload.
- Setup for CVP monitoring includes a central line, a water manometer ($10), and IV tubing.
- Normal CVP (via water manometer) is 0–5 cm H_2O.
- CVP monitoring will allow the veterinarian to titrate fluid therapy appropriately.
- A low CVP may reflect a hypovolemic state, while a high CVP may indicate fluid overload, right-sided heart failure, increased right atrial filling pressure, pericardial disease, or cranial mediastinal masses.
- CVPs can be falsely elevated with pleural space disease (such as pneumothorax) or with positive-end expiratory pressure, and should be evaluated subjectively based on trends. The reflection of HR, BP, and CVP together should be used in conjunction with physical exam findings, UOP, PCV/TS, etc. to aid in adequate volume resuscitation.
- CVP monitoring is useful in the poisoned patient that is in ARF from nephrotoxins such as ethylene glycol, lilies, grapes/raisins, NSAIDs, etc.

Urine Output (UOP)

- Normal urine output is 1–2 mL/kg/hour.
- UOP should be monitored and fluid therapy directed toward achieving normal UOP, particularly with nephrotoxic drugs (e.g., NSAIDs, grapes/raisins, ethylene glycol, lilies, amikacin, ACE inhibitors, etc.).
- Assess dehydration by evaluating the volume and specific gravity of urine:
  - Hypersthenuria may suggest ongoing dehydration (dog >1.025; cat >1.040), and aggressive fluid resuscitation may still be indicated.
  - Patients on IV fluids should be isosthenuric, so urine specific gravity should ideally be assessed prior to fluid administration.
  - If UOP is decreased (particularly in azotemic patients), fluid therapy and vasopressor support (to increase renal blood flow) should be initiated to prevent anuria or oliguria. Ensure adequate hydration prior to instituting medications to increase UOP (e.g., furosemide, mannitol); otherwise, these products will just result in increased UOP while dehydrating the patient.
- Increasing renal blood flow
  - IV fluids first! If concerned about hydration and renal function, measure UOP carefully. If ≤0.5 mL/kg/hour of UOP *and adequately hydrated or volume resuscitated*, consider the following:
    - Dopamine: 1–5 µg/kg/min IV CRI (dose for dopaminergic effect)

☐ Dobutamine: dogs: 5–15 µg/kg/min IV CRI
☐ Furosemide (if patient becoming oliguric): 0.1–1 mg/kg/hour IV CRI or intermittent 2 mg/kg IV boluses q 4–6 hours PRN
- Due to the complexity of this topic, readers are referred to a critical care book (see "Suggested Reading") for further information.

Pulse Oximetry

■ Pulse oximeters are noninvasive, easy-to-use bedside monitors that measure SpO_2 rather than SaO_2 (oxygen saturation). A pulsatile tissue bed is required for an accurate reading. Measurements can be taken on the lip, tongue, pinnae, base of tail, toe web, vulva, prepuce, or rectum (with a rectal probe).

■ Reliable pulse oximetry readings are affected by ambient light, hypotension, poor perfusion, pigmentation, icterus, and nail polish.

■ An accurate HR and strong signal *must* correlate with the pulse oximeter before a reliable reading can be taken.

■ Normal pulse oximetry (without oxygen supplementation) is ≥94%–100%. A pulse oximetry reading of 90% correlates with a PaO_2 of 60 mm Hg (normal 80–100 mm Hg), consistent with *severe* hypoxemia.

■ A pulse oximeter (with the aid of the oxygen dissociation curve) and venous blood gas (VBG) may alternatively be used *together* to help identify the severity of hypoxemia and hypoventilation. Venous $PvCO_2$ is, on average, 5 mm Hg higher than arterial $PaCO_2$ with the exception being if the patient (or the limb that the sample was drawn from) was severely hypotensive and peripherally vasoconstricted.

■ Pulse oximetry is useful in the poisoned patient when dyspnea, tachypnea, abnormal lung sounds, or respiratory distress is evident. Toxins that may result in these clinical signs include LAACs (multilobular pulmonary hemorrhage, pleural effusion), phosphide rodenticides (pulmonary edema), essential oils (ARDS or ALI), or hydrocarbons (aspiration pneumonia). Any poisoned patient that is vomiting may also have secondary aspiration pneumonia.

End-Tidal CO_2 (ETCO$_2$)

■ Canography is a noninvasive way of continuously measuring $PaCO_2$. $ETCO_2$ is an effective way of measuring the ability to adequately ventilate. In veterinary medicine, the use of $ETCO_2$ typically is used in sedated, intubated patients.

■ With the poisoned patient, the use of $ETCO_2$ may be beneficial to assess the severity of hypercapnea (or hypoventilation). Examples include toxicosis with ivermectin, baclofen, anticonvulsant medications, opioids, benzodiazepines, and others.

■ Patients who are excessively sedate benefit from $ETCO_2$ monitoring to determine if PPV needs to be implemented.

■ When in doubt, a VBG ($PvCO_2$) can be used to estimate $PaCO_2$. Normal $PaCO_2$ is approximately 35 mm Hg, and a $PvCO_2$ will be approximately 5–10 mm Hg higher on the venous side.

- In patients with an $ETCO_2$ >40–50 mm Hg, appropriate PPV may be warranted or respiratory arrest may occur.

Blood Gas Analysis

- Venous (VBG) or arterial (ABG) blood gas analysis is the determination of the pH, paO_2 (arterial), pCO_2, base excess (BE), and bicarbonate (HCO_3) of blood. Blood gases allow clinicians to evaluate the acidity of the blood, the overall acid-base status, the respiratory and metabolic contributions, and the pulmonary function.
- The bicarbonate (HCO_3) is a measure of the metabolic component, while the pCO_2 is a measure of ventilation and is the respiratory component of a patient's acid-base status. The reader is referred to an acid-base source for more information.
- In general, the steps for interpretation of blood gas analysis should be the following:
  1. **pH.** Is the pH acidemic or alkalemic?
  2. **BE.** As this is the truest assessment of the metabolic component, a more negative number (e.g., −15) represents a severe metabolic acidosis, while a positive number (e.g., +15) represents a severe metabolic alkalosis.
  3. **pCO_2.** This evaluates the respiratory component. A high pCO_2 indicates a respiratory acidosis. A lower pCO_2 indicates a respiratory alkalosis.
  4. **Compensation.** Is there compensation occurring? For example, an animal with a severe metabolic acidosis should be hyperventilating and blowing off its extra acid (pCO_2). Keep in mind that an animal will never overcompensate.
  5. **Hypoxia.** If this is an ABG sample, evaluate if the paO_2 is <80 mm Hg to rule out hypoxemia.
  6. Do these changes correspond to the clinical picture?
- The use of VBG analysis with pulse oximetry interpretation can be used together and is oftentimes as beneficial as ABG results. For the evaluation of acid-base parameters, a VBG is an attractive alternative as it does not require arterial sampling. Venous samples can be interpreted as previously described for an arterial sample, with three known exceptions:
  - The PCO_2 is approximately 5–10 mm Hg higher in the venous versus the arterial system.
  - One cannot assess PO_2 on a VBG, only an ABG. Only an arterial PO_2 can provide information regarding the oxygenation function of the lungs. With pulse oximetry, SpO_2 (oxygen saturation) can be correlated with an oxygen-hemoglobin dissociation curve and the pO_2 can then be deduced. Pulse oximeter + VBG = ABG.
  - When peripheral vasoconstriction, severe shock, hypovolemia, or low flow states (e.g., saddle thrombus, tourniquet application) occur, a peripheral venous sample may not accurately reflect the patient's acid-base status.

- VBG analysis is beneficial in the poisoned patient to evaluate the severity of acid-base imbalances. Metabolic acidosis can be caused with 4–5 main causes, including:
  - Ethylene glycol (EG) toxicosis
  - Lactic acidosis
  - Uremic acidosis (e.g., ARF)
  - Diabetic ketoacidosis
  - Salicylate toxicity
- VBG analysis can be used in conjunction with other diagnostic testing (e.g., EG testing) to confirm ingestion. For example, a dog presenting to a clinic 3 hours after possibly ingesting EG should have an EG blood test and VBG done simultaneously if possible. The absence of a metabolic acidosis in the face of a weak (or false) positive result makes it unlikely that true exposure occurred, as the presence of a metabolic acidosis would be expected. Likewise, measurement of a VBG may be useful with iron toxicosis to determine the severity of metabolic acidosis. Treatment would include aggressive IV fluid resuscitation and monitoring. VBG analysis may titrate therapy; for example, if a severe metabolic acidosis (pH <7.0, BE −18, HCO_3 11 mm Hg) is present, the use of sodium bicarbonate therapy may be indicated.

Fluid Therapy

- Fluid therapy is one of the cornerstone therapies of emergency management of the poisoned patient:
  - Corrects dehydration
  - Maintains perfusion at a cellular level
  - Vasodilates the renal vessels (particularly with nephrotoxic toxins like NSAIDs, lilies, etc.)
  - Treats hypotension (particularly with drugs like beta-blockers, calcium channel blockers, ACE inhibitors, others)
- Fluid therapy can also be used to aid in detoxification of the patient by increasing renal excretion of toxicants by forced diuresis. Refer to chapter 1 on the use of forced diuresis.
- Patients should be evaluated for dehydration based on skin turgor, tacky mucous membrane, and the presence of sunken eyes. Depending on the severity of dehydration and illness, patients should be treated with IV fluid replacement.
- Monitor hydration status by assessing weight gain (or loss), PCV/TS (as evidence of hemoconcentration), and BUN (which gives a gross estimate of decreased renal perfusion and glomerular filtration rate, resulting in a prerenal azotemia). Evidence of hypersthenuria (cat >1.040; dog >1.025) is consistent with dehydration.
- Crystalloids
  - Any balanced, isotonic buffered solution can be used (e.g., NormR, LRS).

- Dose: The dose of IV fluids to administer is dependent on the clinical state and physical examination findings of the patient.
- In a healthy patient, fluid rates of 4–6 mL/kg/hour can be used to force renal clearance of the toxicant.
- Neonates have a higher maintenance fluid rate (80–100 mL/kg/day), and fluid rates should be adjusted accordingly.
- Patients with cardiac disease, respiratory disease, or those who have ingested toxins that may increase the patient's risk toward pulmonary edema (e.g., TCA antidepressants, phosphide rodenticides) should have judicious fluid administration.
- Careful assessment of hydration should be made based on PCV/TS, weight gain, CVP, and physical examination findings.

- Colloids
  - Colloids are large molecules that stay in the intravascular space for a longer duration of time.
  - The use of colloids (e.g., Hetastarch) should be considered for those patients having a low colloid osmotic pressure (normal reference range 18–20 mm Hg). In general, hypoproteinemic (TS <6) or persistently hypotensive patients may benefit from the added effective of a colloid.
    - Hetastarch
      - Bolus 5 mL/kg IV over 20 minutes, titrate to effect, repeat if needed.
      - Maintenance 1 mL/kg/hour, IV CRI thereafter with concurrent crystalloid therapy.

Cardiovascular Support

- Please see "Circulation," "Fluid Therapy," and "Continuous ECG" for more information.
- In patients with cardiovascular collapse (e.g., hypotension, tachycardia, bradycardia, etc.), the appropriate use of IV fluids ± antiarrhythmic therapy is warranted. In persistently hypotensive patients not responding to boluses of crystalloids, colloids, or blood products, the use of positive inotropes may be necessary to increase cardiac contractility or blood pressure. Due to the complexity of this topic, readers are directed toward the references listed at the end of this chapter.
  - Dopamine:
    - 3–10 μg/kg/min IV CRI to effect (dose for beta effect)
    - >10 μg/kg/min IV CRI to effect (dose for alpha effect)
  - Dobutamine: (not to be used for more than 24 hours, ideally)
    - Dogs: 5–20 μg/kg/min IV CRI
    - Cats: 2.5–10 μg/kg/min IV CRI (observe closely for seizure activity!)
  - Norepinephrine: 0.1–1.0 μg/kg/min IV CRI

- Epinephrine: 0.1–0.4 µg/kg/min IV CRI
- Vasopressin: Start with 0.8 U/kg IV bolus, then 0.5–1 mU/kg/min IV CRI
- Digoxin
    - This is reserved for those patients with abnormal heart function (e.g., DCM) or decreased cardiac contractility (e.g., beta-blocker toxicity, calcium channel blocker toxicity).
    - Dogs: 0.005–0.01 mg/kg PO q 12 hours
    - Cats: Generally not recommended and contraindicated if cat has HCM; 0.007–0.015 mg/kg PO q 24 hours.

Gastrointestinal Support

- Certain toxins result in severe gastric ulceration (corrosive agents, iron, human NSAIDs [e.g., naproxen, ibuprofen, aspirin, diclofenac], veterinary NSAIDS [e.g., carprofen, deracoxib, firocoxib]).
- Patients should be monitored closely for signs of gastric ulceration, including the presence of vomiting, hematemesis, coffee-ground appearance to vomitus, diarrhea, bloody diarrhea, or black, tarry stool (melena). Dogs should have a rectal exam performed daily while hospitalized, if possible.
- As the shock organ in the dog is the GIT, appropriate fluid resuscitation is necessary to aid in perfusion of the gut.
- Treatment should be initiated promptly and includes the use of the following antiulcer drugs:
    - H_2 antagonists
        - Famotidine 0.5–1.0 mg/kg, PO, SQ, IM, or IV q 12–24 hours
        - Ranitidine 1–2 mg/kg, PO, IV, SQ q 8–12 hours
        - Cimetidine 5–10 mg/kg, PO, IM, IV q 6–8 hours
    - Proton pump inhibitors
        - Omeprazole 0.5–1.0 mg/kg, PO q 24 hours in dogs; 0.7 mg/kg, PO q 24 hours in cats
        - Pantoprazole 1 mg/kg, IV q 24 hours in dogs
    - Sucralfate 0.25–1 g, PO q 24 hours
    - Antiemetic therapy
        - Maropitant 1 mg/kg, SQ q 24 hours (not labeled for cats)
        - Ondansetron 0.1–0.2 mg/kg, SQ, IV q 8–12 hours
        - Metoclopramide 0.2–0.5 mg/kg, PO, IM, SQ q 8 hours or 1–2 mg/kg/day, CRI IV
        - Dolasetron mesylate 0.6 to 3.0 mg/kg, IV q 24 hours
- Adequate nutritional support should be provided to critically ill patients whose calories have been restricted for more than 3–4 days, provided risks of aspiration pneumonia have resolved.
- If patients are vomiting despite antiemetic therapy, alternate nutrition such as TPN should be initiated.

- Nutrition is important to help reduce intestinal villous atrophy or bacterial translocation, prevent gastric ulceration, increase gastric or intestinal blood flow, increase GI mucous production, and preserve normal GI flora, all which aid to speed recovery and decrease risk for sepsis and morbidity.
- Patients should not be force-fed, as this is stressful to the patient and increases the risk of aspiration pneumonia.

Neurologic Support

- Certain toxicants may result in mild signs of agitation, CNS depression, or refractory seizures. Examples include 5-FU, amphetamines, SSRIs, baclofen, ivermectin, bromethalin, benzodiazepines, lamotrigine, pyrethrins, organo-phosphates, metaldehyde, cocaine, mushrooms, salt, blue-green algae, and others.
- In the poisoned patient, it is imperative that appropriate drug therapy be used to stop tremors and seizures immediately. Persistent tremoring and seizuring can result in rhabdomyolysis with secondary ARF, lowering of the seizure threshold, secondary hyperthermia, and DIC. The use of muscle relaxants and anticonvulsant therapy is imperative:
  - Methocarbamol 55–220 mg/kg, IV or PO, PRN to effect
  - Diazepam 0.25–0.5 mg/kg, IV, PRN to effect, followed by CRI if indicated
  - Phenobarbital 4 mg/kg, IV q 4 hours × 4 doses to load; additional doses may be necessary
  - Pentobarbital 2–15 mg/kg, IV, PRN to effect
  - Propofol 1–4 mg/kg, IV slow, PRN to effect, followed by CRI if indicated
  - General anesthesia (inhalant therapy)
- Severely neurologically impaired poisoned patients should be monitored and treated as if they have cerebral ischemia or edema with the following supportive care, if needed:
  - 15°–30° head elevation
  - Oxygen therapy
  - Fluid therapy to maintain perfusion, blood pressure, UOP
  - ECG, pulse oximetry, or $ETCO_2$ monitoring
  - Frequent neurologic examination (PLR, mentation, etc.)
  - Treatment for cerebral edema:
    - Furosemide 2–4 mg/kg, IV, SQ, IM q 6–8 hours
    - Mannitol 1–2 g/kg, IV slowly over 20–30 minutes PRN
  - Patients should be monitored for increased intracranial pressure (ICP), which may be evident by Cushing's reflex (different from Cushings' disease). Cushing's reflex is seen secondary to increased ICP, and clinical signs include: progressive lethargy, nonresponsiveness, acute bradycardic (HR <60 bpm dog, <140 bpm cat), and concurrent hypertension (>190–

200 mm Hg systolic). This reflex is indicative of *severe cerebral edema* and imminent herniation.

Analgesics/Sedatives

- Certain toxicities may result in severe agitation, where sedation may be necessary. Common toxicities include beta-agonist toxicity (e.g., albuterol), SSRIs, TCAs, benzodiazepines, non-benzodiazepines, amphetamines, methamphetamines, metaldehyde, tremorgenic toxins, and others.
- Sedatives and analgesics should be used when appropriate. For agitation and hypertension, higher doses of sedatives may be required.
  - Acepromazine
    - Dog: 0.05–0.2 mg/kg, IV, IM, SQ PRN to effect. Doses of up to 1 mg/kg may be necessary in severe cases, but in general more than 3 mg total per dog is not recommended.
    - Cat: 0.05–0.1 mg/kg IV, IM, SQ PRN. Doses of up to 1 mg/kg may be necessary in severe cases, but it is generally not recommended to give more than 1 mg total per cat.
  - Chlorpromazine
    - Dog: 0.5–1 mg/kg, IV, IM, SQ PRN to effect
    - Cat: 0.5 mg/kg, IV, IM PRN to effect
  - Torbugesic 0.1–0.8 mg/kg, IV, IM, SQ PRN to effect
  - Diazepam 0.1–0.5 mg/kg, IV only, PRN to effect. Contraindicated with SSRI, benzodiazepine, or non-benzodiazepine toxicosis (e.g., sleep aids). See the specific chapter for further information.
- In patients with oral corrosive injury (e.g., ultra-bleach cleaning products, essential oils/liquid potpourri), the use of topical analgesics should be avoided in the mouth. While analgesic therapy is important, further self-mutilation or trauma may occur with the use of products such as lidocaine gels or numbing oral rinses. Rather, the use of analgesics should be considered:
  - Buprenex 11–22 µg/kg sublingual, IV, IM, SQ q 6 hours as needed
  - Torbugesic 0.2–0.8 mg/kg, IV, SQ, IM, PRN to effect
  - Tramadol 1–5 mg/kg, PO q 6–8 hours to effect

Miscellaneous

- Cyproheptadine, a serotonin antagonist, can be given for toxicants that result in serotonin syndrome (e.g., SSRI, TCAs, amphetamines, etc.).
  - Cats: 2–4 mg total dose q 4–6 hours as needed until resolution of clinical signs
  - Dogs: 1.1 mg/kg q 4–6 hours as needed
- N-acetylcysteine (NAC) can be used to limit formation of toxic metabolites (e.g., NAPQI with acetaminophen toxicity) by maintaining glutathione and sulfate concentrations and providing glutathione substrates.

- 10% to 20% solutions should be diluted to a 5% solution prior to IV administration.
- Initial loading doses of 140 mg/kg, followed by 70 mg/kg PO or IV every 4–6 hours for 7–17 doses.
- Oral formulation may be given IV (off-label) slowly over 15–20 minutes through a 0.2-micron bacteriostatic filter.
- S-adenosyl-methionine (SAMe) can be used as a hepatoprotectant and antioxidant, and may help with glutathione production and maintenance.
  - 18 mg/kg/day PO may reduce oxidative damage.
- Ascorbic acid (vitamin C) can be used as an antioxidant and to help reduce MetHb to Hb.
  - 30 mg/kg PO, SQ, IV q 6 hours

CONCLUSIONS

- With toxicosis, the majority of toxins do not have a readily available antidote. Symptomatic and supportive care remains the primary goal of emergency management of the poisoned patient.

Abbreviations

2-PAM = pralidoxime
5-FU   = fluorouracil
ABG   = arterial blood gas
ACE   = angiotensin-converting enzyme
ALI   = acute lung injury
ARDS   = acute respiratory distress
ARF   = acute renal failure
BP   = blood pressure
bpm   = breaths per minute or beats per minute
BE   = base excess
BUN   = blood urea nitrogen
CBC   = complete blood count
cECG   = continuous electrocardiography
CNS   = central nervous system
CO_2 = carbon dioxide
CRI   = continuous rate infusion
CRT   = capillary refill time
CVP   = central venous pressure
DIC   = disseminated intravascular coagulation
EG   = ethylene glycol
$ETCO_2$ = end-tidal CO_2
ETT   = endotracheal tube

GI	= gastrointestinal	
GIT	= gastrointestinal tract	
Hb	= hemoglobin	
HCM	= hypertrophic cardiomyopathy	
HCO_3	= bicarbonate	
HR	= heart rate	
ICP	= intracranial pressure	
IM	= intramuscular	
IV	= intravenous	
LAAC	= long-acting anticoagulant	
MAP	= mean arterial pressure	
MetHb	= methemoglobin	
NAC	= N-acetylcysteine	
NAPQI	= N-acetyl-p-benzoquinone imine	
NSAIDs	= nonsteroidal anti-inflammatory drugs	
PCV	= packed cell volume	
paO_2	= arterial partial pressure of oxygen	
pCO_2	= partial pressure of carbon dioxide	
PLR	= pupillary light reflex	
PO	= *per os* (by mouth)	
PPV	= positive pressure ventilation	
PRN	= *pro re nata* (as needed)	
PT	= prothrombin	
PTT	= partial thromboplastin time	
q	= every	
SAMe	= S-adenosyl-methionine	
SaO_2	= arterial oxyhemoglobin saturation	
SpO_2	= saturation of oxyhemoglobin	
SQ	= subcutaneous	
SSRI	= selective serotonin reuptake inhibitor	
SVT	= supraventricular tachyarrhythmia	
TCA	= tricyclic antidepressants	
TPN	= total parenteral nutrition	
TS	= total solids	
UA	= urinalysis	
UOP	= urine output	
VBG	= venous blood gas	
VPC	= ventricular premature complex	

Suggested Reading

Drellich S, Aldrich J. Initial management of the acutely poisoned patient. In: Peterson ME, Talcott PA, eds. Small Animal Toxicology, 2nd ed. St. Louis: Elsevier Saunders, 2006, pp. 45–59.

Hopper K. Basic mechanical ventilation and advanced mechanical ventilation. In: Silverstein DC, Hopper K, eds. Small Animal Critical Care Medicine. St. Louis: Elsevier Saunders, 2009, pp. 900–903.

Hopper K. Advanced mechanical ventilation. In: Silverstein DC, Hopper K, eds. Small Animal Critical Care Medicine. St. Louis: Elsevier Saunders, 2009, pp. 904–909.

Pypendop BH. Capnography. In: Silverstein DC, Hopper K, eds. Small Animal Critical Care Medicine. St. Louis: Elsevier Saunders, 2009, pp. 875–877.

Sorell-Raschi L. Blood gas and oximetry monitoring. In: Silverstein DC, Hopper K, eds. Small Animal Critical Care Medicine. St. Louis: Elsevier Saunders, 2009, pp. 878–882.

Waddell LS, Brown AJ. Hemodynamic monitoring. In: Silverstein DC, Hopper K, eds. Small Animal Critical Care Medicine. St. Louis: Elsevier Saunders, 2009, pp. 859–864.

Author: Justine A. Lee, DVM, DACVECC
Consulting Editor: Justine A. Lee, DVM, DACVECC; Lynn R. Hovda, DVM, MS, DACVIM

Antidotes and Other Useful Drugs

DEFINITION/OVERVIEW

- Antidotes are remedies used to counteract poisons. Specifically, antidotes are defined as any substance used to relieve or prevent the effects associated with a toxicant.
- Very few antidotes exist in medicine, and those that do are generally not approved for veterinary use. Any use associated with non-veterinary-approved antidotes is considered extralabel. The doses used are often extrapolated from human literature with very little scientific animal data available. Veterinarians are allowed to legally use medications in an extralabel manner but when doing so assume all the responsibility associated with their use.
- Little effort has been made by manufacturers to produce antidotes approved for use in veterinary medicine. There is little financial incentive for them to do this as the use of antidotes is limited, making research and manufacturing cost prohibitive.
- Antidotes can be divided into three broad categories:
  - *Chemical or causal antidotes* are those that work directly on the toxicant. They bind with the toxicant to yield an innocuous compound that is excreted from the body.
  - *Functional antidotes* have no chemical or physical interaction with toxicants but work to lessen the clinical signs associated with intoxication.
  - *Pharmacological or physiological antidotes* work in the body by several different mechanisms. Most commonly they work directly at the receptor site, generally counteracting toxicosis by producing opposing clinical signs. They may also prevent the formation of toxic metabolites, facilitate a more rapid elimination of a toxicant, or aid in the restoration of normal body function.

Chemical Antidotes

- **Antivenom.** IV antivenom can be used in dogs and cats to prevent paralysis, coagulopathies, and thrombocytopenia from snake or black widow spider bites. They have no effect on tissue necrosis. Early administration is preferred as it not only lessens the severity of signs but attenuates the need for a large number of doses at a later date.

- Both anaphylactoid and anaphylactic reactions can occur, especially if the animal has received antivenom at a prior time.
- Elapid antivenin (coral snakes)
  - Specific *M. fulvius* antivenin is no longer readily available in the USA, but antivenins from other countries may sometimes be obtained from zoos. The manufacturer's guidelines for dilution and administration should be followed closely.
  - Protective cross reactivity occurs with the following antivenins:
    - Coralmyn Fab$_2$ (equine derived); Instituto Bioclon, Mexico
    - Costa Rican coral snake antivenin; Instituto Clodomiro Picado, Costa Rica
    - Australian tiger snake (*Notechis scutatus*) antivenin; CSL Limited, Parkville, Victoria, Australia
- Crotalid Antivenin (pit vipers)
  - Antivenin Crotalidae Polyvalent (veterinary antivenin)—IgG (equine derived); Boehringer-Ingelheim, St. Joseph, MO
    - Dose varies from 1 to 5 vials IV depending on severity of clinical signs.
    - 95% of cases are controlled with a single vial.
  - CroFab (human antivenin)—Crotalidae Polyvalent Immune Fab$_1$ (ovine derived); BTG, Brentwood, TN
    - Currently not licensed as a specific veterinary product
    - The dose is not precisely determined for veterinary use.
    - Veterinary trial has been completed and is pending publication; average dose needed is expected to be one vial (personal communication, ME Peterson).
  - Antivipmyn (human antivenin)—Polyvalent antiviper serum—Fab$_2$ (equine derived); Instituto Bioclon, SA, Mexico
    - Available through many zoos in USA
    - Currently undergoing veterinary trials
  - Costa Rican pit viper antivenin (human antivenin)—Polyvalent Fab$_2$ (equine derived); Instituto Clodomino Picado, Costa Rica
    - Not cross-reactive to all species of North American rattlesnakes
- Black widow spider antivenin
  - Reserved for high-risk patients (e.g., pediatric, geriatric, or metabolically compromised)
  - Lycovac Antivenin Black Widow Spider (human antivenin, equine origin), Merck, West Point, PA
    - 1 vial mixed with 100 mL crystalloid solution; administer IV slowly with monitoring of the inner ear pinna for evidence of hyperemia (an indicator of allergic response)
    - One dose is usually sufficient with response evident within 30 minutes.

□ New antivenin (Aracmyn; Instituto Bioclon, Mexico) has completed human phase three trials but has not yet been approved for human use. This is an equine-origin Fab$_2$ antivenin product and may be less likely to trigger an allergic reaction.

- **Chelating Agents**. These antidotes are generally used to remove heavy metals from the body. The chelating agent combines with a metal ion to form a complex that is then excreted.
  - Calcium disodium ethylenediaminetetraacetic acid or CaNa$_2$EDTA (Calcium Disodium Versenate, 3M Pharmaceuticals)
    □ Labeled for use in pediatric and adult human beings with acute and chronic lead poisoning. The use has declined over the years due to side effects and decreased incidence of lead toxicosis in human beings.
    □ Still widely used in veterinary medicine to chelate lead, zinc, inorganic mercury, and perhaps cadmium, particularly in birds.
    □ Calcium disodium EDTA and NOT disodium EDTA must be used. These two should not be confused.
    □ Should not be used while lead remains in the GIT as it may enhance the systemic absorption of lead
    □ Should be used in conjunction with dimercaprol to increase lead excretion and prevent acute neurological signs
    □ Dose (dogs and cats): 25 mg/kg IV or SQ every 6 hours. Maximum recommended daily dose of 2 g/day. Treat for 5 days; rest for 5–7 days; and repeat if needed. Dilute product in 5% dextrose to a final concentration of 2–4 mg/mL prior to use.
    □ IM injection is painful and not recommended.
    □ It is very nephrotoxic so caution needs to be taken to ensure hydration; should not be used in animals with chronic renal failure.
  - D-penicillamine (Cuprimine, Merck)
    □ Labeled for use in human beings for copper, lead, iron, and mercury poisoning.
    □ Used in veterinary medicine for acute cadmium, inorganic mercury, lead, and zinc toxicosis, and with chronic copper toxicosis in dogs with inherited copper storage disease
    □ Often difficult to obtain and may be expensive, depending on source
    □ Dose (dogs) for at-home therapy after CaNa$_2$EDTA lead treatment: 110 mg/kg/day divided, PO q 6–8 hours for 1–2 weeks.
    □ Dose (cats) for at home therapy after CaNa$_2$EDTA lead treatment and in the presence of elevated blood levels: 125 mg *total* dose, PO q 12 hours for 5 days.
  - Deferoxamine (Desferal, Novartis Pharmaceutical Corporation)
    □ Labeled in human beings for the treatment of acute iron intoxication and chronic iron overload due to transfusion-dependent anemia

- □ Contraindicated in patients with severe renal disease or anuria and those with high circulating levels of aluminum
- □ Complexes with iron; deferoxamine chelated complex is water soluble and excreted primarily in urine.
- □ Dose (dogs and cats): 40 mg/kg IM q 4–8 hours. In critical situations, an IV infusion of 15 mg/kg/hour can be used, but the cardiovascular system must be monitored closely during this time. The excreted complex turns the urine pink or salmon colored and is sometimes referred to as the "vin rose" of iron poisoning. Continue treatment until the urine is clear or serum iron levels are within normal limits.
- □ Deferoxamine is most effective if used within the first 24 hours while iron is still in circulation and has not been distributed to tissues.
- □ Ascorbic acid: 10–15 mg/kg IM, IV, SQ, PO q 4–6 hours can be used in acute situations *after* all iron has been removed from the GIT to increase the efficacy of deferoxamine, but should be used cautiously in chronic iron poisoning as it can cause adverse cardiac effects.
- Dimercaprol (BAL in oil, Taylor)
  - □ Labeled in human beings for use in the treatment of arsenic, gold, and mercury poisoning. Can also be used in acute lead poisoning concomitantly with $CaNa_2EDTA$ and for treatment of high copper levels in those animals with copper storage disease.
  - □ Complex is water soluble and excreted in urine
  - □ Dose (dogs and cats):
    - ○ For arsenic toxicosis: 5 mg/kg IM × one dose followed by 2.5 mg/kg IM q 4 hours for 2 days, q 8 hours for 1 day, and q 12 hours until recovered.
    - ○ For lead toxicosis: 2.5–5 mg/kg IM as 10% solution q 4 hours on days 1 and 2, then q 6 hours on day 3
  - □ IM injections are painful (peanut oil carrier) and should only be given deep IM.
  - □ Dimercaprol is nephrotoxic so limit use and monitor BUN and creatinine. Be sure patients are adequately hydrated while product is used.
- Dimercaptosuccinic acid (DMSA or succimer; Chemet, Ovation)
  - □ Labeled for use in pediatric human beings for lead poisoning when the blood levels are >45 µg/mL. Unlabelled use includes mercury and arsenic toxicosis. It has not been shown to be effective for iron poisoning.
  - □ Used in veterinary medicine for lead or zinc toxicosis
  - □ Advantages over other chelators:
    - ○ Can be given PO or rectally if GI signs are severe
    - ○ Incidence of adverse GI signs is much lower
    - ○ Can be used while lead is still present in the GIT
    - ○ Has less of an effect on systemic zinc concentrations

  □ Disadvantages
    ○ Cost—expensive
    ○ Availability—often difficult to find
    ○ Postchelation lead level rebound can occur.
    ○ May have a transient increase in AST and ALT
  □ Dose (dogs and cats): 10 mg/kg PO or rectal q 8 hours × 10 days; retreat only if clinical signs are present
- Digoxin immune Fab fragments (Digibind, Glaxo Smith Kline)
  - Specific antidote used for digoxin toxicosis. It may also protect from poisoning associated with *Bufo* toads and cardiac glycoside–containing plants.
  - Fab fragments should be reserved for the treatment of life-threatening cardiac arrhythmias that do not respond to conventional antiarrhythmic therapy.
  - They are expensive and will likely have to be obtained from a human hospital.
  - Dose depends on the amount ingested and serum digoxin level
    □ Serum digoxin level available
      ○ Number of vials = serum digoxin level (ng/mL) × BW (kg)/100.
    □ If serum digoxin levels are not available or if one is treating *Bufo* toad or cardiac-containing plant toxicosis, start therapy with 1–2 vials and reassess as needed.
- Pralidoxime (2-PAM—Protopam Chloride, Wyeth)
  - Pralidoxime is used in organophosphate (OP) toxicosis to reactivate cholinesterase enzymes inactivated by the insecticide. It binds to the enzyme, attaches to the OP, and forms a pralidoxime-OP complex that detaches (reactivating the enzyme) and is excreted.
  - Helps prevent nicotinic signs and should be used in conjunction with atropine
  - Limited benefits with carbamate toxicosis
  - Generally, pralidoxime should be used within 24 hours of exposure, but may still be effective when given at 36–48 hours. There is some evidence that it is also effective when used for treatment of the intermediate syndrome of OP toxicosis.
  - Dose (dogs and cats): 20 mg/kg IM or slow IV (over 30 minutes) for first dose. Repeat dose q 8–12 hours, IM or SQ.
  - Rapid IV administration has resulted in tachycardia, neuromuscular blockade, laryngospasm, muscle rigidity, and death.

Functional Antidotes

- Acetylcysteine (Acetadote, Cumberland)
  - Acetylcysteine (NAC) is used to prevent hepatic necrosis that occurs secondary to acetaminophen toxicosis. It is most effective when used within 8 hours of exposure and should be used within 24 hours to be of value.

- It has also been used successfully as a liver protectant for other hepato-toxins, including *Amanita* mushroom toxicosis.
- It is a sulfhydryl compound that acts to increase glutathione synthesis in the liver, providing an alternate substrate for conjugation of acetamino-phen metabolites and restoring glutathione levels.
- Specifics of use:
  - ▢ Dose (dog and cat): 140 mg/kg IV or PO × 1 dose, then 70 mg/kg IV or PO q 6 hours for 7 doses. The product should be diluted to a 5% solution prior to use.
  - ▢ Variety of other doses have been suggested; most based on extrapola-tion from human literature. Some recommend higher doses (280 mg/kg) and others additional doses (up to 17 doses) for massive ingestions.
  - ▢ Emesis frequently occurs with oral dosing, especially after the initial dose, and an antiemetic may be required prior to starting NAC therapy.
- Bisphosphonates (Pamidronate—Aredia, Novartis)
  - Used as the current and specific antidote for vitamin D_3 (cholecalciferol) toxicosis, including cholecalciferol rodenticides and calcipotriene, a human prescription medication for psoriasis.
  - Bisphosphonates are a group of compounds that lower serum calcium levels by binding to hydroxyapatite crystals in the bone.
  - It is expensive and generally must be obtained from a human hospital or drug warehouse.
  - Due to the poor prognosis with hypercalcemia and secondary mineraliza-tion, the use of pamidronate, despite the cost, is highly recommended early in the treatment of hypercalcemia.
  - Aredia dose (dogs and cats):
    - ▢ 1.3–2 mg/kg diluted in 0.9% NaCl, IV over several hours
    - ▢ Monitor serum calcium levels every 12–24 hours and adjust ancillary treatment as needed. If hypercalcemia is still present, a repeated dose of pamidronate may be necessary 5–7 days after the initial dose.
    - ▢ Very large overdoses of cholecalciferol may require a second dose in 3–4 days.
- Calcitonin (Micalcin, Sandoz; Salmonine, Lennod)
  - Infrequently used to treat hypercalcemia associated with cholecalciferol toxicosis.
  - Salmon calcitonin has a number of physiological effects that result in a lowering of serum calcium. Calcitonin is used less often since pamidro-nate became commercially available, but may be effective when pamidro-nate is unavailable or in cases where the serum calcium is resistant to conventional treatment. The rapid development of resistance may limit its use.

- In general, it should not be used in conjunction with a bisphosphonate as there is some evidence that it may increase the risk of soft tissue mineralization.
  - Dose: 4–6 IU/kg, SQ q 8–12 hours
- Cyproheptadine (various manufacturers)
  - Used for the treatment of serotonin syndrome (e.g., excitation or depression, vocalization, ataxia, hyperthermia, seizures, tremors, vomiting, diarrhea) associated with ingestions of baclofen, SSRIs, and other medications
  - Antihistamine with serotonin antagonistic properties
    - Dose (dogs): 1.1 mg/kg PO or rectally q 4–8 hours PRN
    - Dose (cats): 2–4 mg *total* dose PO or rectally q 4–8 hours PRN
- Intravenous fat emulsion (IFE-Intralipid, Baxter; Liposyn, Hospira)
  - Promising use as an antidote for toxicosis associated with fat soluble drugs
    - IFE was initially used in human medicine to resuscitate patients undergoing cardiac arrest from severe local anesthetic drug toxicosis.
    - It has recently been used in veterinary medicine to treat toxicosis associated with lipid-soluble drugs such as baclofen, beta antagonists, calcium channel antagonists, ivermectin, and moxidectin.
  - The exact mechanism of how IFE works is unknown, but possible mechanisms include the following:
    - IFE may create a "pharmacological sink" for fat-soluble drugs.
    - IFE may provide an additional fatty acid supply to improve cardiac performance.
    - IFE may increase intracellular calcium via direct activation of voltage-gated calcium channels. This may restore myocyte function in the drug-depressed myocardium.
  - Adverse effects of IFE may include hyperlipidemia, hepatosplenomegaly, jaundice, seizures, hemolytic anemia, prolonged clotting time, thrombocytopenia, and fat embolism.
  - IFE dosing information is based on human dosing using a 20% solution.
    - 1.5 mL/kg IV bolus over 1 minute. Follow immediately with an IV CRI of 0.25 mL/kg/min PRN for 30–60 minutes.
    - May repeat an IV bolus q 3–5 minutes as needed up to a maximum total dose of 3 mL/kg.
    - If blood pressure continues to drop, may increase infusion up to 0.5 mL/kg/min.
    - It is recommended not to exceed a total dose of 8 mL/kg (human).
- Phytonadione (various manufacturers)
  - Used for the treatment of anticoagulant rodenticide toxicity
  - Analog of systemic vitamin K_1, which is required for the synthesis of clotting factors II, VII, IX, and X

- Dosing information:
  - □ 2–5 mg/kg PO every 24 hours or divided twice a day
  - □ SQ or IM dosing can be used if need be; IM injection may cause injection site bleeding, especially early in therapy. IV administration is not recommended due to incidence of anaphylactoid reactions.
- Skeletal muscle relaxants
  - Methocarbamol (various manufacturers)
    - □ Used for the treatment of tremors associated with pyrethrins and pyrethroids, tremorgenic mycotoxins, strychnine, and CNS stimulant toxicosis
    - □ Centrally acting skeletal muscle relaxant
    - □ Dose:
      - ○ Dogs: 55–220 mg/kg slow IV. Do not exceed 330 mg/kg/day. Monitor for CNS and respiratory depression when using high doses.
      - ○ Cats: 44 mg/kg slow IV, up to 330 mg/kg/day. Monitor for CNS and respiratory depression when using high doses.
  - Dantrolene (Dantrium, Procter and Gamble Pharmaceuticals)
    - □ Used for the treatment of malignant hyperthermia reactions associated with hops (*Humulus lupulus*) or as an adjunct therapy for black widow spider bites
    - □ Direct-acting skeletal muscle relaxant
    - □ Dose (dogs):
      - ○ Black widow spider bites: 1 mg/kg IV followed by 1 mg/kg PO q 4 hours as needed
      - ○ Hops toxicosis: 2–3 mg/kg IV or 3.5 mg/kg PO

Pharmacological or Physiological Antidotes

- Atipamezole, yohimbine
  - Atipamezole (Antisedan, Pfizer) is an alpha$_2$-adrenergic antagonist labeled for reversal of medetomidine and dexmetdetomine. It is used off-label to reverse other alpha-2-adrenergic agonists, including amitraz, clonidine, and xylazine. The half-life is short (2–3 hours) and the drug may need to be repeated if used to reverse longer acting agonists.
    - □ Dose (dogs): 50 μg/kg IM
    - □ Dose (cats): 25–50 μg/kg IM
  - Yohimbine (Yoban, Lloyd) is an alpha$_2$-adrenergic antagonist indicated to reverse the effects of xylazine. The half-life is short (1.5–2 hours) and the drug will likely need to be repeated if used to reverse longer acting agonists. Yohimbine has more side effects at lower doses than atipamezole, including CNS excitation, tremors, and hypersalivation.
    - □ Dose (dogs and cats): 0.11 mg/kg IV slowly

- Atropine (various manufacturers)
  - Antimuscarinic agent used for treatment of SLUDGE (salivation, lacrimation, urination, defecation, and gastroenteritis) that accompanies OP and carbamate insecticide toxicity
  - Competes with acetylcholine at the postganglionic parasympathetic sites
  - Dose (dogs and cats): 0.2–2 mg/kg. One quarter of the dose should be given IV and the remainder IM or SQ. The dose will likely need to be repeated; heart rate and secretions should be used to guide redosing.
  - It is important that enough atropine be provided, especially in large overdoses of OP or carbamates. Atropine should be given despite initial tachycardia, in order to adequately compete with acetylcholine. Without adequate therapy for OP toxicosis, patients may drown in their own secretions.
- Ethanol (various manufacturers)
  - Used as a second-line treatment for ethylene glycol toxicosis. Fomepazole is the preferred treatment.
  - The mechanism of action is similar to fomepizole (inhibits alcohol dehydrogenase), but side effects including CNS depression, metabolic acidosis, and hyperosmolality limit the use.
  - Many different IV treatment recommendations have been made.
    - Preferred method: using 7% ethanol (70 mg/mL), load with 8.6 mL/kg (600 mg/kg) slow IV × 1 dose and follow with 1.43 mL/kg/hour (100 mg/kg/hour) IV CRI for 24–36 hours or until ethylene glycol (EG) test is negative.
    - Other methods can be used depending on source and concentration of ethanol source.
      - 5.5 mL/kg IV of a 20% ethanol solution every 4 hours × 5 doses; follow with 5.5 mL/kg every 6 hours for 4 more doses OR
      - CRI 5.5 mL/kg/hour of 5% ethanol solution until EG test is negative OR
      - 12 mL/kg IV of 5% ethanol solution slow IV followed by 2 mL/kg/hour as CRI until EG test is negative
- Fomepizole or 4-MP (Antizol Vet, Orphan Medical)
  - Indicated as the specific antidote for EG toxicosis
  - 4-MP is a competitive inhibitor of alcohol dehydrogenase. The mechanism of action is similar to ethanol, as it prevents the conversion of EG to toxic metabolites. Unlike ethanol, fomepizole does not result in CNS depression, metabolic acidosis, or hyperosmolality.
  - Labeled for use in dogs; used off-label in cats
    - Dogs: May be treated as late as 8 hours after ingestion and still survive.
    - Cats: Must be treated within 3 hours after ingestion. Cats treated greater than 4 hours after ingestion have a reported mortality rate of 100%.

- Dose (dogs): 20 mg/kg IV over 15–20 minutes as loading dose; 15 mg/kg IV at 12 and 24 hours; 5 mg/kg IV at 36 hours. Repeat EG test. If positive, continue 5 mg/kg IV every 12 hours until negative.
  - Dose (cats): 125 mg/kg slow IV as a loading dose; 31.25 mg/kg IV at 12, 24, and 36 hours.
- Flumazenil (Romazicon, Hoffman, LaRoche)
  - Reversal agent for benzodiazepine overdoses with marked CNS and respiratory depression that are nonresponsive to conventional therapy
  - Competitive antagonist at the benzodiazepine receptor site
  - Use needs to be carefully balanced against the side effects—lowering of seizure threshold, vomiting, and ataxia
  - The duration of action is very short (1–2 hours) and often needs to be repeated, especially when longer acting benzodiazepines have been ingested.
  - Dose (dog and cat): 0.01 mg/kg IV
- Naloxone (Narcan, DuPont Pharmaceuticals)
  - Used for the reversal of CNS and respiratory depression associated with opiate and opioid intoxication
  - Pure opioid antagonist with no analgesic activity
  - Rapid onset of action (1–5 minutes) and short duration of action (approximately 90 minutes). The dose will likely have to be repeated, especially with longer acting opioids.
  - Dose (dogs and cats): 0.01–0.02 mg/kg, IV or IM; may need to use 0.04 mg/kg with larger overdoses

 COMMENTS

- Antidotes, in and of themselves, are not free of side effects and should never be used indiscriminately. Each case needs to be evaluated on an individual basis and the antidote used with knowledge and forethought.
- Many toxicants lack a true antidote, and symptomatic and supportive care is imperative for survival of the poisoned patient. Refer to the previous chapter, "Emergency Management of the Poisoned Patient," for more information on specific supportive care and treatment.
- Many other useful drugs are not mentioned in this chapter, and the reader is directed to the references below for further information.

Abbreviations

4-MP   = 4-methylpyrazole
ALT   = alanine aminotransferase
AST   = aspartate aminotransferase
BAL   = British anti-Lewisite
BUN   = blood urea nitrogen

BW   = body weight
CNS   = central nervous system
CRI   = continuous rate infusion
Fab   = fragment antigen binding
EG   = ethylene glycol
GI   = gastrointestinal
GIT   = gastrointestinal tract
IM   = intramuscular
IV   = intravenous
IFE   = intravenous fat emulsion
IM   = intramuscular
IU   = international units
NAC   = N-acetylcysteine
OP   = organophosphate
PO   = *per os* (by mouth)
PRN   = *pro re nata* (as needed)
q   = every
SLUDGE = salivation, lacrimation, urination, defecation, gastroenteritis
SQ   = subcutaneous
SSRI   = selective serotonin reuptake inhibitor

Suggested Reading

Dalefield RR, Oehme F. Antidotes for specific poisons. In: Peterson ME, Talcott PA, eds. Small Animal Toxicology, 2nd ed. St. Louis: Elsevier, 2006; pp. 459–474.

Gwaltney-Brant S, Rumbeiha W. Newer antidotal therapies. Vet Clin North Am Small Anim Pract 2002; 32(2):323–339.

Plumb DC. Plumb's Veterinary Drug Handbook, 6th ed. Ames, IA: Blackwell, 2008.

Wismer T. Newer antidotal therapies. Proc Int Vet Emerg Critical Care Symp 2004; 812–815.

Author: Lynn R. Hovda, RPH, DVM, MS, DAVCIM
Consulting Editor: Justine A. Lee, DVM, DACVECC

Laboratory Diagnostics for Toxicology

INTRODUCTION

- Diagnosis of poisoning depends on fulfilling five major diagnostic criteria:
  - History
  - Clinical signs
  - Clinical laboratory evaluation
  - Necropsy lesions
  - Chemical analysis
- Used properly, they are an effective combination for detecting and understanding clinical poisoning.

Historical Information

- Knowledge of a known exposure to toxicants and the circumstances surrounding an exposure are essential to an effective toxicological diagnosis.
- One must refrain from basing a diagnosis exclusively on history of exposure. The Post Hoc Fallacy (*Post hoc ergo propter hoc*) as translated from the original Latin admonishes, "After the fact, therefore because of the fact."
- To avoid this, history is used only as a starting point in the diagnostic process.
- The presence of poisons such as rodenticides, insecticides, drugs, paints, household products, over-the-counter and prescription drugs, drugs of abuse, fertilizers, feed additives, and poisonous plants on the premises or a history of their availability or use should be determined.
- Concurrent with this, the adage "Dosage makes the poison" means exposure alone without knowing the amount or dosage encountered is not sufficient for a diagnosis. An attempt should be made to estimate the amount or degree of exposure.
- The food and water supply should be examined carefully for algae, fungi, toxic plants, and foreign matter as well as odors or physical changes that suggest contamination.
- A thorough history will lead to a more informed clinical examination and choice of diagnostic tests. Fundamental information should include patient identification and characteristics, important demographic factors about the environment, and group or individual issues for affected animals.
- Table 4.1 provides a guide for systematic evaluation of history, environment, and clinical effects.

Table 4.1. Checklist for information collection in suspect poisoning of small animals.

Owner data:

Date:_____

Owner:_____

Manager:_____

Address:_____

Phone:_____

FAX:_____

E-mail:_____

Health History:

- Illness past 6 months:
- Exposure to other animals last 30 days:
- Vaccination history:
- Medications: sprays, dips, hormones, minerals, wormers past 6 months— administered by owner or veterinarian?
- Last exam by a veterinarian:

Environmental Data:

- Location: pasture, woods, near river or pond, confined indoors; recent location changes
- Housing: indoors, outdoors, or combination
- Approximate age of home or kennel
- Type of construction (wood frame, metal, concrete)
- Recent changes in access to trash or garbage; pesticides, flower garden, treated wood, old construction materials; recent burning of materials?
- Confined to fenced yard?
- Allowed to roam free?
- If yes, is animal always supervised?
- Businesses or commercial structures accessible?
- Other (describe): _____

_____

Patient data:

Species:_____

Breed:_____

Sex:_____

Pregnancy:_____

Weight:_____

Age:_____

Current Clinical and Environmental History:

- Housing: indoors/outdoors/with other animals
- Are other similar groups on the same premises?
- Common feed or water among groups?
- If a group, what is:
  - morbidity___ mortality ___
- When first observed sick?
- How long has problem existed in this animal?
- If dead, when last seen alive and healthy
- Any recent malicious threats; if yes, describe.
- Recent losses at home or in neighborhood?
- Pesticide use (insecticides, rodenticides, herbicides) and specific types or names if available (ask for tags or bags to ID)
- Materials used for construction/renovation
- Services: e.g., lawn care, seeding, tree planting, fertilization, pest control
- Access to automotive products, cleaning agents, hobby materials, flower gardens, ornamental trees?
- OTC and prescription medications in the home?
- Interactions with wildlife?

Dietary Data:

- Diet components: Dry food only, canned food only, combination? Access to snacks or table foods?
- Recent changes in total diet or specific diet component(s): List any OTC or prescribed supplements.
- Method of feeding: hand feeding, free choice? Is feeding supervised? Food bowl outside?
- Access to molded or spoiled food, mushrooms, bulbs, flower garden plants, indoor plants?
- Recent changes in home/yard: painting, remodeling, pest control, weed sprays, burning trash?
- Any evidence of digging in yard or garden, evidence of damage to plants?
- Water source (flowing stream, pond, well, county or city water):

(Continued)

Table 4.1. *Continued*

Clinical Signs (Check all that apply)	GI Signs	Cardiovascular	Blood
Nervous System	Anorexia	Arrhythmia	Anemia
Ataxia	Colic	Bradycardia	Hemorrhage
Salivation	Vomiting	Hypotension	Icterus
Blindness/vision impaired/ pupil response	Diarrhea	Tachycardia	Hemoglobinuria
	Melena	Other	Methemoglobinemia
Depression	Constipation	**Pulmonary**	**Other**
Excitement	Polyphagia	Cyanosis	Straining
Seizures	**Urinary-Renal**	Dyspnea	Fever
Cerebellar signs	Polydipsia	Hyperpnea	Weakness
Paraparesis or tetraparesis	Polyuria	Rales	
Dysphonia	Hematuria		
Syncope			
Other (describe):			

Clinical Signs

- Clinical signs are of prime importance to the clinician and toxicologist.
  - Both the nature of the signs and sequence of occurrence are important.
    - Did the signs begin explosively and taper off, or did they begin as mild events and worsen with time?
    - Is one body system primarily affected, or are major signs present in several systems?
- Details are often important.
  - For example, a wide range of CNS signs exists and a general description of "seizures" or "tremors" is less useful than an explicit description.
    - Are the signs a typical cranial-to-caudal epileptiform seizure?
    - Is the animal ataxic with cerebellar, vestibular, or peripheral nerve signs?
  - Are there parasympathetic signs such as vomiting, salivation, urination, diarrhea, and dyspnea?
  - Are there parasympatholytic signs such as bloat, dry mouth, mydriasis, hallucinations, or bradycardia?
- Careful attention to changes in heart rate and rhythm can help define several cardiotoxins.
- The attending veterinarian may see only one phase of a toxicological response, so the owner or caretaker should be queried for more information.
- There are dangers in making a toxicological diagnosis based solely on clinical signs as there are thousands of toxic agents but only a limited range of clinical responses that can be expressed by an animal.

Clinical Laboratory

- Evaluation of clinical laboratory changes can help refine associations with specific toxicants or toxicant groups, as well as suggest potential mechanisms of action and alterations in homeostasis that need correction to save the animal.
- Some changes are very characteristic of certain toxicants, while the absence of organ damage is typical of other toxicants.
- CBC and serum chemistries are useful tools for evaluating clinical signs and formulating a treatment plan.
- Table 4.2 provides some typical clinical chemistry and hematologic changes that help define various poisons.

Necropsy Lesions

- Loss of one or more animals in a group or a single animal at risk provides an invaluable opportunity to increase diagnostic information for the science of toxicology.
  - Necropsy may help improve diagnosis and therapy in the remainder of a kennel, herd, or flock.
  - It can also provide guidance to the owner/manager in planning ahead and eliminating the risk for toxicosis.
- Necropsy and microscopic lesions may be invaluable in supporting insurance claims or actions where liability is involved.
  - Lesions are typically absent in certain toxicoses, while the presence of lesions may correlate with other toxicoses.
    - ◻ Pyrethroid toxicosis, strychnine poisoning, and lead poisoning often cause few or very subtle lesions.
    - ◻ Ethylene glycol, copper poisoning, monensin poisoning, and many other toxicoses provide defined lesions helpful for making a diagnosis.
- Necropsy should include the brain (and a rabies exam) if neurological signs are present.
- A thorough selection of lesions at necropsy is easier and more inclusive if consistently performed.
- Should legal or insurance claims be likely, a necropsy is usually essential. In this instance, photographs and detailed notes regarding the necropsy and premise examination should be taken and preserved.
- Table 4.3 summarizes recommended necropsy specimens.

Chemical Analysis

- Chemical analysis is an indispensible aid in forming a toxicological diagnosis. When used properly, and in the right context, chemical analysis may be the single best diagnostic criterion.

Table 4.2. Selected clinical laboratory tests supporting toxicological diagnosis.

Clinical Laboratory Assay	Example Toxicants
Ammonia (serum)	NPN toxicosis, hepatic encephalopathy
aplastic anemia	Phenylbutazone, chloramphenicol, gasoline, petroleum solvents, trichothecene mycotoxins
AST, ALT, LDH increase	Aflatoxin, blue-green algae, fumonisins, pyrrolizidine alkaloids, *Lantana* spp., *Amanita* mushrooms, Sago Palm, xylitol
Azotemia (BUN, creatinine)	Arsenic, cadmium, antifreeze, oak, oxalate plants (e.g., lilies), NSAIDs, grapes, raisins, ACE-inhibitors, beta-blockers, calcium channel antagonists mercury
Basophilic stippling	Lead, zinc
Bile acids	Aflatoxin, other hepatotoxicants (e.g., blue-green algae, *Amanita* mushrooms, xylitol)
Bilirubin	Aflatoxin, fumonisins, zinc toxicosis other hepatotoxicants (e.g., blue-green algae, *Amanita* mushrooms, xylitol)
Carboxyhemoglobin	Carbon monoxide (buildings, trailers), smoke inhalation
Cholinesterase	Organophosphates; blue-green algae; *Solanum* plants
CK increase	Ionophores (monensin, lasalocid), white snake root, *Cassia* spp. toxicants resulting in tremoring or seizuring (causing secondary increased CK)
Coagulopathy (PT, PTT)	Anticoagulant rodenticides, hepatotoxicants, DIC secondary to toxicants resulting in hyperthermia (e.g., Hops, amphetamines, SSRIs)
Crystalluria	Antifreeze, oxalate plants
GGT increase	Aflatoxin, fumonisins, pyrrolizidine alkaloids; glucocorticoids, other hepatotoxicants
Hemolysis	Copper, garlic, onion, red maple, phenothiazine wormers, zinc
Hypercalcemia	Vitamin D_3, day-blooming jessamine, calcium supplements, calcipotriene
Hyperkalemia	Digitalis glycosides, oleander, nephrotoxicants (e.g., ethylene glycol, NSAIDS, grapes, raisins, calcium oxalate containing plants, etc.).
Hyperosmolarity	Antifreeze, aspirin, ethanol, propylene glycol
Hypocalcemia	Antifreeze, oxalate poisoning, nephrotoxicants resulting in renal secondary hyperparathyroidism
Hypoproteinemia	Aflatoxins, chemotherapy, blood loss (e.g., secondary to anticoagulant rodenticides, DIC, NSAID-induced gastric ulceration, etc.)
Iron (serum) and TIBC	Iron toxicosis
Methemoglobin	Acetaminophen, copper, nitrites, chlorates, methylene blue, smoke inhalation red maple
Urinary casts	Nephrotoxicants (e.g., aminoglycosides, NSAIDS, ethylene glycol, grapes, lilies, beta blockers, ACE inhibitors, etc.), arsenic, cadmium, mercury, oak

Table 4.3. Necropsy specimen collection recommended for toxicology.
Brain ½ frozen, ½ formalin. *Leave midline in formalin for pathologist orientation.*
Ocular fluid (2–4 mL) chilled
Injection site (100 g) frozen
Stomach and intestinal contents (1 kg) frozen
Colon contents (1 kg) frozen
Liver (200 g) frozen
Kidney (200 g) frozen
Urine if present (100 mL) ½ chilled, ½ frozen

- Limitations to chemical analysis:
  - Chemical tests should not be relied upon without supporting historical and/or clinical data.
  - Time course of the intoxication, changes since death, or limitations on testing methodology can render a chemical analysis less useful or ineffective for diagnostic confirmation.
  - Chemical tests for all possible poisons are rarely available.
  - Broad spectrum screens using gas chromatography and/or high performance liquid chromatography coupled with mass spectrometry provide more latitude for analysis but often are not quantitative and may be less sensitive than more focused assays.
  - More generalized tests that include ELISA or other immunological technology can be very sensitive but sometimes suffer from cross-reactions or low specificity.
  - Identify a laboratory in advance and be familiar with its reputation and performance prior to the time when rapid or critical testing is needed.
- Most laboratories welcome inquiries about appropriate sampling and test limitations.
- A good laboratory will inform you when a received sample is inadequate or the test requested is not part of their routine and approved offerings.
- For some toxicoses, chemical analysis may not be developed, or a toxic principle may be unknown, so reliance must be on clinical and pathological confirmation of your diagnosis.

Getting the Most from Your Diagnostic Effort

- The principles and approaches described here provide your clients a combination of your best efforts, their best management and information, and the best value you can obtain from laboratory assistance. Not all acute or chronic poisonings become a positive diagnosis.

- In some cases, perhaps many, the poisoning suspect is actually something else that may never be identified.
- The approach outlined is widely accepted and provides a standard of diagnosis that should be supportable and acceptable in veterinary practice.

Abbreviations

ACE	= angiotensin converting enzyme
ALT	= aspartate transferase
AST	= alanine transferase
BUN	= blood urea nitrogen
CK	= creatine kinase
CNS	= central nervous system
DIC	= disseminated intravascular coagulation
ELISA	= enzyme linked immunosorbent assay
GI	= gastrointestinal
LDH	= lactate dehydrogenase
NPN	= non protein nitrogen
NSAIDS	= nonsteroidal anti-inflammatory drugs
OTC	= over the counter
PT	= prothrombin time
PTT	= partial thromboplastin time
SSRI	= selective serotonin reuptake inhibitors

Suggested Reading

Galey FD, Puschner B. Approach to diagnosis and initial treatment of the toxicology case. In: Peterson ME, Talcott, eds. Small Animal Toxicology, 2nd ed. St. Louis: Saunders Elsevier, 2006; pp. 142–153.

Galey FD, Talcott PA. Effective use of a diagnostic laboratory. In: Peterson ME, Talcott, PA, eds. Small Animal Toxicology, 2nd ed. St. Louis: Saunders Elsevier, 2006; pp. 154–164.

Osweiler GD. Diagnostic toxicology. In: Toxicology. Philadelphia: Williams & Wilkins, 1996; pp. 37–46.

Puschner B, Galey FD. Diagnosis and approach to poisoning in the horse. Vet Clin No Amer 2001; 17(3):399–409.

Author: Gary D. Osweiler, DVM, PhD, DABVT
Consulting Editor: Lynn R. Hovda, RPH, DVM, MS, DACVIM

Alcohols and Glycol Ethers

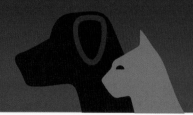

Alcohols (Ethanol, Methanol, Isopropanol)

chapter **5**

DEFINITION/OVERVIEW

- Volatile alcohols are short chain hydrocarbons with a hydroxyl group—methanol has one carbon group, ethanol has two, and isopropanol has three carbons in its hydrocarbon chain.
- Alcohols are commonly used in medicinal, cleaning, and automotive products and as fuels.
- Common sources of exposure for small animals:
  - Ethanol from alcoholic beverages and raw bread dough
  - Isopropanol from rubbing alcohol and antiseptic hand gels
  - Methanol from automotive windshield washer fluid
- Clinical signs and management of toxicosis for volatile alcohols are similar in small animals.
  - CNS depression, ataxia, lethargy, metabolic acidosis, and hypoglycemia are commonly observed.
  - Treatment is primarily supportive with IV fluids to correct dehydration and acid-base status.

ETIOLOGY/PATHOPHYSIOLOGY

Conditions of Exposure and Prevalence

- Ethanol
  - The most common exposure source for ethanol in small animals is alcoholic beverages.
  - The percentage of ethanol in alcoholic beverages is ½ of the value of the drink's proof value (e.g., 100 proof = 50% alcohol).
  - Used in numerous commercial or household products
  - Manufacturing component of paints and varnishes
  - Carrier in various medications
  - Disinfectant in hand antiseptic gels
  - Some types of thermometers
  - Fuel substitute
  - Some forms of antifreeze

- Less commonly used therapeutically to treat ethylene glycol poisoning in dogs and cats (see chap. 3 on antidotes and chap. 6 on ethylene glycol)
- Poisoning has occurred following ingestion of fermented garbage, bread dough, and rotten apples in dogs.
■ **Methanol**
- Methanol is commonly found in automotive windshield washer fluid.
- Present in some gasoline additives
- Solvents and household cleaning products
■ **Isopropanol**
- Commonly found in rubbing alcohol and antiseptic hand gels
- Also found in many everyday products such as paints, inks, general-purpose cleaners, disinfectants, room sprays, and windshield deicing agents

Mechanism of Action

- The neurotoxic effects of volatile alcohols are thought to be due to nonspecific interactions with biomembranes. The mechanism of action probably involves interference with ion transport, such as sodium flux, at the cell membrane rather than at synapses, similar to the action of anesthetic agents.
- Although methanol causes severe acidosis and blindness in humans, other primates, and a few laboratory animals, clinical signs in most domestic animals are less severe and similar to ethanol toxicosis.

Pharmacokinetics/Absorption, Distribution, Metabolism, and Excretion

- Volatile alcohol compounds can be absorbed orally, by inhalation, or by dermal exposure, with oral exposure occurring most commonly.
- The highest blood levels are seen after oral dosing, with lower levels after inhalation and lowest levels after dermal application.
- Volatile alcohols are all rapidly absorbed from the GIT.
- Alcohols rapidly distribute throughout the body and cross the BBB and the placenta.
- Ethanol, methanol, and isopropanol are metabolized by hepatic alcohol dehydrogenase.
  - Ethanol is metabolized to acetaldehyde
  - Methanol to formaldehyde
  - Isopropanol to acetone
- In methanol toxicosis, formaldehyde is rapidly oxidized to formic acid, which is metabolized to carbon dioxide and water in nonprimate species.
- In isopropanol toxicosis, acetone is metabolized to acetic acid, formic acid, and carbon dioxide. The metabolites can be excreted in the urine along with unmetabolized parent compound.
- Volatile alcohols are also excreted via exhaled air.

Toxicity

- Ethanol
  - The LD_{LO} intravenous route for ethanol in dogs is 1.6 ml/kg.
  - The LD_{LO} oral is 5–8 mL/kg.
  - The oral LD_{50} of ethanol in rats is 9 mL/kg.
- Methanol
  - The oral LD_{50} for methanol in dogs is reported to be 4–8 mL/kg.
  - Toxic doses for methanol in canines and felines are approximately the same as for ethanol.
- Isopropanol
  - The oral LD_{50} for isopropanol in dogs is reported to be approximately 2 mL/kg of a 70% isopropanol solution (rubbing alcohol).
  - In general, isopropanol is considered to be twice as potent a CNS depressant than ethanol.

Systems Affected

- Nervous—CNS depression, ataxia, lethargy, sedation
- Gastrointestinal—nausea, vomiting
- Endocrine/metabolic—metabolic acidosis, hypothermia

 # SIGNALMENT/HISTORY

- Canines are more commonly reported to ingest alcoholic products than felines.
- Younger animals tend to chew and drink articles not intended for their consumption.

Risk Factors

- A seasonal effect is seen with alcohol toxicosis. Ethanol toxicosis often occurs during holiday seasons (e.g., Christmas, Easter), when pet owners may be baking desserts more frequently. Methanol toxicosis often occurs during the spring and summer, when windshield wiper fluid is more readily available in the garage.

Historical Findings

- Witnessed ingestion by the owner; chewed bottle found by the pet owner
- Clinical symptoms of ataxia, CNS depression, and lethargy noted by the pet owner

Location and Circumstances of Poisoning

- Ethanol toxicity often occurs in the kitchen, where baked goods are being made.

- Dogs housed in the garage may be at higher risk for ingestion.
- Chewed bottles may be found in the garage or outdoor environment.

 # CLINICAL FEATURES

- Ethanol
  - CNS depression, ataxia, lethargy, and sedation
  - Hypothermia
  - Metabolic acidosis
  - Clinical signs (ataxia and depression) would be expected rapidly (within an hour) if the animal ingested a toxic dose.
  - Excessive gas accumulation in the gut, flatulence, bloating, abdominal pain, vomiting, retching, and nausea can occur in animals ingesting fermented bread dough. The smell of ethanol may be prevalent on the pet's breath.
- Methanol and isopropanol
  - Clinical signs of intoxication are similar to ethanol toxicosis.
  - Isopropanol intoxications may be more prolonged compared to ethanol and methanol intoxications because the acetone metabolite is also a CNS depressant.

 # DIFFERENTIAL DIAGNOSIS

- Other toxicants with sedative and/or CNS depressant effects
  - 2-butoxyethanol
  - Amitraz
  - Barbiturates
  - Benzodiazepines
  - Ethylene glycol
  - Macrolide antiparasitics
  - Marijuana
  - Other volatile alcohols
- Primary neurologic disease (e.g., inflammatory, infectious, infiltrative, etc.)
- Primary metabolic disease (e.g., hypoglycemia, hepatic encephalopathy)
- Hypoglycemia (e.g., juvenile hypoglycemia, xylitol toxicosis, hypoadrenocorticism, insulinoma, hepatic tumor, hunting dog hypoglycemia)

 # DIAGNOSTICS

Clinical Laboratory

- A PCV/TS, blood glucose, and venous blood gas should be performed to evaluate severity of dehydration and electrolyte and acid-base status.

- In isopropanol toxicosis, an osmole gap may develop.
- Most laboratories are capable of determining ethanol, methanol, or isopropanol levels in blood although ethanol determination is most commonly available as a routine test.
- The PRN ethylene glycol test should not be used to test for the presence of ethanol and methanol, as these alcohols will not be detected by that test.

Pathological Findings

- There are no specific gross or histological lesions observed in alcohol-poisoned animals and in methanol poisoning in nonprimate animals.

THERAPEUTICS

Detoxification

- Alcohols in general are absorbed very quickly from the GIT. If recent ingestion of ethanol (e.g., desserts, alcoholic drinks, bread dough, etc.) has occurred (e.g., witnessed, <15 minutes), emesis induction should promptly occur provided the patient is asymptomatic and able to protect its airway.
- Since alcohols can cause CNS depression, inducing emesis in a symptomatic animal may result in aspiration of vomitus and is contraindicated. If a large amount of gastric contents is present in a symptomatic patient, gastric lavage may need to be performed under sedation and with an inflated endotracheal tube to prevent aspiration.
- Activated charcoal has been shown not to be effective with alcohol overdoses and is not recommended.

Appropriate Health Care

- If respiratory function is compromised, a cuffed endotracheal tube should be placed and ventilation supported mechanically as required.
- If dermal exposure to volatile alcohols has occurred, rinse the affected area with water.

Drugs and Antidotes of Choice

- A balanced, isotonic crystalloid IV fluid should be used in symptomatic patients to aid in correction of dehydration and to enhance renal excretion.
- In the presence of a severe metabolic acidosis (e.g., pH <7.0, BE < −15 mm Hg, HCO_3 <11 mm Hg), the judicious use of sodium bicarbonate can be considered.
  - Dose: 0.3 × BW in kg × base deficit
  - Give ⅓–½ this amount of sodium bicarbonate slowly IV over 20–30 minutes; repeat as needed, pending recheck venous blood gas analysis.
- Yohimbine

- Give 0.1–0.2 mg/kg IV, beginning with lower dosage. Yohimbine's half-life is short (<2 hr), so repeat therapy may be important. This drug is not specifically cleared for treatment of ethanol toxicosis but is reported effective for that purpose.

Nursing Care

- Alcohol toxicosis can result in severe obtundation, and appropriate nursing care is imperative. Patients should be in a bedded cage and should be turned every 6 hours to prevent atelectasis. Ophthalmic lubrication may be necessary every 6 hours. Keeping the patient clean and dry is imperative.
- Monitor temperature, heart rate, and respiratory rate.
- Monitor blood pressure and blood glucose frequently and treat appropriately.

Follow-up

- Follow-up is generally unnecessary, as patients are clinically normal once signs resolve.

Activity

- Patients should be restricted from activity until clinical signs resolve, as ataxia and CNS depression will be apparent. Once clinical signs resolve, no exercise restriction is necessary.

Prevention

- Prevent access of pets to obvious or potential sources of alcohol.

 COMMENTS

Client Education

- Advise and reinforce that alcohol products are dangerous for pets, and review the atypical sources of alcohol available in the home (e.g., kitchen).
- Recommend exposures resulting in severe depression and/or GIT signs be examined by a veterinarian.

Patient Monitoring

- Acid-base monitoring is recommended in symptomatic animals.

Expected Course and Prognosis

- Most cases involving mild signs usually resolve with close monitoring and supportive care within a 24-hour period.

■ No long-term effects are expected.
■ The prognosis is fair to guarded in cases involving metabolic acidosis, severe CNS or respiratory system depression, or aspiration pneumonia.

Abbreviations

BBB = blood brain barrier
BE   = base excess
BW   = body weight
CNS = central nervous system
GI   = gastrointestinal
GIT = gastrointestinal tract
IM   = intramuscular
IV   = intravenous
LD_{LO} = lowest observed lethal dose
LD_{50} = median lethal dose
PCV = packed cell volume
PRN = *pro re nata* (as needed)
TS   = total solids

See also

Ethylene Glycol

Suggested Reading

Means C. Bread dough toxicosis in dogs. J Vet Emerg Crit Care 2003; 13(1):39–41.
Valentine WM. Short-chain alcohols. Vet Clin North Am Small Anim Pract 1990; 20(2):515–523.

Author: Anita M. Kore, DVM, PhD, DABVT
Consulting Editor: Gary D. Osweiler, DVM, PhD, DABVT; Justine A. Lee, DVM, DACVECC

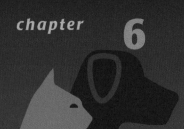

chapter **6**

Ethylene Glycol

DEFINITION/OVERVIEW

- Ethylene glycol (EG) is a sweet-tasting and odorless liquid used for its antifreeze properties to lower the freezing point of water.
- The most common source of EG exposure in small animals is automotive antifreeze (95% EG).
- EG is also found in windshield deicing agents, solvents, paints, hydraulic brake fluid, motor oil, inks, wood stains, and in developing solutions for photography.

ETIOLOGY/PATHOPHYSIOLOGY

Mechanism of Action

- EG is biotransformed into highly toxic metabolites leading to acute renal failure (ARF) and severe metabolic acidosis.
- Oxalic acid, a primary metabolite of EG, binds to serum calcium resulting in calcium oxalate crystal formation. Crystals are then deposited in the kidneys resulting in crystalluria, ARF, and death.

Pharmacokinetics/Absorption, Distribution, Metabolism, and Excretion

- Absorption
  - EG is rapidly absorbed from the GIT.
  - Food in the stomach delays absorption.
- Distribution
  - Distribution through blood and tissues occurs quickly.
  - The plasma half-life is about 3 hours.
  - Calcium oxalate deposition in the tissues (primarily renal) will remain much longer.
- Metabolism
  - Metabolism occurs primarily in the liver within 2–4 hours of ingestion.
  - EG is largely metabolized by alcohol dehydrogenase (ADH) to glycoaldehydes and organic acids, the most notable of which is oxalic acid.

- Calcium oxalate crystals are formed when calcium binds to oxalic acid. They may be deposited in many tissues but cause severe damage in the kidneys.
- Excretion
    - Excretion of the parent compound and the metabolites is usually complete within 24–48 hours via the kidneys.

Toxicity

- The minimum lethal dose of undiluted ethylene glycol is 4.2–6.6 mL/kg for the dog (the equivalent of about 1 teaspoon/kg) and 1.5 mL/kg for the cat (the equivalent of about ¼ teaspoon/kg).

Systems Affected

- Gastrointestinal—EG is a gastric irritant.
- Nervous—Glycoaldehyde causes CNS dysfunction secondary to glucose and serotonin metabolism depression.
- Metabolic—Glycolic acid accumulation is the primary cause of metabolic acidosis.
- Cardiovascular—tachycardia
- Respiratory—tachypnea
- Renal—ARF is the primary cause of death from EG toxicity. EG metabolites are cytotoxic resulting in calcium oxalate crystalluria, swollen and painful kidneys, and oliguria progressing to anuria.

 SIGNALMENT/HISTORY

- Any pet with access to ethylene glycol is at risk for toxicosis.
- Diagnosis is based on history, clinical signs, and specific diagnostic testing.

Risk Factors

- EG is thought to have a mildly sweet flavor that intrigues and is palatable to dogs.
- Cats are generally affected by walking through the spilled product, then grooming their paws.

Historical Findings

- Owners may report "drunken" behavior such as ataxia, stupor, vomiting, and lethargy.
- Witnessed ingestions of automotive antifreeze (spilled puddles, leaking radiators, straight from the container) are the most commonly reported finding with EG exposures.
- Cases of malicious poisoning have been reported.

Location and Circumstances of Poisoning

- Most exposures occur in the garage or driveway.
- Most cases occur in the fall, winter, and spring.

Interactions with Drugs, Nutrients, or Environment

- There is a higher incidence of toxicity in colder areas of the country where ethylene glycol is used more frequently as antifreeze.

 CLINICAL FEATURES

- There are typically three stages of EG toxicity.
- Stage 1 and stage 2 are difficult to distinguish from each other.
  - Stage 1: occurs within 30 minutes to 12 hours and appears as alcohol intoxication.
    - □ Nausea, vomiting, PU/PD, CNS depression, ataxia, compromised withdrawal and righting reflexes, pronounced hypothermia, osmotic diuresis, seizures, coma, and death (rarely)
    - □ Cats are primarily depressed and do not show polydipsia.
    - □ Metabolic acidosis
    - □ Calcium oxalate crystalluria
  - Stage 2: occurs 12–24 hours postingestion
    - □ CNS signs may abate and dogs appear "recovered"; cats typically remain depressed
    - □ Dehydration
    - □ Tachycardia and tachypnea
  - Stage 3: occurs 12–24 hours postingestion in cats and 36–72 hours postingestion in dogs and is a result of the metabolites.
    - □ Oliguric renal failure (increases in BUN and creatinine, decrease in urine output) progressing to anuric renal failure
    - □ The kidneys can be swollen and painful, especially in cats.
    - □ Severe depression, lethargy, or coma
    - □ Anorexia, continuous vomiting, oral ulcers, and hypersalivation.
    - □ Seizures, coma, death

 DIFFERENTIAL DIAGNOSIS

- Other toxins: ethanol, methanol, marijuana
- Increased anion gap: DKA and lactic acidosis
- Hypoglycemic shock
- Pancreatitis
- Gastroenteritis (viral, bacterial, garbage can toxicity)
- Rabies
- Acute renal failure secondary to:

- Infectious causes (leptospirosis)
- Inflammatory causes (nephritis)
- Renal ischemia (hypoperfusion)
- Drugs (aminoglycoside antibiotics, cyclosporine, acetaminophen, aspirin, others)
- Grapes/raisins
- Plants (lilies ingested by cats)
- Heavy metals

 DIAGNOSTICS

- Blood EG concentration—depending on the test, very helpful in establishing diagnosis
  - Veterinary diagnostic labs and human hospitals can accurately determine blood (and sometimes urine) EG concentrations using enzymatic assays, HPLC or GC-MS. Turnaround times vary but may be quick enough to aid in diagnosis.
  - Inexpensive, bedside, commercially available tests estimate blood EG concentrations ≥20 mg/dL (at the time of publication, only the Kacey Diagnostics KCEGT test remained on the market; the PRN Pharmacal REACT Ethylene Glycol Test Kit was discontinued in 2010).
    - □ Bedside tests measure the parent compound (EG) and do not test for EG metabolites. Thus, they must be used within the first few hours after ingestion. Late use may result in false negatives.
    - □ False positive test results may occur with propylene glycol (carrier of diazepam), glycerol, mannitol, sorbitol (common cathartic in activated charcoal preparations), and isopropyl alcohol. (Do not swab the venipuncture site prior to sampling.)
    - □ Ethanol and methanol do not typically cause false positive tests results.
    - □ Cats may suffer toxicosis below 50 mg/dL. Some bedside tests may be sensitive enough to measure below this point. Consultation with the manufacturer is recommended.
- Blood gases—very helpful in establishing diagnosis
  - Total CO_2, plasma bicarbonate concentration, and blood pH are all decreased by 3 hours postingestion. All are markedly decreased by 12 hours postingestion.
  - Thus, a severe metabolic acidosis combined with a positive bedside test (above) is consistent with EG exposure.
- Chemistry panel and serum osmolality—very helpful in establishing diagnosis
  - Serum osmolality is very useful in early diagnosis. Serum osmolality and osmole gap are dose related and are increased by 1 hour postingestion. Results up to 450 mosm/kg may be seen 3 hours postingestion, and both remain elevated for 18 hours postingestion.

- Anion gap is increased by 3 hours postingestion. It peaks at 6 hours postingestion and remains increased for approximately 48 hours.
- Elevated BUN and creatinine (occurs about 24–48 hours postingestion in dogs and about 12 hours postingestion in cats)
- Hyperkalemia if oliguric or anuric
- Hypocalcemia occurs in about half of the patients because of chelation of calcium by oxalic acid, and is occasionally observed secondary to acidosis.
- Hyperglycemia occurs in about half of the patients because of inhibition of glucose metabolism by aldehydes, increased epinephrine, and endogenous corticosteroids. It may also occur because of uremia.
- Hyperphosphatemia occurs transiently about 3–6 hours postingestion because of phosphate rust inhibitors in some antifreeze products.
  - ☐ Absence of elevated BUN and creatinine may be due to ingestion of the rust inhibitor and should not necessarily be considered a result of renal failure.
  - ☐ Hyperphosphatemia seen later in the course of the toxicity is secondary to decreased glomerular filtration.
- Urinalysis—helpful in establishing diagnosis
  - Isosthenuria (1.008–1.012) occurs in dogs by 3 hours postingestion. It may occur in later stages of toxicosis because of renal dysfunction.
  - Cats may also show decreased urine specific gravity, but it may be above the isosthenuria range.
  - Calcium oxalate crystalluria may show as early as 3 hours postingestion in cats and 6 hours postingestion in dogs. The monohydrate form is more common.
  - Urine pH consistently decreases.
  - Hematuria, proteinuria, glucosuria are inconsistent findings.
  - May see granular and cellular casts, WBCs, RBCs and renal epithelial cells in the sediment.
- CBC—not useful to establish diagnosis
  - PCV and TP are often elevated secondary to dehydration.
  - Stress leukogram
- Other
  - Use Wood's lamp examination of urine, face, paws, vomitus, etc. to note fluorescein dye (often added to automotive antifreeze). Dye is excreted in the urine for up to 6 hours after ingestion.

Pathological Findings

- Focal hemorrhage in gastric lining, intestinal mucosa, heart, brain, liver
- Swollen kidneys (gross)
- Proximal tubular degeneration and necrosis with intraluminal calcium oxalate deposition in the kidneys

- Interstitial fibrosis and inflammation in the kidneys, primarily in chronic renal failure cases

 THERAPEUTICS

- Treatment must be instituted quickly.
- The goal of therapy is to prevent absorption, increase excretion, and prevent conversion of EG to highly toxic metabolites.

Detoxification

- Very early emesis or gastric lavage may help limit absorption, but absorption occurs quickly, so decontamination will be of benefit only if instituted early.
- AC does not bind well to EG (and *does* bind well to oral ethanol, so if oral ethanol is to be used as a treatment, AC should definitely *not* be used).

Appropriate Health Care

- See "Drug(s) and Antidotes of Choice"
- Additional treatments include the following:
  - IVF at 2–3 × maintenance if using the antidote of ethanol
  - IVF at 2 × maintenance if using the antidote of fomepizole
  - IV sodium bicarbonate added to IVF if blood gas analysis indicates a severe metabolic acidosis (if pH <7.1, HCO_3 <11, base excess <–15)
  - If treating with ethanol, monitor blood glucose q 4–6 hours because of risk of hypoglycemia.
    - □ Administer IV 2.5%–5 % dextrose as IV CRI to maintain blood glucose.
  - Antiemetics if needed (e.g., maropitant 1 mg/kg SQ q 24 hours). Not labeled for cats.
  - GIT protectants if needed
    - □ H_2 blockers (e.g., famotidine 0.5–1 mg/kg PO, SQ, IM, IV q 12 hours) (Do not use IV in cats.)
    - □ Proton pump inhibitors (e.g., omeprazole 0.5–1 mg/kg PO q 24 hours)
    - □ Sucralfate (0.25–1 g PO q 8 hours) if evidence of gastric erosion/ ulceration
  - Phosphate binders if needed:
    - □ Aluminum hydroxide 2–10 mL PO every 6 hours
  - Monitor urine output. If becoming oliguric (0.5 mL urine/kg/hour) or anuric (<0.5 mL urine/kg/hour), consider the following:
    - □ First increase the fluid rate, but monitor hydration, weight, and respiration carefully to avoid volume overload.
    - □ If no improvement in urine output, add intermittent boluses of furosemide (2–4 mg/kg IV for dogs and cats), 20–25% mannitol (0.25– 0.5 gm/kg IV over 5–10 minutes), or dopamine CRI (2–5 mcg/kg/min).

- Vitamin B$_1$ (100 mg/day PO)
- 10% calcium gluconate (50–150 mg/kg, dogs), (94–140 mg/kg, cats) can be added over 20–30 minutes to effect for severe clinical hypocalcemia (tremors, seizures). Monitor heart rate and rhythm, respiratory rate during infusion.
- If no vomiting, offer food and water throughout care, especially if ethanol is used as an antidote (to help avoid hypoglycemia).

Drug(s) and Antidotes of Choice

- Fomepizole and ethanol are both antidotes for EG toxicity. Fomepizole is strongly preferred. Use only one, not both.
- Fomepizole (4-metylpyrazole, Antizole-Vet) should be used within the first 3–8 hours to be effective. It inhibits ADH, which stops the formation of oxalic acid.
    - Antizole-Vet is available as 1.5 g fomepizole/1.5 mL solution. The small vial must be reconstituted with 30 mL 0.9% NaCl (large vial in box) resulting in a final concentration of 50 mg/mL.
        - Dogs:
            - Loading dose of 20 mg/kg IV
            - 15 mg/kg IV at 12 and 24 hours
            - 5 mg/kg IV at 36 hours
            - Can continue to treat with 3 mg/kg IV q 12 hours until serum EG is undetectable or animal is clinically normal
        - Cats:
            - Not labeled for use in cats, as very large doses may be needed to obtain results.
            - If cat has ingested a very high dose, use within the first 6 hours. For the greatest chance of survival, use within the first 3 hours following ingestion is strongly recommended.
            - 125 mg/kg IV slowly to load
            - 31.25 mg/kg IV at 12, 24, and 36 hours after initial loading
        - Adverse reactions:
            - Approximately 1% of dogs will develop an anaphylactic reaction after the second IV dose.
            - Other side effects are trembling, salivation, tachypnea.
            - CNS depression, serum hyperosmolarity, or osmotic diuresis does not occur at therapeutic doses.
            - If large nontherapeutic doses are used, CNS depression may be severe.
        - Advantages:
            - Advantages over the use of ethanol as an antidote include fewer CNS effects, fewer renal effects, and no need for continuous infusions.

Alternative drugs

- If fomepizole is not available, ethanol may be used as an antidote.
- Ethanol needs to be given within the first few hours of ingestion to be effective.
- Ethanol needs to be diluted to the appropriate concentration and dextrose must be added to prevent hypoglycemia. Various acceptable IV fluids include D5W, LRS plus dextrose, etc.
  - In the U.S., alcoholic proof is twice the percentage of alcohol (i.e., 100 proof = 50% ethanol = 500 mg/ mL).
- Different IV treatment recommendations have been made.
  - Preferred method
    - Using 7% ethanol (70 mg/ mL), load with 8.6 mL/kg (600 mg/kg) slow IV × 1 dose. Then follow with 1.43 mL/kg/hour (100 mg/kg/hour), IV CRI for 24–36 hours or until EG test is negative.
  - Other methods can be used depending on source and concentration of ethanol source:
    - 5.5 mL/kg IV of a 20% ethanol solution every 4 hours × 5 doses; follow with 5.5 mL/kg every 6 hours for 4 more doses, *OR*
    - CRI 5.5 mL/kg/hour of 5% ethanol solution until EG test is negative, *OR*
    - 12 mL/kg IV of 5% ethanol solution slow IV followed by 2 mL/kg/ hour as CRI until EG test is negative.

Precautions/Interactions

- Use only *one* of the antidotes, fomepizole *OR* ethanol.
- Fomepizole may contribute to CNS depression in cats (not seen in dogs).
- Intermittent ethanol can cause fluctuations in treatment and side effects.
- Hypoglycemia, CNS depression, respiratory depression, and hypothermia may occur as side effects to use of ethanol as an antidote.

Surgical Considerations

- Kidney transplantation has been accomplished successfully in cats with renal failure following ethylene glycol toxicity.

Prevention

- Keep pets away from areas of leaking antifreeze.
- Clean leaks immediately with use of kitty litter or copious flushing.
- Use antifreeze containing propylene glycol instead of ethylene glycol.

COMMENTS

Client Education

- Educate clients about the risk of toxicity and about preventive measures.
- Educate clients about early intervention and treatment if exposure occurs.

Patient Monitoring

- Monitor urine output, blood pressure, hydration, awareness often.
- Monitor BUN/creatinine/venous blood gas daily (at minimum).

Expected Course and Prognosis

- Renal tubular damage by EG may be reversible, but complete recovery may take weeks to months, and some animals may not regain concentrating ability for a year or more.
- Prognosis is excellent for dogs treated with fomepizole within 5 hours of EG ingestion.
- Most dogs treated with fomepizole within 8 hours of ingestion will recover.
- Prognosis is good for cats treated within 3 hours of ingestion.
- Prognosis is poor for patients in oliguric renal failure.

Synonym

Antifreeze toxicity

Abbreviations

AC	= activated charcoal
ADH	= alcohol dehydrogenase
ARF	= acute renal failure
BUN	= blood urea nitrogen
CBC	= complete blood count
CNS	= central nervous system
CO_2	= carbon dioxide
CRI	= continuous rate infusion
DKA	= diabetic ketoacidosis
EG	= ethylene glycol
GC-MS	= gas chromatography–mass spectrometry
GI	= gastrointestinal
GIT	= gastrointestinal tract
HCO_3	= bicarbonate
HPLC	= high pressure liquid chromatography
IM	= intramuscular

IV   = intravenous
NaCl   = sodium chloride
PCV   = packed cell volume
PO   = *per os* (by mouth)
PRN   = *pro re nata* (as needed)
PU/PD   = polyuria/polydipsia
q   = every
RBC   = red blood cell
SQ   = subcutaneous
TP   = total protein
WBC   = white blood cell

See Also

Alcohols (Ethanol, Methanol, Isopropanol)
Propylene Glycol

Suggested Reading

Connally HE, et al. Inhibition of canine and feline alcohol dehydrogenase activity by fomepizole. Am J Vet Res 2000; 61:450–455.
Dalefield R. Ethylene glycol. In: Plumlee K, ed. Clinical Veterinary Toxicology. St. Louis: Mosby Elsevier, 2004; pp. 150–154.
Thrall MA et al. Ethylene glycol. In: Talcott P, Peterson M, eds. Small Animal Toxicology, 2nd ed. Philadelphia: Elsevier Saunders, 2005; pp. 702–726.

Authors: Catherine M. Adams, DVM; Mary Anna Thrall, DVM, MS
Consulting Editors: Ahna G. Brutlag, DVM; Gary D. Osweiler, DVM, PhD, DABVT

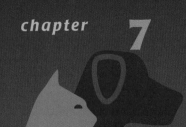

chapter 7

Propylene Glycol

DEFINITION/OVERVIEW

Description

- Propylene glycol (PG) is a dihydroxy alcohol that is miscible with water, so frequently is used as a carrier for hydrophobic compounds usually insoluble in water.
- It is colorless, nearly odorless, and tasteless. After consumption by animals, it is metabolized to L- and D-lactic acid, which results in acidosis as a part of its mechanism of action.

Uses

- Propylene glycol is a component of many consumer products that require humectant, emollient, or hydroscopic properties.
- PG is found in consumer products such as solvents and preservatives for room deodorants, disinfectants, hair dyes/colorants, suntan lotions, cosmetic creams, dentrifices, food coloring, moist pet foods, medicines, and paints and varnishes.
- Major component of safer alternative automotive antifreeze fluids
- Industrial products use PG in lubricants, heat-transfer fluids, and corrosion inhibitors.
- Metabolism of PG produces excessive D-lactic acid leading to metabolic acidosis.
- Acute clinical effects of oral exposure include depression or narcosis that is primarily related to the agent itself and enhanced by the depressive effect of acidosis from excessive metabolism to D-lactic acidosis. For cats, exposure can result in Heinz body anemia.

ETIOLOGY/PATHOPHYSIOLOGY

Mechanism of Action

- After consumption, PG can accumulate in the brain at high concentrations and result in CNS depression and narcosis similar to the early effects of ethylene glycol or the depressant effects of ethanol.

- Metabolized by similar hepatic enzymes as for ethylene glycol (e.g., alcohol dehydrogenase and aldehyde dehydrogenase)
- D and L isomers of lactic acid are produced.
- L-lactic acid is utilized for energy in the TCA cycle, but D-lactic acid is not and accumulates in blood.
- Result of D-lactic acid accumulation in blood is metabolic acidosis due to lactic acid.
- Prolonged exposure to PG can denature susceptible Hb of cats and lead to RBC membrane damage, resulting in Heinz body anemia.

Pharmacokinetics/Absorption, Distribution, Metabolism, and Excretion

- Rapidly absorbed from the GIT after oral administration
- Negligible absorption from application to intact skin
- Volume of distribution is approximately 0.6 L/kg in humans; information for dogs or cats not available.
- Plasma levels peak approximately one hour postingestion.
- Metabolized by alcohol dehydrogenase to pyruvic acid, D-lactic acid, and L-lactic acid
- Pyruvic and D-lactic acid are utilized in the TCA cycle.
- Aldehyde dehydrogenase further metabolizes PG to intermediates which are excreted as CO_2 and water.
- An average of approximately 28% of PG is excreted unmetabolized in urine.
- Metabolites may be conjugated with glucuronides and excreted in urine.
- Dogs excrete nearly all of dosed PG within 24 hours.

Toxicity

- Toxicity values for dogs and cats are relatively sparse.
- The acute LD_{50} for dogs is reported as low as 9 mL/kg.
- Dosage of 5 g/kg daily to dogs caused hemolytic anemia, reticulocytosis, and hyperbilirubinemia.
- Canine dosage of 2 g/kg/day caused no effects.
- Cats administered 1.6 g/kg and 8 g/kg PG PO daily had dose-related increases in Heinz bodies of 28% and 92%, respectively after 2–4 weeks.
- Moist-soft food containing >5% PG caused Heinz body anemia in kittens.
- PG at 6% of the diet caused increased reticulocyte counts in adult cats.

Systems Affected

- Neurologic—depression to narcosis resulting from alcohol-like effects of the parent compound early and by lactic acidosis later in toxicosis
- Respiratory—increased respiratory rate and effort secondary to metabolic acidosis (more prominent in dog versus cat)

- Musculoskeletal—muscle twitching (cats)
- Cardiovascular—hypotension (cats), circulatory failure (dogs)
- Renal/urologic—PU/PD secondary to PG's osmotic diuretic effect
- Hemic/lymphatic/immune—hemolytic anemia from large overdoses; Heinz body anemia (primarily cats)

 ## SIGNALMENT/HISTORY

Risk Factors

- Accidental exposure to large dosages such as solvents and carriers results in acute CNS depression and hemolytic anemia.
- Prolonged contamination at lower dosages (e.g., contaminated foods) is likely to result in Heinz body anemia in cats when fed at >5% PG for more than 2–4 weeks.

Historical Findings

- Acute onset of depression, ataxia, or narcosis after exposure to commercial or industrial products
- Onset of Heinz body anemia and/or hyperbilirubinemia with no other explanation

Location and Circumstances of Poisoning

- Has been associated with contaminated moist foods in cats
- Animals exposed to environments high in contaminated commercial products or home care products

Interactions with Drugs, Nutrients, or Environment

- Presence of or exposure to CNS depressants (e.g., alcohols, narcotics, barbiturates)
- Consumption of other oxidant drugs or foods (e.g., acetaminophen, onions)
- Diabetes mellitus and hyperthyroidism are reported to increase susceptibility to Heinz body anemia, potentially worsening the severity of PG toxicosis.

 ## CLINICAL FEATURES

- Initial signs of depression, weakness, ataxia followed by severe depression to narcosis
- Some species are reported to have seizures as well (e.g., cats).
- Hypotension and/or cardiovascular collapse can occur.

- Continuing lactic acidosis may be manifest as depression that compounds the early PG narcotic effects.
- Renal—PU/PD

 DIFFERENTIAL DIAGNOSIS

- Primary neurologic disease
- Primary metabolic disease (e.g., hepatic encephalopathy, hypoglycemia, hypoadrenocorticism)
- Hypoglycemia (e.g., insulinoma, hepatic neoplasia, iatrogenic insulin therapy, hunting dog hypoglycemia)
- Metabolic acidosis (e.g., diabetic ketoacidosis, uremic acidosis, lactic acidosis, ethylene glycol toxicity, etc.)
- Toxicosis:
  - Acetaminophen toxicosis
  - Ethanol toxicosis
  - Ethylene glycol poisoning—phase I
  - Heinz body anemia
  - Onion/garlic
  - Zinc toxicosis

DIAGNOSTICS

Clinical Laboratory

- Baseline CBC, chemistry panel, UA, and venous blood gas analysis to rule out underlying metabolic disease and acid-base/electrolyte disorders
  - Cats
    - Decreased RBC is variable
    - Increased reticulocyte count
    - Reduced RBC survival time
    - Elevated mean corpuscular hemoglobin concentration
    - Increased anion gap which correlates with increased D-lactic acidemia
  - Dogs
    - No specific laboratory effects reported
    - Acute high-dose exposure might increase D-lactic acidemia

Pathological Findings (Cats)

- Nodular spleen
- Mottled liver

- Periportal hepatocyte vacuolation with positive staining for glycogen
- Slight increase in iron pigmentation after chronic exposure to PG

 ## THERAPEUTICS

Detoxification

- Acute poisoning from single ingestions is less likely than prolonged subacute or chronic exposure.
  - Therefore, activated charcoal or emesis is not always effective unless recent ingestion occurred or large dosages were ingested.
- Because of the hydrophilic nature of PG, it may cause diarrhea from acute ingestion, and the use of cathartics with activated charcoal should be considered carefully before proceeding.
- PG is poorly absorbed through skin, but very large dermal exposure can be reduced by a warm soap and water bath.

Appropriate Health Care

- The usual course for affected animals will involve a combination of CNS, GI and hematological effects.
- Treat depression or narcosis medically if severe enough to threaten life functions.
  - Provide CNS supportive care (e.g., respiratory support, mechanical ventilation, etc.) as needed.
  - As PG is metabolized, neurologic effects should regress.
- Assess conditions such as vomiting, diarrhea, and aspiration.
- Monitor blood pressure and ECG to rule out underlying arrhythmias and hypotension; treat accordingly.
- Hypoglycemia and metabolic acidosis should be treated appropriately with IV supplementation and IV fluids.

Drug(s) and Antidotes of Choice

- There is no antidote.
- IV fluid therapy with a balanced, maintenance, isotonic fluid to maintain hydration, perfusion, and correct metabolic acidosis
- Ascorbic acid can be used as an antioxidant. However, research with cats indicates that common antioxidants (e.g., NAC, d-l α tocopherol, ascorbic acid) are not effective in reducing the hematological effects of PG.
- For severe metabolic acidosis (e.g., pH <7.0, BE <−15 mm Hg, HCO_3 <11 mm Hg), consider sodium bicarbonate therapy.
  - Sodium bicarbonate dose: $0.3 \times BW$ (kg) $\times$ base deficit

- Give ⅓–½ of calculated dose, slow IV over 20 minutes; recheck venous blood gas analysis, clinical condition, and response to therapy as needed.
■ Assess need to treat for Heinz body anemia.
    - PCV may not be significantly decreased when Heinz body anemia is present.
    - Half-life of RBCs in cats is reduced by 50% with Heinz body anemia.
    - Evaluate PCV, reticulocyte count, extent of Heinz bodies, and clinical symptoms for hemorrhagic shock. Treat as necessary with pRBCs or hemoglobin-binding oxygen carriers (e.g., Oxyglobin).

Precautions/Interactions

■ Fish-based or soft-moist diets are associated with increased RBC damage from PG.
■ Of the common antioxidants (e.g., NAC, vitamin E, ascorbic acid), only NAC was modestly beneficial to improved erythrocyte status during PG toxicosis.

Nursing Care

■ Continue to monitor acid-base status and RBC indices.
■ Treat symptomatically for continuing vomiting or diarrhea.

Follow-up

■ Recheck red cell indices 1–2 weeks after discharge, sooner if patient develops symptoms.
■ Heinz bodies should resolve in 6–8 weeks after exposure stops.

Diet

■ High-quality dry diet, free of fish products and low in fat

Activity

■ Normal activity is likely if acute acidosis and anemia have resolved.

Prevention

■ Avoid potential exposures, especially in cats.

Public Health

■ Humans are susceptible to overdose of PG.

Environmental Issues

■ Improper disposal of PG or PG-containing products in water or soil should be avoided.

COMMENTS

Client Education

▪ Inform clients of caution with high-fat, fish-based, low-quality moist diets.

Patient Monitoring

▪ Monitor RBC morphology, which should return to normal 6–8 weeks postexposure.

Prevention/Avoidance

▪ Avoid common sources of PG in diet or commercial products.
▪ Note that alternative automotive antifreeze is primarily PG.
▪ Nursing queens and growing kittens are considered more susceptible to PG effects.

Expected Course and Prognosis

▪ Recovery after acute phase should be uncomplicated.

Abbreviations

BE   = base excess
BW   = body weight
CBC   = complete blood count
CNS   = central nervous system
CO_2 = carbon dioxide
ECG   = electrocardiogram
GI   = gastrointestinal
GIT   = gastrointestinal tract
Hb   = hemoglobin
HCO_3 = bicarbonate
IM   = intramuscular
IV   = intravenous
NAC   = N-acetylcysteine
PCV   = packed cell volume
PG   = propylene glycol
PO   = *per os* (by mouth)
pRBC   = packed red blood cells
PU/PD   = polyuria/polydypsia
RBC   = red blood cell
TCA   = tricarboxylic acid
TS   = total solids
UA   = urinalysis

See Also

Acetaminophen
Alcohols (Ethanol, Methanol, Isopropanol)
Ethylene Glycol
Onions and Garlic
Zinc

Suggested Reading

Bauer MC, Weiss DJ, Perman V. Hematologic alterations in adult cats fed 6% or 12% propylene glycol. Am J Vet Res 1992; 53(1):69–72.

Bischoff K. Propylene glycol. In: Peterson ME, Talcott PA, eds. Small Animal Toxicology, St. Louis: Elsevier Saunders, 2006; pp 996–1001.

Christopher MM, Perman V, Eaton JW. Contribution of propylene glycol–induced Heinz body formation to anemia in cats. JAVMA 1989; 194(8):1045–1056.

Dalefield R. Propylene glycol. In: Plumlee KH, ed. Clinical Veterinary Toxicology, St. Louis: Elsevier Mosby, 2004; pp 168–170.

Hickman MA, Rodgers QR, Morris JG. Effects of diet on Heinz body formation in kittens. Am J Vet Res 1990; 50(3):475–478.

Author: Gary D. Osweiler, DVM, PhD, DABVT
Consulting Editors: Gary D. Osweiler, DVM, PhD, DABVT; Justine A. Lee, DVM, DACVECC

Construction and Industrial Materials

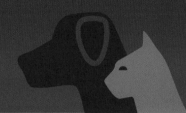

Glues/Adhesives

DEFINITION/OVERVIEW

- Cyanoacrylate glues or adhesives, also called "instant glues," have multiple uses ranging from consumer/home use to medical/tissue adhesives. Common brand names include Super Glue and Krazy Glue.
- Cyanoacrylate glue ingestion or dermal exposure can result in instant local tissue adhesions and mild skin or GI irritation. Gastroenteritis is usually self-limiting and adhesions are often easily treated.
- Diisocyanate glues include the popular Gorilla Glue, some types of wood glue, construction glues, and other high-strength glues.
- Diisocyanate glue ingestions can result in GI irritation or a large foreign body obstruction due to glue expansion. Often, diisocyanate glue ingestions necessitate surgical intervention. Inhalation may cause irritation or obstruction of the airways.
- Polyvinyl acetate (PVA or PVAc) glues or adhesives are typically rubbery, water-soluble glues used for crafts, paper, and children's activities. Elmer's school glue products often fall into this category. While these glues may cause minor gastroenteritis, severe toxicosis is not a concern.
- Glue traps used to trap insects or rodents do not typically contain insecticides or rodenticides (though they may contain a small amount of eugenol) and do not pose a toxicity concern.

ETIOLOGY/PATHOPHYSIOLOGY

Mechanism of Action

- Cyanoacrylate: On contact with the skin or moist surfaces (mucus membranes), the glue hardens and adheres.
- Diisocyanate: Moisture in the GI tract results in significant expansion of the product. Inhalation causes irritation to the lungs.

Pharmacokinetics/Absorption

- No significant systemic absorption occurs with the glues described in the Definition/Overview section.

Toxicity

- Ingestion of all listed glues is considered a nontoxic ingestion.
- Small amounts (1–2 tsp) of ingested diisocyanate can result in a foreign body obstruction.

Systems Affected

- Cyanoacrylate
  - Gastrointestinal: gastroenteritis
  - Skin: adhesions, dermal irritation
  - Respiratory: irritation, obstruction (rare)
  - Ophthalmic: corneal irritation, eyelid adhesions
- Diisocyanate
  - Gastrointestinal: gastroenteritis, foreign body obstruction (common)
  - Skin: dermal irritation, adhesion
  - Respiratory: tachypnea, coughing, sneezing, obstruction (rare)

 SIGNALMENT/HISTORY

- Dogs are affected more than cats due to chewing behaviors. There is no breed predilection.
- Younger dogs (<3 years) are more commonly affected, but exposure can occur at any age.

Historical Findings

- Owners frequently report a chewed product container or ingestion of other materials that had been recently glued. They may also note glue adherence to skin or teeth, vomiting, and anorexia.

Location and Circumstances of Poisoning

- Most exposures occur in the home, garage, or utility area/workshop.

 CLINICAL FEATURES

- Cyanoacrylate
  - Clinical signs occur within seconds to minutes of exposure to glue.
  - The most common signs include glue adherence to the fur, teeth, tongue or gums, and local tissue adhesions.
  - Cyanosis can occur if there is an oropharyngeal obstruction.
  - Vomiting may occur if a significant amount is ingested.

- Diisocyanate
  - Clinical signs occur within 15 minutes to 20 hours after ingestion.
  - The most common clinical signs are consistent with a GI foreign body obstruction and include vomiting, lethargy, abdominal distention, or firm stomach.
  - Diarrhea may be noted on rectal exam.
  - Tachypnea can occur with inhalation or may be secondary to pain and discomfort.
  - Dehydration can develop with prolonged clinical signs.

 ## DIFFERENTIAL DIAGNOSIS

- Cyanoacrylate
  - Respiratory signs: laryngeal paralysis, upper airway obstruction, lower airway disease
  - Gastrointestinal signs: foreign body obstruction, gastroenteritis, pancreatitis, inflammatory bowel disease
- Diisocyanate
  - Gastrointestinal signs: food bloat, foreign body obstruction, gastroenteritis, pancreatitis, inflammatory bowel disease, GDV

 ## DIAGNOSTICS

- CBC: No significant changes, can see WBC count elevation with prolonged illness
- Serum biochemistry profile: Usually normal or mild elevation in albumin due to dehydration
- Abdominal radiographs for diisocyanate ingestion often show a mottled gas and soft tissue opacity in the stomach with gastric distention. This often resembles food ingestion. See figure 8.1.

Pathologic Findings

- Cyanoacrylate: No specific gross or histopathologic findings (aside from gross tissue adhesion)
- Diisocyanate: Gross findings would be related to a foreign body present in the GIT. No specific histopathologic findings anticipated.

 ## THERAPEUTICS

- Treatment of nonobstructive ingestions involves removal of glue and supportive care for GI symptoms. Surgery often needed for foreign body removal in diisocyanate ingestion.

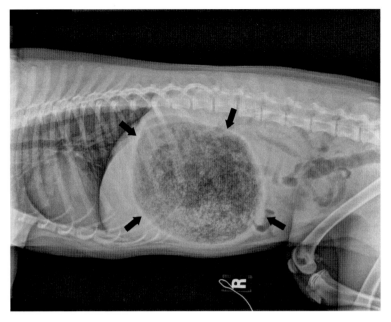

■ **Fig. 8.1.** Abdominal radiograph from a 9-month-old female Pit Bull Terrier after the ingestion of approximately 1.5 oz of Gorilla Glue 12 hours earlier. Surgery was performed and a large, firm, glue obstruction was removed (approximately 7–8 inches diameter). Note the similarity of the glue to food or other ingesta. (Photo by Catherine A. Angle)

Detoxification

- Induce emesis only if immediately after ingestion. Inducing vomiting is generally not recommended due to risk of foreign body obstruction, potential for esophageal obstruction, or lung aspiration with diisocyanate glue and is typically not needed for nonobstructive ingestion.
- Gastric lavage can be attempted; however, due to rapid expansion of diisocyanate glue, may not be beneficial.
- Activated charcoal is not recommended.
- Respiratory
  - Sedated oral exam for glue removal as needed for airway obstruction
  - Oxygen therapy as needed
- Ocular
  - Irrigate for 15 minutes with room-temperature water.
  - Fluorescein stain if indicated
  - May need anesthesia or heavy sedation to safely disarticulate adhered eyelids. An Elizabethan collar may be needed until the eye opens.
- Skin
  - Warm, soapy water or vegetable oil rubbed on fur or teeth will aid in loosening glue adhesions. Remove fur with clippers to remove glue from the coat as needed.

- Glue adhered to surfaces not causing significant morbidity or agitation to the animal does not need to be removed and will wear off with time.

Drug(s) and Antidotes of Choice

- H₂ blocker (e.g., famotidine 0.5 mg/kg PO, SQ, IV, IM q 12–24 hours) can be used to decrease gastric irritation.
- Sucralfate, 0.25–1.0 g PO q 8 hours, can be used if evidence of a gastric ulcer is present.
- Antiemetic such as ondansetron, 0.1–0.2 mg/kg IV q 6–12 hours or 0.1–1 mg/kg PO q 12–24 hours, once an obstruction is ruled out.

Precautions/Interactions

- Avoid prokinetics such as metoclopramide or cisapride until a foreign body obstruction is ruled out.

Appropriate Health Care

- Exploratory laparotomy and gastrotomy needed for dogs with evidence of a gastric obstruction
- IV fluids as needed for supportive care in dehydrated or postsurgical patients
- Postsurgical analgesia (i.e., hydromorphone, 0.05–0.2 mg/kg IV, IM, SQ q 2–6 hours)

Nursing Care

- Surgical site care
- Nutrition supplementation if needed

Follow-up

- Animals should be monitored until clinical signs are controlled. Recheck should be done in 10–14 days in surgery patients for suture removal.

 COMMENTS

Client Education

- Owners should be educated about the dangers of glue expansion and the high risk for foreign body obstruction.

Patient Monitoring

- Monitor hydration, appetite, and for evidence of pain, especially postoperatively.

Prevention/Avoidance

▪ Keeping pets out of areas where the products are being used/stored

Possible Complications

▪ Surgical dehiscence and postoperative ileus can occur.
▪ Gastric rupture can occur if there is an obstruction present and it is left untreated.

Expected Course and Prognosis

▪ Symptoms generally resolve within 24 hours with mild, nonobstructive ingestion.
▪ Prognosis is generally good with either glue ingestion (if treated appropriately).
▪ Up to 75% of patients need surgery after diisocyanate ingestion. Surgery for foreign body removal can prolong recovery and may affect prognosis depending on surgical complications.

Synonyms

▪ Cyanoacrylate glues are also known as "instant glue" and fall under a variety of brand names such as Super Glue and Krazy Glue.
▪ Diisocyanate glues include chemical names such as 4,4'-diphenyl methane diisocyanate, diphenylmethyl diisocyanate, diphenylmethane diisocyanate (MDI), and methylenedi-p-phenyl diisocyanate.

Abbreviations

CBC = complete blood count
GDV = gastric dilatation volvulus
GI   = gastrointestinal
IM   = intramuscular
IV   = intravenous
MDI = diphenylmethane diisocyanate
PO   = *per os* (by mouth)
q   = every
SQ   = subcutaneous
WBC = white blood cell

See Also

Foreign Bodies

Suggested Reading

Bailey T. The expanding threat of polyurethane adhesive ingestion. Vet Tech 2004; 426–428.

Horstman CL, Eubig PA, Khan SA, et al. Gastric outflow obstruction after ingestion of wood glue in a dog. JAAHA 2003; 47–51.

Lubich C, Mrvos R, Krenzelok EP. Beware of canine *Gorilla glue* ingestions. Vet Human Toxicol 2004; 153–154.

Yilmaz T, Ylimaz G. Accidental cyanoacrylate glue ingestion. Internal Journal of Pediatric Otorhinolaryngology 2005; 853–855.

Author: Katherine L. Peterson, DVM
Consulting Editor: Ahna G. Brutlag, DVM

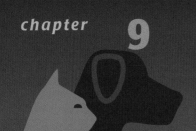

chapter **9**

Hydrocarbons

DEFINITION/OVERVIEW

- Hydrocarbons encompass a large group of chemical entities that contain hydrogen and carbon as their main constituents.
- Hydrocarbons include liquid fuels such as gasoline and diesel as well as household products such as paint solvents, wood stains, wood strippers, turpentine, "tiki-torch" fuels, kerosene, engine oil, roofing tar/asphalt, and liquid lighter fluids.
- Many constituents are often generically referred to as "petroleum distillates" and are categorized based on their viscosity, lipid solubility, and carbon chain length.
- Toxicity, depending on the specific agent, involves route of exposure, dose, and duration of exposure, which can result in a spectrum of problems, including dermal irritation or burns, respiratory irritation or pneumonia-like lung infections, CNS depression, and cardiovascular problems, including arrhythmias or hypotension.

ETIOLOGY/PATHOPHYSIOLOGY

Mechanism of Action

- Hydrocarbons predominantly act as irritants to the GI tract as well as the skin, eyes, and respiratory tract.
- Low-viscosity hydrocarbons (kerosene, gasoline) carry the risk of aspiration when swallowed, which can result in respiratory injury or lung infections.
- Systemic effects, especially to the liver and kidneys, can occur through an unknown mechanism though this is rare.
- Arrhythmias may occur due to cardiac sensitization following exposure to highly volatile hydrocarbons (e.g., gasoline or kerosene).

Toxicity

- Because hydrocarbons represent a wide variety of compounds, the relative toxicity can vary.

- Oral LD_{50} data in rat models show wide variability between specific agents:
  - Methylene chloride: 1,600 mg/kg
  - Gasoline: 13,600 mg/kg
  - Kerosene: 15,000 mg/kg
  - Mineral spirits: >5,000 mg/kg

Systems Affected

- Skin—Most hydrocarbons are poorly absorbed though intact skin in cases involving brief exposures. Injury most frequently results in redness, irritation, or dermatitis. Caustic injury or systemic effects are rare but can occur with prolonged dermal exposure to some compounds.
- Gastrointestinal—Self-limiting gastroenteritis may occur. Caustic injury to the GI tract is very rare. Vomiting increases the risk for aspiration of the stomach contents. End organ damage is unexpected from small ingestions of hydrocarbons.
- Nervous—Inhalation may cause CNS depression.
- Respiratory—Inhalation of the vapors from hydrocarbons can be irritating to the respiratory tract. Aspiration pneumonia and hypoxemia may occur.
- Ophthalmic—Ocular irritation, ulceration (rare), and injury secondary to self-mutilation.
- Cardiovascular—Inhalation may cause nonspecific arrhythmias.
- Renal—ARF and RTA with chronic exposure to halogenated hydrocarbons (carbon tetrachloride and others). End organ damage is typically unexpected from small ingestions of hydrocarbons.
- Hepatobiliary—Nonspecific liver injury usually with halogenated hydrocarbons (carbon tetrachloride and others). End organ damage is typically unexpected from small ingestions of hydrocarbons.

SIGNALMENT/HISTORY

Risk Factors

- No specific breed sensitivities are expected.
- Pediatrics, geriatrics, and those with underlying organ dysfunction are at greatest risk of significant problems following exposure.

Historical Findings

- Witnessed exposure
- Access to storage areas (basement, garage) with evidence of spilled or chewed on hydrocarbon containing products
- Owners report a strong "fuel" or "chemical" odor on the pet's breath, coat, or in the vomitus or stool.

Location and Circumstances of Poisoning

- Animals are frequently found in the garage or basement with spilled or chewed open containers (i.e., spilled can of gasoline or chewed bottle of motor oil).
- Inhalation exposure commonly occurs in two scenarios:
  - Animals left in poorly ventilated spaces following the spill of volatile hydrocarbons (gasoline)
  - Animals with significant dermal exposure continue to inhale the product off their fur.

Interaction with Drugs, Nutrients, or Environment

- Warm environments (e.g., garage or shed in summer months) may increase the volatility of the hydrocarbon resulting in higher ambient air concentrations.

 # CLINICAL FEATURES

- Clinical signs will begin minutes to hours after exposure (depending on route).
- Animals may smell strongly of the hydrocarbon.
- Dermal exposure—red, irritated, dry, or cracked skin; thermal injury from hot oils/tars.
- Ocular exposure—red, irritated, or swollen ocular tissue
- Oral exposure—oral irritation, salivation, nausea/vomiting, and self-limiting gastroenteritis are common. Vomiting may lead to aspiration. HGE and caustic injury are very rare.
- Inhalation exposure—CNS depression, ataxia, agitation, respiratory irritation, coughing, wheezing, or rales on auscultation. Aspiration may lead to pneumonia.
  - CNS signs typically resolve soon after decontamination/exposure to fresh air.
- Cardiac arrhythmias may occur following exposure to low-viscosity hydrocarbons (gasoline).
- The core body temperature may be elevated in the event of an infectious disease process.

 # DIFFERENTIAL DIAGNOSIS

- Primary or infectious respiratory disease
- Primary dermal disease, hypersensitivity reactions (drug eruptions), external parasites, exposure to other household chemicals/cleaning agents
- Primary GI disease, ingestion of other GI irritants such as plants, cleaning products, foreign material, essential oils, etc.
- Toxicities: CNS depressants, acetaminophen (liver), ibuprofen (kidneys and GIT)

DIAGNOSTICS

- Injury to the kidneys and/or liver may be evident on laboratory tests.

Radiologic Findings

- Radiographs of the lungs may reveal pneumonia or evidence of pulmonary edema.
- Radiographic evidence of pulmonary injury may be delayed by several hours following exposure.

Laboratory and Other Diagnostic Findings

- Chemistry panel: Increased BUN, creatinine, AST, or ALT
  - Not expected with small exposures. Possible with large exposures.
- ECG: Nonspecific tachyarrhythmias

Pathological Findings

- Postmortem findings often reveal pulmonary edema as the primary finding.
- Other infrequent postmortem findings have included renal cell degeneration and necrosis or fatty hepatic changes.

THERAPEUTICS

Detoxification

- Bathe the animal with a nonmedicated, degreasing shampoo or a hand-dishwashing detergent. Multiple baths may be needed.
- Clip the fur to remove thick or dried substances such as tar/asphalt. The use of solvents (e.g., mineral spirits) is not recommended.
- Emesis or gastric lavage is typically not recommended due to the increased risk of aspiration.
- Activated charcoal does not bind with hydrocarbons and is not recommended.
- Forced diuresis with IV fluids is not expected to hasten excretion.

Appropriate Health Care

- Evaluation and initial management should focus on any needed dermal decontamination and symptomatic and supportive care.
- Specific care should focus on support of vital functions, including airway or lung issues.
- Some animals presenting with respiratory problems need aggressive airway management, including the use of ventilator support.
- Transfer of critically ill animals to a referral care center should be considered.
- Critically ill animals may develop significant cardiovascular problems such as arrhythmias or hypotension.

- Ocular Exposure
  - Prompt eye irrigation
  - Fluorescein stain/slit lamp examination
- Skin Exposures
  - Treat minimal redness or irritation with topical antibiotic agents, vitamin E oil, or similar skin protectants.
  - Dermatitis-type injury can be treated with topical steroids if needed.
  - Burns, blistering, or more serious dermal involvement may require oral or IV antibiotics, depending on the severity.
- Oral Exposures
  - Examination and careful irrigation of the oral cavity
  - IV fluids to correct dehydration and/or electrolyte imbalances and maintain tissue perfusion
  - GI protectants such as sucralfate (0.25–1 g PO q 6–8 hours) or an H_2 blocker (famotidine, 0.5 mg/kg PO, SQ, IM, IV q 12–24 hours) as well as a bland diet for several days may be of benefit.
  - Caustic injury is not typically seen following ingestion. If present, consider endoscopy to determine the extent of the injury and consider analgesics and broad-spectrum antibiotics.
  - Any animal with respiratory distress following ingestion or inhalation should be admitted to the hospital or clinic and aggressively managed. Ventilation support may be needed.
  - Prophylactic use of antibacterial agents or steroids remains controversial.
- Inhalation/Respiratory Exposure
  - Thoracic radiographs to determine extent of injury and lung involvement in symptomatic animals.
  - Supplement oxygen or $beta_2$ agonists (e.g., albuterol) may be required depending on their condition.
  - Blood gases may be needed to manage acid/base status.
  - Broad spectrum antibiotics for aspiration pneumonia (ampicillin, 5 mg/kg IV q 8 hours with enrofloxacin, 5–20 mg/kg IV q 12 hours)
- Renal impairment can be managed supportively with IV fluids.
- Hepatoprotective agents such as s-adenosyl-methionine (SAMe; 18–20 mg/kg PO q 24 hours) if liver injury is identified. N-acetylcystine (NAC) should be considered in more profound cases.

Drug(s) and Antidote of Choice

- No antidote exists for exposure to hydrocarbons.

Precautions/Interactions

- Use sympathomimetic agents cautiously if an arrhythmia is detected due to sensitization of the myocardium.

Nursing Care

- Periodic reevaluation of the animal's condition throughout any hospitalization should occur. Special attention to any respiratory or airway issues should be promptly evaluated.

Follow-up

- Owners should be instructed to return to the clinic if any change to the animal occurs in the days following exposure. They should be especially watching for any respiratory problems.

Diet

- A bland diet may be needed for several days if the animal has developed significant GI distress.

Activity

- No specific changes in activity are needed, though the animal may be less active during the convalescent stages immediately following the event.

Prevention

- Encourage animal owners to inspect the animal's environment and to store such products correctly to prevent future events.

 COMMENTS

Client Education

- Encourage animal owners to inspect the animal's environment to prevent future exposures.
- Advise that such products are stored correctly in original containers with tight seals.

Expected Course and Prognosis

- Expected course and prognosis largely dependent on presentation and severity of symptoms.
- Animals that remain free of respiratory problems for 12–24 hours following exposure are unlikely to develop such issues.
- Animals with underlying disease to the organ involved may have a worse prognosis.

Abbreviations

ALT = alanine aminotransferase
ARF = acute renal failure

AST   = aspartate aminotransferase
BUN   = blood urea nitrogen
CNS   = central nervous system
ECG   = electrocardiogram
GI   = gastrointestinal
GIT   = gastrointestinal tract
HGE   = hemorrhagic gastroenteritis
IM   = intramuscular
IV   = intravenous
NAC   = N-acetylcystine
PO   = *per os* (by mouth)
q   = every
RTA   = renal tubular acidosis
SAMe = s-adenosyl-methionine
SQ   = subcutaneous

See Also

Essential Oils/Liquid Potpourri
Phenols/Pine Oils

Suggested Reading

Dorman DC. Petroleum distillates and turpentine. Vet Clin North Am Small Anim Pract 1990; 20(2):505–513.

Owens JG, Dorman DC. Common household hazards for small animals. Vet Med 1997; 92(2):140–148.

Goodwin SR, Berman LS, Tabeling BB, Sundlof SF. Kerosene aspiration: Immediate and early pulmonary and cardiovascular effects. Vet Hum Toxic 1988; 30(6):521–524.

Author: Stephen H. LeMaster, PharmD, MPH
Consulting Editor: Ahna G. Brutlag, DVM

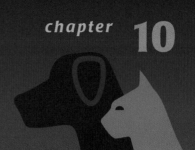

chapter **10**

Hydrofluoric Acid

DEFINITION/OVERVIEW

- Highly concentrated hydrofluoric acid (HF) is used in glass etching, polishing of metals, and as an alkylating agent in industrial production. Household products (rust removers and automotive cleaning products) may contain lower concentrations of HF.
- Hydrofluoric acid is a weak acid with most of its toxicity resulting from the fluoride anion.
- HF is corrosive and can cause serious burns to the eye, skin, and GI tract as well as systemic effects including electrolyte disturbances, respiratory problems, cardiac toxicity, and death.
- Any product containing HF should be considered potentially toxic.

ETIOLOGY/PATHOPHYSIOLOGY

Mechanism of Action

- There are several proposed toxicologic mechanisms:
  - HF penetrates deep into tissue and then dissociates.
  - Free fluoride ions chelate with calcium and magnesium to form insoluble complexes that precipitate in tissue leading to pain, necrosis, and bone decalcification.
  - In bone, fluoride replaces the hydroxyl group of hydroxyapatite.
  - Depletion of serum calcium and magnesium disrupts metabolism and may lead to severe hypocalcemia with resulting potassium efflux and hyperkalemia. These disruptions in potassium and magnesium can lead to myocardial irritability and dysrhythmias.
- Fluoride ions bind and inhibit multiple enzyme systems, including acetyl cholinesterase, adenyl cyclase, and Na+ -K+ ATPase, which results in excessive cholinergic stimulation and further potassium efflux.

Pharmacokinetics/Absorption, Distribution, Metabolism, Excretion

- HF is readily absorbed via any route of exposure. Systemic absorption occurs readily from the stomach because of its acidic environment.

- Corrosive effect of HF is almost immediate, but symptoms may be delayed 12–24 hours.
- Fluoride volume of distribution is 0.5 to 0.7 L/kg.
- Fluoride is not metabolized by the body.
- It is excreted by the kidney—approximately 90% of fluoride is excreted unchanged in urine.
- A small percentage (5%–10%) of absorbed fluoride is excreted in the feces.
- Fluoride elimination half-life is 2–9 hours.

Toxicity

- Systemic toxicosis is possible with low to moderately concentrated products (i.e., even <10% can be harmful).
- Systemic toxicosis is the most common cause of death following ingestion.
- Human fatalities have been reported in cases of dermal exposures with highly concentrated HF (100%) affecting 2.5% body surface area.
- LC_{50} (inhalation) rat: 1278 ppm/1 hr
- LC_{50} (inhalation) mouse: 500 ppm/1 hr
- LC_{50} (inhalation) guinea pig: 4372 ppm/15 min
- LC_{50} (inhalation) monkey: 1780 ppm/1 hr

Systems Affected

- Dermatologic—pain (which is often severe), erythema, burns, and necrosis
- Gastrointestinal—nausea, vomiting, diarrhea, abdominal pain, gastritis (may be hemorrhagic), corrosive burns to the mouth, throat, esophagus, and stomach
- Respiratory—cough, dyspnea, bronchospasm, chemical pneumonitis, pulmonary edema (often hemorrhagic), and burns to the upper airways. The onset of lung injury may be delayed for several days.
- Cardiovascular—QTc prolongation, torsade de pointes, ventricular fibrillation, ventricular tachycardia, dysrhythmias, asystole, and cardiac arrest
- Electrolyte and acid/base—hypocalcemia, hypomagnesemia, metabolic acidosis, and hyperkalemia
- Bone—decalcification and corrosion
- Eye—pain, conjunctival injection, corneal burns, necrosis, and opacification. Conjunctivitis may persist for several months with moderately concentrated solutions.

 # SIGNALMENT/HISTORY

- Any age or breed of animal can be affected.

Risk Factors

- Preexisting renal impairment may lead to further toxicity.

- Preexisting cardiac arrhythmias/disease may increase risk of cardiotoxicity.

Historical Findings

- Exposure (witnessed or suspected) to rust removers, automotive cleaning products, or other products containing HF.
- Symptoms following topical exposure are often delayed. As a result, HF exposure in animals may not be reported until toxic damage is quite severe.

 # CLINICAL FEATURES

- Initial signs of vomiting postingestion; cough, labored breathing, or bronchospasm postinhalation; watery or red eyes following ocular exposure and pain
- As toxicosis progresses, corrosive GI or respiratory injury may result from ingestion or inhalation, respectively. Electrolyte abnormalities and cardiovascular toxicity may appear due to systemic absorption. Death has occurred within 1–2 hours following ingestion.
- Pain and erythema from dermal exposure may be delayed:
  - Up to 24 hours if HF concentration is <20%
  - Up to 8 hours if HF concentration is between 20% and 50%
  - No delay if HF concentration is >50%
- HF penetrates deeply into tissue causing widespread necrosis, ulcerations, and scarring.
- In dog studies, fatalities were most often caused by delayed cardiovascular collapse, ventricular fibrillation, and irreversible hyperkalemia.
- Hyperkalemia has been identified as a primary cause of ventricular arrhythmias in dogs. Potassium levels begin to rise slowly at 2 hours postexposure and exponentially at 6 hours.

 # DIFFERENTIAL DIAGNOSIS

- Toxicities
  - Ammonium bifluoride toxicosis
  - Aspirin toxicosis
  - Beta-blocker or calcium channel blocker ingestion
  - Corrosive injury from other products (acids, alkaline agents, etc.)
  - Tricyclic antidepressant toxicosis
- Primary cardiac disease
- Primary respiratory disease
- Primary metabolic disease
- Primary mineral deficiencies

DIAGNOSTICS

- Diagnosis should be made based on history, physical examination, and clinical suspicion.
- Serum electrolyte levels—hypocalcemia, hypomagnesemia, and hyperkalemia
- ECG—QTc prolongation, torsade de pointes, ventricular fibrillation, and ventricular tachycardia
- Arterial or venous blood gases may reveal metabolic acidosis.
- Endoscopy should be performed within 12–24 hours after ingestion of large quantities and/or highly concentrated HF products (>20%) or if symptoms (e.g., drooling, stridor, repeated vomiting) persist.
- Thoracic radiographs should be considered in symptomatic animals postinhalation.
- Urine or serum fluoride levels may be used to confirm HF exposure (serum normal: 0.001–0.047 mg/L) but should not be the only determining factor. Limited availability in veterinary medicine.

Pathological Findings

- Gross examination at necropsy may reveal GI erosion following ingestion of HF, hemorrhagic pulmonary edema and/or burns to the pulmonary tree following inhalation, and severe deep necrotic damage following dermal exposure.
- Corneal erosion, necrosis, and opacification may follow ocular exposure.

 ## THERAPEUTICS

- Goals of treatment for HF toxicosis include removal from the source of contamination, aggressive decontamination and prevention of additional absorption, assessing the potential for systemic toxicosis monitoring for cardiac signs preventing and correcting electrolyte imbalances (especially Ca, Mg and K) and acidosis, and providing supportive and symptomatic care.
- Treatment and care should be directed at potential toxic signs and symptoms.

Detoxification

- Dermal: irrigate affected area(s) with copious amounts of lukewarm tap water for at least 30 minutes followed by liberal application of a fluoride-binding calcium gluconate or carbonate 2.5% gel.
- Ingestion: immediately administer a fluoride-binding substance (containing Ca or Mg) such as milk, chewable calcium carbonate tablets, milk of magnesia, or a liquid antacid. If a large volume of fluid was ingested, consider removal via a nasogastric tube if within 1 hour of exposure.
- Ocular: irrigate with water, normal saline, or LRS for at least 15 minutes (calcium solutions have not been shown more effective than saline for ocular irrigation).

Continue irrigation until ocular pH is normal (check with litmus paper). Consult with a veterinary ophthalmologist if initial symptoms persist.
- Inhalation: administer humidified oxygen and assist with ventilation as needed. Administer 2.5% calcium gluconate by nebulizer to help control respiratory symptoms.

Drug(s) of Choice

- Initially treat arrhythmias by assessing and correcting for hypocalcemia, hypomagnesemia, and hyperkalemia. Because of its potassium channel blocking activity, amiodarone (10–25 mg/kg PO q 12 hours) is a preferred agent for ventricular arrhythmias. Otherwise, standard cardiac protocols may be used, avoiding agents that may increase the QTc interval (e.g., propranolol and certain calcium channel blockers)
- Hypomagnesemia should be treated with IV magnesium sulfate (0.15–0.3 mEq/kg over 5–15 minutes) followed by a CRI (0.75–1.0 mEq/kg/day).
- Initial doses of calcium can be given while waiting for labs to return.
  - Calcium gluconate 10% (0.50–1.50 mL/kg) can be given as a slow IV bolus over 5–10 minutes. An infusion (0.50–1.50 mL/kg/hr) can be initiated after the bolus to maintain its effect.
  - Calcium chloride 10% (0.15–0.50 mL/kg) may be preferred over calcium gluconate due to a greater concentration of calcium (13.4 mEq vs. 4.5 mEq per 10 mL of 10% calcium if this chloride or gluconate, respectively). Tissue injury secondary to drug extravasation of calcium chloride can be significant. Therefore, calcium gluconate is preferred if a central line cannot be established.
- Administrate sodium bicarbonate at 1–3 mEq/kg IV over 30 minutes to shift K^+ intracellularly and/or to treat acidosis.
- Provide adequate analgesia.

Precautions/Interactions

- Do not induce vomiting as this may cause further esophageal erosion.
- Avoid administering large amounts of liquid or activated charcoal postingestion as this may induce vomiting.
- Do not perform ocular irrigation more than once since this has been shown to increase corneal damage.
- Intradermal and subcutaneous administration of 10% calcium chloride solution may be damaging to tissues and should be avoided.

Alternative Drugs

- Topical agents such as Epsom salt (magnesium sulfate), Mylanta (magnesium hydroxide), and benzalkonium or benzethonium chloride solution are additional detoxification options. Calcium acetate soaks and iodine preparations have also shown effectiveness at reducing dermal injuries.

- A 0.5-mL/cm^2 subcutaneous infiltration of 10% calcium gluconate solution is an option if pain continues for >30 minutes after applying calcium gluconate gel.
- Topical corticosteroids can be applied in cases of severe dermal inflammation.
- Hexafluorine optical rinse has been shown useful in cases of ocular exposure with apparent advantages over saline in diminishing HF absorption into the eye. Consult with an ophthalmologist if prolonged symptoms.
- In canine studies, quinidine sulfate 5–10 mg/kg IV has shown efficacy in stopping K+ efflux and preventing hyperkalemia and resultant cardiotoxicity.
- Oral or IV corticosteroids and inhaled beta-2 agonists may help control bronchospasms.
- Cation exchange resins may be useful for hyperkalemia.
- Hemodialysis may be considered as a last-line option to remove fluoride anions in critical cases of systemic toxicosis or to treat hyperkalemia, although execution in the unstable, compromised patient will be difficult.

Nursing Care

- The animal should be given frequent opportunities to urinate to help excrete fluoride ions if catheterization is not feasible.

Diet

- If oral ingestion or altered level of consciousness, temporarily hold food and water.

Activity

- Base on symptoms and severity of exposure

Surgical Considerations

- In cases of severe dermal necrosis with refractory hypocalcemia, surgical debridement of affected skin region(s) or packing with benzalkonium chloride solution may be necessary.
- Amputation of affected limb(s) may be considered a last resort if animal fails to respond to other treatment methods.

 COMMENTS

Client Education

- Readmit the animal if symptoms reappear or worsen even after proper treatment.

Patient Monitoring

- Continuous cardiac monitoring is recommended during hospitalization (even if initial ECG is normal) and for up to 48 hours postexposure depending on the

severity of exposure. QTc prolongation commonly precedes dysrhythmias and indicates the presence of hypocalcemia.
- Monitor respiratory function for up to 72 hours after inhalation of HF.
- Serum electrolyte levels (especially serum Ca) should be obtained every 30 minutes in cases of systemic toxicosis or large dermal exposures.
- Animals with well-controlled pain, normal electrolyte levels and ECG readings, and insignificant burns can be sent home after 6 or more hours.

Prevention/Avoidance

- Prevent access to HF-containing products in the home, particularly while cleaning.

Possible Complications

- Pulmonary edema and chronic lung disease
- Ocular damage, changes in vision, and blindness
- Scarring
- Esophageal and GI strictures

Expected Course and Prognosis

- Prognosis depends on HF concentration, route and duration of exposure, and quantity exposed to or ingested.
- Single, small exposures are linked to good prognosis with low risk of long-term effects.
- Larger, multiple, or more severe exposures may require up to 72 hours of monitoring with potential systemic and long-term effects.

Synonyms

hydrogen fluoride solution, hydrofluoric acid solution, aqueous hydrofluoric acid, fluoric acid solution

Abbreviations

CRI = continuous rate infusion
ECG = electrocardiogram
HF = hydrofluoric acid
GI = gastrointestinal
IV = intravenous
LC_{50} = median lethal concentration
PO = *per os* (by mouth)
q = every

See Also

Acids
Aspirin

Beta-Blockers
Calcium Channel Blockers

Suggested Reading

Cummings CC, McIvor ME. Fluoride-induced hyperkalemia: The role of Ca2+-dependent K+ channels. Am J Emerg Med 1988; 6:1–3.

Dünser MW, Ohlbauer M, Rieder J, Zimmermann I, Ruatti H, Schwabegger AH, et al. Critical care management of major hydrofluoric acid burns: A case report, review of the literature, and recommendations for therapy. Burns 2004; 30(4):391–398.

Flomenbaum, Goldfrank, Hoffman, et al. Hydrofluoric Acid and Fluorides. In: Su M, ed. Goldfrank's Toxicologic Emergencies, 8th ed. New York: McGraw-Hill, 2006.

Greenberg MI, Hamilton RJ, Phillips SD, et al. Occupational, Industrial, and Environmental Toxicology, 2nd ed. Philadelphia: Mosby, 2003; pp. 100–101.

Spoler F, Frentz M, Forst M, et al. Analysis of hydrofluoric acid penetration and decontamination of the eye by means of time-resolved optical coherence tomography. Burns 2008; 34(4):549–555.

Sullivan JB Jr., Krieger GR. Hydrofluoric acid. In: Krenzelok EP, ed. Hazardous Materials Toxicology: Clinical Principles of Environmental Health. Baltimore: Williams & Wilkins, 1992.

Authors: Leo J. Sioris, PharmD; Lauren E. Haak, PharmD
Consulting Editor: Ahna G. Brutlag, DVM

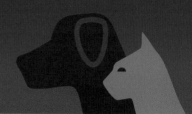

Drugs: Human Prescription

chapter 11

5-Fluorouracil

DEFINITION/OVERVIEW

- 5-fluorouracil (5-FU) is a pyrimidine analog of the uracil nucleotide, and is a chemotherapeutic agent used to treat a variety of different neoplasias in both human and veterinary medicine.
- 5-FU is prepared as either a 1% or 5% topical cream, or as an IV preparation.
- Most common signs from toxicosis are related to the GIT, CNS, and bone marrow.
- Onset of toxicosis is rapid (30 minutes to 6 hours), with death reported in as little as 7 hours.

ETIOLOGY/PATHOPHYSIOLOGY

- The efficacy of 5-FU as a chemotherapeutic agent is due to the conversion of the uracil nucleotide into one of three metabolic pathways, all resulting in programmed cell death.
- In humans, 5-FU is used to treat GI carcinomas, breast carcinomas, and superficial malignancies of the head and neck.
- It has been used in dogs to treat cutaneous lymphoma, but due to its unpredictable response rate it is rarely used.
- 5-FU is contraindicated for use in cats due to severe neurotoxicity, even at therapeutic doses.

Mechanism of Action

- 5-FU is metabolized to fluoroacetate, which then enters the tricarboxylic acid (TCA) cycle as fluoracetyl-coenzyme A.
- Generation of fluorocitrate through continued metabolism blocks the TCA cycle, causing inhibition of citric acid uptake.
- Accumulation of citrate occurs, affecting hepatic function.
- Increased amounts of circulating citrate enter the CNS, resulting in neurotoxicity.
- Inhibition of thiamine pyrophosphate production by 5-FU may result in decreased production of thiamine, contributing to the neurotoxic effects.

113

- Rapidly dividing cell lines are affected, resulting in bone marrow suppression and intestinal mucosal damage.

Pharmacokinetics/Absorption, Distribution, Metabolism, and Excretion

- Rapidly absorbed and distributed to tissues
- Metabolized to several metabolites
- In humans, the elimination time is approximately 20 hours.

Toxicity

- The nadir for maximal bone marrow suppression is 7–20 days in humans.
- The oral LD_{50} is reported to be 100 mg/kg in rats and 500 mg/kg in mice.
- Dogs
  - 6.8 mg/kg minimum reported toxic dose
  - 20 mg/kg minimum reported lethal dose
  - 46 mg/kg—one case report of a dog surviving this dose with very aggressive treatment and supportive care
- Cats
  - No reported mg/kg dose; very small amounts are associated with CNS signs

Systems Affected

- Nervous—seizures often develop within 30–45 minutes.
- Gastrointestinal—persistent vomiting (±blood) secondary to mucosal damage
- Hemic/lymphatic/immune—dose-dependent myelosuppression
- Cardiovascular—arrhythmias

 SIGNALMENT/HISTORY

- There is no age or breed disposition.
- Most reported cases occurred from accidental ingestion of a 5-FU-based product.
- Toxicosis can also occur due to intentional but inappropriate use of a topical 5-FU product applied to the skin.

 CLINICAL FEATURES

- Dogs
  - Cerebellar ataxia, seizures, hyperesthesia, hyperexcitability, muscle tremors, vomiting, diarrhea, hematochezia, mucositis, cardiac arrhythmias
- Cats
  - Severe cerebellar neurotoxicity and dementia, even at therapeutic doses

DIFFERENTIAL DIAGNOSIS

- Primary neurologic diseases including meningitis, CNS neoplasia, idiopathic epilepsy, GME, and congenital structural CNS abnormalities
- Primary metabolic diseases (e.g., hepatic failure, renal failure), hypoglycemia, hepatic encephalopathy
- Toxins including strychnine, bromethalin, metaldehyde, ethylene glycol, and medications

 ## DIAGNOSTICS

- Minimum database (CBC, serum chemistry profile, urinalysis) should be performed to try to eliminate other causes of neurologic abnormalities, including metabolic disease or electrolyte abnormalities.
- Venous blood gas analysis
- Bile acids test or blood ammonia level to rule out hepatic encephalopathy
- Advanced imaging, including MRI or CT of the brain, can be performed to exclude primary CNS disease as a cause for the neurologic signs.
- Bone marrow aspirate—consistent with marrow aplasia at day 9 and recovery of hematopoesis by day 15

Pathological Findings

- GI lesions of hemorrhage, ulcers, and mucosal sloughing
- Histopathological findings include complete bone marrow aplasia with only stromal elements present. Neurological lesions include vacuolization, myelin lamellar splitting, and separation between the axon and innermost myelin fibers.

 ## THERAPEUTICS

Detoxification

- Emesis not advised due to rapid onset of neurological signs
- Gastric lavage if early after ingestion

Appropriate Healthcare

- Intensive monitoring should be employed in these patients, particularly if the patient is heavily sedated for seizure control. Respiratory rate and effort, heart rate and rhythm, blood pressure monitoring, pulse oximetry monitoring, and, if intubated, end-tidal carbon dioxide ($ETCO_2$) monitoring should be performed.

- If an ETCO$_2$ monitor is not available, intermittent blood gas analysis can be performed to assess ventilation (pCO$_2$ levels, arterial or venous sample) and oxygenation (pO$_2$, arterial sample).
- Monitor for hypotension and cardiac arrhythmias and treat appropriately
- Monitor PCV, TP, and blood glucose 3–4 x a day

Drug(s) and Antidotes of Choice

- IV fluids—treat aggressively to maintain perfusion and hydration; titrate according to physical examination findings, PCV and TP, urine output, weight gain.
- Colloids or blood products as needed
- Antiemetics
    - Maropitant 1 mg/kg, SQ q 24 hours
    - Ondansetron 0.1–0.2 mg/kg, IV q 8–12 hours
- GI protectants
    - H$_2$ blockers
        - Famotidine 0.5–1 mg/kg, PO, SQ, IM, IV q 12–24 hours
        - Ranitidine 1–2 mg/kg, PO, SQ, IM, IV q 8–12 hours
        - Cimetidine 5–10 mg/kg, PO, SQ, IM, IV q 6 hours
    - Omeprazole 0.5–1 mg/kg, PO q 24 hours
    - Sucralfate 0.25–1 gram, PO q 8 hours x 5–7 days if evidence of active ulcer disease
- CNS support
    - In general, seizures seen with 5-FU toxicosis are severe and often refractory to diazepam; additional aggressive anticonvulsant therapy should be initiated.
    - Seizures should initially be controlled using loading doses of phenobarbital (4–16 mg/kg IV to effect).
    - Status epilepticus can also be controlled with the following:
        - Propofol 2–6 mg/kg IV or a CRI of 0.6 mg/kg/min
        - Pentobarbital 3–15 mg/kg, IV to effect
        - General anesthesia may also be required.
- Severe diarrhea or hematochezia
    - Metronidazole 10 mg/kg, IV or PO q 12 hours
- Leukopenia: Broad-spectrum antibiotics should be administered if severe leukopenia is diagnosed.
- Bone marrow stimulation: Neupogen 4.2–6 µg/kg, SQ q 3–5 days for severe leukopenia

Follow-up

- Because of the bone marrow suppression caused by 5-FU, serial CBCs should be monitored (see "Patient Monitoring") aggressively.

COMMENTS

Patient Monitoring

- Because of the bone marrow suppression caused by 5-FU, serial CBCs should be monitored every 24 hours during hospitalization, and weekly thereafter for a total of 4 weeks.
- Leukopenia typically occurs by day 7, worsens by day 9, and continues through day 13.
- Thrombocytopenia occurs by day 7, worsens by day 9, and continues through days 18–21.
- Anemia occurs by day 9 and continues through days 18–21.
- Pancytopenia occurs through day 13.
- All cell lines tend to return to normal by day 25.

Prevention/Avoidance

- Keep topical creams well away from pets and wipe up even small spills before they have time to lick them up.

Expected Course and Prognosis

- No dog with a reported intoxication of greater than 43 mg/kg survived in one study; however, a separate case report described a dog that survived an estimated dose of 46 mg/kg.
- If dogs survive the acute toxicosis, full resolution of both neurologic abnormalities and bone marrow suppression can occur.

Abbreviations

5-FU   = 5 fluorouracil
CBC   = complete blood count
CNS   = central nervous system
CRI   = continuous rate infusion
CT   = computed tomography
$ETCO_2$ = end tidal carbon dioxide
GI   = gastrointestinal
GIT   = gastrointestinal tract
GME   = granulomatous meningoencephalitis
IM   = intramuscular
IV   = intravenous
MRI   = magnetic resonance imaging
PCV   = packed cell volume
PO   = *per os* (by mouth)

q   = every
SQ   = subcutaneous
TCA   = tricarboxylic acid
TP   = total protein

See Also

Bromethalin
Ethylene Glycol

Suggested Reading

Dorman DC, Coddington KA, Richardson RC. 5-fluorouracil toxicosis in the dog. J Vet Int Med 1990; 4:254–257.

Fry MM, Forman MA. 5-fluorouracil toxicity with severe bone marrow suppression in a dog. Vet Human Tox 2004; 48(4):278–280.

Roberts J, Powell LL. Accidental 5-fluorouracil exposure in a dog. J Vet Emerg Crit Care 2001; 11(4):281–286.

Author: Lisa L. Powell, DVM, MS, DACVECC
Consulting Editor: Lynn R. Hovda, RPH, DVM, MS, DACVIM

chapter 12

Albuterol

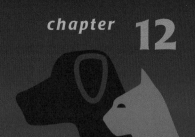

DEFINITION/OVERVIEW

- Albuterol, a beta-2 receptor agonist, is commonly used for relief of broncho-spasm caused by conditions such as asthma and chronic obstructive pulmonary disease in humans.
- Although not FDA-approved for use in veterinary patients, albuterol is commonly used as a bronchodilator in cats, dogs, and horses.
- Accidental exposure occurs when pets gain access to albuterol in its various formulations: aerosolized canisters (metered-dose inhalers), tablets, extended release tablets, powders, and solutions.
- Albuterol overdose typically results in tachycardia, weakness, and tachypnea; hypokalemia and agitation may also occur.

ETIOLOGY/PATHOPHYSIOLOGY

Mechanism of Action

- Albuterol relaxes bronchial, vascular, and uterine smooth muscle by stimulating beta-2 receptors.
- Beta-2 receptor agonism leads to a conformational change triggering the conversion of ATP into cyclic adenosine monophosphate (cAMP) and subsequent activation of cellular $Na^+K^+ATPase$. This can result in profound systemic hypokalemia.
- At high plasma levels, beta-2 receptor agonists lose selectivity, resulting in agonism at both beta-1 and beta-2 receptors.
- Activation of beta-1 receptors results in tachycardia and positive inotropy.
- Activation of beta-2 receptors results in peripheral vasodilation that may cause hypotension and a reflex tachycardia.
- The fluorocarbon and chlorofluorocarbon propellants present in older aerosol-ized formulations sensitize the myocardium and may contribute to arrhythmias. For the most part, they have been replaced with water-based formulations.

Pharmacokinetics/Absorption, Distribution, Metabolism, and Excretion

- Albuterol is rapidly absorbed after oral administration.

- Effects can occur within 5 minutes after inhalation and 30 minutes after oral administration.
- Drug effects persist for 3–6 hours after inhalation and up to 12 hours (depending on dosage form) after oral administration.
- The drug is metabolized in the liver.

Toxicity

- A toxic dose has not been established for companion animals.
- The LD_{50} in rats is reported to be more than 2 g/kg.
- In human pediatric patients, 1 mg/kg has been identified as a dose associated with three or more signs of toxicity.
- Adverse effects are possible even at therapeutic doses.

Systems Affected

- Cardiovascular
  - Arrhythmias can result from excessive stimulation of beta-1 and beta-2 receptors and may be worsened by hypokalemia.
  - Excessive beta-2 stimulation may lead to vasodilation, hypotension, and reflex tachycardia.
- Endocrine/metabolic
  - Hypokalemia results from intracellular translocation of potassium due to activation of $Na^+K^+ATPase$.
  - Hyperglycemia from sympathetic stimulation may cause insulin secretion.
- Nervous
  - Anxiety, restlessness, and seizures may be seen.
- Respiratory
  - Increased respiratory rates may be due to sympathetic stimulation or anxiety.
- Musculoskeletal
  - Tremors may occur from beta-2 stimulation of muscles and excessive sympathetic activity.
- Neuromuscular
  - Weakness may result from hypokalemia or arrhythmias.

 # SIGNALMENT/HISTORY

- There is no known breed, age, or gender predilection.

Historical Findings

- Clinical signs may be seen within minutes of exposure, or delayed by hours if extended release tablets were ingested.

- Owners may report an elevated heart rate, panting, excessive thirst, vomiting, weakness, blood-shot or glazed eyes, agitation, and shaking.
- Use of albuterol or other beta-2 agonists by pets or household members may be reported.

Location and Circumstances of Poisoning

- Exposure is usually accidental.
- Pressurized inhalers, if punctured, may deliver the entire contents directly into the oral cavity.

Interactions with Drugs, Nutrients, or Environment

- Concurrent administration of other sympathomimetic drugs may exacerbate the effects of albuterol.
- Tricyclic antidepressants and monoamine oxidase inhibitors may worsen hypotension, and digitalis may exacerbate arrhythmias.

CLINICAL FEATURES

- Patients may appear apprehensive, agitated, or hyperactive; others can present with depression.
- Cardiac arrhythmias may be present and include sinus tachycardia, ventricular premature contractions, atrioventricular block, and ventricular tachycardia.
- Pulse deficits or weak pulse quality may be palpated.
- Muscle tremors may be evident.
- Patients may be tachypneic.
- Muscle weakness, collapse, and paresis may be present due to cardiovascular effects or due to severe hypokalemia.
- Vomiting, hyperthermia, and hypertension may also be noted.
- Conjunctivitis and scleral injection may result from exposure to a punctured canister.

DIFFERENTIAL DIAGNOSIS

- Differentials include shock, cardiac disease, exposure to sympathomimetic medications, thyroid medication overdose, or thyroid storm.
- Severe hypokalemia may result from insulin overdose, primary hyperaldosteronism, chronic renal failure, and administration of loop diuretics.

DIAGNOSTICS

- Continuous ECG monitoring is recommended, and may reveal the presence of arrhythmias.

- Blood pressure monitoring
- Baseline laboratory work should include an electrolyte panel, PCV/TS, and blood glucose measurement. CBC, serum chemistry panel, and urinalysis should be performed if indicated.
- Common electrolyte and chemistry abnormalities include the following:
  - Hypokalemia
  - Hypophosphatemia
  - Hypomagnesemia
  - Elevated lactate
  - Hyper- or hypoglycemia
  - Elevated AST
- Thoracic radiographs are indicated if a patient is tachypneic, to rule out evidence of pulmonary edema and to assess cardiac size.

 # THERAPEUTICS

- Clinical signs should be treated symptomatically.
- Sinus tachycardia and tachyarrhythmias may be treated with beta blockers such as esmolol or propranolol when rates exceed 160 bpm in large dogs and 180 bpm in small dogs. Calcium channel blockers may also be used to slow tachyarrhythmias. Ventricular arrhythmias may be treated with lidocaine.
- Serum potassium levels should be monitored every 4–6 hours and potassium supplemented as needed.
- Hyperactivity and tremors can be treated with benzodiazepines.

Detoxification

- Asymptomatic patients that have ingested tablets should have emesis induced immediately.
- If large quantities of tablets were ingested within 2 hours of presentation, gastric lavage may be indicated.
- Emesis should *not* be induced if exposure was to a pressurized canister, powder, or liquid formulations, due to quick absorption and rapid onset of effects.
- A single dose of activated charcoal (1–3 g/kg) with a cathartic is warranted in patients that ingest albuterol tablets.

Appropriate Health Care

- Continuous cardiovascular monitoring (heart rate and rhythm, blood pressure) should be performed.
- Serial measurement of potassium should be performed, with appropriate adjustments made to the fluid therapy regimen.
- Restrict activity until asymptomatic.

Drug(s) and Antidotes of Choice

- No specific antidote
- Intravenous fluid therapy is necessary to alleviate signs of hypotension associated with vasodilation.
- In hypokalemic patients, potassium chloride should be supplemented appropriately in intravenous fluids, with a rate not to exceed 0.5 mEq/kg/hour of potassium chloride.
- Sinus tachycardia and tachyarrhythmias
  - Propranolol 0.02 mg/kg IV slowly q 8 hours (maximum of 1 mg/kg)
  - Esmolol 0.1–0.5 mg/kg IV slowly, followed by a CRI of 0.05–0.1 mg/kg/min
  - Diltiazem 0.1–0.2 mg/kg slow IV bolus, followed by an IV CRI of 0.005–0.02 mg/kg/min
- Ventricular arrhythmias
  - Lidocaine 2 mg/kg slow IV bolus followed by 30–50 µg/kg/min IV CRI
- Diazepam
  - 0.2–0.5 mg/kg IV (to effect) for agitation

Follow-up

- Monitor for signs of weakness over the first 12–24 hours after hospital discharge.
- If weakness is observed, cardiovascular and electrolyte status should be reevaluated.

Prevention

- Prevent access to pills or pressurized inhalers.

 COMMENTS

Client Education

- Monitor for adverse effects even if prescribed at therapeutic doses.

Patient Monitoring

- Frequent or continuous heart rate and rhythm monitoring
- Frequent blood pressure monitoring
- Serial potassium measurement

Prevention/Avoidance

- Prevent access
- Report any adverse reactions that occur in pets prescribed therapeutic doses of albuterol

Possible Complications

- Beta-blocking drugs may cause bronchoconstriction in animals with allergic airway disease or asthma.
- Dextrose-containing fluids may stimulate insulin release, which may further decrease serum potassium levels.

Expected Course and Prognosis

- Prognosis is good for healthy animals with prompt veterinary care.
- Animals with preexisting heart disease may have a more guarded prognosis.
- Most treated animals recover completely within 12 hours of exposure. Some require 24–48 hours of therapy if severe arrhythmias are present.

Abbreviations

ATP	= adenosine triphosphate
AST	= aspartate aminotransferase
BPM	= beats per minute
cAMP	= cyclic adenosine monophosphate
CBC	= complete blood count
CRI	= continuous rate infusion
ECG	= electrocardiogram
FDA	= Federal Drug Administration
IV	= intravenous
$Na^+K^+ATPase$	= sodium potassium adenosine triphosphatase
q	= every
PCV	= packed cell volume
TS	= total solids

See Also

Diuretics

Suggested Reading

McCown JL, Lechner ES, Cooke KL. Suspected albuterol toxicosis in a dog. J Am Vet Med Assoc 2008; 232(8):1168–1171.

Mensching D, Volmer PA. Breathe with ease when managing beta$_2$ agonist inhaler toxicosis in dogs. Vet Med 2007; 2:369–345.

Vite CH, Gfeller RW. Suspected albuterol intoxication in a dog. J Vet Emerg Crit Care 2007; 4(1):7–13.

Wiley JF, Spiller HA, Krenzelok EP, et al. Unintentional albuterol ingestion in children. Pediatr Emerg Care 1994; 10(4):193–196.

Authors: Danielle M. Babski, DVM; Benjamin M. Brainard, VMD, DACVA, DACVECC
Consulting Editor: Lynn R. Hovda, RPH, DVM, MS, DACVIM

chapter 13

Amphetamines

DEFINITION/OVERVIEW

- Amphetamines can be either prescription medications (ADHD, weight loss, etc.) or illegal drugs (methamphetamine, ecstasy).
- Intoxication with amphetamines stimulates the CNS and cardiovascular systems.

ETIOLOGY/PATHOPHYSIOLOGY

- Amphetamines are sympathomimetic amines. They stimulate the medullary respiratory center and reticular activating system.
- Amphetamines cause stimulation of the α and β receptors and release of norepinephrine and serotonin. This increases the amount of catecholamines found in the synapse.
- Clinical signs are stimulatory (agitation, tachycardia, tremors, seizures).
- Amphetamine intoxication in animals is not uncommon, especially in households with ADHD children.

Mechanism of Action

- Amphetamines are stimulants of the CNS and cardiovascular system. They stimulate the medullary respiratory center and reticular activating system.
- Amphetamines increase the concentration of catecholamines at nerve endings by increasing their release and inhibiting their reuptake and metabolism.
- There is also an increase in the presynaptic release of serotonin.

Pharmacokinetics/Absorption, Distribution, Metabolism, and Excretion

- Amphetamines are quickly absorbed orally.
- Depending on the formulation, signs can be seen almost immediately, or they can be delayed for several hours (extended release formulations).
- Amphetamines are highly lipid soluble leading to high concentrations in the liver, kidneys, and lungs. Amphetamines cross the blood brain barrier.
- Metabolism is minimal and most are excreted as the parent compound.
- Amphetamines are eliminated in the urine. Urinary elimination is pH dependent. The half-life varies from 7 to 34 hours (shorter with acidic urine).

Toxicity

- The oral lethal dose in dogs for most amphetamines ranges from 10 to 23 mg/kg.

Systems Affected

- Nervous—stimulation resulting in agitation and nervousness
- Neuromuscular—stimulation resulting in tremors and seizures
- Cardiovascular—stimulation resulting in tachycardia and hypertension
- Respiratory—stimulation resulting in tachypnea
- Gastrointestinal—stimulation resulting in vomiting, hypersalivation, and diarrhea
- Ophthalmic—dilation of the pupils

 SIGNALMENT/HISTORY

- All species and breeds can be affected.
- The owner may report agitation, tachycardia, panting, tremors, hyperthermia, seizures, and/or death.

Risk Factors

- Animals with preexisting cardiac disease may be more at risk for developing severe signs and fatal arrhythmias.

Historical Findings

- Owners may have evidence of exposure to amphetamines.
- Owners often report agitation (running around), tremors (shaking), and tachy-cardia (heart racing).

Location and Circumstances of Poisoning

- Most poisonings occur within the home.
- Animals may be given the wrong medication by mistake or may have access to prescription medications.

Interactions with Drugs, Nutrients, or Environment

- Acetazolamide and sodium bicarbonate alkalinize the urine causing increased renal tubular reabsorption of amphetamines.
- Tricyclic antidepressants (amitriptyline, amoxapine, clomipramine, desipramine, doxepin, imipramine, nortriptyline, protriptyline, trimipramine) enhance release of norepinephrine (hypertension, CNS stimulation).

- Monoamine oxidase inhibitors (clorgyline, isocarboxazide, meclobemide, nialamide, pargyline, phenylzine, procarbazine, rasagiline, selegiline, toloxatone, tranylcypromine) and furazolidone when ingested with amphetamines result in more norepinephrine being made available through inhibition of catecholamine degradation. Greater amounts of norepinephrine increase sympathetic activity.
- Sibutramine when ingested with amphetamines increases blood pressure and heart rate.

 # CLINICAL FEATURES

- Neurologic—acute onset of restlessness and hyperactivity, followed by tremors and seizures
- Cardiovascular—tachycardia
- Respiratory—acute onset of tachypnea
- Ophthalmic—mydriasis
- Signs can begin within minutes (methamphetamine) or may be delayed for several hours. If signs have been present for a while, hyperthermia and myoglobinuria may be noted.

 # DIFFERENTIAL DIAGNOSIS

- Other stimulants, including the following:
  - Methylxanthines (caffeine, theobromine, theophylline)
  - Nicotine
  - Serotonergic medications

 # DIAGNOSTICS

- Illicit drug urine test: Amphetamines will show up positive on amphetamine and/or methamphetamine tests, although these tests have not been validated in animals.
- Amphetamines can be detected in urine or stomach contents by human hospital laboratories.
- ECG—sinus tachycardia, ventricular arrhythmias
- Blood gas—metabolic acidosis
- Blood pressure—hypertension
- Urinalysis—myoglobinuria secondary to rhabdomyolysis

Pathological Findings

- There are no specific histopathologic lesions consistent with this toxicosis.

THERAPEUTICS

- Treatment is aimed at controlling life-threatening CNS and cardiovascular signs.

Detoxification

- Emesis if <15 minutes and asymptomatic
- Gastric lavage if large amounts of pills have been ingested
- Activated charcoal (may need to be repeated with extended release medications) to reduce absorption
- Acidifying urine to 4.5–5.5 pH with either ammonium chloride (100–200 mg/kg/day PO divided QID) or ascorbic acid (20–30 mg/kg PO, SQ, IM or IV) to enhance elimination

Appropriate Health Care

- Monitor body temperature, respirations, and heart rate.
- Monitor blood pressure.
- Monitor acid/base status.
- ECG for arrhythmias

Drug(s) and Antidotes of Choice

- No specific antidote
- IV fluids to help regulate body temperature and to protect kidneys from myoglobinuria
- Agitation
  - Phenothiazine
    - □ Acepromazine 0.05 mg/kg IV or IM, titrate to effect as needed
    - □ Chlorpromazine 0.5 mg/kg IV, IM or SQ, titrate up as needed
  - Cyproheptadine
    - □ Dogs: 1.1 mg/kg PO or rectally; serotonin antagonist
    - □ Cats: 2–4 mg total dose per cat
- Tachycardia
  - Beta-blockers
    - □ Propranolol 0.02–0.06 mg/kg IV
- Tremors
  - Methocarbamol 50–100 mg/kg IV, titrate up as needed
- Seizures
  - Barbiturates to effect
    - □ Phenobarbital 3–4 mg/kg IV

Precautions/Interactions

- Diazepam can increase the dysphoria and lead to increased morbidity. It is not recommended for use in amphetamine toxicosis.

Alternative Drugs

- Seizures—inhalant anesthetics (isoflurane, sevoflurane), propofol CRI

Nursing Care

- Thermoregulation
- Minimize sensory stimuli

Follow-up

- No long-term problems are expected in most cases.

Diet

- No diet change is needed, except NPO during severe CNS signs.

Prevention

- Keep all medications out of the reach of pets.

 COMMENTS

- Treatment in most cases is very rewarding.
- These animals tend to require large doses of phenothiazines to control their clinical signs.

Client Education

- Monitor appetite and urine color for 24 hours.

Patient Monitoring

- Monitor HR, BP, and urine color, hourly at first and then less often if the animal remains clinically normal.

Prevention/Avoidance

- Keep all medications out of the reach of pets.
- Do not store human and animal drugs in the same area to decrease medication errors.

Possible Complications

- DIC secondary to severe hyperthermia
- Rhabdomyolysis and secondary renal failure

Expected Course and Prognosis

- If CNS and cardiac signs can be controlled, prognosis is good.
- Signs may last up to 72 hours with extended release products.

Abbreviations

ADHD = attention deficit hyperactive disorder
CNS   = central nervous system
CRI   = continuous rate infusion
DIC   = disseminated intravascular hemolysis
ECG   = electrocardiogram
IM   = intramuscular
IV   = intravenous
NPO   = *nil per os* (nothing by mouth)
PO   = *per os* (by mouth)
q   = every
QID   = four times a day
SQ   = subcutaneous

See Also

Club Drugs
Methamphetamine
Selective Serotonin Reuptake Inhibitors (SSRIs)

Suggested Reading

Bloom FE. Neurotransmission and the central nervous system. In: Brunton LL, Lazo JS, Parker KL, eds. Goodman & Gilman's The Pharmacological Basis of Therapeutics, 11th ed. New York: McGraw-Hill Professional, 2006.
Plumb DC. Plumb's Veterinary Drug Handbook, 6th ed. Ames, IA: Wiley-Blackwell, 2008.

Author: Tina Wismer, DVM, DABVT, DABT
Consulting Editor: Lynn R. Hovda, RPH, DVM, MS, DACVIM

Angiotensin-Converting Enzyme (ACE) Inhibitors

chapter 14

DEFINITION/OVERVIEW

- ACEIs are a group of medications that lower blood pressure by decreasing peripheral vascular resistance.
  - Several are used in veterinary medicine in cases of heart failure or hypertension.
  - They may also be of benefit in the treatment of chronic renal failure or protein-losing enteropathies.
  - Included are benazepril, captopril, enalapril, imidapril, lisinopril, and ramipril.
- Primary concern in overdose situations is development of hypotension.
- Hypotension, lethargy, hypersalivation, and tachycardia are the most common clinical signs, followed by GI distress and renal dysfunction.

ETIOLOGY/PATHOPHYSIOLOGY

Mechanism of Action

- ACEIs block the conversion of angiotensin I to angiotensin II, resulting in a decrease in aldosterone production, decrease in sympathetic nervous system output, and an increase in vascular smooth muscle vasodilation. The net result is lowered blood pressure.
- ACEIs also block the breakdown of bradykinin, which contributes to lowering blood pressure but may also be responsible for the risk of angioedema.

Pharmacokinetics/Absorption, Distribution, Metabolism, and Excretion

- All ACEIs have rapid oral absorption and are well distributed (except to the CNS), metabolized in the liver, and primarily excreted by the kidneys.
- In general, healthy dogs with no underlying cardiovascular or renal issues are unlikely to experience hypotension at doses less than 20 mg/kg.
- Benazepril
  - Peak plasma levels occur about 75 minutes after dosing (dogs).
  - Metabolized in the liver to the active metabolite benazeprilat (age or hepatic compromise does not seem to alter metabolite levels)

- T½ in healthy dogs is 3.5 hours, but there may be an additional elimination slow phase, which may increase the half-life to 55–60 hours.
- T½ in healthy cats is 16–23 hours.
- Captopril
  - Rapid absorption in dogs
  - Food in the stomach decreases bioavailability by 30%–40%.
  - T½ in dogs is about 2.8 hours, but duration of effect may persist for 4 hours. Renal dysfunction can greatly extend the T½.
- Enalapril
  - Enalapril is converted in the liver into enalaprilat, an active metabolite.
  - Onset of action in dogs is 4–6 hours.
  - Duration of action in dogs is 12–14 hours.
  - 40% is excreted through the kidneys; 35% is excreted in the feces.
  - T½ enalaprilat in dogs is about 11 hours.
  - Severe cardiac disease or renal insufficiency will prolong the T½.
- Lisinopril
  - Peak plasma levels in dogs occur about 4 hours after ingestion.
  - T½ in dogs is 3 hours.
  - Effects last 24 hours.
- Ramipril
  - Ramipril is converted to the active metabolite ramiprilat by the liver.
  - Effects last 24 hours.
- Imidapril
  - T½ is 18–20 hours.

Toxicity

- ACEIs have a fairly wide margin of safety.
- Hypotension is the primary complication of overdose but is usually mild.
- Other adverse effects reported with use include angioedema, proteinuria, hyperkalemia, bronchospasm, pancreatitis, hepatotoxicity, renal insufficiency, and leukopenia.
  - Benazepril
    - Long T½ may require prolonged monitoring.
  - Captopril
    - 6.6 mg/kg every 8 hours may cause renal failure in dogs.
  - Enalapril
    - 200 mg/kg is lethal in dogs.
    - 100 mg/kg requires prolonged monitoring.
  - Lisinopril, Ramipril, Imidapril
    - No data available, but the long duration of action necessitates prolonged monitoring in overdose cases.

Systems Affected

- Renal/urologic—renin-angiotensin system is affected, causing a decrease in blood pressure; acute renal failure
- Cardiovascular—hypotension resulting in tachycardia
- Gastrointestinal—vomiting, diarrhea
- Respiratory—bronchospasm

 SIGNALMENT/HISTORY

- No specific breed or age predilection

Risk Factors

- Animals with severe CHF or renal insufficiency may be at higher risk.

 CLINICAL FEATURES

- Most common signs of overdose are hypotension followed by lethargy, salivation, and tachycardia.
- Secondary signs include vomiting, diarrhea, weakness, cough/bronchospasm, and dysfunction of the renal system.
- Rare potential for skin rashes and neutropenia
- The onset and duration of signs depends on the particular ACEI ingested.

 DIFFERENTIAL DIAGNOSIS

- Autonomic insufficiency
- Acute hypovolemia
- Benzodiazepine compounds including flunitrazepam
- Opiate or opioid ingestions

 DIAGNOSTICS

- Serum ACEI values are of little use in veterinary medicine.
- Presence of hypotension (systolic BP <90 mm Hg or MAP <60 mm Hg)
- Baseline laboratory work to include:
  - CBC (rare neutropenia or leukopenia)
  - Electrolytes (e.g., hyperkalemia)
  - Serum chemistry including liver enzymes, BUN and creatinine, lipase, and amylase
  - Urinalysis for early signs of renal disease

Pathological Findings

■ Nonspecific findings

 # THERAPEUTICS

Detoxification

■ Induce emesis only if early after ingestion and animal is asymptomatic. Potential for hypotension-induced aspiration pneumonia is high.
■ Gastric lavage in large ingestions
■ Activated charcoal with a cathartic x one dose, if no risk of aspiration and GI motility is normal

Appropriate Health Care

■ Monitor blood pressure and vital signs every 4 hours. Repeat more often if animal is hypotensive (MAP <60 mmHG).
■ Monitor BUN, creatinine, and electrolytes, especially if there is evidence of hypotension or if there is preexisting renal insufficiency.

Drug(s) and Antidotes of Choice

■ No specific antidote is available.
  • IV fluid therapy to maintain renal blood flow. Maintain urine output and hydration status appropriately.
  • Furosemide CRI at 1–2 mg/kg/hr
  • Mannitol bolus at 1–2 g/kg IV slowly
■ Persistent hypotension
  • IV crystalloids at 20–30 mL/kg in aliquots. Repeat 2–3 times as needed for volume expansion.
  • Colloids or blood products as needed
  • Vasopressors
    □ Dopamine 5–20 µg/kg/min IV CRI
    □ Norepinephrine 0.1–1.0 µg/kg/min IV CRI
    □ Epinephrine 0.1–0.4 µg/kg/min IV CRI
■ Antiemetics
  • Maropitant 1 mg/kg SQ q 24 hours, not labeled for cats
  • Ondansetron 0.1–0.2 mg/kg IV q 8–12 hours

 # COMMENTS

Expected Course and Prognosis

■ Prognosis is good with appropriate decontamination, monitoring, and treatment.

Abbreviations

ACEI = angiotensin-converting enzyme inhibitor
BP   = blood pressure
BUN = blood urea nitrogen
CBC = complete blood count
CHF = congestive heart failure
CNS = central nervous system
CRI   = continuous rate infusion
GI   = gastrointestinal
Hg   = mercury
IV   = intravenous
MAP = mean arterial pressure
q   = every
SQ   = subcutaneous
T½   = half-life

See Also

Opiates and opioids

Suggested Reading

Atkins CE, Brown WA, Coats JR, et al. Effects of long-term administration of enalapril on clinical indicators of renal function in dogs with compensated mitral regurgitation. J Am Vet Med Assoc 2002; 221(5):654–658.

Atkins CE, Keene BW, Brown WA, et al. Results of the veterinary enalapril trial to prove reduction in onset of heart failure in dogs chronically treated with enalapril alone for compensated, naturally occurring mitral valve insufficiency. J Am Vet Med Assoc 2007; 231(7):1061–1069.

Hamlin RL, Nakayama T. Comparison of some pharmacokinetic parameters of 5 angiotensin-converting enzyme inhibitors in normal beagles. J Vet Intern Med 1998; 12:93–95.

Schlesinger DP, Rubin SL. Potential adverse effects of angiotensin-converting enzyme inhibitors in the treatment of congestive heart failure. Comp Contin Ed 1994; 16(3):385–387.

Author: Catherine M. Adams, DVM
Consulting Editor: Lynn R. Hovda, RPH, DVM, MS, DACVIM

chapter 15

Atypical Antipsychotics

DEFINITION/OVERVIEW

- Atypical antipsychotics are a relatively new class of drugs for use in human medicine.
- Included are aripiprazole (Abilify), olanzapine (Zyprexa), paliperidone (Invega), quetiapine (Seroquel), risperidone (Risperdal), and ziprasidone (Geodon).
- While these medications are commonly used in psychiatric disorders in humans, there is no current labeled use for them in veterinary medicine. Several of them have been used off-label in a limited manner for canine aggression.
- Hypotension, tachycardia, and sedation or agitation are the most common clinical signs resulting from overdose.

ETIOLOGY/PATHOPHYSIOLOGY

Mechanism of Action

- The exact mechanism of action of the atypical antipsychotics is unknown, but it is postulated that they are strong antagonists at serotonin ($5\text{-}HT_2$) and dopamine (D_2) receptors.
- All of the atypical antipsychotics exhibit antagonism at α_1 and H_1 receptors, which explains why they may cause orthostatic hypotension and somnolence, respectively.
- Risperidone, quetiapine, and paliperidone exhibit antagonism at α_2 receptors.
- Quetiapine and olanzapine exhibit antagonism at muscarinic receptors and may cause anticholinergic signs.

Pharmacokinetics/Absorption, Distribution, Metabolism, Excretion

- Based primarily on human literature; very little animal information is available.
- All of the atypical antipsychotics have good oral absorption.
- All undergo hepatic metabolism through the CYP450 isoenzymes.
- All of the atypical antipsychotics are excreted in the urine.

Toxicity

- Aripiprazole
  - A toxic dose in animals has not been established.
  - Overdose data in humans is limited and a toxic dose has not been established.
- Olanzapine
  - A toxic dose in animals has not been established.
  - Acute study of dogs given 15 mg olanzapine/day PO for 4–6 weeks showed the following:
    - Increase in adipose stores and total body fat
    - Insulin resistance
  - There have been reported deaths in adult humans at 600 mg, but there have also been patients who have ingested more than 1 g and survived with supportive care.
- Paliperidone
  - A toxic dose in animals and in humans has not been established.
- Quetiapine
  - A toxic dose in animals has not been established.
  - Ingestion of 1300 mg in an 11-year-old child resulted in mild toxicosis and no cardiac abnormalities.
  - Adults have survived ingestions of 1,200–24,000 mg.
  - One reported fatality in an adult human who ingested 10,800 mg
- Risperidone
  - Oral LD_{50} in dogs is 14–24 mg/kg
  - 0.05 mg/kg in dogs—ataxia, weakness, tachycardia, agitation, hypotension, tremors, seizures have been observed
  - Studies in the literature have revealed that animals should be able to survive a total dose of at least 5 mg with supportive care.
- Ziprasidone
  - 6–12 mg/kg in dogs—hypotension or hypertension, tachycardia, hyperesthesia, ataxia
  - A 30-month-old human infant developed coma and respiratory depression after an ingestion of 40 mg.
  - In adult humans, ingestions of up to 4480 mg have not resulted in serious toxicity.
  - Extrapyramidal syndrome (EPS) developed in an adult human after ingesting 12,800 mg.

Systems Affected

- Cardiovascular—hypotension, tachycardia, QTc prolongation, QRS widening, arrhythmias

- Nervous—sedation, anxiety, agitation, insomnia, tremor, seizure, akathisia, tardive dyskinesia, somnolence, CNS depression, EPS
- Endocrine/metabolic—serotonin syndrome
- Ophthalmic—congested conjunctiva

 # SIGNALMENT/HISTORY

- All breeds or veterinary species can be affected.

Risk Factors

- Animals with the following underlying conditions are at risk:
  - Seizure disorders
  - Cardiovascular disease
  - Pregnant or nursing

Historical Findings

- Signs typically develop within an hour but may be delayed for up to a few hours, due to the lag in time to peak plasma concentrations.
- These drugs have long half-lives, so prolonged supportive care may be needed if early decontamination does not occur.

Interaction with Drugs, Nutrients, or Environment

- Drugs that also prolong the QTc interval or widen the QRS interval (i.e., amiodarone, phenytoin, others)

 # CLINICAL FEATURES

- The most common signs are hypotension, tachycardia, ataxia, and agitation or lethargy.
- Other signs, occurring less often and drug dependent, include the development of a serotonin syndrome, cardiac arrhythmias, and perhaps a neuroleptic malignant-like syndrome.

 # DIFFERENTIAL DIAGNOSIS

- Clomipramine
- SSRIs

 # DIAGNOSTICS

- Patient history and clinical signs should be used for diagnosis.

- Serum electrolytes may show hyponatremia and hypokalemia.

Pathological Findings

- No specific findings

 THERAPEUTICS

- The goals of treatment are to prevent absorption, address neurological and cardiovascular status, and provide supportive care.

Detoxification

- Induce emesis if ingestion occurred within the past 30 minutes and the dog is asymptomatic.
- If emesis was not induced at home, perform in DVM's office within 60 minutes of ingestion.
- Activated charcoal with a cathartic may be given for one dose.
- Multidose activated charcoal without a cathartic should be given to animals ingesting sustained-release formulations.

Appropriate Healthcare

- If clinical signs are present, hospitalize until asymptomatic, generally about 12–24 hours.
- Maintain hydration and monitor for hyponatremia if using multiple-dose activated charcoal.
- Monitor blood pressure and heart rate.
- Monitor for temperature alterations and treat appropriately.
- ECG for arrhythmias
- Observe closely for development of serotonin syndrome.

Drug(s) of Choice

- IV fluids for renal perfusion and correction of hypotension. Run at 1.5–2 times maintenance until blood pressure improves, and then decrease as needed.
- Pressor agents only after well hydrated and when hypotension is severe and does not respond to IV fluids
- Agitation and CNS stimulation
  - Diazepam 0.25–0.5 mg/kg IV
  - Phenobarbital 3–5 mg/kg IV PRN
- EPS
  - Diphenhydramine 2–4 mg/kg IM or PO

- Serotonin syndrome
  - Cyproheptadine is generally given orally but can be administered rectally, at the same dose, in animals with severe clinical signs.
    - □ Cats: 2–4 mg total dose every 4–6 hours as needed until resolution of clinical signs
    - □ Dogs: 1.1 mg/kg BW every 4–6 hours as needed

Precautions/Interactions

- Refrain from using sodium channel–blocking or potassium-blocking antiarrhythmics.
- There is some controversy about whether true neuroleptic malignant syndrome, found in human beings and other species, occurs in dogs and cats. Some veterinarians agree; some disagree.

Nursing Care

- Ensure urine output
- Frequent TPRs

Prevention

- Pet owners should be advised to keep medications out of the reach of pets, preferably stored in locked cabinets or cabinets located high off the ground.

 COMMENTS

Client Education

- Ensure the home environment is safe for the pet's return.
- Readmit if clinical signs recur or worsen even after proper treatment.

Patient Monitoring

- Serum chemistry for renal and hepatic values
- Electrolytes, especially potassium and sodium
- ECG as needed

Prevention/Avoidance

- Store medications in locked cabinets or difficult-to-reach cabinets.
- Keep purses and full shopping bags off of the floor and away from easy-to-reach places.
- Do not leave medications on countertops that may be accessible by a pet.

Possible Complications

- Rhabdomyolysis if seizures occur and are left untreated

Expected Course and Prognosis

- Clinical signs typically develop within 1 hour, but may take up to several hours.
- Signs resolve in 12–24 hours but may be prolonged when sustained-release products have been ingested.
- Prognosis for recovery is excellent, especially with early treatment. Appropriately treated animals rarely die after ingestion of atypical antipsychotics.

Abbreviations

CNS = central nervous system
EPS = extrapyramidal syndrome
ECG = electrocardiogram
IM   = intramuscular
IV   = intravenous
PO   = *per os* (by mouth)
PRN = *pro re nata* (as needed)
TPR = temperature, pulse, respiration

See Also

Selective Serotonin Reuptake Inhibitors (SSRIs)

Suggested Reading

Ader M, Kim SP, Catalano KJ, et al. Metabolic dysregulation with atypical antipsychotics occurs in the absence of underlying disease: a placebo-controlled study of olanzapine and risperidone in dogs. Diabetes 2005; 54(3):862–871.

Juurlink D. Antipsychotics. In: Flomenbaum NE, Goldfrank LR, Hoffman RS, et al., eds. Goldfrank's Toxicologic Emergencies, 8th ed. New York: McGraw-Hill, 2006; pp. 1039–1051.

Author: Kelly M. Sioris, PharmD
Consulting Editor: Lynn R. Hovda, RPH, DVM, MS, DACVIM

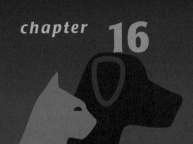

chapter 16

Baclofen

DEFINITION/OVERVIEW

- Baclofen is a centrally acting skeletal muscle relaxant that mimics gamma-aminobutyric acid (GABA) within the spinal cord.
- Baclofen is used to control spasticity and pain in people with multiple sclerosis and spinal disorders.
- It is used extralabel in dogs to treat urinary retention by reducing urethral resistance.
- The most common clinical signs of an overdose are vocalization, disorientation, vomiting, and ataxia.
- The most life-threatening clinical signs are dyspnea, respiratory depression, respiratory arrest, and nonresponsive seizures.

PATHOPHYSIOLOGY

Mechanism of Action

- Baclofen binds to GABA$_b$ receptors and inhibits the influx of calcium, which prevents the release of the excitatory neurotransmitters glutamate and aspartate. The GABA$_b$ receptor also opens selective K$^+$ channels allowing an outward ion flux. Stimulation of GABA results in hyperpolarization and increased inhibitory tone.
- Baclofen can cause excitatory stimulation that may result in seizure activity.

Pharmacokinetics/Absorption, Distribution, Metabolism, and Excretion

- Baclofen is rapidly and completely absorbed from the GIT.
- Clinical signs after acute oral exposure may be rapid, occurring within minutes, or delayed for several hours.
- The duration of clinical signs can vary from several hours to several days due to the slow clearance from the CNS.
- Baclofen has low protein binding and a wide volume of distribution. Approximately 80% of the drug is eliminated unchanged in the urine with 20% undergoing

deamination in the liver and biliary excretion. There is also some deamination in the renal tubules.
- Baclofen's plasma half-life is 2 to 6 hours.

Toxicity

- Doses as low as 1.3 mg/kg may cause vomiting, depression, and vocalization.
- Deaths have occurred with doses between 8 and 16 mg/kg.

Systems Affected

- Respiratory—dyspnea, respiratory depression, respiratory arrest
- Nervous—ataxia, vocalization, disorientation, seizures
- Gastrointestinal—vomiting
- Cardiovascular—bradycardia, hypotension
- Endocrine/metabolic—hypothermia

 # SIGNALMENT/HISTORY

- Any breed or age of dog is susceptible.
- Cats are especially susceptible to toxicity.
- Toxicosis most commonly occurs when the animal ingests the owner's medication.

Risk Factors

- Pet owners with medical conditions (e.g., multiple sclerosis and spinal disorders) are more likely to have baclofen in the house, propagating potential pet ingestion.

Historical Findings

- Evidence of a chewed bottle, witnessed ingestion, inadvertent or accidental administration by pet owner
- Generally, the diagnosis is made based on the history of ingestion coupled with clinical signs.

 # CLINICAL FEATURES

- Common clinical signs—vocalization, vomiting, ataxia, disorientation, salivation, depression, coma, weakness, generalized flaccid paralysis, recumbency, seizures, and hypothermia
- Life-threatening signs—dyspnea, respiratory depression, and respiratory arrest secondary to paralysis of the diaphragm and intercostal muscles

- Less frequent signs—hypotension, bradycardia, hypertension, cardiac arrhythmias, tachycardia, hyperactivity, agitation, tremors, panting, hyperesthesia, mydriasis, miosis, diarrhea, pulmonary edema, and death

 # DIFFERENTIAL DIAGNOSIS

- Neuromuscular disease such as lower motor neuron disease (e.g., botulism, polyradiculitis, tick paralysis, *Toxoplasma*, and *Neospora*)
- Primary metabolic disease (renal, hepatic, hepatic encephalopathy, hypoglycemia, hypoadrenocorticism)
- Toxicants
  - Benzodiazepines
  - Opiates and opioids
  - Barbiturates
  - Sedatives

 # DIAGNOSTICS

- Baseline CBC, chemistry, UA
- Arterial blood gas analysis to evaluate for hypoxemia, oxygenation, and ventilation
- Pulse oximetry to evaluate for hypoxemia
- End-tidal CO_2 to evaluate for hypercapnea or hypoventilation
- Thoracic radiographs to evaluate for aspiration pneumonia secondary to severe sedation

Pathologic Findings

- No specific lesions associated. May see secondary aspiration pneumonia or atelectasis.

 # THERAPEUTICS

Detoxification

- Emesis if animal presents within one hour of ingestion. Emesis is contraindicated in symptomatic animals.
- Gastric lavage should be considered with large ingestions but should be done with the patient intubated with an inflated endotracheal tube to prevent secondary aspiration pneumonia.
- One dose of activated charcoal with a cathartic may be given. Baclofen does not undergo enterohepatic circulation, so repeated dosing of activated charcoal is unnecessary.
- Elimination may be enhanced with fluid diuresis.

Appropriate Health Care

- Monitor for cardiac arrhythmias and hypothermia.
- Monitor for hypoventilation and aspiration pneumonia and treat appropriately with mechanical ventilation, oxygen support, IV antibiotic therapy, nebulization and coupage, and appropriate hydration.
- Ventilatory support may be required in those animals with severe respiratory depression and is required with respiratory failure.
- Hemodialysis and hemoperfusion can be used to shorten the serum elimination half-life to baclofen and decrease time to recovery. Hemodialysis is useful for the removal of drugs and toxins with a molecular weight of <1500 Daltons, a low volume of distribution, and minimal (<80%) plasma protein binding. It is the unbound portion of the drug that is removed via dialysis.

Drugs(s) and Antidotes of Choice

- No specific antidote is available.
- Atropine 0.02–0.04 mg/kg IM, IV, or SQ as needed for bradycardia.
- Diazepam is used to treat baclofen-induced seizures. The lowest effective dose should be used, due to profound sedation from both drugs. Diazepam may be given intermittently (0.25–0.5 mg/kg, IV, to effect, PRN) or as a CRI (0.5–1 mg/kg/hr, IV, to effect if needed).
- Refractory seizures may require treatment with propofol or general anesthesia.
  - Propofol 1–8 mg/kg, IV to effect, followed by CRI dose of 0.1–0.6 mg/kg/hr if uncontrolled seizures.
- During drug withdrawal profound agitation may occur, which may necessitate treatment with acepromazine, diazepam, or midazolam.
  - Acepromazine 0.05–0.2 mg/kg, IV, SQ, IM q 4–6 hours PRN
  - Diazepam 0.1–0.25 mg/kg, IV to effect, PRN
  - Midazolam 0.1–0.5 mg/kg, IV or IM to effect, PRN
- Cyproheptadine hydrochloride
  - Dogs: 1.1 mg/kg, PO or rectally q 4–6 hours as needed may help reduce vocalization or disorientation
  - Cats: 2–4 mg *total* dose q 4–6 hours PRN
- Intravenous fat emulsion (IFE) is considered a new, experimental antidote for fat-soluble drugs (e.g., baclofen, ivermectin, bupivicaine).
  - The exact mechanism of action through which IFE acts as an antidote and helps augment conventional resuscitation efforts is unknown; however, four potentially complementary mechanisms exist.
    - Augmentation of cardiac performance through provision of myocytes energy substrates
    - Restoration of myocardial function by increasing intracellular calcium concentration
    - Sequestration of lipophillic compounds into the newly created lipid compartment within the intravascular space (a lipid or pharmaco-

logical sink). Compartmentalization of the drug into the lipid phase results in lesser free drug concentration available to tissues.
  - ☐ Lipid emulsion increases the overall fatty acid pool and overcomes bupivicaine inhibition of mitochondrial fatty acid metabolism.
- Dosing for IFE (extrapolated from human medicine)
  - ☐ Using the 20% emulsion, administer 1.5 mL/kg IV bolus followed by 0.25 mL/kg/min for 30–60 minutes.
  - ☐ The initial bolus could be repeated 1–2 times if no response to the initial bolus is obtained, with a goal of not to exceed 8 mL/kg/day.

Alternative Drugs

- Flumazenil has been used with limited success in baclofen overdoses but may potentially precipitate seizures. Dose 0.01 mg/kg IV, to effect.

Nursing Care

- Close patient monitoring with blood gas analysis, pulse oximetry, and $ETCO_2$ may be necessary to evaluate for hypoxemia or hypercapnea; the patient may need to be intubated and ventilated.
- Nursing care, including turning q 6 hours, lubricating eyes, keeping the patient dry and clean, passive range of motion of limbs, and soft bedding may be necessary for intubated or very sedate patients.

Follow-up

- Thoracic radiographs may be warranted to asses for development of aspiration pneumonia.

Client Education

- Clients should be made aware that even though baclofen is used in humans for muscle relaxation, it can be a severe toxin in pets and can lead to serious complications and potential death of the animal.

Possible Complications

- Aspiration pneumonia is a common complication due to clinical signs of vomiting, seizures, and paralysis of the diaphragm and intercostal muscles.

Expected Course and Prognosis

- Hospitalized animals may require 5–7 days for a full recovery. Recovery occurs with no residual CNS effects.
- Prognosis is generally good with early and appropriate care but becomes poor with an extended period of time prior to veterinary care. Animals with seizures or aspiration pneumonia have a much more guarded prognosis.

Abbreviations

BUN   = blood urea nitrogen
CBC   = complete blood count
CNS   = central nervous system
CRI   = continuous rate infusion
ETCO$_2$ = end-tidal carbon dioxide
GABA = gamma-aminobutyric acid
GIT   = gastrointestinal tract
IFE   = intravenous fat emulsion
IM   = intramuscular
IV   = intravenous
PO   = *per os* (by mouth)
PRN   = *pro re nata* (as needed)
q   = every
SQ   = subcutaneous
UA   = urinalysis

See Also

Benzodiazepines
Opiates and Opioids

Suggested Reading

Hecht DV, Allenspach K. Presumptive baclofen intoxication in a dog. J Vet Emerg Crit Care 1998; 8:49–54.
Scott NE, Francey T, Jandrey K. Baclofen intoxication in a dog successfully treated with hemodialysis and hemoperfusion coupled with intensive supportive care. J Vet Emerg Crit Care 2007; 17:191–196.
Torre DM, Labato MA, Rossi T, et al. Treatment of a dog with severe baclofen intoxication using hemodialysis and mechanical ventilation. J Vet Emerg Crit Care 2008; 18:312–318.
Wismer T. Baclofen overdose in dogs. Vet Med 2004; 99:406–408.

Author: Jane Quandt, DVM, DACVA, DACVECC
Consulting Editors: Lynn R. Hovda, RPH, DVM, MS, DAVCIM; Justine A. Lee, DVM, DACVECC

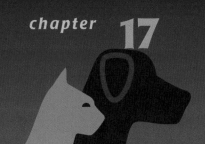

chapter 17

Benzodiazepines

DEFINITION/OVERVIEW

- Three benzodiazepines are commonly used in veterinary medicine—diazepam (Valium), midazolam (Versed), and zolazepam found in combination with tiletamine, a dissociative agent (Telazol).
- Many other benzodiazepines are used in human medicine (see table 17.1).
- Benzodiazepines are used as a tranquilizing sedative and provide anxiolytic, muscle relaxant, and anticonvulsant properties.
- Benzodiazepines have a wide margin of safety.
- Common clinical signs of overdose are related to the CNS and include confusion, ataxia, and depression.

ETIOLOGY/PATHOPHYSIOLOGY

Mechanism of Action

- Benzodiazepines interact with the benzodiazepine receptors that modulate GABA, an inhibitory neurotransmitter.
- Chronic use of benzodiazepines in cats can result in fulminant hepatic failure through an unknown mechanism. Toxicity may relate to the cat's inherent deficiency in glucuronide conjugation and glutathione detoxification of reactive intermediates.

Pharmacokinetics/Absorption, Distribution, Metabolism, and Excretion

- Benzodiazepines are well absorbed orally.
- All are highly protein bound and lipid soluble.
- Peak plasma levels generally occur between 30 and 120 minutes.
- Widely distributed to brain, liver, and spleen; poorly to fat and muscle
- Metabolized in liver to active and inactive metabolites
  - Half-life elimination of diazepam (cat) after IV dosing—5.46 hours
  - Half-life elimination of nordiazepam (active diazepam metabolite) (cat) after IV dosing—21.3 hours

TABLE 17.1. Benzodiazepine drugs currently on the market.

Generic Name	Trade Name	Peak Plasma Level in Hours (Human Data)	T ½ in Hours (Human Data)	Speed of Onset
Alprazolam	Xanax	1–2	6.3–26.9	Intermediate
Chlordiazepoxide	Librium	0.5–4	5–30	Intermediate
Clonazepam	Klonopin	1–2	18–50	Intermediate
Clorazepate	Tranxene	1–2	40–50	Fast
Diazepam	Valium	0.5–2	20–80	Very Fast
Estazolam	Prosom	2	8–28	Fast
Flurazepam	Dalmane	0.5–1	2–3	Fast
Lorazepam	Ativan	2–4	10–20	Intermediate
Midazolam	Versed	0.28–0.83	2.2–6.8	Very Fast
Oxazepam	Serax	2–4	5–20	Slow
Quazepam	Doral	1–2	41	Fast
Temazepam	Restoril	1.6–2	3.5–18.4	Fast
Triazolam	Halcion	1–2	1.5–5.5	Fast

- Conjugated with glucuronide and excreted in urine
- Duration of action is specific for each benzodiazepine compound

Toxicity

- Overdose as a single exposure is rarely life-threatening in healthy animals.
- Oral exposure of more than one dose may be life-threatening in the cat.

Systems Affected

- Nervous—CNS depression, dysphoria, ataxia, excitement, aggression
- Respiratory—respiratory depression
- Cardiovascular—bradycardia, hypotension
- Endocrine/metabolic—hypothermia from sedation
- Hepatic—fulminant hepatic necrosis (cats only); appears as anorexia, lethargy, vomiting, dehydration, hypothermia, icterus, increased liver enzymes, coagulopathy, hypoglycemia

 SIGNALMENT/HISTORY

- Any age or breed of dog or cat can be affected.

- Overdose usually occurs due to iatrogenic administration of an improper dose or ingestion of a human medication.

Risk Factors

- Benzodiazepines present in the household may pose an increased risk of exposure to pets.
- Pediatric, geriatric, or debilitated patients with underlying metabolic disease may have prolonged duration of effects from toxicosis, or even from therapeutic dosing.
- Cats given oral, chronic diazepam for behavior modification treatment may develop acute fulminant hepatic necrosis.

Historical Findings

- Witnessed exposure by pet owner
- Pet owner may find chewed pill vial.
- Clinical symptoms of ataxia, sedation, agitation, and dysphoria may be noted by the pet owner.

 # CLINICAL FEATURES

- Common clinical signs include CNS depression, ataxia, confusion, disorientation, and aggression.
- As ingested dose increases, risks for hypotension, hypothermia, coma, and seizures occur.
- In approximately 40%–50% of cases, paradoxical stimulation and excitation occurs in both dogs and cats.

 # DIFFERENTIAL DIAGNOSIS

- Primary metabolic disease (hepatic encephalopathy, hypoglycemia)
- Primary neurologic disease
- Toxicants:
  - Acetaminophen
  - Barbiturates
  - Ethylene glycol
  - Marijuana
  - Opioids
  - Phenothiazines
  - Xylitol

DIAGNOSTICS

- Baseline CBC, chemistry, UA to evaluate underlying metabolic disease
- The Quick Screen Pro Multi Drug Screening Test is a human testing kit that has been validated by GC/MS for use in animals. It may provide a rapid and accurate diagnosis if the drug is present in high enough concentrations and the time frame is appropriate.
- Urine or serum can be submitted specifically for GC/MS or LC/MS, but the results will take several days to be returned and will only indicate exposure.
- In cats suspected of having acute hepatic necrosis, a coagulation panel should be done to evaluate PT/PTT.

Pathological Findings

- Histology of the feline liver shows severe, acute to subacute, lobular to massive hepatic necrosis.

 # THERAPEUTICS

- Treatment consists of general supportive measures, early decontamination, and if necessary, administration of the reversal agent, flumazenil.

Detoxification

- Emesis if early after ingestion
- Activated charcoal with a cathartic x one dose

Appropriate Health Care

- Monitor body temperature and blood pressure; support appropriately with warming methods and IV fluid therapy. Monitor for severe CNS or respiratory depression; if indicated, consider the use of flumazenil.
- Cats suffering from hepatic failure due to oral diazepam need aggressive treatment.

Drugs and Antidotes of Choice

- Flumazenil (Romazicon) is the specific antidote for benzodiazepine overdose but should be used only in cases where CNS depression is severe. Flumazenil rapidly reverses the sedative and muscle relaxant effects of the benzodiazepine agonists. Effects are usually seen within 5 minutes.
  - Dose: flumazenil 0.01 mg/kg IV to effect, repeat PRN. If a long-acting benzodiazepine has been ingested, repeated doses of flumazenil may be necessary, due to its short duration of action (1–2 hours).

- IV fluids as needed to treat hypotension, maintain perfusion, and correct dehydration. A balanced crystalloid should be used. If evidence of hepatic failure, LRS should be avoided.
- If the animal is experiencing paradoxical stimulation (e.g., agitation, aggression), treatment with additional benzodiazepines (e.g., diazepam) is contraindicated. An alternative sedative or anxiolytic should be used:
  - Acepromazine 0.05–0.2 mg/kg, IV, SQ, IM PRN
  - Medetomidine 1–10 μg/kg, IV, SQ, IM PRN
  - Diphenhydramine 2–4 mg/kg IM or PO
- Treatment for hepatic failure consists of IV fluid therapy, antibiotic therapy, glucose and potassium supplementation, administration of both water-soluble vitamins (e.g., vitamin B) and vitamin K, nutritional support, hepatoprotectants (SAMe), and potentially, blood-plasma transfusions (if coagulopathic or evidence of hemorrhagic shock).

Precautions/Interactions

- CNS stimulants such as caffeine should be avoided.
- Diazepam is not water soluble, and the parenteral formula contains 40% propylene glycol and 10% ethanol. It is very irritating, painful, and poorly absorbed when given IM.

Follow-up

- Cats that survive diazepam-induced acute hepatic necrosis should have liver enzymes checked every 5–7 days until clinically normal.

 COMMENTS

Client Education

- Owners should be advised not to use their own medicines to treat their pets and to keep them out of the reach of pets.

Patient Monitoring

- While hospitalized, excessively sedate patients should have blood pressure, ECG, TPR, and ventilatory status closely monitored.

Prevention/Avoidance

- Owners should be informed about the risks of benzodiazepines in pets, and keep them out of reach, particularly in the bedroom (sleep aid medication placed on bedroom table).

Expected Course and Prognosis

- Once decontaminated, animals generally only need to be monitored for 4–8 hours. If no clinical signs develop, the patient can be monitored at home. If signs develop, they should be monitored until clinical signs have resolved (typically 8–24 hours depending on the drug involved).
- In those animals experiencing a single overdose exposure, the prognosis is excellent.
- In those cats experiencing idiosyncratic hepatic failure due to repeated doses of oral diazepam, the prognosis is poor to guarded. Based on this, oral chronic use of benzodiazepines should be avoided in cats.

Abbreviations

CNS   = central nervous system
ECG   = electrocardiogram
GABA   = gamma aminobutyric acid
GC/MS = gas chromatography/mass spectrometry
IM   = intramuscular
IV   = intravenous
LC/MS = liquid chromatography/mass spectrometry
LRS   = lactated Ringers solution
PO   = *per os* (by mouth)
PRN   = *pro re nata* (as needed)
PT   = prothrombin time
PTT   = partial thromboplastin time
q   = every
SAMe   = S-adenosyl-methionine
SQ   = subcutaneous
TPR   = temperature, pulse, respiration
UA   = urinalysis

See Also

Ethylene Glycol
Opiates and Opioids

Suggested Reading

Center SA, Elston TH, Rowland PH, et al. Fulminant hepatic failure associated with oral administration of diazepam in 11 cats. J Am Vet Med Assoc 1996; 209:618–625.
Lemke KA. Anticholinergics and sedatives. In: Tranquilli WJ, Thurmon JC, Grimm KA, eds. Lumb & Jones Veterinary Anesthesia and Analgesia 4th ed. Ames, IA: Blackwell, 2007; pp. 203–239.

Malouin A, Boiler M. Sedatives, muscle relaxants, and opioids toxicity. In: Silverstein DC, Hopper K, eds. Small Animal Critical Care Medicine, St. Louis: Elsevier, 2009; pp. 350–356.

Author: Jane Quandt, DVM, MS, DACVA, DACVECC
Consulting Editors: Lynn R. Hovda, RPH, DVM, MS, DACVIM; Justine A. Lee, DVM, DACVECC

chapter 18

Beta-Blockers

DEFINITION/OVERVIEW

- Beta receptor antagonists are class II antidysrhythmics commonly used in humans to treat hypertension, tachydysrhythmia, essential tremors, glaucoma, anxiety, migraine headaches, and to prevent heart disease.
- In animals, beta receptor antagonists are most commonly used to treat hypertrophic or hypertrophic-obstructive cardiomyopathy in cats and tachydysrhythmias in dogs.
- In 2007, the American Association of Poison Control Centers (AAPCC) reported 86,122 human exposures to cardiovascular agents. Cardiovascular drugs were cited as number five on the list of substances most frequently involved in human exposures with the largest number of fatalities. In fact, among the top 25 human fatality–causing categories reported by the AAPCC, cardiovascular agents accounted for 24% of all deaths.
- The current standard treatment for patients presenting with beta antagonist overdose uses traditional vasopressor agents, often in high doses. However, recent findings suggest this may not only be ineffective, it may actually increase mortality. Thus, the treatment of beta-blocker overdose has changed significantly in the last few years.

ETIOLOGY/PATHOPHYSIOLOGY

Mechanism of Action

- Beta adrenergic antagonists work primarily by blocking the beta adrenergic receptors.
- B_1 receptors are primarily located in the heart, eye, and kidney and may result in significant bradycardia with B_1 blockade.
- B_2 receptors are found in bronchial smooth muscle, the gastrointestinal tract, pancreas, liver, skeletal muscle, and blood vessels. Blockade of B_2 receptors may result in bronchospasm (more likely to occur in cats or dogs with underlying airway disease) and peripheral vasodilation resulting in hypotension.

Pharmacokinetics

- See table 18.1.

TABLE 18.1. Pharmacologic properties of the β-adrenergic antagonists.

	Adrenergic Blocking Activity	Partial Agonist Activity (ISA)	Membrane Stabilizing Activity	Vasodilating Property	Lipid Solubility	Protein Binding	Oral Bioavailability	Half-Life (h)	Metabolism	Volume of Distribution (L/kg)
Acebutolol	β_1	Yes	Yes	No	Low	25%	40%	2–4	Hepatic/renal	1.2
Atenolol	β_1	No	No	No	Low	<5%	40%–50%	5–9	Renal	1
Betaxolol (ophthalmic and tabs)	β_1	No	Yes	Yes (calcium channel blockade)	Low	50%	80%–90%	14–22	Hepatic/renal	NA
Bisoprolol	β_1	No	No	No	Low	30%	80%	9–12	Hepatic/renal	NA
Bucindolol	β_1, β_2	β_2 agonism		Yes (β_2 agonism)	Moderate		30%	8 ± 4.5	Hepatic	NA
Carteolol (ophthalmic)	β_1, β_2	Yes	No	Yes (β_2 agonism and nitric oxide mediated)	Low	30%	85%	5–6	Renal	NA
Carvedilol	$\alpha_1, \beta_1, \beta_2$	No		Yes (α_1 blockade)	Moderate	~98%	25%–35%	6–10	Hepatic	115
Celiprolol	α_2, β_1	β_2 agonism		Yes (β_2 agonism)	Low	22%–24%	30%–70%	5	Hepatic	NA
Esmolol	β_1	No	No	No	Low	50%	NA	~8min	RBC esterases	2
Labetalol	$\alpha_1, \beta_1, \beta_2$	No	Low	Yes (α_1 antagonism)	Moderate	50%	20%–33%	4–8	Hepatic	9

Drug	Receptor		ISA	Vasodilation	Lipid solubility	Protein binding	Bioavailability	Half-life (h)	Elimination	
Levobunolol (ophthalmic)	β₁, β₂	No	No	No	NA	NA	NA	6	NA	NA
Metipranolol (ophthalmic)	β₁, β₂	No	No	No	NA	NA	NA	3–4	NA	NA
Metoprolol (long-acting form available)	β₁	No	Low	No	Moderate	10%	40%–50%	3–4	Hepatic	4
Nadolol	β₁, β₂	No	No	No	Low	20%–30%	30%–35%	10–24	Renal	2
Nebivolol	β₁	No		Yes (nitric oxide mediated?)	Moderate	98%	12%–96%	8–32	Hepatic	10–40
Oxprenolol	β₁, β₂	Yes	Yes	No	Moderate	80%	20%–70%	1–3	Hepatic	1.3
Penbutolol	β₁, β₂	Yes	No	No	High	90%	~100%	5	Hepatic/renal	NA
Pindolol	β₁, β₂	Yes	Low	No	Moderate	50%	75%–90%	3–4	Hepatic/renal	2
Propranolol (long-acting form acting)	β₁, β₂	No	Yes	No	High	90%	30%–70%	3–5	Hepatic	4
Sotalol	β₁, β₂	No	No	No	Low	0%	90%	9–12	Renal	2
Timolol (ophthalmic)	β₁, β₂	No	No	No	Moderate	60%	75%	3–5	Hepatic/renal	2

Note: Agents in italics are *not* FDA approved. The notation "NA" indicates that information is not available. ISA = intrinsic sympathomimetic activity.
Source: Goldfrank's Toxicologic Emergencies, 2nd ed. (New York: McGraw-Hill, 2006), table 59-1.

Toxicity

- Some beta antagonists (primarily propranolol) may inhibit fast sodium channels, resulting in prolongation of PR and QRS intervals.
- Seizure activity has been reported in beta antagonist overdoses. This primarily occurs with propranolol toxicosis secondary to its significant lipophilicity and entrance into the CNS.
- Despite aggressive IV fluids and therapies (e.g., calcium, glucagon, and atropine), cardiogenic shock may ensue secondary to the negative inotropic effects of beta antagonists on the myocardium.
- Propranolol may inhibit catecholamine-induced glycogenolysis, resulting in hypoglycemia.

Systems Affected

- Cardiovascular—bradycardia, hypotension
- CNS—decreased mental status, seizures
- Endocrine/metabolic—hypoglycemia, metabolic acidosis secondary to hypotension, and decreased perfusion
- Respiratory—bronchospasm

 ## CLINICAL FEATURES

- Bradycardia
- 1st, 2nd, and 3rd degree heart block
- Myocardial depression/negative inotropic effects
- Hypotension/cardiogenic shock
- Seizures
- Hypoglycemia
- Prolongation of the PR, QRS, and QT complexes
- Respiratory compromise/bronchospasm
- Altered mental status/coma

 ## DIFFERENTIAL DIAGNOSIS

- Baclofen or opiate/opioid toxicosis
- Calcium channel blocker overdose
- Cardiac disease with secondary arrhythmias
- Other cardiovascular agent overdose (e.g., clonidine, digoxin toxicosis)
- Sick sinus syndrome of miniature schnauzers

DIAGNOSTICS

- Measurement of serum or urine beta-blocker concentrations is not readily available. Serum and urine concentrations do not correlate well with the degree of toxicosis. Therefore, obtaining urine or serum concentrations is not routinely performed.

THERAPEUTICS

Detoxification

- Emesis is *NOT* recommended in beta antagonist overdose secondary to rapid decreases in mental status and possible seizure activity. Emesis may also result in a vagal response exacerbating beta antagonist induced bradycardia.
- Consider gastric lavage for significant ingestions of immediate-release beta antagonist preparations presenting within 1 hour of ingestion.
- Activated charcoal should be administered (1–2 g/kg) for significant ingestions of immediate-release beta antagonist preparations presenting within 1 hour of ingestion.
- Whole bowel irrigation with GoLytely may be considered for ingestions of extended- or sustained-release preparations of beta antagonists.

Appropriate Healthcare

- Airway protection and ventilatory support (e.g., intubation and positive pressure ventilation) as needed for decreased mental status, respiratory depression, or seizure activity
- Blood pressure monitoring: Hypotension is a noted side effect of beta antagonists in overdose.
- ECG monitoring: Monitoring for the presence of bradycardia or AV conduction blockade (1st, 2nd and 3rd degree block), which occur commonly in overdose. Prolongation of QRS intervals may also occur.
- Baseline blood work and electrolyte monitoring: Basic metabolic panel to monitor for hypoglycemia and potassium shifts secondary to acidosis or if using high dose insulin (HDI) therapy
- Venous blood gas analysis: Monitor for the presence of metabolic acidosis due to secondary hypoperfusion.
- Urine output: Monitor urine output as an indicator of renal perfusion.
- Central line placement: Beneficial for frequent blood glucose monitoring (particularly if using HDI therapy) and for guidance of fluid therapy with CVP monitoring

Drugs and Antidotes of Choice

- No specific antidote is available.
- Volume resuscitation with IV fluid administration for hypotension
  - 10–15 mL/kg for cats over 15–30 minutes
  - 20 mL/kg for dogs given over 15–30 minutes
- Atropine may be used to treat sinus bradycardia (heart rate ≤50 in dogs, ≤120 in cats).
  - Atropine dose 0.02–0.04 mg/kg IV
  - Bradycardia is frequently resistant to atropine.
- 10% calcium chloride or gluconate for hypotension and increased efficacy of HDI therapy
  - 10% calcium chloride 0.2 mL/kg IV bolus. May repeat as needed to maintain an ionized calcium level of 1–2 mmol/L (Therapeutic ionized calcium levels are 1.13–1.33 mmol/L). The goal is to maintain ionized calcium levels at 1–2 x therapeutic levels.
  - 10% calcium gluconate may be substituted for calcium chloride, but it only provides ⅓ the amount of calcium. Therefore, 3 times the dose (0.6 mL/kg) of calcium gluconate is required.
- HDI therapy/glucose administration for increased inotropy and treatment of hypoperfusion
  - The exact mechanism by which HDI works is unknown.
  - HDI is *NOT* a vasopressor.
  - HDI appears to promote the uptake and utilization of carbohydrates as an energy source.
  - HDI has potent inotropic effects and increases perfusion by increasing cardiac output. It does not increase SVR, and therefore large increases in BP or MAP are not seen, but clinical improvement in tissue perfusion occurs.
  - HDI may increase cytosolic calcium in myocardial cells, thus enhancing cardiac contractility and cardiac output.
  - Recommended dose
    - Check blood glucose (BG) concentration first. Administer glucose if BG is <100 mg/dL for dog or <200 mg/dL for cat.
    - Administer regular insulin at 1 unit/kg IV bolus. Follow with a CRI IV infusion of regular insulin at 2 units/kg/hr. May increase infusion by 2 units/kg/hr every 10 minutes up to a maximum dose of 10 units/kg/hr.
    - Carefully monitor BG every 10 minutes while titrating insulin dosing. A concentrated IV infusion of dextrose (often >5% dextrose, possibly upwards of 15%–30%) will be needed to maintain BG concentrations and should be administered through a central line. Once insulin dosing is stabilized, check BG concentrations every 30–60 minutes.
    - Monitor potassium concentrations every hour. Keep potassium concentrations in low therapeutic range. Administer potassium chloride if K^+ ≤ 3.0 mmol/L.

□ When beta antagonist toxicosis has resolved, decrease insulin by 1–2 units/kg/hr. Glucose administration will likely need to be continued for up to 24 hours after the insulin infusion has been stopped.

□ Monitor calcium and potassium levels every hour while decreasing insulin infusions.

■ Intravenous fat emulsion (IFE) for severe dysrhythmias, hypotension, and cardiac arrest.

• IFE was initially used to resuscitate patients after severe local anesthetic drug toxicity (cardiac arrest).

• IFE has recently been used to treat toxicity from other lipid-soluble drugs such as baclofen, beta antagonist, calcium channel antagonist, and ivermectin overdose.

• The exact mechanism of how IFE works is not known, but possible mechanisms include the following:

□ IFE may create a "pharmacological sink" for fat-soluble drugs.

□ IFE may provide an additional fatty acid supply to improve cardiac performance.

□ IFE may increase intracellular calcium via direct activation of voltage-gated calcium channels. This may restore myocyte function in the drug-depressed myocardium.

• Adverse effects of IFE may include hyperlipidemia, hepatosplenomegaly, jaundice, seizures, hemolytic anemia, prolonged clotting time, thrombocytopenia, and fat embolism.

• IFE dose: 1.5 mL/kg IV bolus of a 20% solution over 1 minute. Follow immediately with a CRI of 0.25 mL/kg/min for 30–60 minutes.

□ May repeat IV bolus every 3–5 minutes as needed up to a maximum total dose of 3 mL/kg

□ If blood pressure continues to drop, may increase CRI infusion up to 0.5 mL/kg/min.

□ It is recommended *not to exceed* a total dose of 8 mL/kg.

□ For further information, refer to Chapter 3 (Antidotes and Other Useful Drugs).

■ Glucagon—traditionally used as an antidote for beta antagonist overdose; increases inotropy by increasing myocardial cAMP levels. HDI or IFE now recommended instead of glucagon as they appear to be more effective. The traditionally recommended dose of glucagon is 0.05–0.2 mg/kg slow IV bolus followed by a continuous infusion of glucagon of 0.1–0.15 mg/kg/hr.

■ Vasopressors: Please see below under "Precautions/Interactions."

Precautions/Interactions

■ Epinephrine/norepinephrine/dopamine/dobutamine: Vasopressors are *NOT* recommended in the treatment of hypotension caused by beta antagonist overdose. Recent literature suggests that vasopressors are less effective than HDI or IFE therapy and may even be potentially harmful.

COMMENTS

Expected Course and Prognosis

- Toxicosis from beta adrenergic antagonists may result in rapid decreases in mental status, seizures, and dysrhythmias.
- Ingestion of immediate-release beta adrenergic antagonist agents can be expected to produce clinical signs within 6 hours of exposure.
- Sustained-release preparations and sotalol may produce delayed toxicity.
- Ingestion of sustained-release preparations requires 24 hours of observation.
- Toxicosis is more likely to occur from beta adrenergic antagonists with higher liphophilicity or membrane stabilizing activity.
- Ingestion or presence of a vasoactive or cardioactive drug can significantly worsen the toxicity of a beta adrenergic antagonist.
- Toxicosis normally results in hypotension, bradycardia, coma, seizures, and apnea.
- If the animal remains asymptomatic for 8 hours postingestion of an immediate-release preparation, 12 hours of sotolol ingestion, or 24 hours of extended-release preparation, the animal may be discharged from the monitored setting.

Abbreviations

ABG = arterial blood gas
ARDS = acute respiratory distress syndrome
BG = blood glucose
BP = blood pressure
CNS = central nervous system
CRI = continuous rate infusion
CVP = central venous pressure
ECG = electrocardiogram
HDI = high-dose insulin
IFE = intravenous fat emulsion
IV = intravenous
MAP = mean arterial pressure
SVR = systemic vascular resistance

See Also

Baclofen
Calcium Channel Blockers
Cardiac Glycosides
Opiates and Opioids

Suggested Readings

Bronstein AC, Spyker DA, Canilena LR, et al. 2007 Annual report of the American Association of Poison Control Centers' national poison data system (DPDS): 25th annual report. Clin Tox 2008; 46(10):930–1057.

Brubacher, J. B-adrenergic antagonists. In: Flomenbaum NE, Goldfrank LR, Hoffman RS, et al, eds. Goldfrank's Toxicologic Emergencies, 2nd ed. New York: McGraw-Hill, 2006; pp. 924–941.

Felice FL, Schumman HM. Intravenous lipid emulsion for local anesthetic toxicity: a review of the literature. J Med Tox 2008; 4(3):184–191.

Holger JS, Engebretsen KM, Fritzlar SJ, et al. Insulin versus vasopressin and epinephrine to treat beta-blocker toxicity. Clin Toxicol 2007; 45(4): 396–401.

Sirianni AJ, Osterhoudt KC, Clello DP, et al. Use of lipid emulsion in the resuscitation of a patient with prolonged cardiovascular collapse after overdose of buproprion and lamotrigine. Ann Emerg Med 2008; 51(4): 412–415.

Authors: Kristin M. Engebretsen, PharmD, DABAT; Rebecca S. Syring, DVM, DACVECC

Contributing Editor: Lynn R. Hovda, RPH, DVM, MS, DACVIM

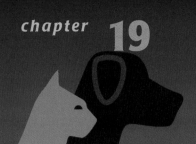

chapter 19

Calcipotriene/ Calcipotriol

DEFINITION/OVERVIEW

- Calcipotriene/calcipotriol is a synthetic analog of calcitriol, the most active metabolite of cholecalciferol (vitamin D_3). It is not the same as cholecalciferol, although the clinical signs and treatment protocol are very similar.
- It is the active ingredient in Dovonex cream, ointment, or scalp solution used to treat human psoriasis.
- Dovonex in a concentration of 0.005% (50 µg/g) is marketed in 30-, 60-, and 100-gram tubes.
- Ingestion of even small amounts results in severe clinical signs.

ETIOLOGY/PATHOPHYSIOLOGY

Mechanism of Action

- Calcipotriene has effects similar to cholecalciferol, ultimately causing significant elevations in serum calcium and phosphorus levels.
- Untreated, these levels quickly lead to acute renal failure and mineralization of soft tissues, in particular the heart, lungs, blood vessels, gastrointestinal tract, and kidneys.

Pharmacokinetics/Absorption, Distribution, Metabolism, and Excretion

- Little kinetic information regarding calcipotriene exists in domestic animals.
- Topical application shows 5%–6% systemic absorption, a transient hypercalcemia, and rapid conversion to inactive metabolites.
- Absorption of ingested topical product is good.
- Enterohepatic circulation occurs.
- The half-life, similar to cholecalciferol, is felt to be extremely long.

Toxicity

- Calcipotriene is highly toxic to dogs and cats.
- Pets become exposed by chewing on the tube but can also show clinical signs if they lick their owner's skin where the product has been applied.

- The minimum acute toxic dose in dogs is 37 μg calcipotriene/kg BW. Many references are even more conservative and list 1.8–3.6 μg/kg BW as toxic to dogs.
- Dogs treated with 3.6 μg/kg/day for 1 week showed an increase in calcium, phosphorus, BUN, and creatinine; acute renal failure developed.
- Soft tissue mineralization occurs when serum calcium (mg/dL) x serum phosphorus (mg/dL) ≥60 in mature animals or ≥70 in growing, immature animals.

Systems Affected

- Renal/urologic—hypercalcemic nephropathy and acute renal failure
- Gastrointestinal—full range of signs including anorexia, vomiting, hypersalivation, constipation, diarrhea, melena, hematemesis, abdominal pain, oropharyngeal erosions
- Endocrine/metabolic—electrolyte imbalances, in particular hypercalcemia and hyperphosphatemia
- Cardiovascular—bradycardia, arrhythmias
- Nervous—decreased neural responsiveness, weakness
- Musculoskeletal—decreased muscle responsiveness

SIGNALMENT/HISTORY

- All breeds and ages of cats and dogs are susceptible to this toxicity.
- Cats and dogs under 6 months of age may be more susceptible.
- Diagnosis is based on history of ingestion and clinical signs.

CLINICAL FEATURES

- Initial signs include vomiting, depression, anorexia, diarrhea, and polyuria within 24 hours of ingestion.
- Hypercalcemia, hyperphosphatemia, and hypercalcemic nephropathy occur between 18 and 72 hours of ingestion.
- Soft tissue mineralization occurs when serum calcium (mg/dL) x serum phosphorus mg/dL) ≥60 in mature animals or ≥70 in growing, immature animals.

DIFFERENTIAL DIAGNOSIS

- Acute or chronic renal failure
- Ethylene glycol intoxication
- Grape-raisin intoxication
- Hypercalcemia of malignancy
- Hypoadrenocorticism
- Idiopathic hypercalcemia of cats

- Ingestion of other vitamin D products (rodenticides, high-dose vitamin D supplements)
- Juvenile hypercalcemia
- Primary hyperparathyroidism

DIAGNOSTICS

- Serum chemistry to include calcium, phosphorous, BUN, and creatinine
- Urinalysis with specific gravity
- Toxicosis is serious when the serum calcium is greater than 12.5 mg/dL, serum phosphorus levels are over 7 mg/dL, and hyposthenuria are documented.
- Radiographs or ultrasound may show calcification of renal, gastrointestinal, respiratory, or vascular tissues.
- There is no specific laboratory test for calcipotriol/calcipotriene.
- Anecdotally, there may be a rise in the neutrophils, but the cause is unknown.

Pathological Findings

- At necropsy, renal tubular degeneration and necrosis; mineralization of the renal tubules, coronary arteries, gastrointestinal wall, and other soft tissues; and hemorrhage of gastric mucosa may all be evident.

THERAPEUTICS

- The goal of treatment is to keep the calcium level at less than 12.5 mg/dL and the phosphorus level at less than 7 mg/dL.

Detoxification

- Early emesis or gastric lavage
- In cases where the product has been licked, rinse the mouth well for 10–15 minutes.
- Activated charcoal with a cathartic initially, followed by activated charcoal without a cathartic q 8 hours for 1–2 days if GI motility is normal

Appropriate Health Care

- Laboratory work as follows:
  - Obtain baseline serum chemistries, including calcium, phosphorus, BUN, creatinine, and liver enzymes.
  - Urinalysis with specific gravity
  - If serum calcium is less than 12.5 mg/dL, begin fluids and repeat lab work in 8–12 hours. If levels are still within normal limits, continue fluid therapy and repeat the lab work daily for 4 days. If normal at that time, wean off fluids.

- • If at any time the serum calcium becomes greater than 12.5 mg/dL, or if the serum calcium x serum phosphorus exceeds 60 (adults) or 70 (growing, immature animals), begin more aggressive therapy.
- Monitor urine output for oliguria or anuria. If urine output is at or less than 0.5 mL/kg/hour, increase fluids or consider other options.
- Monitor blood pressure and treat accordingly.

Drug(s) and Antidotes of Choice

- No specific antidote is available for calcipotriene toxicity.
- Aggressive 0.9% NaCl diuresis at 2–3 times maintenance until calcium levels decrease
- If urine output decreases in face of adequate hydration, one or both of the following may be used:
  - • Furosemide CRI at 1–2 mg/kg/hr
  - • Mannitol bolus at 1–2 g/kg IV slowly
- To increase calcium excretion:
  - • Furosemide 0.5 mg/kg/hr IV or 2.5–4.5 mg/kg PO TID
  - • Dexamethasone 0.2 mg/kg IV q 12 hours *or* prednisone 2–3 mg/kg PO BID
- Phosphate binders to keep the calcium x phosphorus product at less than 60 or 70.
  - • Aluminum hydroxide 2–10 mL PO q 6 hours if phosphorus levels are high
- Bisphosphonates to inhibit bone reabsorption and minimize hypercalcemia
  - • Currently, pamidronate is the most widely used, although others have been suggested.
  - • Pamidronate disodium (Aredia)
    - □ 1.3–2 mg/kg IV diluted in saline and infused over 2 hours for one dose only
    - □ Expect serum calcium and phosphorus levels to decrease in 24–48 hours.
    - □ If levels decrease and then rebound, a second dose may be needed in 5–7 days. Anecdotally, extremely large ingestions have needed redosing in just 3–4 days.
- Antiemetics as needed for persistent vomiting
  - • Dolasetron 0.5–1.0 mg/kg IV q 24 hours
  - • Maropitant 1 mg/kg SQ q 24 hours, not labeled for cats
  - • Ondansetron 0.1–0.2 mg/kg IV q 8–12 hours
- GI protectants
  - • H$_2$ blockers
    - □ Famotidine 0.5–1 mg/kg PO, SQ, IM, IV q 12–24 hours (Do not use IV in cats.)
    - □ Ranitidine 1–2 mg/kg PO, SQ, IM, IV q 8–12 hours
    - □ Cimetidine 5–10 mg/kg PO, SQ, IM, IV q 6 hours

- Omeprazole 0.5–1 mg/kg PO daily
- Sucralfate 0.25–1 g PO TID x 5–7 days if evidence of active ulcer disease

Precautions/Interactions

- Thiazide diuretics are contraindicated as they decrease clearance of calcium.
- Bisphosphonates should be used cautiously in combination with calcitonin and then only in refractory cases. There is some evidence that the combined use may increase soft tissue mineralization.
- Excessive doses of pamidronate can cause hypocalcemia, and treatment with calcium carbonate may be needed. In severe cases, IV calcium gluconate may be used.

Alternative Drugs

- Salmon calcitonin (Calcimar, Micalcin) at 4–7 IU/kg SQ q 8–12 hours
  - Currently used less often than pamidronate due to inconsistencies in treatment and development of resistance after several days of treatment
  - Used instead of pamidronate. All other treatment recommendations remain the same.

Follow-up

- Calcium and phosphorous levels every 3rd day as needed, then weekly for 3–4 weeks.

Prevention

- Owners should be educated about keeping medications out of reach of pets.

 COMMENTS

Patient Monitoring

- Calcium and phosphorus levels should be checked in all exposed animals regardless of amount ingested.
- Repeat calcium, phosphorus, BUN, creatinine q 12–24 hours, depending on dose ingested and response to therapy.
- Repeat until normal, then daily, then every 3rd day as needed, then weekly for 3–4 weeks.

Prevention/Avoidance

- Medications should be kept well out of a pet's reach.
- Do not allow the pet to lick this product.

Possible Complications

- Reproductive
  - Spontaneous abortion has occurred in humans.
  - Product can be secreted in breast milk in small amounts.
- Cardiac insufficiency and chronic renal failure secondary to calcification

Expected Course and Prognosis

- The prognosis is good if serum calcium x serum phosphorus is <60 (mature animals) or <70 (growing, immature animals) and aggressive treatment is provided in a timely manner. Soft tissue mineralization is unlikely.
- The prognosis is much more guarded if the serum calcium x serum phosphorus is ≥60 (mature animals) or ≥70 (growing, immature animals) and prolonged for even a few days. The risk of soft tissue mineralization is high.
- Death from cardiac calcification may occur weeks after a presumed recovery.

Abbreviations

BID = twice a day
BUN = blood urea nitrogen
BW = body weight
CRI = continuous rate infusion
GI   = gastrointestinal
IM   = intramuscular
IU   = international units
IV   = intravenous
PO   = *per os* (by mouth)
q   = every
SQ   = subcutaneous
TID = three times a day

See Also

Cholecalciferol

Suggested Reading

Hostutler R, Chew DJ, Jaeger JQ, et al. Uses and effectiveness of pamidronate disodium for treatment of dogs and cats with hypercalcemia. J Vet Intern Med 2005; 19(1):29–33.
Martin TM, De Lorimer LP, Fan TM, et al. Pharmacokinetics and pharmacodynamics of a single dose of zoledronate in healthy dogs. J Vet Pharmacol Therap 2007; 30:492–495.
Saedi N, Horn R, Muffoletto A, et al. Death of a dog caused by calcipotriene toxicity. J Amer Acad Derm 2007; 56(4):712–713.
Torley D, Drummond A, Bilsland DJ. Calcipotriol toxicity in dogs. Br J Derm 2002; 147(6):1270.

Author: Catherine M. Adams, DVM
Consulting Editor: Lynn R. Hovda, RPH, DVM, MS, DACVIM

chapter *20*

Calcium Channel Blockers

DEFINITION/OVERVIEW

- Calcium channel blockers (CCBs) are medications commonly used in both human and veterinary medicine to treat underlying cardiac disease, tachyarrhythmias, systemic hypertension and, more recently, oliguric/anuric renal failure.
- CCB intoxication is one of the leading toxicosis reported to human poison control centers, and its incidence in veterinary medicine is increasing.
- Common side effects of toxicosis include vomiting, bradyarrhythmias, hypotension, and weakness.

ETIOLOGY/PATHOPHYSIOLOGY

Mechanism of Action

- CCBs inhibit intracellular movement of calcium through L-type voltage-gated slow calcium channels, located predominantly in cardiac (atrial) muscle, vascular smooth muscle, and beta cells of the pancreas.
- There are three different classes of CCBs (phenylalkylamines, benzothiazepines, and dihydropyridines) and at least ten different approved CCB agents.
- CCBs result in reduced cardiac automaticity, conduction, contractility, and loss of vascular tone. The degree to which a particular CCB affects these functions of the heart and vasculature depends on the class of CCB (see table 20.1).
- Automaticity and conduction: Sinoatrial (SA) node depolarization and atrioventricular (AV) node conduction are dependent on activation of L-type calcium channels. Blockade of these channels reduces SA node firing and delays AV conduction.
- Contractility: Blockade of L-type calcium channels impairs phase 2 of the action potential in cardiac muscle, ultimately resulting in reduced excitation-contraction coupling of cardiac muscle and reduced force of cardiac contractility.
- Vascular tone: Blockade of L-type calcium channels impairs vascular smooth muscle contraction, resulting in vasodilation.
- Pancreas: Hypoinsulinemia and hyperglycemia may occur secondary to CCB administration/overdose because of impaired beta-cell function.

170

TABLE 20.1. Relative effects of the three classes of calcium channel blockers (phenylalkylamines, benzothiazepines, and dihydropyridines) on cardiac automaticity, conduction, contractility, and vascular tone.

Class	Drugs	Automaticity	Conduction	Contractility	Vessel Tone
Phenylalkylamine	Verapamil	+++	+++	+++	+++
Benzothiazepine	Diltiazem	++++	+++	+	++
Dihydropyridine	Amlodipine Nifedipine Nisoldipine Nimodipine Nicardipine Felodipine Isradipine Clevidipine	+	0	+	++++

Note: Plus signs signify an increasing response, with more plus signs denoting a more inhibitory response. The zero denotes no response.

Pharmacokinetics/Absorption, Distribution, Metabolism, and Excretion

- Verapamil
  - Elimination half-life in humans 3–7 hours. Serum half-lives ranging from 0.8–2.5 hours have been reported in dogs.
  - Distribution—large volume of distribution; extensively protein bound
  - Metabolism—large first pass effect, only 15%–30% of absorbed drug available to systemic circulation
  - Excretion—renal with 96% as metabolites; 3%–4% excreted unchanged as parent compound
- Diltiazem
  - Immediate release formulations
    - Absorption—peak plasma concentrations occur within 1.5–4.25 hours of ingestion of a normal dose of a diltiazem; may be delayed with toxic doses. If a toxic dose was ingested, clinical signs should be evident within no more than 6 hours following ingestion.
    - Distribution—in humans, approximately 75% of CCBs are protein bound.
    - Metabolism
      - Rapidly metabolized by the liver
      - Large first-pass effect, such that only a small amount of the drug is absorbed following oral ingestion by dogs.
      - In humans, approximately 80% of a diltiazem dose is absorbed following oral dosing. In cats, only 50%–80% is absorbed.
      - Serum half-life for diltiazem is approximately 3.5–10 hours. In cats, the serum half-life is shorter at 2 hours.

- □ Excretion—metabolites are excreted through the urinary system. Renal impairment will minimally prolong the half-life of CCB.
- Sustained-release (SR), extended-release (XR), controlled-release (CR) formulations
    - □ With SR/XR/CR formulations, development of clinical signs of toxicosis may be delayed by as much as 6–12 hours following toxic ingestions.
    - □ Distribution, metabolism, and excretion are similar to immediate release formulations.
- Amlodipine
    - Amlodipine has a much different pharmacokinetic profile than other CCBs, as it is absorbed slowly following oral dosing. Peak plasma concentrations, and clinical effects, are reported 6–9 hours after oral dosing. Terminal half-life reports to be approximately 35 hours in humans.
    - Distribution—highly protein bound (>90%)
    - Metabolism—slowly metabolized to inactive compounds by the liver
    - Excretion—renal excretion of inactive metabolites

Toxicity

- Diltiazem
    - The therapeutic dose for immediate-release formulations of diltiazem in dogs and cats is 0.5–1.5 mg/kg PO every 8 hours.
    - Therapeutic doses for SR/XR/CR formulations in dogs and cats vary depending on the formulation used.
    - The lowest reported LD_{50} for diltiazem is 50 mg/kg in dogs.
    - In humans with diltiazem toxicosis, the mean toxic dose was 30 mg/kg.

Systems Affected

- Gastrointestinal—vomiting, diarrhea, ileus
- Cardiovascular—bradycardia, AV dissociation, AV conduction blockade (1st-, 2nd-, or 3rd-degree AV block), and hypotension
- Musculoskeletal—diffuse weakness/recumbency secondary to reduced cardiac output/hypotension
- CNS—depressed mentation/level of consciousness related to decreased cardiac output, hypotension, and reduced cerebral perfusion. Seizures have been reported.
- Respiratory—pulmonary edema has been reported secondary to increased pulmonary hydrostatic pressure (cardiogenic), secondary to increased vascular permeability (noncardiogenic), and neurogenic pulmonary edema.

 # SIGNALMENT/HISTORY

- There are no specific breed or sex predilections for this toxicosis.

- Dogs may be at increased risk for toxicosis, given their propensity to chew into and ingest large quantities of owner's medications.
- Cats may be at increased risk when CR or SR formulations are prescribed to treat underlying hypertrophic cardiomyopathy and dosing errors occur by pet owners.

Risk Factors

- CCB medication in animal's environment; pet owner or pet with filled prescription in household.
- Co-administration with beta-blocker medications
- Dosing errors by owner (particularly with cats on SR/XR/CR formulations)
- Liver dysfunction will result in higher serum concentrations and delayed metabolism of the drug.

Historical Findings

- Known dosing error
- Known ingestion of owner's medications by pet (chewed/empty pill vials)
- Acute onset of weakness, lethargy, syncopal episodes

 CLINICAL FEATURES

- 1st-, 2nd-, or 3rd-degree AV block
- AV dissociation
- Bradycardia
- Cardiogenic pulmonary edema
- Depressed mentation
- Diarrhea
- Hyperglycemia
- Hypotension
- Ileus
- Lactic acidosis
- Noncardiogenic pulmonary edema
- Recumbency, weakness
- Respiratory distress
- Syncope, collapse
- Vomiting

 DIFFERENTIAL DIAGNOSIS

- Beta adrenergic antagonist toxicosis
- Intrinsic cardiac conduction defects—sick sinus syndrome, AV block, and atrial standstill
- Atrial standstill secondary to hyperkalemia

- Baclofen toxicosis
- Opiate and opioid toxicosis

 # DIAGNOSTICS

- ECG: Sinus bradycardia, 1st-, 2nd-, or 3rd-degree AV block, AV dissociation, junctional escape rhythms, idioventricular rhythms, or asystole may be noted following CCB toxicosis.
- Serum ionized/total calcium concentrations: It is important to note that calcium concentrations will remain normal despite CCB intoxication.
- Serum glucose concentrations: Hyperglycemia may be noted with toxicosis as a result of suppressed insulin release from beta-cells of the pancreas; the extent of hyperglycemia is associated with degree of intoxication.
- Serum lactate concentrations: Hyperlactatemia may be noted with toxicosis as a result of impaired cardiac output and glucose entry into cells for aerobic metabolism; the extent of hyperlactatemia is associated with degree of intoxication.
- Thoracic radiographs should be considered, particularly if any signs of respiratory distress, to assess for intravascular volume status and risk for congestive heart failure.
- Serum drug concentrations: Concentrations of specific drugs can be measured via high-performance lipid chromatography (HPLC).
  - Serum drug concentrations results take, on average, about 3 days to obtain and therefore are not clinically useful in the management of toxicities.
  - Therapeutic verapamil concentrations of 300–500 ng/mL are reported for cats and dogs.

 # THERAPEUTICS

Detoxification

- Emesis should be induced if the animal is presented within 2 hours of ingestion and is relatively normal with respect to neurologic and cardiovascular systems.
- If the animal is deemed too unstable with respect to the neurologic system to induce vomiting, and the animal is presented within 2 hours of ingestion, gastric lavage should be performed.
- Activated charcoal should be given to adsorb any residual medication in the GI tract. Because of the abundance of SR and XR CCBs on the market, emesis, gastric lavage, and activated charcoal administration may be useful beyond the first 1–2 hours of ingestion, and the use of these therapies with delayed hospital presentations should be considered on a case-by-case basis. This is controversial though and may be of little benefit.

- Whole bowel irrigation with GoLytely is used when SR and XR formulations are involved in CCB toxicity and may be more effective than gastric lavage at removing intact tablets from the intestinal tract.
- CCBs are extensively protein bound, making hemodialysis or hemofiltration ineffective tools for expediting drug elimination following intoxication.
- Temporary transvenous pacing has been used to increase heart rate (and therefore cardiac output) in human CCB overdoses and was recently reported in a dog with diltiazem intoxication. Pacing could be considered when therapies fail to improve heart rate and cardiac output/peripheral tissue perfusion remains impaired.

Appropriate Health Care

- Close monitoring for fluid overload: frequent assessment of respiratory rate/effort, auscultation of the lungs, pulse oximetry/arterial blood gas analysis
- Continuous ECG monitoring for assessment of conduction abnormalities
- Blood pressure monitoring (indirect or direct) for development of hypotension

Drug(s) and Antidotes of Choice

- No specific antidote available
- Intravascular fluid therapy: IV fluid therapy, with a balanced electrolyte solution, should be used as needed to maintain hydration status and support cardiovascular function, particularly in animals with inappetence, vomiting, diarrhea, and altered mentation. An initial fluid bolus of 20 mL/kg should be considered in dogs with hypotension secondary to toxicosis. Because of the risk for impaired cardiac function, care should be taken to avoid fluid overload.
- Atropine (0.02–0.04 mg/kg IV) can be used to treat bradycardia; however, heart rate is rarely responsive to atropine with CCB toxicity.
- Calcium
  - Calcium infusion should be used as the first line of therapy for animals with signs of CCB toxicosis. Despite normocalcemia, calcium administration may increase the amount of calcium available for normal cardiac and smooth muscle function.
  - Calcium helps improve myocardial contractility but has little effect on cardiac conduction.
  - Calcium gluconate 10% (0.50–1.50 mL/kg) can be given as a slow IV bolus over 5–10 minutes. A CRI with doses up to 0.50–1.50 mL/kg/hr can be initiated after the bolus and titrated as needed to maintain its effect. During the bolus infusion, an ECG should be monitored for bradycardia or worsening of conduction blockade.
  - Calcium chloride 10% (0.15–0.50 mL/kg) may be preferred over calcium gluconate 10% due to a greater concentration of calcium (13.4 mEq vs. 4.5 mEq per 10 mL of 10% calcium chloride or gluconate, respectively). Tissue injury secondary to drug extravasation of calcium chloride can be

significant. Therefore, calcium gluconate is preferred if a central line cannot be established.
- Serum ionized calcium levels should be monitored during infusion with the goal to maintain ionized calcium at approximately 1.5–2.0x the normal range (normal range 1.1–1.33 mmol/L).
- Glucagon
    - Glucagon has a positive inotropic and chronotropic effect on myocardial cells via stimulation of adenyl cyclase.
    - Glucagon is expensive and may be cost prohibitive in some situations.
    - Dose at 0.05–0.2 mg/kg slow IV bolus; an increase in heart rate should be noted within a few minutes of the initial bolus. If a positive response is noted, the bolus should be followed by a continuous infusion of glucagon at 0.05–0.10 mg/kg/hr.
    - Adverse effects of glucagon—nausea and vomiting may be noted at higher doses; transient hyperglycemia should be expected and does not require treatment.
- High-dose insulin (HDI) therapy/dextrose infusion
    - Also referred to as hyperinsulinemia-euglycemia therapy
    - The exact mechanism by which HDI works is unknown, but it is thought to improve cardiac inotropy and improves perfusion by increasing cardiac output, rather than affecting vascular tone.
    - HDI appears to promote the uptake and utilization of carbohydrates as an energy source.
    - HDI may increase intracellular calcium concentrations in myocardial cells, thus enhancing cardiac contractility and cardiac output.
    - Recommended dose
        - Check blood glucose (BG) concentration first. Administer glucose if BG is ≤100 mg/dL for dog or ≤200 mg/dL for cat.
        - Administer regular insulin at 1 unit/kg IV bolus. Follow with an intravenous CRI of regular insulin at 2 units/kg/hr. May increase infusion by 2 units/kg/hr every 10 minutes up to a maximum dose of 10 units/kg/hr.
        - NOTE: BG must be carefully monitored every 10 minutes while titrating insulin dosing. A concentrated IV infusion of dextrose (often >5% dextrose, possibly upwards of 15%–30%) will be needed to maintain BG concentrations. Therefore, the dextrose infusion should be administered through a central line. Once the insulin infusion dose is stabilized, check BG concentrations every 30–60 minutes.
        - Monitor K^+ concentrations every hour. Keep K^+ concentrations in low therapeutic range. Administer potassium chloride if K^+ ≤ 3.0 mmol/L.
        - When signs of CCB toxicosis have resolved, decrease insulin by 1–2 units/kg/hr. Glucose administration will likely need to be continued for up to 24 hours after the insulin infusion has been stopped.

- ▫ Monitor calcium, glucose, and potassium concentrations hourly while decreasing insulin infusions.
- ■ Intravenous Fat Emulsion (IFE)
  - IFE was initially used in human medicine to resuscitate patients after severe local anesthetic drug toxicity.
  - IFE has been recently used in veterinary medicine to treat toxicosis from other lipid-soluble drugs such as baclofen, beta antagonist, calcium channel antagonist, and ivermectin overdose.
  - The exact mechanism of how IFE works is not known, but possible mechanisms include the following:
    - ▫ IFE may create a "pharmacological sink" for fat-soluble drugs.
    - ▫ IFE may provide an additional fatty acid supply to improve cardiac performance.
    - ▫ IFE may increase intracellular calcium via direct activation of voltage-gated calcium channels. This may restore myocyte function in the drug-depressed myocardium.
  - Adverse effects of IFE may include hyperlipidemia, hepatosplenomegaly, jaundice, seizures, hemolytic anemia, prolonged clotting time, thrombocytopenia, and fat embolism.
  - IFE dose: 1.5 mL/kg IV bolus over 1 minute. Follow immediately with a CRI of 0.25 mL/kg/min as needed until clinical signs of toxicity resolve.
    - ▫ May repeat IV bolus every 3–5 minutes as needed up to a maximum total dose of 3 mL/kg.
    - ▫ If blood pressure continues to drop, may increase infusion up to 0.5 mL/kg/min.
    - ▫ It is recommended *not to exceed* a total dose of 8 mL/kg.
- ■ Vasopressor therapy (dopamine 5–15 µg/kg/min; dobutamine 3–15 µg/kg/min; norepinephrine 0.05–0.3 µg/kg/min) should only be considered when blood pressure has failed to respond to other treatments such as calcium, IFE, or HDI. The aforementioned treatments should be strongly considered in place of vasopressors.

Precautions/Interactions

- ■ Beta-blockers: Coadministration of beta-blockers and CCB may increase the risk for bradyarrhythmias and conduction blockade. Diltiazem may increase the bioavailability of propranolol.
- ■ Digoxin: CCBs may increase serum concentrations of digoxin, increasing the risk for digoxin toxicosis.
- ■ Cimetidine (and/or ranitidine) may impair hepatic metabolism of CCBs, slowing elimination.
- ■ Coadministration with cyclosporine will result in increased cyclosporine drug levels.

Abbreviations

AV   = atrioventricular
BG   = blood glucose
CCB   = calcium channel blocker
CNS   = central nervous system
CR   = controlled release
ECG   = electrocardiogram
GI   = gastrointestinal
HDI   = high-dose insulin therapy
HPLC   = high-performance lipid chromatography
IFE   = intravenous fat emulsion
IV   = intravenous
PO   = *per os* (by mouth)
SA   = sinoatrial
SR   = sustained release
XR   = extended release

See Also

Beta-Blockers

Suggested Reading

Costello M, Syring RS. Calcium channel blocker toxicity. J Vet Emerg Crit Care 2008; 18:54–60.

DeWitt C, Waksman J. Pharmacology, pathophysiology and management of calcium channel blocker and beta-blocker toxicity. Toxicol Rev 2004; 23:223–238.

Kerns W. Management of beta-adrenergic blocker and calcium channel antagonist toxicity. Emerg Med Clin N Am 2007; 25:309–331.

Lheureux PER, Zahir S, Gris M, et al. Bench-to-bedside review: Hyperinsulinaemia/euglycaemia therapy in the management of overdose of calcium-channel blockers. Crit Care 2006; 10:212–218.

Syring RS, Costello MF. Temporary transvenous pacing in a dog with diltiazem intoxication. J Vet Emerg Crit Care 2008; 8(1):75–80.

Authors: Rebecca S. Syring, DVM, DACVECC; Kristin M. Engebretsen, PharmD, DABAT

Consulting Editor: Lynn R. Hovda, RPH, DVM, MS, DACVIM

chapter 21

Diuretics

DEFINITION/OVERVIEW

- Diuretic toxicosis is generally confined to plasma volume depletion, with consequent hypoperfusion of critical organs, mostly the kidneys.
- Rehydration is normally sufficient to correct acute diuretic overdosing.

ETIOLOGY/PATHOPHYSIOLOGY

- Diuretics are primarily used in management of congestive heart failure. Aggressive administration can result in prerenal azotemia, and if renal perfusion pressure drops sufficiently, intrinsic renal damage.
- Less common complications include electrolyte depletion or excess (diuretic dependent).

Mechanism of Action

- Commonly used diuretics in veterinary medicine all affect electrolyte transfer (and water) across the nephron. Diuretics work in specific sites along the renal tubule.
- Table 21.1 describes the mechanism and site of action of most known diuretics.

Pharmacokinetics/Absorption, Distribution, Metabolism, and Excretion

- Hydrochlorothiazide is administered orally and, in humans, approximately 70% is absorbed (no data for dogs or cats). In dogs, it has an onset of action within 2 hours, peaks at 4 hours, and lasts 12 hours. It is excreted in urine unchanged. No data are available for cats.
- Furosemide can be administered parenterally or orally. After intravenous administration, furosemide is highly protein bound (90%) and is concentrated in the kidneys, with an elimination half-life of 60 minutes. Approximately 50% of the drug is excreted in bile, while 50% is excreted in urine, mostly unchanged. Oral administration results in 40%–50% bioavailability. Onset of action is rapid (within 30 minutes), and duration of action is approximately 6 hours. Few data

TABLE 21.1. Mechanism of action of various diuretics.

Classification	Examples	Mechanism	Location
No specific classification	Ethanol, water	Inhibit vasopressin secretion	———
Acidifying salts	$CaCl_2$, NH_4Cl		———
Aquaretics	Goldenrod, juniper	Increase plasma volume	———
Xanthines	Caffeine, theophylline	Inhibit reabsorption of Na^+, increases GFR	Proximal tubule
Osmotic diuretics	Glucose (especially in uncontrolled diabetes), **mannitol**	Promote osmotic diuresis	Proximal tubule, descending limb
Na-H exchange antagonists	**Dopamine**http://en.wikipedia.org/wiki/Diuretic-cite_note-boron875-7#cite_note-boron875-7	Promote Na^+ excretion, increase GFR	Proximal tubulehttp://en.wikipedia.org/wiki/Diuretic-cite_note-boron875-7#cite_note-boron875-7
Carbonic anhydrase inhibitors	Acetazolamide, dorzolamide	Inhibit H^+ secretion, resultant promotion of Na^+ and K^+ excretion	Proximal tubule
Loop diuretics	Bumetanide, ethacrynic acid, **furosemide,** torsemide	Inhibit the Na-K-2Cl symporter	Loop of Henle
Thiazides	Bendroflumethiazide, **hydrochlorothiazide**	Inhibits reabsorption by Na^+/Cl^- symporter	Distal convoluted tubules
Arginine vasopressin receptor 2 antagonists	Amphotericin B, lithium citrate	Inhibit vasopressin	Collecting duct
Potassium-sparing diuretics	Amiloride, **spironolactone**, triamterene, potassium canrenoate	Inhibition of Na^+/K^+ exchanger: Spironolactone inhibits aldosterone action, amiloride inhibits epithelial sodium channels	Cortical collecting ducts

Note: Diuretics of veterinary importance are highlighted in bold. Dashes signify that there is no renal location of action.

exist for cats. However, cats generally require lower doses than dogs for comparable degrees of CHF, suggesting an increased sensitivity to furosemide.

■ Spironolactone is administered orally, has modest bioavailability (60% absorbed), and has a slow onset of action (2–3 days) in dogs and a duration of action of several days after stopping medication. It is metabolized to canrenone (active metabolite) and other metabolites in plasma, which are excreted mainly in urine.

TABLE 21.2. **Adverse effects and clinical signs associated with diuretics.**		
Adverse Effect	Diuretics	Clinical Signs
Hypovolemia	Loop diuretics, thiazides	Thirst, hypotension, azotemia/uremia, oliguric acute renal failure
Hypokalemia	Loop diuretics, thiazides	Muscle weakness, arrhythmias
Hyperkalemia	Spironolactone	Arrhythmias
Hyponatremia	Thiazides, furosemide	Potentially CNS symptoms if severe hyponatremia. Not clinically reported in small animals
Metabolic alkalosis	Loop diuretics, thiazides	Rarely a clinical problem
Hypercalcemia	Thiazides	Only a problem if administered to hypercalcemic patients
Hyperuricemia	Thiazides, loop diuretics	Uric acid retention (dalmatians)
Ototoxicity	Furosemide	Only at supraphysiological doses (20 mg/kg)
Dermatopathy	Spironolactone	Excoriative dermatopathy in cats

Toxicity

- Most clinically applicable diuretics are not intrinsically nephrotoxic.
- Furosemide can potentiate aminoglycoside nephrotoxicity and can cause sufficient decrease in renal perfusion that, if left uncorrected, can result in nephron death.

Systems Affected (see table 21.2)

- Cardiovascular—arrhythmias
- Endocrine/metabolic—electrolyte disturbances
- Gastrointestinal—vomiting, anorexia due to azotemia/uremia
- Musculoskeletal—weakness due to hypokalemia, hypomagnesemia
- Skin/exocrine—pruritic excoriative dermatitis with spironolactone in cats

 # SIGNALMENT/HISTORY

- There are no specific breed or species predispositions to diuretic intoxication.

Risk Factors

- Severe heart failure, especially output failure. Anorexia, hypodipsia

Historical Findings

- Vomiting, anorexia, anuria, depression are the most common signs of excessive diuresis.

Location and Circumstances of Poisoning

- Generally due to continued administration in CHF patients that have stopped eating and drinking.
- Hypokalemia/hypomagnesemia is more likely when combination loop and thiazide diuretics are administered.

Interactions with Drugs, Nutrients, or Environment

- Furosemide can increase the potential for aminoglycoside ototoxicity and nephrotoxicity.
- Clinically relevant hyperkalemia is extremely unlikely with potassium-sparing diuretics, even if coadministered with ACE inhibitors.
- Hypokalemia/hypomagnesemia is more likely with coadministration of loop and thiazide diuretics, or in hyporexic patients.

 # CLINICAL FEATURES

- Depression, weakness, lethargy
- Dehydration
- Vomiting if severely uremic
- Arrhythmias on auscultation if severely hypokalemic/hypomagnesemic, or severely hyperkalemic

 # DIFFERENTIAL DIAGNOSIS

- Primary acute renal failure
- Other drugs that can cause primary renal failure (e.g., NSAIDs)
- Digoxin toxicosis
- Gastroenteritis (vomiting)
- Allergic dermatopathy in cats administered spironolactone

 # DIAGNOSTICS

- General biochemical analysis should be sufficient to identify dehydration or electrolyte imbalances.
- Electrocardiography is required to evaluate possible arrhythmias.

Pathological Findings

- No significant lesions

THERAPEUTICS

- Correction of dehydration generally resolves most of the major adverse effects of diuretics.

Detoxification

- No specific antidote is available.
- Early emesis followed by activated charcoal/cathartic in acute situations

Appropriate Health Care

- Care should be taken when rehydrating patients that have severe cardiac disease.
- Hourly monitoring of the patient's respiratory rate can help determine if the fluid therapy is precipitating CHF recurrence.
- Severe dehydration is best counteracted by judicious fluid administration and cessation of drug administration.

Drug(s) and Antidotes of Choice

- No specific antidote is available.
- Intravenous fluid administration, preferably with an electrolyte/dextrose solution to avoid excessive sodium and chloride administration. This will assist with increasing plasma volume, resulting in increased diuresis and drug excretion.
  - Electrolyte administration might be required in some cases, especially with severe hypokalemia.
  - In severely hyperkalemic patients, furosemide and sodium bicarbonate administration can help reduce the hyperkalemia (rarely required).

Precautions/Interactions

- Aminoglycosides should be used cautiously with furosemide therapy.
- Overly aggressive fluid replacement can precipitate CHF in patients with severe heart disease.
- Furosemide can increase the toxicity of digoxin due to hypokalemia and hypomagnesemia.
- Spironolactone can increase digoxin half-life, resulting in increased digoxin concentrations.

Nursing Care

- Monitor respiratory rate
- With most electrolyte disturbances, oral supplementation suffices to correct deficits.

Diet

- In cases of hypokalemia, a high-potassium supplement can help minimize recurrence.

Prevention

- Use caution when administering diuretics. Use the lowest effective dose.
- Extra vigilance is required when combining diuretics, as the risk of dehydration increases.

 COMMENTS

Client Education

- Clients should be advised to watch for changes in appetite, thirst, or urination while the patient is receiving diuretics. If the patient becomes anorexic or hypodipsic, then the diuretic administration should be suspended and the veterinarian consulted.
- Continued administration of diuretics in anorexic or adipsic patients substantially increases the risk of severe dehydration. Consumption of regular pet food generally provides sufficient electrolytes to avoid electrolyte depletion.

Patient Monitoring

- Urine output should be monitored.
- Patient demeanor
- BUN/creatinine

Expected Course and Prognosis

- Treatment of dehydration due to diuretics is generally straightforward, and if done carefully in heart disease patients, usually results in complete resolution of clinical signs in a few days.

Abbreviations

ACE-I = angiotensin-converting enzyme inhibitors
BUN   = blood urine nitrogen
CHF   = congestive heart failure
GFR   = glomerular filtration rate
NSAIDs = nonsteroidal anti-inflammatory drugs

See Also

Veterinary NSAIDs

Suggested Reading

Aldactazide. Available at: http://www.rxlist.com/aldactazide-drug.htm. Accessed November 23, 2009.

Furosemide. Available at: http://www.rxlist.com/lasix-drug.htm. Accessed November 23, 2009.

Kittleson MD. Management of heart failure-drugs used in treating heart failure. Part 2. In: Kittleson MD, ed. Small Animal Cardiovascular Medicine, 2nd ed. Veterinary Information Network. Available at http://www.vin.com/Members/proceedings/Proceedings.plx?CID =SACARDIO&PID=12499&O=VIN. Accessed November 23, 2009.

MacDonald KA, Kittleson MD, Kass PH, et al. Effect of spironolactone on diastolic function and left ventricular mass in Maine coon cats with familial hypertrophic cardiomyopathy. J Vet Intern Med 2008; 22(2):335–41.

Author: Mark Rishniw, BVSc, MS, PhD, DACVIM
Consulting Editor: Lynn R. Hovda, RPH, DVM, MS, DACVIM

chapter 22

Opiates and Opioids

 DEFINITION/OVERVIEW

- Opiate and opioid drugs drugs are commonly used to provide analgesia to human and animal patients.
- Technically opiates are natural occurring while opioids are semisynthetic or synthetic. Much blurring occurs and the entire group is often referred to as "opioids".
- Many different opioids with a variety of actions are commercially available (table 22.1).
- Opioids are a common drug of abuse such as with prescribed drugs or with illicit drugs such as heroin. See Chapter 30 on illicit opioids for more information.

 ETIOLOGY/PATHOPHYSIOLOGY

Mechanism of Action

- Opioids exert their effects on different opioid receptors.
- Opioid receptors, designated mu (μ_1 and μ_2), kappa (κ), sigma (σ), delta (δ), and epsilon (ε) are found throughout the body including the adrenal glands, ANS, CNS (multiple locations), GIT, heart, lymphocytes, kidneys, pancreas, and vas deferens.
- The action of each drug varies depending on the affinity and activity at the opioid receptor, particular receptor, location of the receptor, and other factors such as lipid solubility.
- Affinity and activity
  - Full agonist (e.g., morphine, codeine, heroin, fentanyl, meperidine, others)—affinity and activity at all important opioid receptors.
  - Full antagonist (e.g., naloxone)—affinity but no activity at opioid receptors; generally used as reversal agents for agonist
  - Agonist/antagonist (e.g., butorphanol, nalorphine)—affinity at all receptors with activity at only some of them
  - Partial agonist (e.g., tramadol, buprenorphine)—affinity for only some of the opioid receptors
- Receptor types

186

TABLE 22.1. Human prescription opioids.

Drug Name (Trade Names)	Opioid Receptor Activity	Routes of Administration
Alfentanil (Alfenta)	Mu agonist Short duration	IV
Buprenorphine (Buprenex, Temgesic, Subutex); Buprenorphine + Naloxone (Suboxone)	Partial mu agonist Dissociates slowly from receptors; long duration of action, difficult to antagonize	IM, IV, sublingual, transdermal patch (Europe)
Butorphanol (Torbugesic)	Mu antagonist Kappa agonist	IM, IV, SQ, nasal spray
Carfentanil (Wildnil)	Mu agonist	IM, PO (if specially prepared)
Codeine (Tylenol with Codeine #3, Robitussin AC)	Mu, delta, and kappa agonist (upon metabolism to morphine)	PO—many combination formulations with acetaminophen for pain and with dextromethorphan or guaifenesin for cough
Diprenorphine (M50–50)	Antagonist—reverses etorphine and carfentanil	IM, IV
Etorphine (M99)	Mu, delta, and kappa agonist (fentanyl analog)	IM
Fentanyl (Duragesic, Actiq, Sublimaze)	Mu agonist Highly lipid soluble Short acting	IM, IV, transdermal patch, PO as lollipop/lozenge or buccal soluble film/tablet
Heroin	Mu, delta, and kappa agonist	Illicit drug
Hydrocodone (Lortab, Lorcet); Hydrocodone + Acetaminophen (Vicodin); Hydrocodone + Ibuprofen (Vicoprofen); Hydrocodone + Aspirin (Lortab-ASA)	Agonist	PO Only available as a combination product in the U.S.
Hydromorphone (Dilaudid)	Mu agonist (morphine derivative)	IM, IV, SQ, PO, rectal suppository
Loperamide (Imodium, Dimor, Lopex)	Act on receptors in myenteric plexus of large intestines only; no CNS effects	PO
Meperidine (Demerol, Pethidine)	Agonist	IM, IV, SQ, PO
Methadone (Dolophine, Methadose)	Mu agonist	IM, IV, SQ, PO

(Continued)

TABLE 22.1. *Continued*

Drug Name (Trade Names)	Opioid Receptor Activity	Routes of Administration
Morphine (Avinza, Kadian, MS Contin)	Mu, delta, and kappa agonist	IM, IV, SQ, PO (often as extended-release forms), epidural, rectal suppository
Nalbuphine (Nubain)	Mu antagonist Kappa agonist	IM, IV
Nalmefene (Revex, disc. 2008)	Antagonist	IV
Naloxone (Narcan); Naloxone + Buprenorphine (Suboxone); Naloxone + Pentazocine (Talwin NX)	Antagonist	IV preferred, IM and SQ acceptable Talwin NX is PO only.
Naltrexone (Vivitrol, Revia); Naltrexone + Morphine sulfate (Embeda)	Antagonist Duration twice as long as naloxone	IM, PO
Oxycodone (OxyContin = controlled release form); Oxycodone + Acetaminophen (Percocet and Roxicet) Oxycodone + Aspirin (Percodan); Oxycodone + Ibuprofen (Combunox)	Agonist	PO
Oxymorphone (Numorphan, Opana)	Mu agonist	IM, IV, SQ, PO
Pentazocine (Talwin); Pentazocine + Naloxone (Talwin NX); Pentazocine + Acetaminphen (Talacen)	Mu antagonist Kappa agonist	IM, IV, SQ Talwin NX and Talacen are PO only.
Remifentanil (Ultiva)	Mu agonist Short duration	IV
Sufentanil (Sufenta)	Mu agonist Short duration	IV, epidural
Tapentadol (Nucynta)	Mu agonist	PO
Thiafentanil (A-3080)	Agonist—faster onset and shorter duration than carfentanil	IM
Tramadol (Ultram, Ultram ER, Ryzolt)	Agonist, weak	PO

- Mu receptors, in particular μ_1 receptors, are responsible for the analgesic effects; μ_2 receptors for respiratory depression. Mu agonists may be responsible for euphoria.
- Kappa receptors produce sedation and dysphoria.
- Delta receptors are responsible for analgesia at the spinal level.
- Sigma receptors were originally thought to be responsible for euphoria and psychoactive effects, but that may no longer be the case.
- Location
  - CNS—location of receptors determines whether excitation or depression occurs.
    - Dog—CNS depression; higher number of opioid receptors in amygdala and frontal cortex
    - Cat—CNS stimulation and excitation; fewer receptors
  - CNS receptors located in CTZ—emesis
  - CNS receptors located in brainstem—cough and respiratory depression
  - GIT—decreased motility and constipation
- Dopamine and norepinephrine concentrations play a role as well.

Pharmacokinetics/Absorption, Distribution, Metabolism, and Excretion

- Opioids are well absorbed by all routes. They undergo extensive first-pass metabolism which results in a bioavailability of about 25% and a less predictable effect when given orally.
- Distribution is variable and depends on the particular opioid.
- Opioids undergo hepatic metabolism via hydrolysis, oxidation, and N-dealkylation.
  - Morphine's major metabolite is morphine-6-glucuronide, which is a pharmacologically active metabolite. Cats are deficient in glucuronyl-S-transferase, so this may account for their sensitivity.
  - Some of the glucuronides undergo enterohepatic recirculation.
- Elimination is renal.

Toxicity

- Morphine
  - The minimum lethal SQ dose in the dog is 210 mg/kg, and for the cat 40 mg/kg.
  - The LD_{50} IV dose for the dog is 133 mg/kg.
- Heroin
  - The minimum lethal SQ dose for the dog is 25 mg/kg.
  - In the cat, the minimum lethal PO dose is 20 mg/kg.
- Codeine
  - The intravenous LD_{50} for the dog is 69 mg/kg.

- Meperidine
  - In the cat, 30 mg/kg has been known to cause seizures.

Systems Affected

- Varies depending on opioid and species involved
- Respiratory—respiratory depression leading to death
- CNS—depression (dogs) or excitation (cats)
- Cardiovascular—instability with hypotension; bradycardia
- Gastrointestinal—decreased GI motility with constipation
- Ophthalmic—miosis (dogs) or mydriasis (cats generally)
- Renal/urologic—urinary retention
- Endocrine/metabolic—meperidine and tramadol have some serotonergic activity

 SIGNALMENT/HISTORY

- Any age or breed of dog or cat
- Cats are particularly sensitive to morphine as at least 50% is metabolized by glucuronidation.
- Opioid overdose is usually through iatrogenic dose miscalculation or accidental ingestion of an oral product or patch.
- Opioid overdose can also occur with accidental ingestion of a human use product.
- Ingestion of spent fentanyl transdermal patches poses a significant risk of toxicosis. Patches worn for three days by humans and then discarded still retain 24%–84% of the original amount of fentanyl.

Risk Factors

- Loperamide should be used with caution in those dogs with the MDR1 gene mutation, now known as the ATP-binding cassette (ABCB1-1Δ) polymorphism. Dogs that may exhibit this gene mutation include collies, Shetland sheepdogs, Old English sheepdogs, and other herding type dogs.

Interactions with Drugs, Nutrients, or Environment

- Tramadol and meperidine should not be used with tricyclic antidepressants, SSRIs, or monoamine oxidase inhibitors as this may lead to serotonin syndrome.

Historical Findings

- Discovery of a chewed pill bottle, fentanyl patch or lollipops, or the loss of a fentanyl patch that the animal has chewed off

CLINICAL FEATURES

- CNS—depression and lethargy (dogs), excitation and aggressiveness (cats), ataxia, frank stupor, seizures, coma, death
- Respiratory—early increasing rate followed by depression; decreased gag response with potential for aspiration pneumonia
- Gastrointestinal—hypersalivation, vomiting, defecation (dogs), constipation (cats), urination or urinary retention
- Cardiovascular—bradycardia, possible vasodilation and hypotension
- Ophthalmic—miosis (dogs) or mydriasis (more common in cats)
- Thermoregulatory center effects include hypothermia as the most common response; in some clinical cases hyperthermia may occur in cats. Panting may be seen in dogs.

 # DIFFERENTIAL DIAGNOSIS

- Marijuana toxicosis
- Other drug related toxicoses:
  - Amphetamines/methylphenidate/methamphetamine/MDMA toxicoses
  - Benzodiazepines
- Primary neurologic disease (e.g., infectious, inflammatory, neoplastic, etc.)
- Primary metabolic disease (e.g., renal, hepatic, hepatic encephalopathy, hypoglycemia, hypoadrenocorticism)
- Toxicities resulting in bradycardia include the following:
  - Alpha$_2$ agonist drugs
  - Barbiturates
  - Beta agonist blocking drugs
  - Calcium channel blocking drugs
  - Cocaine

 # DIAGNOSTICS

- Detection of opioids can be done from urine or serum samples at human hospitals or be submitted to a laboratory for GC/MS or LC/MS.
- The Quick Screen Pro Multi Drug Screening Test is a human testing kit that has been validated by GC/MS for use in animals. It may provide a rapid and accurate diagnosis if the drug is present in high enough concentrations and the time frame is appropriate.
- Baseline CBC, chemistry, and UA, particularly in neonatal and geriatric patients, or those with underlying metabolic disease
- Blood gas analysis to evaluate adequate oxygenation and ventilation

THERAPEUTICS

Detoxification

- If there was recent ingestion and the animal is alert, vomiting should be induced followed by activated charcoal with a cathartic x one dose.
- Gastric lavage if large doses ingested
- Performing decontamination, even several hours post-ingestion, is often effective due to decreased GI motility.
- Removal of fentanyl patches via endoscopy or surgery

Appropriate Health Care

- Monitor closely for signs of respiratory depression, as this is the most common cause of death with opioid overdoses. If the animal is exhibiting severe respiratory depression leading to hypoxemia and hypercarbia, intubation, oxygen therapy, and positive pressure ventilation via orotracheal intubation may be required. Intubation will also protect the airway from possible aspiration of gastric contents.
- Close patient monitoring of heart rate, blood pressure, body temperature, and ventilation
  - In cats demonstrating hyperthermia >105.5°F, active cooling may be required.
- Be aware of the potential for the development of aspiration pneumonia.
- Monitor for normal urination.

Drugs(s) and Antidotes of Choice

- Naloxone is an antidote of choice.
  - The dose is 0.01–0.02 mg/kg IM, IV, SQ. Doses up to 0.04 mg/kg may be required in serious intoxications, but monitor closely for CNS excitement.
  - The effect of naloxone has a duration of 30–60 minutes, so repeat doses of naloxone may be necessary. A continuous IV infusion may be needed to help maintain ventilation.
- If naloxone is not available, butorphanol, 0.1 to 0.2 mg/kg IV, can be used to partially reverse pure mu agonists.
- IV fluid therapy to support blood pressure and treat hypotension
- Bradycardia is vagally mediated and can be treated with an anticholinergic such as atropine or glycopyrrolate given IM, IV, or SQ.
  - Atropine: 0.02–0.04 mg/kg IV, IM, or SQ
  - Glycopyrrolate: 0.01–0.02 mg/kg SQ, IM, or IV

Precautions/Interactions

- Buprenorphine is not reliably reversible with naloxone or butorphanol, due to its high affinity for the mu receptor.

Nursing Care

- Turn frequently, use eye lubricant as needed.
- Monitor TPR and urine output.

Surgical Considerations

- Ingested fentanyl transdermal patches should be removed by endoscopy or surgery. Sticks from fentanyl lollipops may become a foreign object requiring surgical removal.

 COMMENTS

Client Education

- Keep all controlled medications out of reach of pets.
- If a pet has had a fentanyl patch placed, the patch should be monitored frequently to ensure that it is still in place. Preventative measures (e.g., E-collar, bandage, tape) should be used to prevent ingestion. If the patch is missing and cannot be found, immediate veterinary attention should be sought.

Patient Monitoring

- Monitor TPR, ventilation, and blood pressure frequently
- Thoracic radiograph to rule out secondary aspiration pneumonia
- Pulse oximetry and arterial blood gas analysis to evaluate oxygenation and ventilation

Possible Complications

- Aspiration pneumonia

Expected Course and Prognosis

- If the respiratory and cardiovascular function can be maintained, the prognosis is good; if seizures develop, the prognosis is guarded.

Abbreviations

ANS   = autonomic nervous system
CBC   = complete blood count
CNS   = central nervous system
CTZ   = chemoreceptor trigger zone
GC/MS = gas chromatography/mass spectrometry
GI   = gastrointestinal
GIT   = gastrointestinal tract
IM   = intramuscular

IV   = intravenous
LC/MS = liquid chromatography/mass spectrometry
LD_{50} = median lethal dose
MDR1   = multidrug resistance
MDMA = methylenedioxymethamphetamine
PO   = *per os* (by mouth)
SQ   = subcutaneous
SSRIs   = selective serotonin reuptake inhibitors
TPR   = temperature, pulse rate, respiratory rate
UA   = urinalysis

See Also

Benzodiazepines
Opiates and Opioids (Illicit)

Suggested Reading

Lamont LA, Mathews KA. Opioids, non-steroidal anti-inflammatories, and analgesic adjuvants. In: Tranquilli WJ, Thurmon JC, Grimm KA, eds. Lumb & Jones Veterinary Anesthesia and Analgesia, 4th ed. Ames, IA: Blackwell, 2007; pp. 241–271.

Malouin A, Boiler M. Sedatives, muscle relaxants, and opioids toxicity. In: Silverstein DC, Hopper K, eds. Small Animal Critical Care Medicine. St. Louis: Elsevier, 2009; pp. 350–356.

Schmiedt CW, Bjorling DE. Accidental prehension and suspected transmucosal or oral absorption of fentanyl from a transdermal patch in a dog. Vet Anaesth Analg 2007; 34:70–73.

Teitler JB. Evaluation of a human on-site urine multidrug test for emergency use with dogs. J Am Anim Hosp Assoc 2009; 45:59–66.

Author: Jane Quandt, DVM, DACVA, DACVECC
Consulting Editors: Lynn R. Hovda, RPH, DVM, MS, DACVIM; Justine A. Lee, DVM, DACVECC
Acknowledgements to Annemarie J. Solon for her assistance with this manuscript.

Selective Serotonin Reuptake Inhibitors (SSRIs)

chapter 23

DEFINITION/OVERVIEW

- SSRIs are a class of medications that are commonly prescribed for depression in human beings.
- In veterinary medicine, they are used (frequently off label) for a wide range of behavioral issues, including feline urine spraying, lick granuloma, and canine separation anxiety.
- Lethargy, CNS stimulation, and anorexia may occur at therapeutic doses.
- Medications included in the SSRI family are fluoxetine (Prozac in human beings; Reconcile in veterinary medicine), citalopram (Celexa), escitalopram (Lexapro), paroxetine (Paxil), and sertraline (Zoloft).
- This class of medication received its name for its selectivity for the serotonin receptor.

ETIOLOGY/PATHOPHYSIOLOGY

Mechanism of Action

- Selective serotonin reuptake inhibitors block the reuptake of serotonin in the presynapse, thus increasing levels of serotonin in the presynaptic membrane.
- An increase in levels of serotonin, even in small doses, may lead to serotonin syndrome.
- As levels of serotonin increase, the development of serotonin syndrome increases.
- Clinical signs of serotonin syndrome include autonomic instability, tremors, seizures, CNS stimulation, vomiting, diarrhea, abdominal pain, and mydriasis.

Pharmacokinetics/Absorption, Distribution, Metabolism, Excretion

- All of the SSRIs are well absorbed orally.
- Fluoxetine, paroxetine, and sertraline are highly protein bound.
- All of the SSRIs are hepatically metabolized.
- Fluoxetine has an active metabolite, norfluoxetine, which has similar pharmacologic effects as fluoxetine.
- Most of the SSRIs are excreted in the urine; sertraline is excreted in the bile (dogs).

Toxicity

- Fluoxetine
  - Dogs
    - LD_{50} >100 mg/kg
    - Beagles treated with 100 mg/kg in a single acute dose developed drooling, vomiting, mydriasis, tremors, and anorexia.
    - Results of a chronic 1-year feeding study showed the following:
      - 1 mg/kg/day x 1 year—tremors, mydriasis, slow PLR
      - 4.5 mg/kg/day x 1 year—tremors, slow PLR, ataxia
      - 20 mg/kg/day x 6 months, then decreased to 10 mg/kg/day x 6 months—tremors, anorexia, slow PLR, mydriasis, aggressive behavior, nystagmus, emesis, lethargy, ataxia
  - Cats
    - Treated with 50 mg/kg: vomiting, mydriasis, tremors, anorexia
    - Results of a chronic 1-year feeding study showed the following:
      - 1 mg/kg/day—few abnormalities
      - 3 mg/kg/day—decreased food consumption, vomiting, decreased PLR
      - 5 mg/kg/day—whole body tremors, seizures, hypoactivity, low food consumption, dehydration, bradycardia
- Citalopram/escitalopram
  - No established dose in veterinary medicine
  - Escitalopram doses >0.3 mg/kg (dogs)—lethargy, ataxia, sedation; increased doses—agitation, hyperactivity, hyperthermia, tremors, vocalization, cardiac arrhythmias
  - In human beings:
    - 600 mg—seizures
    - 200 mg—QTc prolongation in pediatric population
- Paroxetine
  - 1 mg/kg—mild sedation (dogs)
  - 10 mg/kg—minor ECG changes (dogs)
  - In human beings:
    - 100–800 mg in adolescents (12–17 years old)—no symptoms
    - 10–120 mg in children 5 years and younger—no symptoms
    - 10–1000 mg in adults—minimal to no effect
    - 3600 mg—resulted in serotonin syndrome
- Sertraline
  - 80 mg/kg BW—minimum lethal oral dose in dogs
  - 10–20 mg/kg—mydriasis and transient anorexia in dogs
  - In human beings:
    - 700–2100 mg—no serious symptoms
    - 4 g in an adolescent—seizures
    - 400–500 mg in children—serotonin syndrome

    □ 2.5 g—one reported death

    □ 13.5 g—developed symptoms, but recovered with treatment

Systems Affected

- Nervous—agitation, tremor, seizures
- Metabolic/endocrine—hyperthermia, serotonin syndrome
- Gastrointestinal—abdominal pain, vomiting, diarrhea, salivation
- Ophthalmic—mydriasis
- Cardiovascular—bradycardia, arrhythmias

 SIGNALMENT/HISTORY

- All breeds and species may be affected. Dogs may be more sensitive to the effects.

Risk Factors

- Animals with known cardiovascular or hepatic impairment as well as those with documented seizure disorders are at increased risk.

Interaction with Drugs, Nutrients, or Environment

- If ingested with any of the following agents, toxicosis may be enhanced.
  - Other serotonergic agents (e.g., buproprion, duloxetine, serzone, dextromethorphan, others)
  - MAO inhibitors (e.g., phenelzine, selegiline)
  - TCAs (clomipramine, others)
  - Drugs that lower the seizure threshold

 CLINICAL FEATURES

- Dose dependent
  - The higher the dose, the greater the risk for development of serotonin syndrome.
- Lower doses—lethargy or agitation, tremors, hypersalivation, vomiting, anorexia
- Higher doses—tremors, seizures, head tilt, aggressive behavior, ataxia, nystagmus, weakness, lethargy, diarrhea, bradycardia

 DIFFERENTIAL DIAGNOSIS

- Clomipramine (specific TCA associated with development of serotonin syndrome)
- Opiate or opioid ingestions

- Other serotonergic agents—buspirone, buproprion, duloxetine. Typically these other agents have different clinical findings as they work at multiple receptor sites, not just serotonin.

 # DIAGNOSTICS

- Patient history and clinical signs should be used for diagnosis.

Pathological Findings

- No specific findings

 # THERAPEUTICS

- The goals of treatment are to prevent absorption, treat serotonin syndrome, support the neurological system, and provide supportive care.

Detoxification

- Induce emesis at home if ingestion occurred within 15–20 minutes and the animal is asymptomatic.
- If not done at home, induce in DVM's office within 60 minutes of ingestion.
- Activated charcoal with a cathartic may be given for one dose.
- IV fluids will not enhance excretion of these medications.

Appropriate Health Care

- Ensure adequate urine output and replace fluids as needed
- Frequent vitals with special attention to temperature
- Observe carefully for development of serotonin syndrome
  - Clinical signs include agitation, restlessness, vocalization, seizures, vomiting, diarrhea, salivation, tremors, hyperreflexia, muscle rigidity, ataxia, tachycardia, hypertension, and hyperthermia.
  - Can develop with any dose
- ECG if cardiac abnormalities develop

Drug(s) of Choice

- No specific antidote is available.
- IV fluids as needed to replace losses, support the cardiovascular system, and maintain perfusion.
- Tremors—methocarbamol 55–220 mg/kg IV slowly to effect.
  - Do not exceed 330 mg/kg/day and monitor for CNS and respiratory depression at high doses.

- Seizures
  - Phenobarbital 3–5 mg/kg IV PRN
  - Diazepam 0.25–0.5 mg/kg IV PRN
  - Propofol 2–6 mg/kg IV or 0.6 mg/kg/min CRI, decrease dose 25% if acepromazine or chlorpromazine have already been used.
  - If nonresponsive to IV phenobarbital, diazepam, or propofol, mask down with isofluorane.
- Agitation
  - Chlorpromazine 0.5–1 mg/kg slow IV or IM, start at low end of dose and gradually increase as needed. Can use larger doses if needed, but use caution especially in dehydrated animals.
  - Acepromazine 0.05–0.1 mg/kg IV, IM, or SQ
- Serotonin syndrome
  - Cyproheptadine is generally given orally but can be administered rectally, at the same dose, in animals with severe clinical signs.
    - □ Cats: 2–4 mg total dose every 4–6 hours as needed until resolution of clinical signs
    - □ Dogs: 1.1 mg/kg BW every 4–6 hours as needed

Precautions/Interactions

- Diazepam and other benzodiazepines are not universally recommended by all for treatment of SSRIs, as some feel they may exacerbate agitation associated with a serotonin syndrome.
- TCAs, in particular clomipramine, should not be used in conjunction with SSRIs.
- Amitraz collars and other forms should not be used for several weeks after this toxicity.
- In theory, S-adenosyl-methionine (SAMe) can cause increased serotonergic effects and the concurrent use is not recommended.
- There is some controversy as to whether a neuroleptic malignant syndrome, found in human beings, actually exists in veterinary medicine. Some veterinarians agree; some disagree.

Nursing Care

- Regulate body temperature.
- Minimize stimulation.

Follow-Up

- Animals should be monitored in the clinic until clinical signs have resolved.

Prevention

- Pet owners should be advised to keep medications out of the reach of pets, preferably stored in locked cabinets or cabinets located high off the ground.

COMMENTS

Client Education

- Ensure the home environment is safe for the pet to return to.
- Ensure all pills have been removed from reachable areas.
- Readmit animal if signs recur or worsen after proper treatment.

Patient Monitoring

- Vitals
- ECG
- Clinical signs associated with serotonin syndrome
- Electrolytes and blood glucose in citalopram overdose

Prevention/Avoidance

- Store medications in locked cabinets or difficult to reach cabinets.
- Keep purses and shopping bags off of the floor and away from easy-to-reach places.
- Do not leave medications on countertops that may be accessible by a pet.

Possible Complications

- Rhabdomyolysis if seizures are untreated

Expected Course and Prognosis

- Clinical signs typically develop within 1 hour.
- Animals that receive frequent monitoring and prolonged care have a good prognosis.

Abbreviations

CNS = central nervous system
CRI = continuous rate infusion
ECG = electrocardiogram
IM = intramuscular
IV = intravenous
LD = lethal dose
MAO = monoamineoxidase
PLR = pupillary light response
PRN = as needed
SAMe = S-adenosyl-methionine
SQ = subcutaneous
SSRI = selective serotonin reuptake inhibitors
TCA = tricyclic antidepressant

See Also

Atypical Antipsychotics

Suggested Reading

Mensching D, Volmer PA. Neurotoxicity. In: Gupta RC. Veterinary Toxicology: Basic and Clinical Principles. New York: Elsevier, 2007; p. 135.

Stork CM. Serotonin reuptake inhibitors and atypical antidepressants. In: Flomenbaum NE, Goldrank LR, Hoffman RS, et al., eds. Goldfrank's Toxicologic Emergencies, 8th ed. New York: McGraw-Hill, 2006; pp. 1070–1082.

Wismer TA. Antidepressant drug overdoses in dogs. Vet Med 2000; 95:520–525.

Author: Kelly M. Sioris, PharmD
Consulting Editor: Lynn R. Hovda, RPH, DVM, MS, DACVIM

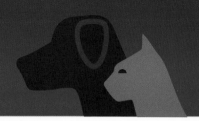

Drugs: Illicit and Recreational

Club Drugs (MDMA, GHB, and Flunitrazepam)

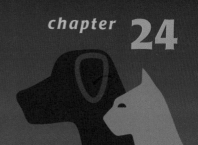

chapter 24

DEFINITION/OVERVIEW

- Toxicosis caused by ingestion of designer drugs methylenedioxymethamphetamine (MDMA; see fig. 24.1), gamma-hydroxybutyric acid (GHB), and flunitrazepam (Rohypnol).
- MDMA and GHB are DEA Schedule I controlled substances; flunitrazepam a DEA Schedule IV controlled substance (under review for rescheduling at a Schedule I).
- MDMA is referred to as "ecstasy"; GHB and flunitrazepam as "date rape drugs."
- Animal cases may be the result of malicious poisonings, accidental ingestion of drugs in the environment, or intentional sharing of drugs with a pet.
- Degree of intoxication depends on how much of the drug has been ingested and what other toxic substances may be present as adulterants or contaminants.
- Most common responses to exposure:
  - MDMA—neurologic stimulant with possible hallucinations
  - GHB—signs of CNS depression
  - Flunitrazepam—sedation, confusion, muscle relaxation, and hallucinations

ETIOLOGY/PATHOPHYSIOLOGY

- The incidence of club drug toxicosis is unknown and probably underreported due to the clandestine nature of the chemicals.
- Club or party drugs are used by young adults at all-night dance parties (raves or trances), dance clubs, and bars. MDMA, GHB, and flunitrazepam are the most commonly abused drugs, but ketamine, PCP, and methamphetamine are also involved.

Mechanism of Action

- MDMA—increases the release of serotonin while also inhibiting the uptake of the neurotransmitter
- GHB—synthetic GABA derivative; modulates dopamine signaling
- Flunitrazepam—benzodiazepine drug; acts on chloride channel of GABA (an inhibitory neurotransmitter) receptor in the CNS and increases the frequency of chloride channel opening

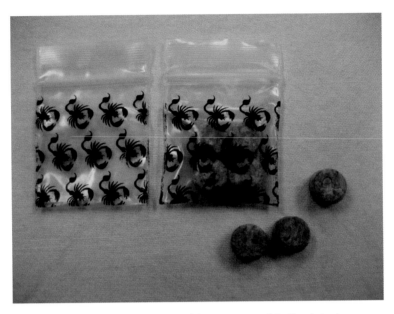

■ Fig. 24.1. MDMA (ecstasy) tablets and baggie. (Photo courtesy of Justine A. Lee)

Pharmacokinetics/Absorption, Distribution, Metabolism, and Excretion

- MDMA—readily absorbed from GI tract and crosses blood brain barrier from plasma; metabolized by the liver and excreted by the renal tract
- GHB—rapidly absorbed from GI tract and distributed across blood brain barrier; excreted as carbon dioxide through respiratory tract
- Flunitrazepam—absorbed well from the GI and metabolized by the liver into two active compounds; excreted by the renal system

Toxicity

- MDMA—Chronic dosing of dogs at 15 mg/kg shows restricted weight gain, testicular atrophy, and damage to serotonin receptors in the brain. A single dose of 18 mg/kg has been shown to be fatal.
- GHB—Doses exceeding 50 mg/kg have been associated with death. There is a slim margin between clinical effect and fatal dosing.
- Flunitrazepam—Extent of toxicosis is a direct continuation of side effects.

Systems Affected

- Central nervous system—MDMA has a stimulatory effect; GHB and flunitrazepam cause CNS depression.
- Hepatobiliary—MDMA may produce liver failure as a result of hyperthermia.
- Renal/urologic—Renal failure may be seen with MDMA toxicosis secondary to hyperthermia and rhabdomyolysis.

- Cardiovascular—MDMA and GHB intoxication may cause cardiac arrhythmias.
- Endocrine/metabolic—MDMA is associated with hyperthermia; GHB with hypothermia.

 SIGNALMENT/HISTORY

- Dogs are the species most commonly affected by ingestion of a club drug.
- Signs associated with MDMA are similar to those with amphetamines and occur within 45 minutes after ingestion. They include the following:
  - Hyperactivity and agitation
  - Mydriasis
  - Hyperthermia
  - Seizures
  - Cardiac arrhythmias
  - Death
- Signs associated with GHB occur within 15–30 minutes after ingestion and include the following:
  - Lethargy
  - Hypotonia
  - Tremors
  - Hypothermia
  - Loss of consciousness
  - Respiratory depression
- Signs associated with flunitrazepam occur 20–30 minutes after ingestion and include the following:
  - Confusion
  - Sedation
  - Muscle relaxation
  - Memory inhibition that may affect training

Risk Factors

- Animals in households with young people who attend raves.
- Drug-sniffing police dogs

Location and Circumstances of Poisoning

- Cases occur anywhere these drugs are available.

 CLINICAL FEATURES

- Onset of clinical signs
  - MDMA signs occur within about 45 minutes after ingestion and may last for 8 hours.

- GHB signs occur within 15–30 minutes of ingestion and resolve within 7 hours.
- Flunitrazepam signs occur within 30–60 minutes and may last up to 8–12 hours.
- Systems most commonly affected include the following:
  - Nervous system
  - Cardiovascular
- Nervous system—MDMA may cause hyperactivity, seizures; GHB and flunitrazepam may cause lethargy, loss of consciousness, and in severe cases seizures.
- Cardiovascular—MDMA-associated signs include tachycardia or bradycardia, hypertension, and AV block.

 # DIFFERENTIAL DIAGNOSIS

- MDMA, GHB, and flunitrazepam
  - Any disease process that would cause CNS signs
    - □ Meningitis or meningioencephalitis
    - □ Severe hepatoencephalopathy
- MDMA
  - Amphetamines or methamphetamine
  - Cocaine
  - MDMA
  - Metaldehyde
- GHB and flunitrazepam
  - Benzodiazepines including diazepam and lorazepam
  - Barbiturates
  - Marijuana
  - Opioids

 # DIAGNOSTICS

- Urine may be sent to human hospital toxicity screening to detect MDMA and, in some cases, flunitrazepam. GHB is metabolized too quickly to be detected.
- The Quick Screen Pro Multi Drug Screening Test is a human testing kit that has been validated by GC/MS for use in animals. It may provide a rapid and accurate diagnosis for flunitrazepam and perhaps MDMA if the drug is present in high enough concentrations and the time frame is appropriate.

Pathological Findings

- Gross findings include icterus; petechial and ecchymotic hemorrhage; dark, tarry ingesta in the stomach (postmortem); and liver damage (postmortem).

- Histopathological findings include hepatic necrosis and evidence of generalized hemorrhagic disease.

 THERAPEUTICS

- Objectives of treatment are to prevent further toxin absorption, provide supportive care, and correct clotting abnormalities.

Detoxification

- Emesis is generally ineffective as the onset of signs is so rapid.
- Activated charcoal with a cathartic x 1 dose

Appropriate Health Care

- MDMA
  - Monitor and treat for hyperthermia with cooling vests, blankets, or fluids. Do not overcool. Stop at 103 to 103.5°F.
  - Keep in darkened area and avoid excess stimulation
  - ECG and frequent cardiac monitoring
  - Observe closely for signs of serotonin syndrome.
- GHB
  - Monitor for hypothermia and use heating methods as needed. Do not overheat.
  - Observe for respiratory depression. Be prepared to intubate and ventilate if needed.
- GHB and flunitrazepam—Monitor closely for signs of excess CNS depression

Drug(s) and Antidotes of Choice

- Flunitrazepam: Flumazenil, a benzodiazepine antagonist, is the antidote. Dose is 0.01 mg/kg IV (dogs and cats). The half-life of flumazenil is about an hour, so the drug, if effective, may need to be repeated several times.
- MDMA and GHB: No specific antidote is available.
- IV fluids at 1.5 to 2 times maintenance
- MDMA is a close analog of methamphetamine and specific treatment is the same. Refer to Chapter 28 (Methamphetamine) for recommendations.
- GHB and flunitrazepam require symptomatic and supportive care until signs resolve.

Public Health

- Substances are scheduled controlled substances.

COMMENTS

Client Education

■ Educate the client on the potential for toxicosis from club drugs.

Prevention/Avoidance

■ Remove drugs from the environment or restrict the dog's access to them.

Possible Complications

■ Contaminants or deliberate adulterants in the drug mixture

Expected Course and Prognosis

■ Will depend on how much drug was ingested and time of presentation
■ At lower doses, recovery is probable.
■ At higher doses, animal may die within 8 hours of ingestion.

Synonyms

MDMA: ecstasy, blue Niles, eve, Scooby snacks, X, XTC
GHB: liquid X, liquid ecstasy, scoop
Flunitrazepam: wolfies, circles, roofies, rophies, rope, forget me pills

Abbreviations

CNS   = central nervous system
DEA   = Drug Enforcement Association
GABA   = gamma-aminobutyric acid
GC/MS = gas chromatography/mass spectrometry
GHB   = gamma-hydroxybutyric acid
IV   = intravenous
MDMA = methylenedioxymethamphetamine

See Also

Cocaine
Amphetamines
MDMA
Methamphetamine
Opiates and Opioids
PCP (Phencyclidine)

Suggested Reading

Climko RP, Roehrich H, Sweeney DR, et al. A review of MDMA and MDA. Int J Psy Med 1986; 18(4):359–365.

Frith CH, Chang LW, Lattin DL, et al. Toxicity of methylenedioxymethamphetamine (MDMA) in the dog and rat. Fundam Appl Toxicol 1987; 9:110–119.

Smith KM, Larive LL, Romanelli F. Club drugs: methylenedioxymethamphetamine, flunitrazepam, ketamine hydrochloride, and γ-hydroxybutyrate. Am J Health-Syst Pharm 2002; 59(11):1067–1076.

Teitler JB. Evaluation of a human on-site urine multidrug test for emergency use with dogs. J Am Anim Hosp Assoc 2009; 45:59–66.

Wisner, T. Drugs of abuse. Proc Int Vet Emer Crit Care 2007; 853–857.

Author: Teresa K. Drotar, DVM
Consulting Editor: Lynn R. Hovda, RPH, DVM, MS, DACVIM

chapter **25**

Cocaine

DEFINITION/OVERVIEW

- Solid white powder containing 12% to 16% cocaine salts and adulterants, which may include lidocaine, caffeine, amphetamines (fig. 25.1)
- Free basic alkaloid of cocaine may also be precipitated into "rocks" of crack to be smoked in a process known as "free basing" (fig. 25.2).
- Schedule II drug for topical anesthesia

ETIOLOGY/PATHOPHYSIOLOGY

- Cocaine is a natural alkaloid from the shrubs *Erythroxylon coca* and *E. monogynum*.
  - Grown in Mexico, South America, Indonesia, and the West Indies
- Historically one of the most commonly abused drugs in the United States

Mechanism of Action

- Sympathomimetic
  - Blocks NE reuptake
  - Blocks serotonin reuptake
  - Blocks dopamine reuptake
  - Increases catecholamine release
- Direct myocardial effect
- NE-mediated hypothalamic effects
  - Regulates appetite, sleep, and body temperature

Pharmacokinetics/Absorption, Distribution, Metabolism, and Excretion

- Peak plasma concentrations 15–12 minutes after exposure
- Readily crosses the blood-brain barrier
- Hydrolyzed by plasma and hepatic esterases to water-soluble metabolites
- Urinary excretion
  - 10%–20% unchanged
  - Rest as metabolites

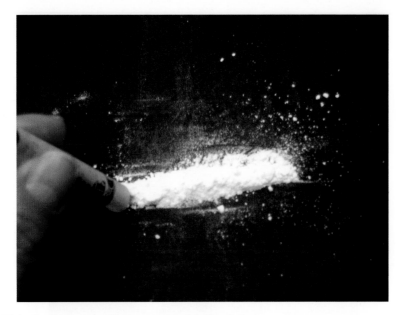

■ Fig. 25.1. Cocaine powder. (Photo courtesy of Justine A. Lee)

Toxicity

- Dog
    - IV LD_{50}: 3 mg/kg
    - Estimated PO LD_{50}: 6–12 mg/kg
    - Lowest LD: 3.5 mg/kg SQ
- Cat
    - Lowest LD: 7.5 mg/kg IV
    - Lowest LD: 16 mg/kg SQ

Systems Affected

- Nervous
- Cardiovascular

 SIGNALMENT/HISTORY

- Dogs most commonly affected
- Police dogs may be predisposed.

Risk Factors

- Ingestion of illegal cocaine or crack
- Police dogs may be predisposed.

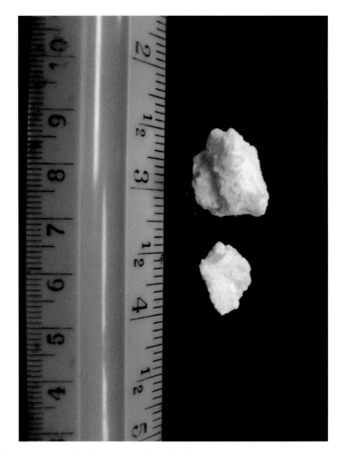

■ **Fig. 25.2.** Crack cocaine. (Photo courtesy of Justine A. Lee)

Historical Findings

- Access to drugs
  - Personal use
  - Guests or party in the home
- Client may be reluctant to give a complete history.

Location and Circumstances of Poisoning

- Animals residing in neighborhoods with known drug use

 CLINICAL FEATURES

- CNS stimulation
- Hyperactivity, tremors, seizures
- Mydriasis

- Hypersalivation
- Vomiting
- Increased heart rate
- Hyperthermia
- Elevated CK

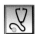 DIFFERENTIAL DIAGNOSIS

- Other stimulant drugs
  - Amphetamines and methamphetamine
  - Caffeine
- Other causes of seizures
  - Strychnine
  - Metaldehyde
  - Penitrem A

 DIAGNOSTICS

- Submit urine, plasma, or stomach contents for laboratory analysis.
  - Thin-layer chromatography
  - Gas chromatography/mass spectrometry
- ECG for cardiac effects

Pathological Findings

- Subendocardial and epicardial hemorrhage
- Myocardial degeneration
- Pericardial effusion
- Pulmonary hemorrhage

 THERAPEUTICS

Detoxification

- Early decontamination if large quantity ingested
- Avoid emesis due to seizure potential
- Sedation and gastric lavage
- Activated charcoal with cathartic x 1 dose
- Endoscopic or surgical retrieval if bagged cocaine ingested

Appropriate Health Care

- Prevent and control hyperthermia; it may become life threatening.
- Maintain an adequate airway and monitor respirations.

- Avoid excess CNS stimulation; keep in a darkened room.
- ECG monitoring for cardiac effects

Drug(s) and Antidotes of Choice

- No specific antidote available
- Seizure control
  - Diazepam 0.25–2.0 mg/kg IV
  - Phenobarbital 2–5 mg/kg IV, can be repeated up to twice at 20 minute intervals
- Propranolol (0.02 mg/kg IV slowly, maximum of 1 mg/kg) for life-threatening arrhythmias only
- Antiemetics as needed
  - Maropitant 1 mg/kg SQ q 24 hours, not labeled for cats
  - Ondansetron 0.1–0.2 mg/kg IV q 8–12 hours
- IV bicarbonate may prevent cardiac arrhythmias.

Surgical Considerations

- Cautious surgical or endoscopic removal required if whole bags of cocaine are ingested.
  - Avoid rupture of the bag.

Prevention

- Proper training of police dogs
- Muzzling of police dogs to avoid ingestion
- Preventing exposure to illegal drugs

Public Health

- This is an illegal drug; therefore, knowledge of laws concerning drug possession and animal welfare may be helpful.

 COMMENTS

Client Education

- Properly train police dogs.
- Prevent exposure to illegal drugs.
  - Keep animals away from illegal drug stash.
  - Keep them confined during parties where drugs may be used.

Prevention/Avoidance

- Avoid access to illegal drugs.
- Keep animals away from parties and other sources of illegal drugs.

- Police dogs can use a muzzle to prevent ingestion of illegal drugs.
- Monitor teenagers, who may intentionally expose companion animals to illegal drugs.

Possible Complications

- Cardiac arrest due to cardiac vasospasm
- Hyperthermia due to seizures and vasoconstriction

Expected Course and Prognosis

- Guarded prognosis

Synonyms

Cocaine: coke, bernies, snow, dust, blow, nose candy, toot, white lady
Crack cocaine: beamers, rock, crank, flake, ice

Abbreviations

CK = creatine kinase
ECG = echocardiogram
IV = intravenous
LD = lethal dose
NE = norepinephrine
PO = *per os* (by mouth)
q   = every
SQ = subcutaneous

See Also

Amphetamines
Methamphetamine

Suggested Reading

Bischoff K. Toxicity of drugs of abuse. In: Gupta RC, ed. Veterinary Toxicology: Basic and Clinical Principles. New York: Academic Press, 2007; pp. 400–401.
Llera RM, Volmer PA. Toxicologic hazards for police dogs involved in drug detection. J Am Vet Med Assoc 2006; 228:1028–1031.

Authors: Karyn Bischoff DVM, MS, DABVT; Hwan Goo Kang DVM, PhD
Consulting Editor: Lynn R Hovda, RPH, DVM, MS, DACVIM

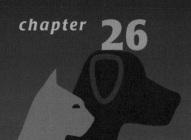

chapter **26**

LSD (Lysergic Acid Diethylamide)

DEFINITION/OVERVIEW

- Lysergic acid diethylamide (LSD) was first synthesized from ergot in 1938.
- Similar compounds are present in other plants.
  - Morning glory seeds (*Ipomea violacia*)
  - Sleepygrass (*Stipa robusta*)
  - Hawaiian baby wood rose (*Agyreia nervosa*)

ETIOLOGY/PATHOPHYSIOLOGY

- LSD is used as a recreational drug.
  - Banned by FDA in 1966; currently DEA Schedule I drug
  - Decline in illegal use over last 20 years
- LSD is dissolved in water and applied to paper, sugar cubes, gelatin cubes, or other substances for ingestion.
- Final product in circulation today contains 0.04 to 0.06 mg.
- Older products (1960s) contained up to 0.25 mg LSD per sugar cube or dose.
- Difficult to predict effects on individuals
  - Altered sensory perceptions (visual, auditory) in humans
  - May cause euphoria or panic.

Mechanism of Action

- Not completely understood
- Predominantly a partial agonist at serotonin receptors in the CNS
- Increases release of glutamate in prefrontal cortex
- Binds dopamine and α-adrenergic receptors

Pharmacokinetics/Absorption, Distribution, Metabolism, and Excretion

- Data from human subjects are available.
- Rapid gastrointestinal absorption
- Peak plasma concentrations within 6 hours

- Highly protein bound
- Hepatic metabolism
  - Hydroxylation
  - Glucuronide conjugation
- Predominantly fecal elimination
- Elimination half-life 2 to 5 hours
- Clinical signs often last a few hours but may persist for up to 12 hours.

Toxicity

- Effective dose in humans—0.05 to 0.20 mg
- Toxic dose in humans—0.70 to 2.80 mg/kg BW.
- Clinical signs seen in cats dosed with IP LSD
  - 0.0025 mg/kg BW—mild signs
  - 0.0500 mg/kg BW—marked signs
- Rat IV LD_{50}—16 mg/kg BW

Systems Affected

- Nervous—ranges from excitation to complete disorientation
- Cardiovascular—tachycardia from stimulation of autonomic nervous system
- Endocrine/metabolic—malignant hyperthermia reported in humans.
- Ophthalmic—mydriasis

 SIGNALMENT/HISTORY

- Young animals, particularly puppies, may be predisposed to ingest foreign material.

Risk Factors

- Police dogs used to detect drugs may be more susceptible.

Historical Findings

- Access to drugs
  - Teenagers in the home
  - Guests or party in the home
- Owner may be reluctant to provide a complete history.
- May be combined with other drugs

Location and Circumstances of Poisoning

- Animals residing in neighborhoods with known drug use

CLINICAL FEATURES

- Disorientation
- Mydriasis
- Vocalization
- Excitation or sedation
- Tachycardia
- Signs reported in cats:
  - Hallucinatory behavior—tracking and pouncing on unseen objects
  - Compulsive scratching in litter
  - Bizarre sitting and standing postures
  - Increased grooming, which may be incomplete
  - Increased play behavior (chasing tails, pawing, biting, sniffing)
  - Vomiting
  - Increased defecation

 DIFFERENTIAL DIAGNOSIS

- Other hallucinogenic or dissociative drugs
  - Ketamine
  - MDMA
  - Mescaline
  - PCP
  - *Psilocybe* spp. mushrooms
  - Salvia (*S. divinorum*)

 DIAGNOSTICS

- No specific serum chemistry abnormalities
- Laboratory analysis to confirm exposure. Results will take several days to be returned and cannot be used to guide therapy.
  - Immunoassays
  - HPLC
  - LC/MC
  - TLC

Pathological Findings

- No specific lesion. LSD is not reported as a direct cause of death.

THERAPEUTICS

- Treatment is generally limited to symptomatic and supportive care with close observation until clinical signs have resolved. Up to 12 hours may be required after a large ingestion.

Detoxification

- Gastrointestinal detoxification is not usually useful due to rapid onset of clinical signs.

Appropriate Health Care

- Keep in a darkened, quiet area
- Avoid excessive restraint, which may result in hyperthermia
- Monitor for tachycardia and hyperthermia; treat appropriately

Drug(s) and Antidotes of Choice

- No specific antidote available
- IV fluids as needed to stabilize cardiovascular system
- Diazepam 0.25–2.0 mg/kg IV for seizures
- Haloperidol has been used successfully in human beings.

Precautions/Interactions

- Phenothiazine tranquilizers may lower seizure threshold.
- Selective serotonin reuptake inhibitors may aggravate CNS effects and should be avoided.

Activity

- Minimize sensory stimulation for 12 hours
  - Dark, quiet room

Prevention

- Avoid access to illegal drugs.
  - Keep animals away from parties and other sources of illegal drugs.
  - Police dogs can wear a muzzle to prevent ingestion of illegal drugs.
- Monitor teenagers, who may intentionally expose companion animals to illegal drugs.

COMMENTS

Client Education

- Most animals will recover within 12 hours if kept in a dark, quiet room.
- This is an illegal drug; therefore, knowledge of laws concerning drug possession and animal welfare may be helpful.

Patient Monitoring

- Monitor heart rate and body temperature regularly over 12 hours postexposure.

Prevention/Avoidance

- Avoid access to illegal drugs.
    - Keep animals away from parties and other sources of illegal drugs.
    - Police dogs can use a muzzle to prevent ingestion of illegal drugs.
    - Monitor teenagers, who may intentionally expose companion animals to illegal drugs.

Possible Complications

- Tachycardia has been reported in humans.
- Hyperthermia has been reported in humans.
    - May be associated with restraint
- Behavioral changes may cause accident or injury to animal or caretaker.

Expected Course and Prognosis

- Deaths have not been attributed directly to LSD abuse.
    - Fatal accidents are possible due to behavioral changes.

Synonyms

acid, blotter, dots, sugar cubes, purple haze, window pane

Abbreviations

HPLC = high performance liquid chromatography
IP   = intraperitoneal
LC/MS = liquid chromatography/mass spectrography
LSD   = lysergic acid diethylamide
MDMA = 3,4-methylene-dioxymethamphetamine
PCP   = phencyclidine
TLC   = thin-layer chromatography

See Also

Club Drugs

Suggested Reading

Bischoff K. Toxicity of drugs of abuse. In: Gupta RC, ed. Veterinary Toxicology: Basic and Clinical Principles. New York: Elsevier, 2007.

Jacobs BL, Trulson ME, Stern WC. Behavioral effects of LSD in the cat: proposal of an animal behavior model for studying the actions of hallucinogenic drugs. Brain Res 1977; 132:301–314.

Volmer PA. Recreational drugs. In: Peterson ME, Talcot PA, eds. Small Animal Toxicology, 2nd ed. Philadelphia: Saunders, 2006.

Authors: Karyn Bischoff, DVM, MS, DABVT; Hwan Goo Kang, DVM, PhD
Consulting Editor: Lynn Rolland Hovda, RPH, DVM, MS, DACVIM

chapter **27**

Marijuana

DEFINITION/OVERVIEW

- Toxicosis caused by ingestion or inhalation of marijuana (*Cannabis sativa*; see figs. 27.1 and 27.2)
- Degree of signs is dependent on the quantity of toxin ingested.
  - Tetrahydrocannabinol (THC), the toxin, is highest in leaves and flowering tops of plants but varies with plant, season, and location.
  - **Marijuana** refers to the dried preparations of flowers and leaves and has varying concentrations of THC.
  - **Hashish** is the resin extracted from flowering tops and is higher in THC.
- Most common effects from exposure are neurological and gastrointestinal.

ETIOLOGY/PATHOPHYSIOLOGY

- The use of marijuana as a human recreational drug is widespread across the country, and therefore cases of marijuana toxicosis may be seen nationwide.

Mechanism of Action

- THC, the toxin, affects CB1 receptors in the brain, altering normal activity of various neurotransmitters.
- Exposure to plant toxins by ingestion causes irritation to the mucosa of the gastrointestinal tract, often resulting in vomiting.

Pharmacokinetics/Absorption, Distribution, Metabolism, and Excretion

- The toxin is ingested orally and absorbed through the gastrointestinal tract or inhaled and absorbed via the respiratory system.
- Absorption is rapid by either route.
- Pharmacokinetic studies in dogs show hepatic production of several metabolites with elimination through the feces (45%), urine (16.5%), and bile (55%). Elimination is complete within 5 days.

224

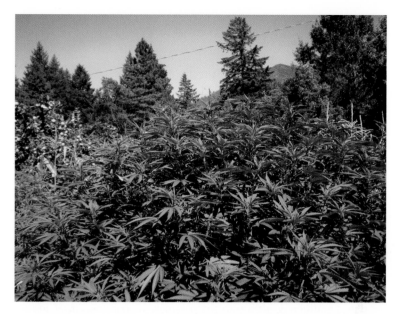

■ **Fig. 27.1.** Marijuana growing wild in a field. (Photo courtesy of Lynn R. Hovda.)

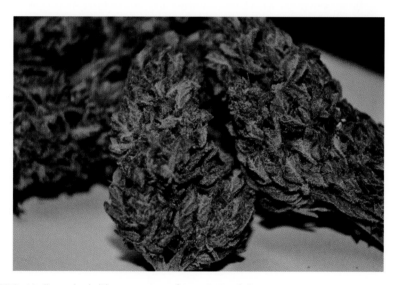

■ **Fig. 27.2.** Marijuana bud. (Photo courtesy of Lynn R. Hovda.)

Toxicity

■ Due to THC
  • Toxicosis may occur by accidental ingestion of cookies or brownies containing marijuana, loose marijuana, marijuana plants, or cigarettes containing marijuana.

- Toxicosis may also occur by inhalation of secondhand smoke from marijuana cigarettes.
- It is difficult to provide a true toxic dose in mg/kg BW because the degree of purity varies substantially with the product and route of exposure.

Systems Affected

- Nervous—varies from depression and disorientation to ataxia or coma; CNS stimulation occurs more rarely.
- Gastrointestinal—primarily vomiting
- Cardiovascular—either bradycardia or tachycardia
- Endocrine/metabolic—hypothermia or hyperthermia

 SIGNALMENT/HISTORY

- Dogs are most often affected but cats are just as susceptible.
- No breed or sex predilection
- Any age may be affected, although the majority of reported dogs are less than 1 year of age.
- Clinical signs associated with this condition include ataxia, weakness, vomiting, depression, disorientation, muscle trembling, hyperexcitability, and coma.

Risk Factors

- Exposure to marijuana by ingestion or inhalation
- Marijuana use by owners or family members
- Police dogs in service

Historical Findings

- History of exposure to or ingestion of marijuana
- Owners are often reluctant to admit this and may need encouragement to help with diagnosis.

Location and Circumstances of Poisoning

- Cases occur throughout the country as use of marijuana by humans is widespread.

 CLINICAL FEATURES

- Onset of clinical signs ranges from 5 minutes to 12 hours, with most clinical signs occurring within 1 to 3 hours of exposure.
- Duration of clinical signs ranges from 30 minutes to 3 days, with 18–24 hours being the average.

- Systems most commonly affected include the following:
  - Nervous system—signs vary from weakness and ataxia to depression and coma; eyes may be glassy with a glazed look with eventual mydriasis; CNS stimulation occurs more rarely and signs include vocalization, hyperactivity, and seizures.
  - Gastrointestinal tract—vomiting is most common clinical sign observed.
  - Other reported signs include bradycardia or tachycardia and hypothermia or hyperthermia.
- Signs of toxicosis often resolve spontaneously without treatment.

 # DIFFERENTIAL DIAGNOSIS

- Hallucinogenic mushrooms
- Recreational plants and drugs
- Human pharmaceuticals with CNS stimulant effects (amphetamines, methylphenidate, and others)
- Human pharmaceuticals with CNS depressant effects (benzodiazepines and others)

 # DIAGNOSTICS

- Not usually performed as owners, with some persuasion, disclose marijuana exposure.
- The use of the human on-site urine tests for marijuana has not shown to be effective in dogs likely due to the large number of metabolites in dog urine.
- Gas chromatography/mass spectrometry (GC/MS) is effective in identifying marijuana but takes several days to perform and is not useful in guiding therapy.

 # THERAPEUTICS

- The objectives of treatment are to prevent further toxin absorption and provide supportive care. In general, animals will require care for 18–24 hours, but this varies depending on clinical signs and route of exposure.

Detoxification

- Remove from source, especially smoke inhalation
- Emesis not rewarding
  - Many animals are already vomiting.
  - In those that don't vomit, THC appears to have a powerful antiemetic effect.
- Activated charcoal with cathartic x 1 for oral exposure
- Gastric lavage if the dog has ingested large quantities of marijuana baked goods.

Appropriate Health Care

- Warming measures for hypothermia; cooling for hyperthermia
- Oxygen therapy if respiratory depression occurs
- Close monitoring of CNS signs
  - Depression occurs most frequently and is generally not treated.
  - If the animal develops CNS stimulation and becomes hazardous to itself or handlers, consider sedation.

Drug(s) and Antidotes of Choice

- No specific antidote is available.
- IV fluids as needed for dehydration secondary to vomiting
- Sedation if needed
  - Diazepam 0.25–0.5 mg/kg IV PRN
  - Chlorpromazine 0.5–1 mg/kg IV PRN
- Antiemetic agents if vomiting persists or is severe
  - Maropitant 1 mg/kg SQ q 24 hours, not labeled for cats
  - Ondansetron 0.1–0.2 mg/kg IV q 8–12 hours

Nursing Care

- Rotate comatose animals every 4 hours.
- Monitor TPR every 2–4 hours until animal has returned to normal mentation.

Prevention

- Eliminate marijuana from the dog's environment.

Public Health

- Marijuana is an illegal street drug and presents human health risks.

 COMMENTS

Client Education

- Educate the client on the toxicity of marijuana in dogs.
- Discuss intentional misuse.
  - Do not intentionally blow smoke in a dog's face or feed marijuana-laced baked goods.
- Muzzle police dogs if they are indiscriminate eaters.

Prevention/Avoidance

- Eliminate marijuana from the environment.
- Keep dogs out of the area where parties occur.

Expected Course and Prognosis

- Recovery time will depend on the quantity of toxin ingested or inhaled but is usually complete within three days.
- Marijuana toxicosis is rarely fatal.

Synonyms

weed, pot, grass, Mary Jane, reefers, hemp, devil week, hashish, and a wide variety of others

Abbreviations

BW   = body weight
CNS = central nervous system
IV   = intravenous
PRN = *pro re nata* (as needed)
q   = every
SQ   = subcutaneous
TPR = temperature, pulse, respiration

See Also

Club Drugs
Opiates and Opioids

Suggested Reading

Garrett ER, Hunt CA. Pharmacokinetics of delta 9-tetrahydrocannabinol in dogs. J Pharm Sci 1977; 66:395–407.
Godbold JC, Hawkins BJ, Woodward MG. Acute oral marijuana poisoning in the dog. J Am Vet Med Assoc 1979; (175):1101–1102.
Janczyk P, Donaldson CW, Gwaltney S. Two hundred and thirteen cases of marijuana toxicoses in dogs. Vet Hum Tox 2004; 46(1):19–21.
Llera RM, Volmer PA. Toxicologic hazards for police dogs involved in drug detection. J Am Vet Med Assoc 2006; 228(7):1028–1031.
Teitler JB. Evaluation of a human on-site urine multidrug test for emergency use with dogs. J Am Animal Hosp Assoc 2009; 45:59–66.

Author: Christy A. Klatt, DVM
Consulting Editor: Lynn R. Hovda, RPH, DVM, MS, DACVIM

28

Methamphetamine

DEFINITION/OVERVIEW

- Toxicosis caused by ingestion, and less frequently, inhalation of methamphetamine
- Degree of toxicosis is dependent upon the quantity of methamphetamine ingested
- Most common effects are neurological with cardiac failure and hyperthermia as secondary effects

ETIOLOGY/PATHOPHYSIOLOGY

- The manufacture and use of methamphetamine (meth = slang or street name) as a human recreational drug is widespread across the country. Cases of methamphetamine intoxication may be seen nationwide; however, due to the illegal nature of the substance, cases may be underreported.
  - Crystal meth (fig. 28.1) is smoked.
  - Powdered meth is ingested, snorted, or administered IV.
- The abuse of methamphetamine is growing rapidly primarily because it can be easily manufactured in basements and other crude laboratories from precursors like ephedrine.
- Pure methamphetamine is rare; it is often cut or adulterated with other potentially harmful substances, including phenylpropanolamine and caffeine.
- Methamphetamine is a DEA Schedule II drug.

Mechanism of Action

- Increased release of catecholamines
- Inhibition of monoamine oxidase (MAO)
- Probable direct action on dopamine and serotonin receptors

Pharmacokinetics/Absorption, Distribution, Metabolism, and Excretion

- Methamphetamine is rapidly absorbed from the gastrointestinal system.
- Peak plasma levels in human beings are reached in 1–3 hours.
- Methamphetamine crosses the blood-brain barrier in high concentrations and is also distributed to the kidneys, liver, and lungs.

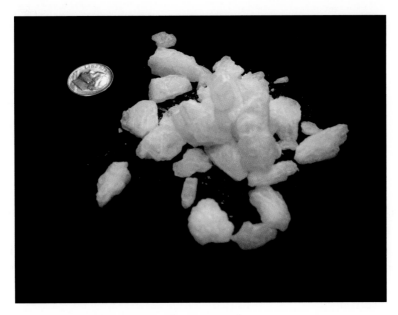

■ **Fig. 28.1.** Crystal meth. (Photo courtesy of Justine A. Lee)

- It is metabolized in the liver by hydroxylation and deamination and excreted in the urine with the rate of excretion increasing with acidification of the urine.

Toxicity

- The LD_{50} in dogs is 9–100 mg/kg when administered orally.
- Toxicosis in animals may occur by accidental ingestion of methamphetamine (oral route) or occasionally by the inhalation of fumes (respiratory route). Adulterants may pose a separate toxicosis.

Systems Affected

- Nervous—hyperactivity, tremors, restlessness, seizures, and occasionally ataxia and depression. Hyperthermia is secondary to peripheral vasoconstriction and seizure activity.
- Cardiovascular—tachycardia and premature ventricular contractions
- Endocrine/metabolic—hyperthermia; liver failure
- Respiratory—failure and death
- Renal/urologic—renal failure from myoglobinuria secondary to rhabdomyolysis

 SIGNALMENT/HISTORY

- Dogs are the species most frequently affected, but cats may also be at risk.
- No breed or sex predilection

- Any age may be affected.
- Signs of exposure to methamphetamine include the following:
  - Hyperactivity, restlessness, muscle tremors
  - Seizures
  - Hyperthermia
  - Tachycardia, ventricular premature contractions
  - Disseminated intravascular coagulation (DIC) secondary to hyperthermia
  - Hypersalivation
  - Hypertension
  - Liver or renal failure
  - Respiratory failure

Risk Factors

- Exposure to methamphetamine by drug-sniffing dogs
- Methamphetamine use or manufacture by family members

Historical Findings

- History of exposure to or ingestion of methamphetamine
- Owners are often reluctant to admit the presence of drugs in the home or environment.

Location and Circumstances of Poisoning

- Cases occur throughout the country as use of methamphetamine by humans is widespread.

 CLINICAL FEATURES

- Onset of clinical signs ranges from 2 minutes to 20 minutes depending on whether intoxication occurred from inhalation or ingestion.
- Duration of acute clinical signs ranges from 3 hours to 8 hours.
- Systems most commonly affected include the following:
  - Nervous system—hyperactivity, long-term neuropsychiatric abnormalities
  - Cardiovascular system—tachycardia to long-term cardiomyopathy
- Fatalities are the result of hyperthermia resulting in cardiomyopathy, respiratory failure, or liver or renal damage.
- In cats, may see signs similar to hallucinations

 DIFFERENTIAL DIAGNOSIS

- Amphetamines, methylphenidate
- Cocaine
- MDMA and other CNS stimulant street drugs

- Ma Huang toxicity
- Metaldehyde
- Other toxins or disease processes that would cause neurologic signs

 # DIAGNOSTICS

- Serum chemistry to measure BUN, creatinine, liver enzymes, CK, glucose, and electrolyte abnormalities
- Urinalysis for evidence of myoglobinuria
- Venous blood gas analysis for metabolic acidosis
- If methamphetamine toxicosis is suspected, a urine sample may be submitted for an illicit drug screen at a human hospital.
- The Quick Screen Pro Multi Drug Screening Test is a human testing kit that has been validated by GC/MS for use in animals. It may provide a rapid and accurate diagnosis if the drug is present in high enough concentrations and the time frame is appropriate.

 # THERAPEUTICS

- Objectives of treatment are to prevent further toxin absorption, control temperature abnormalities by supplying cooling measures, correct hyponatremia, control neurological effects, and provide supportive care.

Detoxification

- Induce emesis if within 2 hours of ingestion and animal is asymptomatic; rapid onset of clinical signs may preclude this.
- Gastric lavage if large dose is ingested
- Activated charcoal with a cathartic x 1 dose

Appropriate Health Care

- Monitor closely for signs of hyperthermia and treat with a cooling vest, cool water baths, fans, or ice packs. Do not overcool. Stop at 103° to 103.5°F.
- ECG for the development of cardiac arrhythmias
- Monitor blood pressure for hypertension.
- Minimize external stimulation; keep in a darkened area.
- Observe closely for signs of serotonin syndrome. If they occur treat as described below.

Drug(s) and Antidotes of Choice

- No specific antidote is available.
- IV fluids at 1.5–2 times maintenance to increase excretion and protect kidneys from myoglobinuria

- Agitation
  - Chlorpromazine (0.5–1 mg/kg IV or IM) is preferred due to its benefit in treating serotonin syndrome. Can go as high as 5 mg/kg but need to titrate use against clinical signs.
  - Acepromazine (0.05–1 mg/kg IV, IM, SQ). Begin at low end of dosage range and increase as necessary. The belief that this drug lowers the seizure threshold is not currently supported by recent literature.
  - Diazepam and other benzodiazepines are generally NOT recommended as they may cause dysphoria or paradoxical stimulation.
- Seizures
  - Chlorpromazine (0.5–1 mg/kg IV or IM) is preferred due to its benefit in treating serotonin syndrome. Can go as high as 5 mg/kg but need to titrate use against clinical signs.
  - Phenobarbital 3–5 mg/kg IV PRN
  - Propofol: Use cautiously in animals with seizures and decrease dose by 25% if animal has already received chlorpromazine or acepromazine.
  - Mask down with isoflurane or sevaflurane if unresponsive to other medications.
  - Avoid diazepam if at all possible and be alert to dysphoria and paradoxical excitation.
- Tremors
  - Methocarbamol 55–220 mg/kg slow IV titrated to effect. Do not exceed 330 mg/kg/day.
- Tachycardia
  - Propranolol 0.02 mg/kg slow IV up to a maximum of 1 mg/kg
- Hypertension: Treat with propranolol.
- Arrhythmias
  - Lidocaine
    - Dogs: 2–8 mg/kg IV to effect while monitoring ECG
    - Cats: 0.25–0.5 mg/kg slow IV while monitoring ECG. Use judiciously in cats!
  - Procainamide
    - Dogs: 2 mg/kg IV over 3–5 minutes (up to 20 mg/kg IV bolus), followed by 25–50 µg/kg/min CRI
    - Cats: 1–2 mg/kg IV once, followed by 10–20 µg/kg IV CRI
- Serotonin syndrome (if occurs)
  - Cyproheptadine 1.1 mg/kg (dogs) and 2–4 mg *total* per cat PO or rectal. Repeat every 4–6 hours as needed.

Public Health

- Methamphetamine and the chemicals used to manufacture meth present human health risks. Amphetamines are controlled substances.
- Residues from the hair may be a risk to animal caretakers.

Environmental Issues

- Remove the animal from the environment where methamphetamines are cooked or stored.

                    # COMMENTS

Client Education

- Educate the client on methamphetamine toxicosis in pets and stress the need to eliminate meth from the animal's environment.

Prevention/Avoidance

- Eliminate methamphetamine from the environment

Expected Course and Prognosis

- Recovery time will depend on the quantity of toxin ingested or inhaled and the chronicity of exposure. Long-term exposure may result in brain and other neurologic damage.

Synonyms

meth, ice, glass, speed

Abbreviations

BUN = blood urea nitrogen
CK   = creatine kinase
CRI   = continuous rate infusion
DEA = Drug Enforcement Administration
DIC = disseminated intravascular coagulation
ECG = electrocardiogram
IM   = intramuscular
IV   = intravenous
LD   = lethal dose
MAO = monoamine oxidase
meth = methamphetamine
PO   = *per os* (by mouth)
PRN = *pro re nata* (as needed)
SQ   = subcutaneous

See Also

Amphetamines
Club Drugs
Cocaine

Suggested Reading

Bischoff K. Toxicity of drugs of abuse. In: Gupta RC, ed. Veterinary Toxicology: Basic and Clinical Principals. New York: Elsevier, 2007: pp. 401–403.

Catravas JD, Waters IW, Hickenbottom JP, et al. The effects of haloperidol, chlorpromazine, and propranolol on acute amphetamine poisoning in the conscious dog. J Pharmacol Exp Ther 1977; 202:230–243.

Dumonceaux GA, Beasley VR. Emergency treatment for police dogs used for illicit drug detection. J Am Vet Med Assoc 1990; 197:185–187.

Street Drugs: A Drug Identification Guide. Minneapolis: Publishers Group, 2010.

Volmer PA. Recreational drugs. In: Peterson ME, Talcott PA, eds. Small Animal Toxicology, 2nd ed. Philadelphia: Saunders, 2006; pp. 273–311.

Author: Teresa K. Drotar, DVM

Consulting Editor: Lynn R. Hovda, RPH, DVM, MS, DACVIM

chapter 29

Miscellaneous Hallucinogens and Dissociative Agents

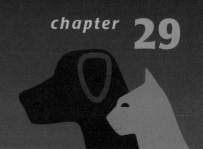

DEFINITION/OVERVIEW

- Several of the remaining hallucinogens and dissociative agents are of concern due to their widespread abuse. They are inexpensive, relatively easy to obtain, and frequently found in parties and homes where pets live.
  - Hallucinogens
    - □ Lysergic acid amide substances (LSAs) are closely related to LSD and provide a similar experience.
      - ○ Seeds from morning glory plant—*Ipomoea violacea* (fig. 29.1)
      - ○ Seeds from Hawaiian baby woodrose plant—*Argyreia nervosa*
      - ○ Salvia—*Salvia divinorum*
  - Dissociative agents
    - □ Ketamine (DEA Schedule III) is a prescription injectable medication often obtained by theft from veterinary clinics. It is gaining popularity as a club drug, and many consider it the ideal substance of abuse as it provides the effects of LSD, opiates, and cocaine in one drug.
- Others worthy of mention but not addressed further in this chapter:
  - Hallucinogens
    - □ Jimson weed (thornapple)
      - ○ Seeds from the *Datura stramonium* plant are chewed or powdered and smoked for hallucinogenic properties. The plant is found in ditches and unimproved land throughout the United States. The powerful anticholinergic alkaloids found in the seeds are responsible for the effects. Clinical signs included diaphoresis, decreased salivation, hyperthermia, and psychoactive effects.
    - □ Nutmeg
      - ○ Seeds from the fruit of an evergreen tree (*Myristica fragrans*) are chewed or powdered and smoked for hallucinogenic properties. The tree is native to the South Pacific, Trinidad, and Grenada. In human beings, the toxic dose is estimated to be three whole nutmegs or 10–15 grams (about one tablespoonful) of the dried spice. Clinical signs include decreased salivation, hypothermia, and vomiting.

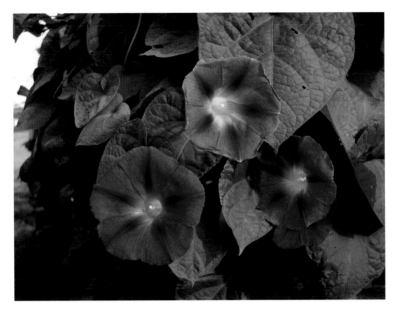

■ **Fig. 29.1.** Morning glory (*Ipomoea violacea*). (Photo courtesy of Tyne K. Hovda)

  □ Peyote (mescaline)
    ◦ The peyote cactus (*Lophophora williamsii*) contains the halluci-
      nogen mescaline. The cactus is found in northern Mexico and
      the southwestern United States. Crowns or tops of the cactus
      are harvested and dried; ingestion is generally by chewing on
      the dried pieces or brewing them and drinking the liquid.
      Clinical signs include early vomiting, diaphoresis, and mydria-
      sis followed by a 12-hour period of psychoactivity resembling
      that seen with LSD.
  □ Psilocybin (magic mushrooms or shrooms)
    ◦ Psilocybin and psilocin are psychoactive agents found in many
      species of hallucinogenic mushrooms. The mechanism of action
      is unknown but may be serotoninergic in nature. Mushrooms
      can be ingested directly, brewed into tea, or dried and chewed.
      Clinical signs are similar to LSD.
• Dissociative Agents
  □ Dextromethorphan (DMX, triple C, skittles [gelatin capsules])
    ◦ Readily available in nonprescription cough syrups and cold
      remedies. The mechanism of action is very similar to ketamine
      and phencyclidine. In human beings, approximately 360 mg
      causes a mild stimulant effect and >1500 mg a completely dis-
      sociative state.

ETIOLOGY/PATHOPHYSIOLOGY

- LSAs
  - Plants are grown throughout the USA and seed packages can be purchased online and in most nurseries.
  - Seeds are germinated, soaked in water, and crushed before ingestion.
- Ketamine
  - DEA Schedule III drug
  - Liquid form is odorless, flavorless, and colorless and often added to party punches or individual drinks.
  - It can also be dried and powdered for smoking and inhalation.
- Salvia
  - Not the same common salvia plant that can be purchased at nurseries and grown in gardens throughout the United States
  - Leafy green plant native to the Sierra Mazateca region of Mexico
  - Seeds generally purchased on the Internet from specific *Salvia divinorum* sites
  - Grown outside in United States in warm, subtropical climates (California and Hawaii); can be grown inside anywhere
  - Most common forms are the dried leaves, which are chewed or smoked, and the fluid extract, which can be ingested or added to drinks.

Mechanism of Action

- LSAs
  - Incompletely understood
  - Structurally similar to serotonin and exert some effects through stimulation of CNS serotonin receptors
- Ketamine
  - Incompletely understood
  - Antagonizes the action of glutamate at the NMDA receptor by binding within the ion channel to block calcium influx
  - Anticholinergic, opiate, alpha adrenergic, and CNS stimulating effects
  - In dogs, ketamine binds to dopamine receptors.
- Salvia
  - Salvorin-A is the active ingredient.
  - Kappa (κ) receptor agonist; no effect on 5-HT_2a receptors

Pharmacokinetics/Absorption, Distribution, Metabolism, and Excretion

- LSAs
  - Little is reported, presumed to follow LSD
  - Clinical signs in 60–90 minutes with a duration of action of several hours

- Ketamine
  - Well absorbed IM and IV
  - Poorly absorbed orally, high first-pass effect
  - Distributed to brain, liver, lung, and other tissues
  - Undergoes hepatic metabolism by demethylation or hydroxylation
  - Renal excretion
  - T ½ cat = 67 minutes after IM dose
- Salvia
  - Smoking
    - Onset time of 20 seconds to 2 minutes (human beings)
    - Duration of action is 30–60 minutes.
  - Oral or chewed
    - Well absorbed through oral mucosa
    - Chew is kept in mouth much like a tobacco chew, and both onset and duration of action depend on potency of leaves.
  - Metabolism unknown
  - T ½ in nonhuman primates is 56 minutes.

Toxicity

- LSAs
  - 1/10 as potent as LSD
  - 150–300 seeds associated with clinical effects in human beings
- Ketamine
  - Species dependent
  - Cats—20 mg/kg IM is recommended dose.
  - Dogs—5–10 mg/kg has resulted in seizures.
- Salvia
  - Not studied in animals

Systems Affected

- LSAs
  - CNS—primarily hallucinations with bizarre behaviors
  - Ophthalmic—mydriasis
  - Musculoskeletal—rhabdomyolysis
- Ketamine
  - CNS—wide variety of signs from ataxia to hallucinations to bizarre or violent behaviors
  - Musculoskeletal—increased muscle tone, spasms, and rigidity
  - Ophthalmic—vertical, horizontal, or rotary nystagmus, fixed stares
- Salvia
  - CNS—purely a "psychedelic" experience

SIGNALMENT/HISTORY

- All species are affected and there is no particular breed predilection.
- Cats and dogs respond differently to ketamine.

Historical Findings

- The owners are often very reluctant to provide any information regarding these substances, although some may discuss salvia freely.

Location and Circumstances of Poisoning

- Homes and parties where illicit drugs are used
- Dogs and cats may be exposed by inhaling smoke, drinking leftover party punch, chewing on seed packages, digging up and mouthing plants, or finding a stash of "chews."

CLINICAL FEATURES

- LSAs
  - Similar to LSD
  - Primarily CNS signs including disorientation, vocalization, depression, or excitation. Cats have exhibited very bizarre postures and behaviors. Onset of signs in 1–2 hours with recovery in 6–8 hours.
- Ketamine
  - Cats—forelimb extensor rigidity, opisthotonus, glazed and dazed staring expression. Hypersalivation with ingestion. Recovery in 10–12 hours.
  - Dogs—CNS excitation with seizures. May develop rhabdomyolysis secondary to seizures.
- Salvia
  - Clinical signs generally include abnormal mentation and vocalization.
  - Very rapid onset of signs with recovery expected in 1–2 hours

DIFFERENTIAL DIAGNOSIS

- Club drugs such as GHB, PCP, and MDMA
- CNS diseases with dissociative effects
- Hepatic encephalopathy
- LSD
- Opiates or opioids

DIAGNOSTICS

- Very limited, difficult to find in serum or urine in routine hospital-based tests
- LC/MS and GC/MS are useful tools but have a long turnaround time.
- Seeds or plant pieces found in emesis may help with diagnosis.

Pathological Findings

- No specific lesions

THERAPEUTICS

Detoxification

- Onset of signs is rapid and emesis is not advised.
- Gastric lavage in large doses, especially when plants or seeds have been ingested
- Activated charcoal plus a cathartic x one dose may be useful.

Appropriate Health Care

- Keep in a dark, quiet area and minimize excess stimulation. Monitor closely for early signs of self-mutilation or psychosis and treat accordingly.
- Monitor body temperature for hyperthermia and treat with cooling vest, cool baths, etc. Do not overcool. Stop when temperature reaches 103°–103.5°F. Rarely, hypothermia may develop.
- Baseline labs should include BUN, creatinine, and CK.

Drug(s) and Antidotes of Choice

- No specific antidote is available.
- IV fluids as needed to replace losses and protect kidneys if rhabdomyolysis occurs.
- Seizures, excitation, muscle rigidity
  - Diazepam 0.25–0.5 mg/kg IV
  - Phenobarbital 3–5 mg/kg IV PRN
  - Mask down with isoflurane or sevoflurane if seizures are severe.

Precautions/Interactions

- SSRIs and clomipramine should not be used as they can aggravate the mental changes that occur with intoxication.

Activity

- Minimize activity and limit restraint until clinically normal.

COMMENTS

Client Education

- Keep these and other illicit substances out of animal's reach and environment.
- Muzzle drug-sniffing dogs if need be.
- Educate users about harmful potential to animals.

Patient Monitoring

- Watch closely for the development of self-mutilation or other bizarre physical behaviors and sedate appropriately.

Possible Complications

- None expected with a single exposure
- Repeated exposures in human beings have resulted in "flashbacks" and permanent psychosis.

Expected Course and Prognosis

- Prognosis is excellent with supportive care. The onset of seizures or rhabdomyolysis complicates treatment and lowers the prognosis for a complete recovery.

Synonyms

LSAs: heavenly blues, flying saucers, pearly gates
Ketamine: special K, cat valium, green K
Salvia: diviner's sage, Shepherdess' herb, Mexican mint, Sally D

Abbreviations

BUN   = blood urea nitrogen
CK   = creatine kinase
GHB   = gammahydroxybutyrate
GC/MS = gas chromatography/mass spectrometry
IM   = intramuscular
IV   = intravenous
LC/MS = liquid chromatography/mass spectrometry
LSAs   = lysergic acid amide substances
LSD   = lysergic acid diamide
MDMA   = methylenedioxymethamphematime
NMDA   = N-methyl-D-aspartic acid
PCP   = phencyclidine
PRN   = *pro re nata* (as needed)

See Also

Antitussives/Expectorants (Dextromethorphan)
LSD
PCP

Suggested Reading

Anonymous. Street Drugs. Long Lake, MN: Publishers Group: Long Lake, 2010; pp. 3–80.
Bischoff K. Toxicity of drugs of abuse. In: Gupta RC, ed. Veterinary Toxicology: Basic and Clinical Principles. New York: Elsevier, 2007; pp. 391–410.
Halpern JH. Hallucinogens and dissociative agents naturally growing in the USA. Pharmacol Ther 2004; 102:131–138.

Author: Lynn R. Hovda, RPH, DVM, MS, DACVIM
Consulting Editor: Ahna G. Brutlag, DVM

chapter 30

Opiates and Opioids (Illicit)

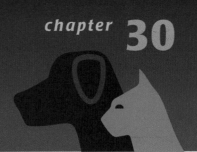

DEFINITION/OVERVIEW

- The opiate and opioid group includes more than 25 different drugs; most are legal prescription drugs.
- Several of these drugs are abused for their psychoactive effects. Among the most frequently abused are opium, morphine, codeine, heroin, oxycodone, hydromorphone, meperidine, and fentanyl.
- Animals can be exposed in a variety of different manners.
  - Drug detecting dogs in active service are at the highest risk for accidental intoxication either by inhalation or ingestion.
  - Puppies have been used as "pack dogs" to transport heroin and cocaine; baggies were surgically placed in their abdomens prior to shipping the dogs into the United States.
  - Sporadic cases of malicious heroin injections exist.
  - Rarely, animal owners want to "share" their experiences with pets.
- Clinical signs vary depending on the species, but death, when it occurs, is generally from respiratory depression and arrest.

ETIOLOGY/PATHOPHYSIOLOGY

- Natural opium, morphine, and codeine are derived from the seeds of the poppy plant (*Papaver somniferum*) and technically classed as opiates.
- Heroin, oxycodone, and hydromorphone are semisynthetic derivatives and considered opioids (see fig. 30.1).
- Meperidine and fentanyl are strictly synthetic drugs and true opioids (see fig. 30.2).
- Exposure, in animals, generally occurs from inhalation or ingestion.

Mechanism of Action

- Varies depending on the particular drug
  - Full agonist—morphine, codeine, heroin, fentanyl, meperidine
  - Full antagonist—naloxone
  - Agonist/antagonist—butorphanol, nalorphine
  - Partial agonist—tramadol, buprenorphine

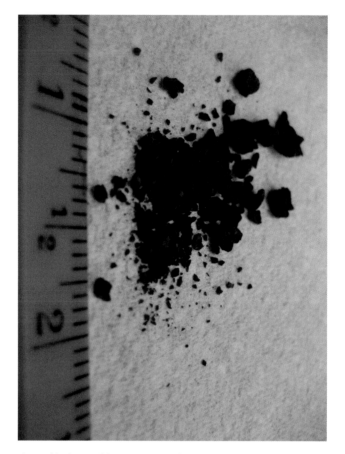

■ **Fig. 30.1.** Heroin or "black tar." (Photo courtesy of Justine A. Lee)

- Both opiates and opioids bind to opioid receptors.
- Opioid receptors, designated mu (μ_1 and μ_2), kappa (κ), sigma (σ), delta (δ), and epsilon (ε) are found throughout the body, including the adrenal glands, ANS, CNS (multiple locations), GIT, heart, lymphocytes, kidney, pancreas, and vas deferens.
  - CNS—location of receptors determines whether excitation or depression occurs
    - Dog—CNS depression; higher number of opioid receptors in amygdala and frontal cortex
    - Cat—CNS stimulation and excitation; fewer receptors
  - CNS receptors located in CTZ—emesis
  - CNS receptors located in brain stem—cough and respiratory depression
  - GIT—decreased motility and constipation
- Mu receptors, in particular $\mu 1$ receptors, are responsible for the analgesic effects; $\mu 2$ receptors for respiratory depression.

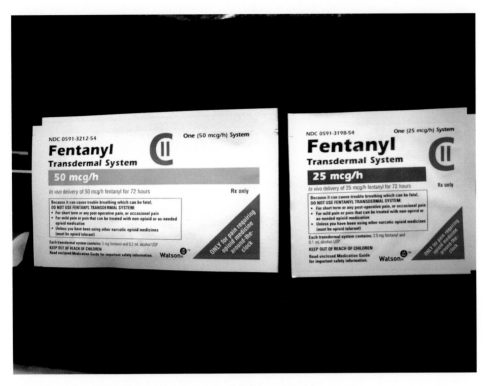

■ Fig. 30.2. Fentanyl patches. (Photo courtesy of Robert N. Hovda)

- Sigma receptors were originally thought to be responsible for euphoria and psychoactive effects, but that may no longer be accurate.
- Dopamine and norepinephrine concentrations are likely to play a role as well.

Pharmacokinetics/Absorption, Distribution, Metabolism, and Excretion

- Absorption
    - Oral absorption is generally rapid and occurs in the small intestine.
- Distribution
    - Well distributed to most organ systems (CNS, intestine, kidney, liver, lungs, placenta, spleen, and skeletal muscle)
    - Liphophilic drugs cross the blood brain barrier (BBB) more efficiently.
- Metabolism
    - Readily metabolized in liver by hydrolysis, oxidation, and N-dealkylation
    - Morphine undergoes glucuronidation to morphine-6-glucuronide, an active metabolite.
    - Enterohepatic recirculation of morphine and its metabolite occurs.
- Excretion
    - Renal, primarily as metabolites
    - Some biliary excretion via feces

Toxicity

- Very limited animal data available
- Codeine
  - IV LD_{50} in dogs—69 mg/kg
- Heroin
  - Minimum lethal dose
    - Dog—25 mg/kg SQ
    - Cat—20 mg/kg PO
- Morphine
  - Minimum lethal dose parenterally
    - Dog—110 to 210 mg/kg SQ
    - Cat—40 mg/kg BW given SQ
- Meperidine
  - >20 mg/kg BW causes excitation in cats
  - 30 mg/kg BW causes seizures in cats

Systems Affected

- Varies depending on drug and species involved
- Respiratory—respiratory depression leading to death
- CNS—depression or excitation
- Cardiovascular—instability with hypotension; heart block and other arrhythmias with propoxyphene overdose
- Gastrointestinal—decreased GI motility with constipation
- Ophthalmic—miosis or mydriasis (species variation)
- Endocrine/metabolic—meperidine and tramadol have some serotonergic activity

 SIGNALMENT/HISTORY

- All breeds and all ages are susceptible.
- Cats and dogs present with different clinical signs when exposed to the same opiate or opioid, primarily due to the location of opioid receptors in the CNS.

Risk Factors

- Age
  - Pediatric animals may have an incomplete BBB and show more severe signs, especially with highly lipophilic substances such as fentanyl.
  - Neonatal animals may have impaired liver systems and be unable to adequately metabolize opiates or opioids.
  - Geriatric animals may have impaired liver and renal systems and be unable to adequately metabolize and excrete them.

- Cats, due to their lack of glucuronyl transferase, may inefficiently metabolize morphine.
- Police dogs, airport dogs, and other narcotic dogs in active service are at a greater risk of exposure.

Historical Findings

- These drugs are illicit and the owners may not provide an accurate history.

Location and Circumstances of Poisoning

- Intoxication can occur anywhere these drugs are found.
- Some dogs have been used as "drug mules" to illegally smuggle heroin or codeine into the country.

Interactions with Drugs, Nutrients, or Environment

- Coingestion/administration with tramadol, tricyclic antidepressants, selective serotonin reuptake inhibitors, or monoamine oxidase inhibitors may lead to serotonin syndrome.

 CLINICAL FEATURES

- Dogs
  - CNS—early excitation followed by lethargy, ataxia, frank stupor, seizures, coma, death
  - Respiratory—early increasing rate followed by depression
  - Gastrointestinal—hypersalivation, vomiting, defecation, urination
  - Cardiovascular—hypotension, arrhythmias related to propoxyphene metabolite
  - Ophthalmic—miosis
  - Endocrine/metabolic—hypothermia, decreased pain response, possible serotonin syndrome
- Cats
  - CNS—aggression, excitation, seizures, or depression
  - Respiratory—variable early on, but eventually depression
  - Gastrointestinal—lack of emesis, constipation
  - Cardiovascular—hypotension and arrhythmias
  - Ophthalmic—mydriasis (more common), miosis
  - Endocrine/metabolic—hypothermia, decreased pain response, possible serotonin syndrome

 DIFFERENTIAL DIAGNOSIS

- Various encephalopathies

- CNS depressants
  - Amitraz
  - Barbiturates
  - Benzodiazepines
  - Ethylene glycol
  - GHB
  - Marijuana
- CNS stimulants
  - Amphetmamines/methylphenidate/methamphetamine/MDMA
  - Cocaine
  - Metaldehyde
  - Strychnine

 # DIAGNOSTICS

- Urine and serum can be submitted to human hospitals for analysis or to a laboratory for GC/MS or LC/MS. Both take several days for results to be returned and will not provide information rapidly enough to guide therapy.
- The Quick Screen Pro Multi Drug Screening Test is a human testing kit that has been successfully used in animals. It may provide a rapid and accurate diagnosis if the drug is present in high enough concentrations and the time frame is appropriate.

Pathological Findings

- No specific findings

 # THERAPEUTICS

- The goal of therapy is to provide early decontamination, careful use of an opioid antagonist, and supportive care.

Detoxification

- Induce emesis either at home or in veterinarian's clinic if no clinical signs have developed. Emesis may be successful for 1–2 hours after ingestion due to decreased GI motility.
- Drug-detecting dogs may have ingested baggies full of narcotics; be careful that these are not ruptured. Surgical removal may be necessary.
- Gastric lavage if large doses ingested or clinical signs preclude emesis.
- Activated charcoal with cathartic x 1 dose. Repeat doses of activated charcoal may be necessary for drugs such as morphine that undergo enterohepatic recirculation.

Appropriate Health Care

- Hospitalize and monitor closely for CNS and respiratory depression. Be prepared to intubate and ventilate if needed.
- Heart monitor with ECG as needed
- Monitor body temperature and treat accordingly. Warm but do not overheat
- Monitor urine output and fluid status.

Drug(s) and Antidotes of Choice

- IV fluids as needed to replace losses and correct hypotension
- Naloxone, a pure opioid antagonist, may be used to reverse CNS and respiratory depression. It has no effects on the GI signs seen in dogs.
  - 0.01–0.04 mg/kg BW IV or IM
  - The high end of the dosage range may be needed in massive overdoses.
  - Duration of action is generally 45–90 minutes.
  - If effective, dose may need to be repeated.
- Diazepam 0.025–0.5 mg/kg IV as needed for seizures
- Arrhythmias
  - Lidocaine
    - Dogs: 2–8 mg/kg IV to effect while monitoring ECG
    - Cats: 0.25–0.5 mg/kg slow IV while monitoring ECG. Use judiciously in cats!
  - Procainamide
    - Dogs: 2 mg/kg IV over 3–5 minutes (up to 20 mg/kg IV bolus), followed by 25–50 µg/kg/min CRI
    - Cats: 1–2 mg/kg IV once, followed by 10–20 µg/kg IV CRI

Precautions/Interactions

- Naloxone is ineffective for seizures caused by normeperidine, tramadol, or propoxyphene toxicity and may exacerbate signs.
- Naloxone will not reverse propoxyphene-induced cardiotoxicity.

Alternative Drugs

- If naloxone is not available, butorphanol 0.1 to 0.2 mg/kg IV can be used to partially reverse pure mu agonists.

Surgical Considerations

- Cautious surgical removal of packets in GIT or abdomen of drug-packing dogs.

COMMENTS

Client Education

- Animals should be kept away from parties where these drugs are used. Personal stashes should be locked up and kept out of reach.
- Party drinks and other goodies should be cleared away before animals have access to the area.
- Police and active drug-detecting dogs that are voracious eaters should wear a muzzle.
- Naloxone should be available for police and drug-detecting dogs in active service.

Patient Monitoring

- Baseline labs with attention to BUN, creatinine, and CK, especially if seizures occur
- Blood gases as needed
- ECG in the event of arrhythmias

Expected Course and Prognosis

- The onset of signs is rapid, occurring within 30–120 minutes. The duration of signs depends on the particular opiate or opioid ingested or inhaled.
- The prognosis is generally excellent, especially when naloxone has been used to reverse the signs.
- Death rarely occurs.

Synonyms

Heroin—dope, Lady Jane, skag, speedball, smack, heaven
Fentanyl—China white, Tango and Cash

Abbreviations

ANS	= autonomic nervous system
BUN	= blood urea nitrogen
BW	= body weight
CK	= creatine kinase
CNS	= central nervous system
CRI	= continuous rate infusion
ECG	= electrocardiogram
GC/MS	= gas chromatography/mass spectrometry
GHB	= gammahydroxybutyrate
GI	= gastrointestinal
GIT	= gastrointestinal tract

IM   = intramuscular
IV   = intravenous
LC/MS = liquid chromatography/mass spectrometry
MDMA = methylenedioxymethamphetamine
PO   = *per os* (by mouth)
SQ   = subcutaneous

See Also

Opiates and Opioids (Human Prescription Drugs section)

Suggested Reading

Anonymous. Major Operations 2006. www.justice.gov/dea/images_major_operations2006.html. Accessed 10 Jan 2010.

Branson KR, Gross ME. Opioid agonists and antagonists. In: Adams R, ed. Veterinary Pharmacology and Therapeutics, 8th ed. Ames: Iowa State University Press, 2001; pp. 268–298.

Hofmeister EH, Herrington J, Mazzaferro EM. Opioid dysphoria in three dogs. J Vet Emerg Crit Care 2006; 16(1):44–49.

Volmer PA. Recreational drugs. In: Peterson ME, Talcott, eds. Small Animal Toxicology, 2nd ed. St. Louis: Saunders, 2006; pp. 273–211.

Author: Lynn R. Hovda, RPH, DVM, MS, DACVIM
Consulting Editor: Ahna G. Brutlag, DVM

chapter **31**

PCP (Phencyclidine)

DEFINITION/OVERVIEW

- PCP (1-[phenylcyclohexyl] piperidine), or phencyclidine, was introduced in the 1950s as a human surgical anesthetic but was discontinued a few years later because of disagreeable and often violent side effects such as hallucination, mania, delirium, and disorientation.
- It was marketed in 1967 as a veterinary anesthetic (Sernylan) but withdrawn in 1978 because of similar side effects, long half-life, and potential as a drug of abuse.
- Currently a DEA Schedule II synthetic drug
- Easily synthesized in clandestine laboratories in both the powder and liquid form
- More than 80 known analogs. Ketamine, one of the analogs, is widely used in veterinary medicine, but it has a shorter half-life and 1/10 to 1/20 potency of PCP.

ETIOLOGY/PATHOPHYSIOLOGY

Mechanism of Action

- Dissociative agent, but the precise mechanism is not fully understood
- Binds with high affinity to receptors in the cerebral cortex, thalamus, and limbic system
  - Acts as a competitive inhibitor of glutamate at the NMDA receptor

Pharmacokinetics/Absorption, Distribution, Metabolism, and Excretion

- PCP is a weak base and poorly absorbed from stomach, but significant intestinal absorption occurs.
- Inhaled PCP is absorbed via the respiratory system.
- Highly lipophilic
  - Crosses the blood brain barrier
  - Partitions to the CNS, which may increase half-life

254

- Metabolism varies with species
  - In dogs, 68% of a single dose is metabolized in the liver and 32% is excreted unchanged by the kidney.
  - In cats, 88% is excreted unchanged by the kidney.

Toxicity

- Oral administration
  - Severe signs of toxicosis
    - Dogs—2.5–10.0 mg/kg BW PO
    - Cats—1.1–12.0 mg/kg BW PO
  - Lethal PO dose in dogs is 25 mg/kg BW
- IV administration—clinical signs can occur in dogs at 1 mg/kg BW IV
- IM administration
  - 2 mg/kg BW—muscle incoordination
  - 5 mg/kg BW—immobilization and seizures

Systems Affected

- Nervous—wide variety of signs from depression to stimulation; may be prolonged for several days
- Neuromuscular—tremors, loss of motor function
- Cardiovascular—tachycardia, hypo- or hypertension, arrhythmias
- Endocrine/metabolic—hyperthermia
- Musculoskeletal—rhabdomyolysis
- Renal/urologic—acute renal failure secondary to myoglobinuria

 # SIGNALMENT/HISTORY

Risk Factors

- Ingestion of illegal PCP
- Police dogs may be predisposed.

Historical Findings

- Access to drugs
  - Teenagers in the home
  - Guests or party in the home
- Owners may be reluctant to give a complete history.

Location and Circumstances of Poisoning

- Animals residing in neighborhoods with known drug use
- May be combined with other drugs

CLINICAL FEATURES

- Acute
  - Behavioral effects vary depending on dosage.
    - Depression at low dose
    - Stimulation at high dose with the potential for seizures
  - General signs include hypertension, tachycardia, nausea, vomiting, hyper-salivation, fever, sweating, and convulsion.
  - Dogs dosed with PCP showed muscular rigidity, facial grimacing, increased motor activity, head weaving, stereotyped sniffing behaviors, jaw snapping, salivation, blank staring, incoordination, nystagmus, coma, tonic-clonic convulsions, and hyperthermia.
  - Cardiovascular effects include tachycardia, hypertension, and cardiac arrhythmias.
- Chronic
  - Not reported

 DIFFERENTIAL DIAGNOSIS

- Hallucinogenic mushrooms
- Ketamine
- LSD
- Marijuana

 DIAGNOSTICS

- Serum chemistry results may show acidosis, hypoglycemia, electrolyte imbalances, and increases in CPK and AST.
- Urine, blood, plasma, or gastric contents for laboratory analysis
  - Urine is the most commonly analyzed sample.
    - PCP may be detected for more than 2 weeks after exposure.
  - Blood levels do not correlate with clinical findings.
- PCP and ketamine may show cross-reactivity on immunoassay.

Pathological Findings

- Nonspecific
- Subendocardial and epicardial hemorrhage

 THERAPEUTICS

- Treatment of poisoning is generally symptomatic and supportive.

Detoxification

- Emesis only in very recent ingestion of large doses
  - Use with caution, as animals develop seizures at any time.
- Activated charcoal with a cathartic x 1 dose

Appropriate Health Care

- Monitor for urine output and adjust IV fluids as needed.
- Monitor for hyperthermia and treat accordingly.
- Monitor blood pressure and treat accordingly.
- Obtain baseline BUN, creatinine, and blood glucose. Repeat as needed.
- Keep animal in a darkened, nonstressful environment and do not overstimulate.

Drug(s) and Antidotes of Choice

- No specific antidote is available.
- IV fluids to correct hypoglycemia and electrolyte abnormalities. IV rate, at a minimum, should be 2 times maintenance to ensure adequate urine output and stabilize the cardiovascular system.
- After rehydrated, forced diuresis with mannitol or furosemide can be used to increase the rate of clearance.
  - Furosemide CRI at 1–2 mg/kg/hour
  - Mannitol bolus at 1–2 g/kg slow IV
- Seizures
  - Diazepam 0.25–2.0 mg/kg IV
  - Phenobarbital 2–5 mg/kg IV, can be repeated up to twice at 20 minute intervals

Precautions/Interactions

- Phenothiazine tranquilizers may decrease the seizure threshold, exacerbate anticholinergic effects, and produce hypotension.

Activity

- Minimize sensory stimulation.
  - Dark, quiet room

 COMMENTS

Client Education

- Police dogs can wear a muzzle to prevent ingestion of illegal drugs.
- Prevent exposure to illegal drugs.
  - Keep animals away from illegal drug stash.
  - Keep them confined during parties where drugs may be used.

Patient Monitoring

- Monitor body temperature regularly over 12 hours postexposure.
- Monitor BUN, creatinine, and blood glucose.

Possible Complications

- Self-induced trauma or rhabdomyolysis may complicate treatment.

Expected Course and Prognosis

- Depends on the clinical condition of the animal at the time of presentation
- Prognosis is generally good with early decontamination, monitoring, and supportive care.
- Dogs injected IM with low dose of PCP
  - 1 mg/kg—recovered in a little over one hour
  - 5 mg/kg—recovered within 2 hours
- Poor prognosis if self-induced trauma or rhabdomyolysis is evident

Synonyms

angel dust, angel hair, boat, dummy dust, jet fuel

Abbreviations

AST   = aspartate transaminase
BUN   = blood urea nitrogen
BW   = body weight
CPK   = creatine phosphokinase
IM   = intramuscular
IV   = intravenous
LD_{50} = median lethal dose
LSD   = lysergic acid diethylamide
NMDA = N-methyl-D-aspartate
PCP   = phencyclidine
PO   = *per os* (by mouth)

See Also

Marijuana
Miscellaneous Hallucinogens and Dissociative Agents

Suggested Reading

Bischoff K. Toxicity of drugs of abuse. In: Gupta RC, ed. Veterinary Toxicology: Basic and Clinical Principles. New York: Elsevier, 2007; pp. 406–409.

Ortega J. Phencyclidine for capture of stray dogs. J Am Vet Med Assoc 1967; 150:772–776.

Volmer PA. Recreational drugs. In: Peterson ME and Talcott PA, eds. Small Animal Toxicology, 2nd ed. Philadelphia: Saunders, 2006; pp. 299–307.

Authors: Hwan Goo Kang DVM, PhD; Karyn Bischoff DVM, MS, DABVT

Consulting Editor: Lynn R. Hovda, RPH, DVM, MS, DACVIM

Drugs:
Over-the-Counter

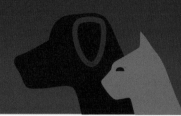

chapter 32

Acetaminophen

DEFINITION/OVERVIEW

- Acetaminophen (N-acetyl-p-aminophenol), also known as Tylenol, paracetamol, and APAP, is an OTC analgesic and antipyretic medication.
- It lacks anti-inflammatory effects.
- Accidental exposure or deliberate administration in dogs and cats can result in toxicosis due to a narrow margin of safety.
- Buildup of toxic metabolites and oxidative injury results when metabolic pathways for glucuronidation and sulfation are absent or depleted.
- Clinical signs are related to methemoglobinemia (MetHb) and hepatoxicity and can result from a single or cumulative dose.
- Common clinical signs include lethargy, respiratory distress, brown mucus membranes, icterus, and vomiting.

ETIOLOGY/PATHOPHYSIOLOGY

Mechanism of Action

- Acetaminophen is a COX-3 inhibitor.
- Although the exact mechanism is unknown, acetaminophen increases the pain threshold by inhibition of chemical mediators that sensitize pain receptors.
- Antipyretic effects are centrally mediated at the level of the hypothalamus due to inhibition of prostaglandin synthesis.

Pharmacokinetics/Absorption, Distribution, Metabolism, and Excretion

- Rapid absorption occurs in the stomach and small intestine after oral administration; peak blood levels are reached within 30 to 60 minutes.
- Poor plasma protein binding leads to wide systemic distribution.
- Metabolism in the liver is completed by three pathways: glucuronidation, sulfation, and cytochrome P-450 mediated oxidation.
- Part of the drug is metabolized into nontoxic conjugates by the glucuronidation and sulfation pathways, while some is excreted unchanged in the urine or metabolized to a toxic metabolite, N-acetyl-para-benzoquinoneimine (NAPQI) via the cytochrome P-450 enzyme pathway.

- NAPQI is normally detoxified by conjugation with glutathione (GSH) in the liver.

Toxicity

- The toxic dose is 75 to 100 mg/kg in dogs and as low as 10 mg/kg in cats.
- In dogs, hepatoxicity may be seen with doses from 75 to 100 mg/kg. MetHb may be seen with doses ≥200 mg/kg.
- Glucuronidation and sulfation elimination pathways become saturated as the drug dose increases and more of the drug is converted in to NAPQI. NAPQI accumulates as cellular stores of GSH are depleted, leading to oxidative injury.
- Cats are more sensitive to the toxic effects due to a deficiency in glucuronyl transferase, an enzyme required to metabolize acetaminophen via the glucuronidation pathway.
- Due to this deficiency, the sulfation pathway is quickly saturated, leaving more drug to be metabolized to NAPQI by the cytochrome P-450 enzyme pathway.

Systems Affected

- Hemic/lymphatic/immune
  - Heinz body and MetHb formation, with subsequent hemolytic anemia, result from binding of NAPQI and associated oxidative injury to the RBCs and Hb molecules.
  - MetHb is most commonly seen in cats but has been reported in dogs.
  - MetHb is a nonfunctional complex formed from Hb by the oxidation of Hb iron from the ferrous to the ferric state.
- Hepatobiliary—binding of NAPQI to hepatocyte membranes leads to hepatocellular death and central lobular necrosis
- Cardiovascular—collapse, shock, death, brown mucous membranes
- Gastrointestinal—vomiting, diarrhea secondary to hepatoxicity
- Nervous—hepatic encephalopathy secondary to hepatotoxicity
- Renal/urologic—renal tubular necrosis
- Respiratory—tachypnea, dyspnea, tissue hypoxia due to MetHb impairing RBC oxygen carrying capacity
- Skin/exocrine—facial or paw edema, icterus

 SIGNALMENT/HISTORY

Risk Factors

- No known risk factors exist.

Historical Findings

- History of exposure to or ingestion of drug
- Lethargy, brown mucus membranes, respiratory distress, edema of the face and paws in cats
- Lethargy, vomiting, diarrhea in dogs
- History may include a nonspecific ailment.
- Acetaminophen may be present with other medications in multisymptom cold and allergy products, and a thorough history must be obtained from the owner about the exact contents/ingredients.

Location and Circumstances of Poisoning

- Intoxication may result from deliberate administration to pets.
- Access to medications may lead to intoxication.

 # CLINICAL FEATURES

- Pets may present with either syndrome; however, cats commonly present with MetHb while dogs present with hepatotoxicity and associated GI and CNS signs.
  - Hepatotoxicity—hepatic failure, anorexia, nausea, vomiting, lethargy, abdominal pain, icterus, hepatic encephalopathy, coma
  - Methemoglobinemia—shock (tachycardia, tachypnea, hypothermia, weakness, collapse), brown mucus membranes, respiratory distress, cyanosis, lethargy, depression, coma, edema of face and paws

 # DIFFERENTIAL DIAGNOSIS

- Anemia
  - Oxidative damage (Heinz bodies) to RBCs may result from other oxidants, such as onion, garlic, and zinc.
    - Zinc toxicosis may also reveal a metallic foreign body on radiographs.
  - IMHA is diagnosed with the presence of spherocytes and/or autoagglutination; blood is not discoloured brown with IMHA.
  - *Mycoplasma felis* may be present on blood smear.
  - Respiratory distress or cyanosis may be due to primary cardiac or respiratory disease.
  - Facial and paw edema may result from hypersensitivity reactions or trauma.
- Hepatic failure (e.g., drug-induced, neoplasia, copper-storage disease, etc).
- Hepatitis, cholangiohepatitis, hepatotoxicity (e.g., *Amanita* mushrooms, NSAIDs, aflatoxins, xylitol, etc.)

DIAGNOSTICS

- CBC, chemistry profile, and UA are indicated. Abdominal imaging may be indicated if other differentials are considered (to rule out primary liver disease).
- CBC may reveal MetHb recognized as dark brown blood and Heinz body anemia.
- Serum chemistry profile may reveal elevated ALT, AST, and total bilirubin.
- Hypoglycemia and a prolonged PT/PTT time may be present in cases of severe hepatic dysfunction.

Pathological Findings

- Centrilobular hepatic necrosis
- Proximal renal tubular necrosis

THERAPEUTICS

Detoxification

- Induce vomiting within 2 hours of ingestion if the patient is asymptomatic.
- Administer activated charcoal (1–3 g/kg) with a cathartic once, if ingestion occurred <1 hour prior. Acetaminophen does not undergo significant enterohepatic recirculation, so multiple doses of activated charcoal are not routinely recommended and may interfere with oral administration of N-acetylcysteine (NAC).

Appropriate Health Care

- Minimize stress.
- Provide supplemental oxygen as indicated.
- Institute IV fluid therapy to provide hemodynamic support and treat for shock.
- Administer packed red blood cells as indicated.

Drug(s) and Antidotes of Choice

- Limit formation of the toxic metabolite, NAPQI, by providing glutathione substrates.
  - N-acetylcysteine (NAC) 140 mg/kg IV initial dose, followed by 70 mg/kg IV q 4–6 hours for 7–17 doses. NAC may be more effective given PO. NAC provides a substrate for sulfation, replenishes glutathione stores, and binds directly to NAPQI, the toxic metabolite.
- Antioxidant therapy
  - S-adenosyl-methionine (SAMe) 18 mg/kg/day PO may reduce oxidative damage.
  - Ascorbic acid (Vitamin C) 30 mg/kg PO, SQ, IV q 6 hours acts as an antioxidant to reduce MetHb to Hb.

- Increase oxygen carrying capacity.
    - Administer pRBC IV, 10–15 mL/kg as needed, or whole blood IV, 20 ml/kg as needed to effect.

Precautions/Interactions

- Activated charcoal may adsorb orally administered NAC, reducing its effect. If treating with oral NAC, separate administration of NAC and activated charcoal by at least 2 hours.

Alternative Drugs

- Cimetidine 5–10 mg/kg, IV, SQ, IM, q 6 hours may reduce metabolism of APAP by the p450 enzyme pathway.
- Oxyglobin 5–15 mL/kg, IV may be administered if pRBCs are unavailable. Caution should be taken to avoid volume overload, particularly when administering to cats.
- FFP 10–15 mL/kg, IV is indicated if a coagulopathy is present (based on PT/ PTT) due to severe hepatic dysfunction.
- Vitamin K 2.5–5 mg/kg/day, SQ or PO, q 12–24 hours can be administered to support productions of factors II, VII, IX, and X.
- Methylene blue, 1.5 mg/kg, IV x 1–2 doses, has been used to treat MetHb, but it can cause Heinz bodies and MetHb particularly in cats. It should be reserved for patients with severe MetHb.

 COMMENTS

Client Education

- Acetaminophen should never be administered to cats, and only to dogs with direct veterinary supervision.

Prevention/Avoidance

- Acetaminophen is commonly available in homes, and appropriate pet proofing and client education is important to prevent inadvertent or iatrogenic intoxication.

Expected Course and Prognosis

- Evidence of improvement includes resolving respiratory distress, normalization of mucus membrane color, improvement of laboratory values, resolving facial and paw edema, and improved mentation.
- Generally, a good prognosis is associated with ingestion of a low dose and prompt medical attention.
- Severe hepatic damage and coma represent a poor prognosis.

Synonyms

Tylenol toxicosis, paracetamol toxicosis

Abbreviations

ALT   = alanine aminotransferase
APAP   = N-acetyl-p-aminophenol
AST   = aspartate aminotransferase
CBC   = complete blood count
CNS   = central nervous system
COX   = cyclooxygenase
FFP   = fresh frozen plasma
GI   = gastrointestinal
GSH   = glutathione
Hb   = hemoglobin
IM   = intramuscular
IMHA   = immune-mediated hemolytic anemia
IV   = intravenous
MetHb = methemoglobinemia
NAC   = N-acetylcysteine
NAPQI = N-acetyl-para-benzoquinoneimine
NSAID = nonsteroidal anti-inflammatory
OTC   = over-the-counter
pRBC   = packed red blood cells
PO   = *per os* (by mouth)
PT   = prothrombin time
PTT   = partial thromboplastin time
q   = every
RBCs   = red blood cells
SAMe   = S-adenosyl-methionine
SQ   = subcutaneous
UA   = urinalysis

Suggested Reading

Alwood AJ. Acetaminophen. In: Silverstein DC and K Hopper, eds. Small Animal Critical Care Medicine. St. Louis: Saunders, 2009.

Aronson LR, Drobatz K. Acetaminophen toxicosis in 17 cats. J Vet Emerg Crit Care 1996; 6:65–69.

Richardson JA. Management of acetaminophen and ibuprofen toxicoses in dogs and cats. J Vet Emerg Crit Care 2000; 10:285–291.

Taylor NS, Dhupa N. Acetaminophen toxicity in cats and dogs. Compend Contin Educ Pract Vet 2000; 22:160–169.

Wallace KP, Center SA, Hickford FH. S-adenosyl-L-methionine (SAMe) for the treatment of acetaminophen toxicity in a dog. J Am Anim Hosp Assoc 2002; 38:246–254.

Authors: Danielle M Babski, DVM; Amie Koenig, DVM, DACVIM, DACVECC
Consulting Editors: Justine A. Lee, DVM, DACVECC; Ahna G. Brutlag, DVM

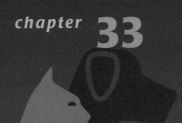

chapter 33

Antitussives/ Expectorants (Dextromethorphan)

DEFINITION/OVERVIEW

- Antitussives include a variety of OTC and prescription medications designed to help reduce coughing in those with upper respiratory infections or other similar illnesses.
- Dextromethorphan (DXM) is the most popular and widely available OTC antitussive.
- Available as a single-agent product or in combination with other OTC cough and cold medications, including analgesics (e.g., acetaminophen, ibuprofen, aspirin), decongestants (e.g., phenylephrine, pseudoephedrine), and antihistamines (e.g., diphenhydramine, chlorpheniramine)
- Available in tablet, capsule, or liquid forms in various dosage strengths between 5 and 40 mg of DXM per dose.
- DXM has been used in veterinary medicine to treat repetitive behavior in dogs. The recommended dose is 2 mg/kg PO q 12 hours.

ETIOLOGY/PATHOPHYSIOLOGY

Mechanism of Action

- Dextromethorphan is the d-isomer of 3-methoxy-N-methylmorphian, a synthetic analogue to codeine and structural analogue to ketamine.
- At therapeutic doses, it exerts antitussive effects by binding to the δ-opiate receptor.
- DXM exhibits no effects on κ or μ opiate receptors that normally impart analgesic effects.
- In overdoses, it, antagonizes N-methyl-D-aspartate (NMDA) glutamate receptors and prevents reuptake of serotonin (SE).

Pharmacokinetics

- Well absorbed orally; extensively (>90%) metabolized
- Serum levels peak approximately 2–4 hours postingestion.
- Undergoes significant first-pass metabolism to the active metabolite dextrorphan and 3-methoxymorphinan in the liver via CYP-450 system

- Volume of distribution varies: 3 L/kg (acute)—160 L/kg (therapeutic)
- Half-life: 2–4 hours, but may be longer with overdose
- Dextrorphan and 3-methoxymorphinan metabolized to 3-hydroxymorphinan
- Dextrorphan and 3-hydroxymorphinan conjugated with sulfate and glucuronide moieties and excreted in urine
- Little of the parent compound (<1%) recovered in urine

Toxicity

- Canine therapeutic dose: 2 mg/kg PO q 12 hours
- No reported canine or feline LD_{50}
- Mouse LD_{50}: 39 mg/kg
- Toxicity is largely dose dependent.
- Primarily affects the CNS
- Resultant behavioral effects can have secondary effects on cardiovascular and other systems.

Systems Affected

- Nervous—highly variable effects including depression or agitation, unprovoked aggressive behavior, apparent hallucinations, tremors, and seizure activity
- Cardiovascular—tachycardia (if agitated) or bradycardia (if sedated)
- Respiratory—tachypnea (if agitated) or hypoventilation (if sedated). Respiratory arrest is uncommon.
- Musculoskeletal—staggering gait, "robot" rigidity to the gait (humans)
- Endocrine/metabolic—hyperthermia secondary to neuromuscular effects
- Renal—renal impairment secondary to prolonged tremors, seizures, and/or hyperthermia
- Gastrointestinal—nausea, vomiting, diarrhea

 SIGNALMENT/HISTORY

Risk Factors

- No breed sensitivities identified
- Brachycephalic breeds may be at greater risk of developing respiratory difficulty due to their anatomy.
- Neonatal or geriatric pets or those with underlying health conditions may have an increased risk for severe toxicity.

Historical Findings

- Witnessed exposure
- Discovery of chewed tablets or spilled bottles of cough and cold products (e.g., cough syrup, decongestants, antihistamines)

- Owners may report behavioral changes such as excessive sedation or agitation (or both). Changes may be abrupt and difficult to predict.
- Unexpected aggressive behavior due to the presumed presence of hallucinations

Locations and Circumstances of Poisoning

- Exposures most likely to occur in the home
- Evidence of exposure often readily identifiable (e.g., spilled bottles, etc.)

Interactions with Drugs, Nutrients, or Environment

- Animals receiving other agents with sedative properties (e.g., antihistamines, tricyclic antidepressants, some analgesics, etc.) may experience more profound sedation due to additive effects.
- If ingested with sedatives, antihistamines, narcotics, illicit substances, etc., toxicity may be enhanced.

 CLINICAL FEATURES

- Clinical features vary widely based on the amount of DXM consumed.
- Effects from intoxication can be gradual, over a period of a few hours.
- Overall neurologic status may vary from sedated to highly agitated.
- Ataxia is common.
- Tremors or seizure activity may occur.
- Tachycardia or bradycardia (depending on level of agitation/sedation)
- Body temperature may be elevated secondary to agitation, tremors, or seizure activity.
- Anticholinergic coingestions (e.g., antihistamines) may result in generalized erythema, dry mucus membranes, and dilated pupils.
- Stimulant coingestions (e.g., decongestants) may result in tachycardia, agitation, or tremors.
- Some animals may develop serotonin syndrome due to DXM's ability to inhibit reuptake of SE. Serotonin syndrome is the overstimulation of SE receptors in the CNS, GIT, cardiovascular, and respiratory system. Clinical signs associated with serotonin syndrome include tremors, seizures, hyperesthesia, hyperthermia, hypersalivation, and death.
- Respiratory arrest is uncommon with DXM alone.

 DIFFERENTIAL DIAGNOSIS

- Other toxicities
  - Recreational/street drugs (e.g., stimulants, sedatives, hallucinogens)

- Other prescription and nonprescription drugs (e.g., antihistamines, amphetamines, benzodiazepines, sedatives), chocolate/caffeine/methylxanthines
- Primary metabolic disorders (e.g., hypoglycemia, hepatic disease resulting in hepatic encephalopathy, renal disease, etc.).
- Primary neurologic disease resulting in ataxia, sedation, behavioral changes, etc.

 # DIAGNOSTICS

- Commercially available urine drug screens may show false positive results for phencyclidine (PCP).
- DXM serum levels are not widely available or helpful in establishing diagnosis.
- Renal indices such as BUN and creatinine should be assessed in any symptomatic animal. Assess upon presentation and repeat 12–18 hours later if tremors, seizures, or severe hyperthermia develop.

 # THERAPEUTICS

- No well-established or accepted antidote exists.
- Overall approach to treatment involves early GI decontamination (if presenting shortly after ingestion) and supportive care for subsequent symptoms that arise.
- Determine if other common cold and flu products were also ingested (e.g., acetaminophen, antihistamines, etc).

Detoxification

- Induce emesis with apomorphine (0.03–0.04 mg/kg IV or 0.04–0.08 mg IM) or hydrogen peroxide (1–3 mL/kg PO) shortly after ingestion (within 15–30 minutes). Emesis initiated later may trigger seizure activity, so judicious decontamination should be performed.
- In asymptomatic patients, a single dose of activated charcoal with a cathartic within the first hour postingestion may be beneficial.
- Decontamination in the symptomatic animal is often not necessary, as the drug is already absorbed. Additionally, it may also put the patient at risk for aspiration pneumonia.
- No evidence that fluid diuresis is specifically beneficial to enhance elimination

Appropriate Health Care

- Treatment is largely symptomatic and supportive following decontamination.
- Symptomatic animals require in-patient hospitalization for 24 hours, or until clinical signs resolve.
- Assess vital signs (including TPR and mental/behavioral status).

- Establish IV access in any symptomatic animal.
- Agitation, hyperactivity, and tachycardia can be treated with phenothiazines.
- Benzodiazepines can also be used in animals not responding to these agents (see Precautions/Interactions).
- Seizure activity can be treated with standard doses of anticonvulsants.
- Closely monitor body temperature in any agitated/hyperactive animal. Hyperthermia should be treated as needed with cooling measures (e.g., water misting and fans, cooling blankets, etc.) if the temperature exceeds 105.5°F. Reassess body temperature frequently. Cooling measures should be discontinued at 103.5°F.
- Metabolic derangement such as acid-base imbalance or glucose metabolism is secondary to overall toxicity and should be managed supportively.
- IV fluids should be used to maintain hydration, perfusion, and ensure adequate urine output.

Drugs and Antidote of Choice

- Naloxone (0.02–0.04 mg/kg IV, IM or SQ) may be beneficial to reverse sedative effects, though effects are not uniform. Duration of effect is 30–60 minutes, necessitating frequent reassessment and possible redosing.
- Acepromazine (0.05–0.1 mg/kg IV, IM, or SQ) to control restlessness and agitation. Start at low end of range and increase as needed to effect. Chlorpromazine may also be used as an alternative.
- Cyproheptadine (1.1 mg/kg, PO or rectally, q 6–12 hours for dogs; 2–4 mg total per cat, PO or rectally q 6–12 hours) for serotonin syndrome. Cyproheptadine is a specific serotonin antagonist. Generally given orally, but can be administered rectally (same dose) in animals with severe signs or those recently administered activated charcoal.

Precautions/Interactions

- Benzodiazepines should generally be avoided if serotonin syndrome is present.

Nursing Care

- Monitor vital signs, including body temperature, HR, RR, and blood pressure routinely.
- Prevent unnecessary agitation by sequestering animal in quiet, dark area to decrease sensory stimulation.
- Monitor hydration status and urine output.
- Mental status of animal may wax and wane. Ensure measures are undertaken to provide for safety of animal and staff.

Follow-up

- Typically not needed unless end organ damage has occurred, requiring monitoring until resolution

Prevention

- Encourage animal owner to store DXM and all other prescription and nonprescription medications out of reach of animals.

 # COMMENTS

- Many cough and cold products contain multiple active ingredients; instruct owner to provide packaging of product to ensure accurate and complete identification.
- Cases can typically be managed with supportive care; ensure animal remains well hydrated and sedated (if signs of agitation are present) as needed until effects pass.
- Observe closely for evidence of serotonin syndrome and treat with sedatives and cyproheptadine as needed if present.

Expected Course and Prognosis

- Symptomatic animals require 24-hour hospitalization until symptoms resolve.
- Animals that present asymptomatic and remain so for 8 hours can be sent home for close observation over the following 24 hours.
- Young and otherwise healthy animals typically do well with symptomatic and supportive care.

Complications

- Renal impairment can occur if agitation or any seizure activity is not addressed quickly and aggressively with IV fluids.

Abbreviations

BP   = blood pressure
BUN   = blood urea nitrogen
CNS   = central nervous system
DMX   = dextromethorphan
GIT   = gastrointestinal tract
HR   = heart rate
IM   = intramuscular
IV   = intravenous
NMDA = N-methyl-D-aspartate
NSAID = nonsteroidal anti-inflammatory
OTC   = over-the-counter
PCP   = phencyclidine
PO   = *per os* (by mouth)
q   = every
RR   = respiratory rate

SE   = serotonin
SQ   = subcutaneous
TPR   = temperature, pulse rate, respiratory rate

See Also

Acetaminophen
Aspirin
Decongestants
Imidazoline Decongestants
Human NSAIDs

Suggested Reading

Barnhart, JW. Urinary excretion of dextromethorphan and three metabolites in dogs and humans. Toxic App Pharm 1980; 55:43–48.

Booth DM. Drugs affecting the respiratory system. In: Adams HR ed. Veterinary Pharmacology and Therapeutics, 8th ed. Ames: Iowa State University Press, 2001.

Dodman NA, Shuster L, Nesbitt G, et al. The use of dextromethorphan to treat repetitive self-directed scratching, biting, or chewing in dogs with allergic dermatitis. J Vet Pharmacol Ther 2004; 27(2):99–104.

Liang IE, Boyer EW. Dissociative agents: phencyclidine, ketamine and dextromethorphan. In: Shannon MW, Borron SW, Burns M, eds. Haddad and Winchester's Clinical Management of Poisoning and Drug Overdose, 4th ed. New York: Saunders, 2007.

Papich MG. Toxicoses from over-the-counter human drugs. Vet Clin North Am Small Anim Pract 1990; 20(2):431–451.

Author: Stephen H. LeMaster, PharmD, MPH
Consulting Editors: Ahna G. Brutlag, DVM; Justine A. Lee, DVM, DACVECC

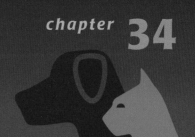

chapter 34

Aspirin

DEFINITION/OVERVIEW

- Aspirin, also known as acetylsalicylic acid (ASA), is a common OTC NSAID and antipyretic medication.
- Therapeutic indications in veterinary medicine include pain management for osteoarthritis and antithrombotic therapy.
- Toxic effects are dose dependent, ranging from GI side effects to multiple organ failure and death.

ETIOLOGY/PATHOPHYSIOLOGY

Mechanism of Action

- Aspirin is a nonselective prostaglandin inhibitor.
- Aspirin causes irreversible inhibition of COX that is needed to produce thromboxane, prostacyclin, and other prostaglandins.
- Inhibition of thromboxane and prostacyclin disrupts platelet aggregation and therefore can alter hemostasis.
- Inhibition of PGE_2 production disrupts normal GI and renal blood flow.
- Salicylates alter the Kreb's cycle, which leads to organ dysfunction from uncoupling of oxidative phosphorylation.

Pharmacokinetics/Absorption, Distribution, Metabolism, and Excretion

- Aspirin is easily and rapidly absorbed in the stomach and proximal small intestine.
- Aspirin is metabolized by the liver, intestines, and RBCs to salicylic acid.
- Salicyclic acid is highly protein bound (70%–90%) and conjugated with glucuronate and glycine.
- Conjugated forms of salicyclic acid are excreted in urine.
- Half-life of aspirin at 25 mg/kg dose: dog 7–8 hours, cat 38–45 hours
  - Cats have a prolonged half-life due to decreased amounts of glucuronate.
- When large quantities of aspirin are ingested, glucuronate conjugation is saturated, thereby decreasing the excretion rate.

- Excreted metabolites of aspirin lower the urinary pH, enabling renal tubular reabsorbtion and therefore prolonging the half-life.

Toxicity

- Intoxication is dose dependent.
- Mild toxicity (≤50 mg/kg) is usually limited to GI side effects.
- Significant toxicity has been reported with doses of 100–500 mg/kg in dogs and multiple doses of 80 mg/kg in cats.
- Exposures to ≥100 mg/kg may have the potential for death.
- Chronic administration of 23 mg/kg PO q 8 hours for ≥6 days produced gastric lesions in an experimental dog model.

Systems Affected

- Gastrointestinal—vomiting, hematemesis, diarrhea, melena, GI ulceration/ erosions
- Hematologic—anemia from GI hemorrhage, primary bone marrow suppression, or Heinz body formation (in cats)
- Renal—azotemia, ARF, anuria, sodium retention, fluid overload
- Hepatic—Hepatopathy induced by aspirin has been documented with high doses in cats.
- Respiratory—respiratory depression secondary to muscle weakness from hypokalemia and CNS depression, pulmonary edema
- Nervous system—CNS depression, seizures, cerebral edema (rare), coma and death

 SIGNALMENT/HISTORY

- Toxicity in small animals occurs by accidental ingestion, complications from prescribed chronic administration, or well-meaning attempts of the pet owner that exceed therapeutic dosages.

Risk Factors

- Cats and pets with coagulation disorders, underlying renal disease, concurrent steroid or NSAID administration, and hypoalbuminemia may be more susceptible.

Historical Findings

- Owners may report that their pet is currently receiving prescription aspirin or concurrent NSAID therapy.
- Owners may report that they self-medicated their pet with OTC medications containing aspirin/aspirin-related products (such as Pepto-Bismol).
- Chewed bottle or other container found by owner at home.

Interactions with Drugs, Nutrients, or Environment

- Animals on steroid therapy or prescription NSAIDs at the time of ingestion will have an increased risk of GI side effects, including vomiting, diarrhea, and ulcer formation.
- Old and/or expired aspirin degrades into salicylic and acetic acid, which does not need to be further conjugated by the liver to have a toxic effect.

 CLINICAL FEATURES

- Usually apparent within several hours after ingestion if acute intoxication; however, some clinical signs may not be apparent for days (e.g., septic peritonitis from GI perforation).
- Dehydration from excessive GI loss (e.g., vomiting, diarrhea, melena) may be noted on exam.
- Abdominal pain may be noted secondary to GI cramping, GI ulceration, or septic peritonitis from GI perforation.
- Pale mucous membranes, prolonged CRT, and poor femoral pulse quality may be present secondary to anemia or hypovolemia.
- Altered mentation from obtundation to severe coma
- Anemia from GIT blood loss
- Elevated anion gap
- Heinz body anemia in cats
- Tachypnea, increased respiratory effort, or dyspnea
- Pulmonary crackles on auscultation if pulmonary edema is present

 DIFFERENTIAL DIAGNOSIS

- Other substances containing salicylate, such as Pepto-Bismol, headache remedies, Bengay, oxycodone with aspirin combinations, and oil of wintergreen may cause salicylate toxicity with similar findings.
- NSAID toxicosis
- Primary or secondary coagulopathy (e.g., thrombocytopenia, etc.)
- Primary gastrointestinal disease
- Metabolic disease (e.g., renal, hepatic, hypoadrenocorticism)

 DIAGNOSTICS

- Baseline blood work (PCV/TS) is recommended to evaluate for anemia secondary to hemorrhage from the GIT. If anemia is present with no evidence of blood loss, a blood smear to screen for the presence of Heinz bodies should be performed, particularly in cats.

- An electrolyte panel should be performed to check for hypokalemia and hypernatremia.
- Increased liver enzymes (e.g., ALP, AST, ALT, and GGT) can be seen with hepatic toxicity.
- Blood gas analysis will usually show a respiratory alkalosis early on with progressive metabolic acidosis as toxicity progresses. An increased anion gap is also commonly seen due to increased lactate and ketone production along with the presence of salicylates themselves.
- Thoracic radiographs are indicated to evaluate for pulmonary edema if dyspnea, tachypnea, or hypoxemia is observed and/or pulmonary crackles are ausculted.
- Blood glucose should be initially evaluated and monitored. Care should be taken when evaluating a patient's glycemic status as neuroglycopenia can be present with a normal glucose reading on blood and/or serum.
- Baseline renal values and urinalysis should be considered, with repeat values done 24–48 hours after presentation to help monitor for development of ARF.
- Patients exhibiting bleeding tendencies and/or liver insufficiency warrant evaluation of the hemostatic system, which may include platelet count, PT, PTT, ACT, BMBT, or rarely, TEG.

 THERAPEUTICS

Detoxification

- Emesis is indicated if ingestion occurred up to several hours before presentation, provided the patient is asymptomatic and able to protect their airway.
- If emesis is unsuccessful, gastric lavage should be considered if ingestion was within 1–2 hours prior and/or an abdominal radiograph confirms the presence of gastric contents.
- Activated charcoal with a cathartic is recommended whether or not emesis or gastric lavage is successful in cases where there has been a massive overdose or ingestion of sustained-release or enteric-coated tablets.
- Repeated doses of activated charcoal without a cathartic should be given orally every 6–8 hours for 24 hours to prevent enterohepatic circulation.

Appropriate Health Care

- Aggressive IV fluids should be used to prevent dehydration, promote renal and GI perfusion, and vasodilate renal vessels.
- Peritoneal and/or hemodialysis should be considered for patients who develop ARF, fluid overload, persistent acidosis, or have deterioration of their neurologic status.

▪ Urine alkalinization therapy, with target urine pH within 7.5–8.0 and systemic pH within 7.35–7.5. This is usually attained by adding 1–2 mEq/kg of sodium bicarbonate, diluted with sterile water in a 1:1 ratio and administered as a bolus slowly IV. Once target range is reached, repeat urine and blood pH q 2–4 hours.

Drug(s) and Antidotes of Choice

▪ No antidote
▪ Treatment consists of decontamination, supportive care, and gastric protectants.
  • Misoprostol (2–5 µg/kg, PO q 8 hours) has been the most effective drug shown to help prevent GI ulcer formation due to NSAID administration and should be part of therapy to treat aspirin toxicosis.
  • GI protectant (e.g., sucralfate 250–1000 mg, PO q 6–8 hours)
  • Proton pump inhibitors (e.g., omeprazole 0.5–1 mg/kg, PO q 24 hours)
  • H$_2$ blockers (e.g., famotidine 0.5 mg/kg, IV or PO q 12 hours)
  • Consider antiemetics such as maropitant (1 mg/kg, SQ q 24 hours) for persistent vomiting if contraindications such as a GI perforation/septic abdomen have been ruled out.

Supportive Care

▪ If hypovolemic, the patient should be volume resuscitated with balanced crystalloid solutions. In severely hypoproteinemic patients, the addition of a synthetic colloid (e.g., Hetastarch) may be necessary.
▪ If the patient has severe blood loss (typically from the GIT), hemoglobin-containing solutions may be necessary, including WB, pRBC, or a hemoglobin-based oxygen carrier (e.g., Oxyglobin).
▪ If presumptive hepatopathy with concurrent coagulopathy is present, consider vitamin K$_1$ supplementation or S-adenosyl-methionine (SAMe) supplementation.
▪ Oxygen supplementation via oxygen cage, nasal cannula, or oxygen mask if hypoxemia present due to pulmonary edema

Monitoring

▪ Electrolytes to monitor for hypokalemia
▪ Blood glucose may be normal with neuroglycopenia.
▪ Acid/base status to help guide alkanization therapy and help offset progressive metabolic acidosis
▪ Monitor respiratory effort/rate in case pulmonary edema develops from toxicity. Pulse oximetry or arterial blood gas monitoring may be useful in determining if hypoxemia is present.
▪ Urine output (UOP) quantification can facilitate decisions for ongoing fluid therapy needs and possibly provide information that may raise a concern for the

development of oliguric (<0.5 mL/kg/hr) or anuric ARF. For those with significant toxicity exposure and concern for ARF, urinary catheter placement should be done to monitor UOP.

- Urinalysis may provide evidence of renal damage (e.g., casts prior to the development of azotemia).
- Monitor neurologic status; if cerebral edema suspected, mannitol should be administered (0.5–1.0 g/kg, IV over 20 minutes).

Precautions/Interactions

- Concurrent NSAIDs or steroid should be avoided.
- Other protein-bound drugs may alter metabolism of aspirin.

Follow-up

- If azotemia is evident during hospitalization, follow-up urinalysis and renal panels are warranted. Aggressive IV fluid therapy should be continued until clinical signs resolve or azotemia improves.

Diet

- A highly digestible bland diet is generally recommended for those patients showing GI signs such as vomiting and/or diarrhea. Once signs have resolved, they can be slowly weaned on to their regular diet.

Surgical Considerations

- If a GI ulcer causing excessive hemorrhage and/or possible associated perforation is suspected, abdominal exploration may be recommended to provide definitive treatment.

 COMMENTS

Prevention/Avoidance

- Prevention of aspirin toxicosis includes refraining from using aspirin for treatment as analgesic/anti-inflammatory in pets and having owners ensure that any aspirin in the house is secured and in out-of-reach locations in cabinets or drawers. This medication should never be left out on nightstands, in purses, or on countertops within reach of pets.

Possible Complications

- Chronic renal damage may be a problem for those dogs and/or cats that develop azotemia after toxic exposure.

Expected Course and Prognosis

- Prognosis varies depending on amount ingested. With lower doses (≤50 mg/kg), prognosis likely good with supportive care for GI side effects. With higher exposures (≥50 mg/kg), prognosis can be poor to guarded if multiple organ dysfunction develops, to fair if patient is treated aggressively and early.

Synonyms

salicylate toxicity, acetylsalicyclic acid toxicity, NSAID toxicity

Abbreviations

ACT = activated clotting time
ALP = alkaline phosphatase
ALT = alanine aminotransferase
ARF = acute renal failure
ASA = acetylsalicylic acid
AST = aspartate aminotransferase
BMBT = buccal mucosa bleeding time
CBC = complete blood count
CNS = central nervous system
COX = cyclooxygenase
CRT = capillary refill time
GI = gastrointestinal
GIT = gastrointestinal tract
GGT = gamma glutamyl transferase
IV = intravenous
NSAID = nonsteroidal anti-inflammatory
OTC = over-the-counter
PCV = packed cell volume
PGE_2 = prostaglandin E_2
PO = *per os* (by mouth)
pRBC = packed red blood cells
PT = prothrombin time
PTT = partial thromboplastin time
q = every
RBCs = red blood cells
SAMe = S-adenosyl-methionine
TEG = thromboelastography
TS = total solids
UOP = urine output
USG = urine specific gravity
WB = whole blood

See Also

Human NSAIDs

Suggested Reading

Alwood AJ. Salicylates. In: Silverstein DC, Hopper K, eds. Small Animal Critical Care Medicine. St. Louis: WB Saunders, 2009.

Curry SL, Cogar SM, Cook JL, Nonsteroidal anti-inflammatory drugs: a review. J Am Anim Hosp Assoc 2005; 41:298–309.

Gfeller RW, Meissonier SP, eds. Handbook of Small Animal Toxicology & Poisonings. St. Louis: Mosby, 1998.

Murphy MJ. Toxin exposures in dogs and cats: drugs and household products. J Am Vet Med Assoc 1994; 205(4):557–560.

Papich MG. An update on nonsteroidal anti-inflammatory drugs (NSAIDS) in small animals. Vet Clin North Am Small Anim Pract 2008; 38(6):1243–1266.

Authors: Megan I. Kaplan, DVM; Sean Smarick, VMD, DACVECC
Consulting Editors: Justine Lee, DVM, DACVECC; Ahna G. Brutlag, DVM

Decongestants (Pseudoephedrine, Phenylephrine)

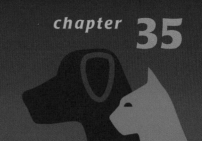

chapter **35**

DEFINITION/OVERVIEW

- Decongestants are commonly used by human beings for their vasoconstrictive effects.
- The most common OTC decongestants are pseudoephedrine (PSE) and phenylephrine.
- PSE is often found in cough/cold preparations, allergy (e.g., Claritin-D, Mucinex-D) and asthma medications, and diet pills.
  - PSE is currently available only from behind the pharmacy counter, as it is commonly used to create the illicit substance methamphetamine.
- Phenylephrine is found in cough/cold preparations (e.g., Benadryl-D), nasal sprays, and hemorrhoid products.
- PSE and phenylephrine are sympathomimetic drugs with alpha-adrenergic properties. Oral PSE and phenylephrine are not typically used in veterinary medicine (historical uses included increasing urethral sphincter tone).
- Clinical signs of toxicity include CNS stimulation, tachycardia, hypertension, decreased appetite, vomiting, mydriasis, and seizures.

ETIOLOGY/PATHOPHYSIOLOGY

Mechanism of Action

- PSE and phenylephrine are sympathomimetics, stimulating both alpha- and beta-adrenergic receptors by increasing levels of norepinephrine.
- PSE is a stereoisomer of ephedrine (from *Ephedra* sp.; see chapter 69, Ephedra/ Ma Huang).
- Phenylephrine typically does not stimulate beta-adrenergic receptors unless it is consumed at higher doses.

Pharmacokinetics/Absorption, Distribution, Metabolism, Excretion

- Absorption
  - Rapid absorption from the GIT with an onset of action generally <30–60 minutes.

285

- Distribution
  - PSE has low protein binding capacity (~20% in humans) and a relatively small distribution. Both PSE and phenylephrine are believed to cross the BBB and placenta.
- Metabolism
  - Both PSE and phenylephrine are metabolized by the liver. PSE is also partially metabolized to the active metabolite norpseudoephedrine.
- Excretion
  - Both drugs are primarily excreted in the urine, largely unchanged (55%–75%).
  - Low urine pH may increase the rate of excretion.
  - Both may be secreted in breast milk.
- Half-life
  - PSE = 2–21 hours (urine pH dependent)
  - Phenylephrine = 2–4 hours

Toxicity

- Phenylephrine
  - No established toxic dose in animals
  - Phenylephrine is less potent than PSE (in humans).
- Pseudoephedrine
  - Historical therapeutic dose: 1–2 mg/kg
  - Moderate to severe clinical signs: 5–6 mg/kg
  - Death: 10–12 mg/kg

Systems Affected

- Cardiovascular—Peripheral vasoconstriction leads to increased systemic vascular resistance and hypertension with tachycardia or reflex bradycardia. Beta-adrenergic stimulation results in tachycardia, increased contractility/output, and tachyarrhythmias.
- Nervous—Stimulation results from endogenous catecholamine release and adrenergic stimulation.
- Metabolic/endocrine—hyperthermia secondary to adrenergic effects (severe)
- Ophthalmic—Alpha-adrenergic stimulation causes mydriasis.
- Hemic—DIC (sequela to prolonged seizure activity and hyperthermia)
- Renal—myoglobinuria (sequela to prolonged seizure activity and hyperthermia)

 SIGNALMENT/HISTORY

- All breeds or species can be affected.

Risk Factors

- Animals with the underlying conditions:
  - Heart disease (including ventricular tachycardia)
  - Seizure disorder
  - Kidney disease (e.g., chronic renal failure, ARF, protein-losing enteropathy, etc.)
  - Diabetes mellitus
  - Glaucoma
  - Concurrent disease predisposing to hypertension (e.g., immune-mediated hemolytic anemia, hyperthyroidism, hyperadrenocorticism)

Historical Findings

- Well intentioned but misinformed owners may unknowingly administer OTC medications containing decongestants (e.g., Benadryl-D instead of plain Benadryl).
- Witnessed ingestion by pet owners, or evidence of chewed containers or pill holders
- Owners may report uncharacteristic behaviors such as restlessness, pacing, and agitation.

Interaction with Drugs, Nutrients, or Environment

- If ingested with any of the following agents, toxicity may be enhanced:
  - Other sympathomimetic agents (e.g., phenylpropanolamine)
  - Methylxanthines
  - MAO inhibitors (e.g., phenelzine, selegiline)

 ## CLINICAL FEATURES

- Initial signs may often occur within 30–60 minutes of ingestion but may be delayed with extended-release products.
- Clinical signs include hyperactivity, agitation, mydriasis, vomiting, tachycardia, hypertension (±reflex bradycardia), ventricular arrhythmias, hyperthermia, cyanosis, hypersalivation, tremors, and possible seizures. Rarely, cerebral hemorrhage may be seen.
- Animals that exhibit severe or sustained CNS signs and hyperthermia typically have a poorer prognosis.

 ## DIFFERENTIAL DIAGNOSIS

- Toxicities:
  - Amphetamines (both prescription and illicit)

- Phenylpropanolamine
- Methylxanthine

 # DIAGNOSTICS

- Minimum baseline blood work, including blood glucose, potassium, and venous blood gas, should be performed.
- Geriatric patients or those with underlying metabolic disease should have more extensive blood work done, including CBC, serum chemistry panel, and creatine kinase.
- Patient history and clinical signs may assist in diagnosis.

Pathological Findings

- None specified

 # THERAPEUTICS

- The goals of treatment are to prevent absorption, support the cardiovascular and neurological systems, and provide supportive care.

Detoxification

- Induce emesis if ingestion occurred within the previous 30 minutes and the pet is asymptomatic.
- If emesis was not induced at home, and the patient is asymptomatic, prompt emesis should be performed by the veterinarian.
- Activated charcoal with a cathartic may be given for one dose in asymptomatic patients.
- Multidose activated charcoal may be given to animals ingesting sustained-release formulations.
- Acidifying the urine may enhance excretion of PSE and phenylephrine.

Appropriate Health Care

- IV fluid therapy should be administered to aid in perfusion and excretion of the drug, maintain hydration, and help cool the patient (if hyperthermic).
- Cooling measures for hyperthermia if temperature >105.5°F; cooling measures should be discontinued at 103.5°F.

Drug(s) of Choice

- In patients demonstrating agitation or anxiety, sedation should be used (see Precautions/Interactions).
  - Acepromazine 0.05–1.0 mg/kg, IV, IM, or SQ PRN to effect; select dose based on severity of signs.

- Chlorpromazine 0.5–1 mg/kg, IV or IM PRN to effect; select dose based on severity of signs. Doses as great as 10–15 mg/kg have been necessary.
- In patients with tachycardia (dog >180 bpm; cat >220 bpm), a fast-acting beta-blocker should be used:
  - Propranolol 0.02 mg/kg IV slowly, up to a maximum of 1 mg/kg
  - Esmolol 0.25–0.5 mg/kg, IV slow load, then 10–200 μg/kg/min CRI
- With severe toxicity, seizures may be seen and should be treated with anticonvulsant therapy (see Precautions/Interactions).
  - Phenobarbital 4 mg/kg, IV x 4–5 doses to affect PRN.

Precautions/Interactions

- Benzodiazepines are not recommended as they may exacerbate signs.

Alternative Drugs

- Urinary acidification in dogs can be used to aid in excretion.
  - Ammonium chloride 50 mg/kg, PO q 6 hours
  - Ascorbic acid 20–30 mg/kg, SQ, IM or IV q 8 hours

Nursing Care

- Regulate body temperature, heart rate, and respiratory rate frequently.
- Ensure appropriate urine output (1–2 mL/kg/hr) and treat accordingly.
- Minimize stimulation or excitement.
- Monitor blood pressure and heart rhythm (with continuous ECG monitoring).

Follow-up

- Animals should be monitored in the clinic for 18–24 hours, or until clinical signs resolve.
- If the product was sustained release, the patient should be monitored for 24–72 hours, or until clinical signs resolve.

Prevention

- Pet owners should be advised to keep medications out of the reach of pets, preferably stored in locked cabinets or cabinets located high off the ground.

 # COMMENTS

Client Education

- Inform clients that medications with similar names contain vastly different ingredients (e.g., Benadryl vs. Benadryl-D).
- Ensure all medications have been picked up/safely stored prior to the pet's return.

Prevention/Avoidance

- Store medications in secured or difficult-to-reach cabinets.
- Keep purses and full shopping bags off of the floor.
- Do not leave medications on countertops that may be accessible by a pet.

Possible Complications

- DIC, rhabdomyolysis, and myoglobinuria (with subsequent ARF) may occur with prolonged, untreated tremors/seizures or hyperthermia.

Expected Course and Prognosis

- The earlier the animal is treated, the better the prognosis.
- Symptoms generally resolve within 1–24 hours for regular formulations, and within 24–72 hours for sustained-release formulations.
- Animals that exhibit severe or sustained CNS signs and hyperthermia typically have a poorer prognosis.
- Animals with DIC or myoglobinuria have a poorer prognosis and will need aggressive therapy, including 24-hour care, aggressive IV fluid therapy, FFP transfusions, and aggressive monitoring.

Synonyms

ephedrine, ephedra; methamphetamine; weight loss supplements

Abbreviations

ARF = acute renal failure
BBB = blood brain barrier
bpm = beats per minute
CBC = complete blood count
CNS = central nervous system
CRI = continuous rate infusion
DIC = disseminated intravascular coagulation
ECG = electrocardiogram
FFP = fresh frozen plasma
GIT = gastrointestinal tract
IM   = intramuscular
IV   = intravenous
OTC = over-the-counter
PO   = *per os* (by mouth)
PRN = *pro re nata* (as needed)
PSE = pseudoephedrine
q   = every
SQ   = subcutaneous

See Also

Amphetamines
Methamphetamine
Phenylpropanolamine (PPA)
Ephedra/Ma Huang

Suggested Reading

Bischoff K. Toxicity of over-the-counter drugs. In: Gupta RC, ed. Veterinary Toxicology: Basic and Clinical Principles. New York: Elsevier, 2007; p. 363.
Means C. Decongestants. In: Plumlee K, ed. Clinical Veterinary Toxicology. St. Louis: Mosby, 2005; p. 309.
Micromedex: MICROMEDEX® Healthcare Series. 2010. Accessed Jan. 2010.

Authors: Kelly M. Sioris, PharmD; Dean Filandrinos, PharmD
Consulting Editors: Justine A. Lee, DVM, DACVECC; Ahna G. Brutlag, DVM

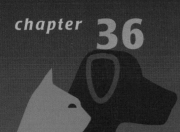

chapter **36**

Human NSAIDs (Ibuprofen, Naproxen)

DEFINITION/OVERVIEW

- NSAIDs have anti-inflammatory, analgesic, and antipyretic properties.
- OTC NSAIDs, such as ibuprofen and naproxen sodium, are a common source of toxicity for dogs, cats, and ferrets.
- Because pet owners are familiar with how NSAIDs affect themselves and these products are readily available, pet owners may administer NSAIDs to their pet when it is exhibiting signs of illness.
- Animals may intentionally ingest these medications in large quantities.
- Effects of NSAID toxicosis in veterinary patients include GI irritation/ulceration/perforation, ARF, and acute CNS impairment.

ETIOLOGY/PATHOPHYSIOLOGY

- Ibuprofen (trade names: Advil, Midol, Nuprin) is available in both OTC and Rx formulations. It comes in 50, 100, 200, 300, 400, 600, and 800 mg tablets and as 40 mg/mL and 100 mg/5 mL oral suspensions. It is also frequently included in several OTC combination flu/cold remedies.
- Naproxen sodium (trade names: Naprosyn, Anaprox, Aleve, and Napralen) is available in both OTC and Rx formulations. It comes in 200, 220, 250, 275, 375, 500, and 550 mg tablets, 375 and 500 mg controlled/delayed release tablets, and as a 25 mg/mL, 40 mg/mL, 125 mg/5 mL, and 375 mg/15 mL oral suspension.

Mechanism of Action

- Ibuprofen (2-[p-Isobutylphenyl] propionic acid) and naproxen sodium have anti-inflammatory, analgesic, and antipyretic properties.
- NSAIDs inhibit the conversion of arachadonic acid to prostaglandins by inhibition of COX enzymes. Prostaglandin inhibition is useful to reduce inflammation.
- Prostaglandins have many other beneficial functions in the body, such as maintaining blood flow to the kidneys and mucosa of the GIT, stimulating intestinal epithelial cell repair and turnover, and stimulating bicarbonate buffer secretion in the stomach.

Pharmacokinetics/Absorption, Distribution, Metabolism, and Excretion

- NSAIDs are well absorbed from the GIT (close to 100% bioavailability) and highly protein bound with a low volume of distribution. Because of the high degree of protein binding, very little of the parent drug is excreted intact through the kidneys.
- NSAIDs are predominantly metabolized in the liver to inactive compounds; however, there is extensive enterohepatic recirculation.
- There are marked differences in clearance and half-life of these drugs between species.
- Ibuprofen: rapidly absorbed after oral dosing (within 30 minutes to 1.5 hours); the plasma half-life in the dog is 2–2.5 hours.
- Naproxen sodium: rapidly absorbed after oral dosing, with 68%–100% bioavailability. It has a very long half-life in dogs (74 hours).

Toxicity

- Ibuprofen
  - GI signs >50–125 mg/kg (dogs); >50 mg/kg (cats). Note: GI irritation or ulceration has been reported in dogs at doses as low as 5–6 mg/kg/day with chronic administration.
  - Renal signs: >175 mg/kg (dogs)
  - CNS signs: >400 mg/kg (dogs)
  - Cats are more sensitive to the toxic effects of ibuprofen and exhibit signs of toxicity at approximately half the doses noted above due to limited hepatic glucuronidation. Renal signs are most commonly reported in cats, with or without GI signs.
  - The toxic dose of ibuprofen is not known in ferrets—acute CNS signs are most commonly reported in ferrets with or without GI or renal signs.
- Naproxen sodium
  - There is little information on the dosages at which clinical signs of toxicity occur; however, it is noted that as little as 5 mg/kg can produce GI signs in dogs. Doses >25 mg/kg can cause ARF.
  - Naproxen has a very long half-life and appears to have a very narrow therapeutic window in animals.

Systems Affected

- Gastrointestinal—anorexia, vomiting (±hematemesis), diarrhea (±melena, hematochezia), GI irritation, GI ulceration, gastric or duodenal perforation, abdominal pain, septic peritonitis
- Renal/urologic—ARF (oliguric or anuric)
- Nervous—acute ataxia, altered mentation, and seizures (with extremely high doses of ibuprofen)

- Cardiovascular—hemorrhagic shock secondary to severe GIT ulceration, septic shock secondary to septic peritonitis from a ruptured GIT ulcer
- Hemic/lymphatic/immune—anemia (with concurrent panhypoproteinemia) secondary to severe GIT ulceration; thrombocytopathia may occur as a result of altered platelet aggregation.

 # SIGNALMENT/HISTORY

- Cats, dogs, and ferrets have been documented to develop signs of toxicosis associated with overdose of these medications. Cats are more sensitive to ibuprofen than dogs.
- There are no breed or sex predilections for this toxicosis.

Risk Factors

- Underlying intestinal or renal pathology
- Animals with liver disease (delays metabolism)
- Geriatric and neonatal animals at higher risk for toxicity
- Hypoalbuminemia increases the risk for toxicity due to degree of protein binding.
- Inappropriate dosing by pet owner

Historical Findings

- Witnessed NSAID ingestion, owner administration of NSAID to pet, chewed container found in household.
- Clinical signs secondary to NSAID administration may be detected by the pet owner, including anorexia, vomiting (±hematemesis), diarrhea (±melena), weakness, abdominal pain, and sudden onset CNS signs (e.g., altered mentation, seizures).

Interactions with Drugs, Nutrients, or Environment

- Coadministration of more than one NSAID, such as an OTC medication, in addition to prescribed NSAID by a veterinarian may result in more severe clinical signs.
- Coadministration of an NSAID with corticosteroids may result in more severe clinical signs.

 # CLINICAL FEATURES

- Gastrointestinal
  - GI signs will usually develop within 2–6 hours of ingestion.
  - Signs of GI hemorrhage, ulceration, or perforation may be delayed 12 hours to 4–5 days following ingestion.

- With ibuprofen, lower doses (50–100 mg/kg in dogs) are usually associated with milder signs (e.g., inappetence, abdominal pain, vomiting, diarrhea), while higher doses (>100 mg/kg) are more likely to cause bleeding, ulceration, and/or perforation.
  - Clinical signs may include anorexia, abdominal pain, hypersalivation/nausea, melena on rectal examination, vomiting, and diarrhea.
- Renal
  - ARF may develop as early as 12 hours following ingestion but may be delayed 3–5 days following exposure.
  - Clinical signs may include depressed mentation, oliguria/anuria, pain on renal palpation (normal to enlarged kidney size), vomiting, uremic breath, and anorexia.
- Neurologic
  - Neurological signs are often noted within 1–2 hours of exposure when extremely high doses are ingested.
  - Clinical signs might include decreased mentation (e.g., obtundation, stupor, coma), respiratory depression, seizures, and delayed or absent PLR.

 DIFFERENTIAL DIAGNOSIS

- Primary GI disease—IBD, neoplasia, gastroenteritis, nonspecific gastritis
- Secondary GI disease:
  - Veterinary prescription NSAID toxicosis
  - Aspirin toxicosis
  - Ethylene glycol toxicosis
  - Gastric ulceration/bleeding secondary to ulcerated gastric masses, thrombocytopenia/thrombocytopathia, gastric foreign bodies
- Primary metabolic disease—renal:
  - Toxins: lily ingestion (cats), ethylene glycol ingestion
  - Chronic renal failure or acute on chronic renal failure
  - ARF secondary to hypoxia, ischemia
  - Ureteral obstruction
  - Urethral obstruction
  - Uroabdomen
  - Pyelonephritis
- Primary metabolic disease—hepatic, hepatic encephalopathy, hypoadrenocorticism, hypoglycemia
- Primary neurologic disease—intracranial disease (e.g., infectious, inflammatory, neoplastic, vascular)
- Secondary neurologic disease—ethylene glycol ingestion, hepatic encephalopathy

DIAGNOSTICS

- Baseline lab work
  - CBC, chemistry profile, UA, and USG (pre-fluid therapy) if >50 mg/kg ibuprofen was ingested
  - Baseline renal values should be obtained on admission. Repeated renal values should be checked at 24 and 48 hours following ingestion of nephrotoxic doses of ibuprofen. With naproxen, renal values should be monitored q 24 hours for 72 hours (minimum).
  - Baseline and serial PCV/TS should be followed daily in hospitalized animals with clinical GI signs, evidence of GI hemorrhage, or cardiovascular instability.
- Radiographs and/or abdominal ultrasound should be considered when abdominal pain or significant GI signs are present to rule out GIT perforation/septic peritonitis.

THERAPEUTICS

Detoxification

- Typically, for emesis to be effective, it should be induced within 30 minutes of ingestion (due to rapid GI absorption).
- If large amounts of tablets were ingested, emesis within 3–6 hours of ingestion may be effective as ibuprofen has been shown to form gastric concretions that may result in delayed breakdown and/or gastric emptying.
- If the animal has CNS signs, emesis should be avoided to prevent aspiration. Instead, secure the airway and perform gastric lavage.
- Administer activated charcoal (2–4 g/kg). A cathartic, such as sorbitol, should be added to the initial dose to increase GI transit time.
- Activated charcoal (1 g/kg) without a cathartic should be repeated q 4–6 hours for 24–48 hours (due to extensive enterohepatic recirculation).

Appropriate Health Care

- Supportive care:
  - Intubation ± mechanical ventilation if acute CNS signs or respiratory depression
  - Urine output should be monitored in animals exposed to a nephrotoxic dose of NSAIDs.
    - An indwelling urinary catheter and closed collection system should be used if oliguric (<1 mL/kg/hr).
    - CVP monitoring is useful to determine extent of volume expansion.

◻ If volume depleted and oliguric, IV fluid boluses (10 mL/kg over 30 minutes) can be used to expand the intravascular volume.

◻ If volume expanded and oliguric, furosemide (1–2 mg/kg IV) and/or mannitol (1 g/kg, IV, over 15 minutes) can be administered to encourage urine production.

Drug(s) and Antidotes of Choice

- Gastroprotection (5–7 days ibuprofen, 2 weeks for naproxen)
  - Misoprostol (2–5 µg/kg, PO q 8 hours)
  - H₂ blockers (e.g., famotidine 0.5 mg/kg, PO, IV, SQ q 12 hours)
  - Proton-pump inhibitors (e.g., omeprazole 0.7–1.4 mg/kg, PO q 12–24 hours or esomeprazole 0.7 mg/kg, IV q 12–24 hours)
  - Sucralfate (0.25–1 g, PO q 6–8 hours)
- IV fluid therapy should be used to maintain euvolemia, hydration, and renal perfusion.
  - Fluid diuresis (at least 6 mL/kg/hr of an isotonic crystalloid) should be performed for 48 hours with ibuprofen ingestions approaching nephrotoxic doses (exceeding 175 mg/kg [dogs] or 50 mg/kg [cats]).
  - Following toxic doses of naproxen, fluid diuresis should ensue for 72 hours.
- If hypoproteinemia results, artificial colloid therapy (e.g., Hetastarch at 1–2 mL/kg/hr) should be considered to maintain colloid osmotic pressure.
- Blood transfusion with pRBC as needed to maintain PCV ≥15%–20% if gastric hemorrhage noted.
- Seizures should be treated with anticonvulsants. Diazepam should be used to stop ongoing seizures (0.25–0.5 mg/kg, IV, to effect PRN). Intravenous phenobarbital loading (4 mg/kg, IV q 2–12 hours x 4–5 doses) should be used when cluster seizures occur.

Precautions/Interactions

- Sucralfate should be dosed at least 2 hours prior to other oral medications.
- Other NSAIDs, aspirin, or corticosteroids should be withheld from any animal with signs of toxicosis for 7–14 days, depending on the severity of toxicity.

Follow-up

- Renal values (e.g., BUN, creatinine, phosphorus) should be determined at time of admission. Recheck blood work should be performed at 24 and 48 hours in dogs ingesting a nephrotoxic dose of ibuprofen and for at least 72 hours following naproxen ingestion.

COMMENTS

Client Education

- Ibuprofen and naproxen sodium are not recommended for use in veterinary patients because of the risk for toxicity.
- Prescription and OTC NSAIDs should be kept out of reach of pets. Care should be taken to find and pick up any dropped medications, since as little as 1 tablet of 200 mg ibuprofen can be toxic to cats, ferrets, and small to moderate-sized dogs.

Patient Monitoring

- Appetite, vomiting, diarrhea, melena
- Renal parameters (e.g., BUN, creatinine, phosphorus)
- Monitor PCV/TS daily to evaluate for severity of blood loss, hemodilution, and hydration status.
- Urine output

Prevention/Avoidance

- Pet owners should be instructed to never administer OTC NSAIDs to their pet(s) unless under direct instruction of their veterinarian.
- There are several NSAIDs that have been specifically formulated and undergone extensive FDA testing and approval for veterinary patients. Veterinary approved COX-selective NSAIDs may reduce the toxic side effects from NSAIDs. Whenever possible, veterinarians should recommend these medications instead of human OTC NSAIDs.

Possible Complications

- Severe gastrointestinal hemorrhage
- Acute renal failure

Expected Course and Prognosis

- Prognosis is variable depending on the dose ingested and the duration of time elapsed from ingestion to admission to a veterinary clinic.

Abbreviations

ARF   = acute renal failure
BUN   = blood urea nitrogen
CBC   = complete blood count
CNS   = central nervous system
COX   = cyclooxygenase

CVP   = central venous pressure
GI   = gastrointestinal
GIT   = gastrointestinal tract
IBD   = inflammatory bowel disease
IV   = intravenous
NSAIDs = nonsteroidal anti-inflammatory drug(s)
OTC   = over-the-counter
PCV   = packed cell volume
PLR   = pupillary light reflexes
PO   = *per os* (by mouth)
pRBC   = packed red blood cells
PRN   = *pro re nata* (as needed)
q   = every
Rx   = prescription
SQ   = subcutaneous
TS   = total solids
UA   = urinalysis
USG   = urine specific gravity

See Also

Aspirin
Veterinary NSAIDs

Suggested Reading

Lees P, Landoni MF, Giraudel J, Toutain PL. Pharmacodynamics and pharmacokinetics of non-steroidal anti-inflammatory drugs in species of veterinary interest. J Vet Pharmacol Therapy 2004; 27:479–490.
Papich M. An update on nonsteroidal anti-inflammatory drugs (NSAIDs) in small animals. Vet Clin Small Anim 2008; 38:1243–1266.

Author: Rebecca S. Syring, DVM, DACVECC
Consulting Editors: Justine A. Lee, DVM, DACVECC; Ahna G. Brutlag, DVM

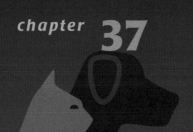

chapter 37

Imidazoline Decongestants

DEFINITION/OVERVIEW

- Imidazolines are a class of drugs that are commonly found in OTC nasal decongestants and ophthalmic preparations for the relief of redness and inflammation due to their topical vasoconstrictive activity.
- They are from a broader class of drugs known as sympathomimetics.
- Examples include oxymetazoline, tetrahydrozoline, naphazoline, and tolazoline.
- While generally safe and well tolerated in adult humans, oral overdoses in children have resulted in significant toxicosis. This is because overdosed amounts of the drug tend to have a central effect.
- The central action of the drug leads to significant CNS depression.

ETIOLOGY/PATHOPHYSIOLOGY

Mechanism of Action

- Imidazolines are sympathomimetic compounds specific to alpha$_2$ adrenergic receptors.
- Oxymetazoline and naphazoline have no effect on histamine H_1 and H_2 receptors.
- Tetrahydrozoline and tolazoline may influence H_2 receptors but not H_1.
- Imidazolines do not influence beta-adrenergic receptors.
- While imidazolines may bind to both central and peripheral receptors, central binding tends to predominate in overdose situations.
  - Central receptor binding will result in the inhibition of norepinephrine, resulting in decreased sympathetic response. Common side effects of this binding are hypotension, bradycardia, and lethargy.
  - Peripheral receptor binding will result in vasoconstriction (topical application) and hypertension.

Pharmacokinetics/Absorption, Distribution, Metabolism, and Excretion

- Information on companion animal pharmacokinetics is limited.

- Systemic absorption may follow topical administration.
- Imidazolines are readily absorbed from the GIT.
- The half-life of most imidazolines is 2–4 hours (humans).
- Widely distributed throughout the body. Though imidazoline receptors have been found in the brain, human studies have shown that their concentrations there were relatively low.
- Metabolism is not well understood but is thought to be (partly) hepatic.
- Imidazolines are eliminated, mostly unchanged, in the urine.

Toxicity

- Imidazolines have a narrow safety margin.
- Oxymetazoline oral LD_{50} (mice): 10 mg/kg
- No therapeutic dose known in veterinary literature

Systems Affected

- Cardiovascular—initial hypertension progressing to severe hypotension, bradycardia, weakness/lethargy, prolonged CRT, and hypoperfusion
- Respiratory—depression
- Nervous—may present as agitated or lethargic. Lethargy can progress to the point of coma.
- Neuromuscular—Animals may develop tremors or seizures.
- Ophthalmic—miotic pupils
- Gastrointestinal—vomiting/GI irritation

 SIGNALMENT/HISTORY

Risk Factors

- Animals with renal insufficiency may have reduced drug clearance, resulting in more severe or prolonged clinical signs.
- Neonates and geriatric animals may be more severely affected.
- Drugs of this class have a narrow safety margin and unknown therapeutic range.

Historical Findings

- Witnessed ingestion or administration
- Discovery of chewed nasal decongestant or "eye-drop" containers
- The owner may find the animal in a state of collapse.

Location and Circumstances of Poisoning

- Exposures generally occur in the home due to unsecured medications.

Interactions with Drugs, Nutrients or Environment

- Potentially fatal in combination with other drugs in this class or those exhibiting adrenoreceptor activity (e.g., clonidine, medetomidine, xylazine, tizanidine, detomidine, etc.). Clinicians should not attempt to induce vomiting in a cat exposed to imidazoline with any of these agents!
- Drugs with the capability of causing CNS depression such as opioids, barbiturates, or other sedatives/anticonvulsants may exacerbate toxicosis.
- Drugs with the capability of causing bradycardia, such as beta blockers, may exacerbate toxicosis.

 ## CLINICAL FEATURES

- Onset of symptoms is generally rapid (within 15 minutes).
- Animals may present with initial hypertension and agitation but will likely progress to depression and bradycardia.
- Cardiovascular collapse may be noted.

 ## DIFFERENTIAL DIAGNOSIS

- Dependent on the stage of toxicosis
- Toxicities—amphetamines, cocaine, other CNS stimulants (early stages)
- Toxicities—sedatives, opioids, tranquilizers (later stages)
- Primary cardiac disease resulting in bradycardia, hypotension, syncope, etc.
- Trauma or blood loss leading to collapse

 ## DIAGNOSTICS

- ECG—may show tachycardia or bradycardia depending on stage of presentation
- Blood pressure monitoring—may vary between hypertension and hypotension, trending toward hypotension
- Chemistry panel—In severe cases, blood glucose and electrolytes (especially potassium) should be monitored.
- As these cases may be critically ill, 24/7 intensive care (along with the ability to perform blood pressure monitoring) is essential.

Pathological Findings

- No specific gross or histopathologic findings

THERAPEUTICS

Detoxification

- It is NOT recommended to induce vomiting due to the rapid onset of CNS depression.
- Activated charcoal with a cathartic may be administered 1x if the animal is asymptomatic and in the early stages of ingestion.

Appropriate Health Care

- Hypotension—Aggressive IV fluids (e.g., a balanced electrolyte crystalloid at 20–30 mL/kg IV over 20–30 minutes, repeat 2–3x as needed) should be used to correct hypotension, as needed to effect. Diuresis does not enhance drug elimination.
- If patient does not respond to crystalloids, consider colloids such as Hetastarch (5 mL/kg IV aliquots—repeat 1–2x as needed).
- If patient is persistently hypotensive, vasopressors may be necessary (e.g., dopamine, 5–20 µg/kg/min IV CRI).
- Frequent monitoring of TPR, HR, blood pressure, mentation, and UOP

Drug(s) and Antidotes of Choice

- No specific antidotes are available; however, alpha$_2$ adrenergic antagonists may be helpful. They may need to be administered multiple times during the course of treatment as their half-life may not be as long as the imidazoline agent.
  - Yohimbine, 0.1 mg/kg IV, to reverse severe sedation and bradycardia
  - Atipamezole, 50 µg/kg IV or IM, to reverse severe sedation and bradycardia
- Atropine, 0.01–0.02 mg/kg IV, IM, SQ, as needed for bradycardia
- Diazepam, 0.5–1 mg/kg IV, as needed for tremors and seizures
- Antiemetics if vomiting is protracted (e.g., maropitant, 1 mg/kg SQ q 24 hours, not labeled for cats)

Precautions/Interactions

- Do not induce vomiting in symptomatic animals.
- Do not attempt to induce vomiting in a cat exposed to imidazolines with xylazine or medetomidine. This may exacerbate toxicosis.
- Any drug that may decrease blood pressure (e.g., beta-blockers, acepromazine, ACE inhibitors) should be used cautiously.

Alternative Drugs

- Naloxone, 0.011–0.022 mg/kg IV or IM q 1 hour or PRN, may also be used. The mechanism is currently unknown so success is unpredictable.

Follow-up

- Generally minimal in uncomplicated cases or cases in which clinical signs are easily controlled.

Diet

- Animal may return to normal diet at discharge or may be given several days of bland diet if GI irritation is persistent.

Activity

- Patient should be kept quiet and secure while symptomatic but may return to normal activity with successful resolution of the case.

Surgical Considerations

- No surgical considerations unless the animal has ingested large amounts of the container, and radiographic evidence or clinical signs of foreign body obstruction are present.

Prevention

- Imidazolines are not intended for use in companion animals.
- Imidazolines are readily available in multiple OTC preparations and their toxicity is widely underestimated for this reason. Owners and clinicians may not make the connection between exposure and symptoms.

 COMMENTS

Client Education

- Secure all medications, even OTCs, so they cannot be accessed by pets or children.
- Imidazolines are readily available in multiple OTC preparations and their toxicity is widely underestimated for this reason. This allows for dogs (most commonly) or cats to chew on bottles out of exploration/curiosity. Owners and clinicians are often unaware of the severity of toxicity, or may not make the connection between exposure and symptoms.
- Do not advise clients to use medicated OTC nasal sprays or eye-drops in their pets without educating them about the dangers of imidazolines.

Patient Monitoring

- Observation may be required for as long as 24–36 hours if the product is a sustained-release formulation.

Expected Course of Prognosis

- Generally good if treated early

Synonyms

oxymetazoline, naphazoline, tetrahydrozoline, tetrizolina, tetryzoline, xylometazoline

Abbreviations

ACE = angiotensin-converting enzyme
CNS = central nervous system
CRT = capillary refill time
ECG = electrocardiogram
GI   = gastrointestinal
GIT = gastrointestinal tract
HR   = heart rate
IM   = intramuscular
IV   = intravenous
OTC = over-the-counter
PRN = *pro re nata* (as needed)
q   = every
SQ   = subcutaneous
TPR = temperature/pulse/respiration
UOP = urine output

Suggested Reading

Daggy A, Kaplan R, Roberge R, Akhtar J. Pediatric Visine (tetrahydrozoline) ingestion: case report and review of imidazoline toxicity. Vet Hum Toxic 2003; 45(4):210–212.

Eddy O, Howell JM. Are one or two dangerous? Clonidine and topical imidazolines exposure in toddlers. J Emerg Med 2003; 25(3):297–302.

Fitzgerald KT, Bronstein AC, Flood AA. Over-the-counter drug toxicities in companion animals. Clin Tech Small Anim Pract 2006; 21(4):215–226.

Giovannoni, MP, Ghelardini C, Vergelli C, Piaz VD. Alpha-2 agonists as analgesic agents. Med Res Rev 2009; 29(2):339–368.

Imidazoline decongestants. Micromedex. Thomson Healthcare Evidence/Healthcare. http://www.thomsonhc.com/hcs/librarian/ND_T/HCS/ND_CPR/ToxicSubstanceLists/NDPR/Toxicology/CS/560128/DUPLICATIONSHIELDSYNC/0BCCE1/ND_PG/PRIH/ND_B/HS/ND_P/Toxicology/PFActionId/hcs.common.RetrieveDocumentCommon/DocId/81/ContentSeId/51>. Accessed, Sept 12, 2009.

Author: Nancy M. Gruber, DVM
Consulting Editors: Ahna G. Brutlag, DVM; Justine A. Lee, DVM, DACVECC

chapter **38**

Nicotine/Tobacco

 DEFINITION/OVERVIEW

- Nicotine is a rapid-onset, dose-dependent nicotinic ganglion depolarizer.
- CNS stimulation followed by depression is the common course of toxicity.
- Clinical signs often develop within 1 hour of ingestion.
- Nicotine is available in many products, including chewing tobacco, cigarettes, cigars, bidis, traditional nicotine replacement therapies (e.g., patches, gum), and newer replacement therapies such as electronic cigarettes, nasal sprays, and inhalers.
    - For nicotine content of common products, see table 38.1.
- Paper wrapping of cigars and bidis may also contain tobacco with nicotine.
    - Ingested cigarette butts may also cause toxicity.
- Some types of nicotine gums contain xylitol, which is also toxic to dogs.
- Although no longer legally used or sold in the United States, 0.05% to 4% nicotine sulfate spray or dust and 40% concentrated nicotine solution (e.g., Black Leaf 40) could be a rare source of nicotine toxicity.

 ETIOLOGY/PATHOPHYSIOLOGY

Mechanism of Action

- Low-dose and early high-dose intoxications result in widespread nervous system excitation due to depolarization and stimulation of nicotinic receptors in autonomic ganglia and neuromuscular junctions, as well as in the CNS, spinal cord, and adrenal medulla.
- Persistent ganglionic and neuromuscular junction depolarization and blockade from high-dose intoxication leads to progressive and pervasive nervous system depression.

Pharmacokinetics/Absorption, Distribution, Metabolism, and Excretion

- Slowly absorbed in the acidic gastric environment
- Much more quickly absorbed in the small intestine
- Eliminated via the kidneys

TABLE 38.1. Average nicotine content of selected products.

Nicotine-Containing Product	Average Nicotine Content (mg/g)	Average Nicotine Content per Typical Unit	Notes
Bidi cigar/cigarettes	15–25	4.7 mg per cigarette	• *Content varies widely*, even within the same brand • Usually flavored (e.g., cherry, mint, chocolate) • Unfiltered rolled tobacco *rolled in tobacco-containing paper* • Usually imported from India
Unfiltered cigarettes	11–30	12 mg per cigarette	• *Content varies widely*, even within the same brand • Average commercial brand product (United States)
Filtered cigarettes	7–30	11.8 mg per cigarette	• *Content varies widely*, even within the same brand • Average commercial brand product (United States)
Cigars	NA	100–444 mg per cigar	• *Wrapped in tobacco-containing paper* • *Cigar size is extremely variable*
Wet chewing tobacco	7–16	NA	• Some products flavored
Nicotine patches	NA	7–114 mg per patch	• Dose absorbed is dependent on whether patch is intact or has been broken or chewed
Nicotine gum	NA	2–4 mg per piece	

Note: NA = not available.

Toxicity

- Canine (oral) LD_{50}: 9–12 mg/kg. However, reports of dogs tolerating significantly higher doses have been made.
- Severe clinical toxicosis is rarely seen, likely due to multiple factors:
  - Central vomition center stimulation soon after ingestion with spontaneous vomiting of the product
  - Nicotine absorption is slow in the acidic gastric environment.
  - Most nicotine-containing products have limited palatability (with the possible exception of flavored chewing tobacco and other products with taste improvement additives such as gum).

Systems Affected

- Gastrointestinal—hypersalivation, vomiting (common shortly after ingestion), diarrhea
- Nervous—stimulation followed by depression, hyperexcitability, agitation, depression, ataxia, tremors, seizures (rare)
- Cardiovascular—tachycardia, hypertension, reflex bradycardia
- Respiratory—tachypnea
- Ophthalmic—mydriasis

 SIGNALMENT/HISTORY

- Seen in any indiscriminant chewers/eaters, especially puppies
- No breed or sex predilection

Risk Factors

- Preexisting cardiovascular or renal disease
- Neonatal and geriatric animals may be more severely affected.
- Presence of nicotine in the environment (e.g., owner is a smoker or trying to quit smoking using gums/patches)
- Access to ashtrays (as cigarette butts can also result in toxicity)

Historical Findings

- Witnessed ingestion
- Discovery of chewed nicotine-containing products (e.g., cigarettes, cigars, smoking-cessation patches or gums, etc.)
- Discovery of nicotine-containing products in the vomitus or stool
- The owners may report vomiting, hyperexcitment, or depression.

CLINICAL FEATURES

- Signs may begin within minutes of ingestion.
- Duration of signs in mild cases is 1–2 hours; in severe cases, 18–24 hours.
- Signs consistent with CNS excitement such as tremors, ataxia, weakness, sensory disturbances, and possibly seizures
- Stimulatory signs acquiesce to progressive CNS depression, descending weakness, and paralysis in high-dose intoxications.
- Simultaneous activation of parasympathetic and sympathetic ganglia at low doses can result in the following clinical signs:
  - Bradycardia, paroxysmal atrial fibrillation, and possible cardiac standstill from profound parasympathetic vagal stimulation

- Tachycardia, hypertension, and ventricular arrhythmias from adrenal and ganglionic sympathetic stimulation
  - Tachypnea and panting from stimulation of the brainstem respiratory center
  - Mydriasis
- Gastrointestinal signs include hypersalivation, vomiting, and diarrhea.
- Ganglionic blockade can lead to death from paralysis of skeletal respiratory muscles, central respiratory depression and subsequent arrest, or cardiovascular collapse.

 # DIFFERENTIAL DIAGNOSIS

- Primary cardiac disease resulting in tachycardia, bradycardia, syncope, etc.
- Primary neurologic disease
- Severe hypoglycemia (e.g., insulin overdose, insulinoma, iatrogenic, hunting dog, sepsis, hepatic disease, etc.)
- Neuromuscular disease (e.g., tick paralysis)
- Toxicities—chocolate/caffeine/methylxanthines, amphetamines, cocaine, carbamates, phenylpropanolamine, pyrethrins/pyrethroids, organophosphates, strychnine, tremorgenic mycotoxins, xylitol

 # DIAGNOSTICS

- Nicotine analysis of serum, gastric contents, or urine is available but rarely clinically useful due to the need for rapid diagnosis and treatment.
- ECG—Monitor symptomatic animals for tachyarrhythmias, ventricular arrhythmias, atrial fibrillation, etc.

Pathological Findings

- Gross and histopathologic findings are nonspecific.

 # THERAPEUTICS

Detoxification

- Gastrointestinal decontamination is the mainstay of therapy.
  - Induction of vomiting (nicotine is an emetic itself so vomiting may already have occurred) with recent ingestion
  - Activated charcoal with a cathartic (given once), provided the patient is asymptomatic and is at low risk for aspiration
  - With sustained-release products (e.g., transdermal patches), multiple doses of activated charcoal may beneficial. Additional doses of activated charcoal should not contain a cathartic.

Appropriate Health Care

- Treatment is symptomatic and supportive.
  - Supplemental oxygen and artificial respiration for respiratory distress
  - IV fluids for hypotension—a balanced electrolyte crystalloid can be administered in small aliquots (i.e., 20–30 mL/kg IV over 20–30 minutes, repeat 2–3x to effect) until blood pressure improves. IV fluids may also speed elimination of nicotine from the kidneys.
  - Antiemetic therapy
    - Maropitant, 1 mg/kg, SQ q 24 hours
    - Ondansetron, 0.1–0.2 mg/kg, IV, IM, SQ q 6–12 hours
  - Acidification of the urine may facilitate excretion.

Drug(s) and Antidotes of Choice

- No antidote available
- Cardiovascular support:
  - Atropine, 0.02–0.04 mg/kg IV or IM, as needed for bradycardia
  - Beta-blockers (e.g., propranolol, 0.02–0.06 mg/kg, IV slowly to effect) for hypertension or tachycardia
- Neurologic support/anticonvulsant therapy:
  - Diazepam, 0.5–1 mg/kg IV to effect
  - Phenobarbital, 2–10 mg/kg IV as needed
- Sedation/anxiolytic
  - Acepromazine at 0.05–0.1 mg/kg IM, SQ, IV as needed

Precautions/Interactions

- Avoid antacids as alkalization of stomach contents hastens absorption.

Nursing Care

- Regular monitoring of heart rate, blood pressure, ECG, and CNS status

Surgical Considerations

- Removal of extended-release nicotine patches from the GIT prevents continuous release and absorption.
- Endoscopy to remove intact transdermal patches in the stomach or proximal intestine
- Surgery to remove intact patches from the distal intestine

Environmental Issues

- Outdoor areas with large numbers of littered cigarette butts may pose a threat for nicotine ingestion as well as a potential foreign body risk.

COMMENTS

Client Education

- Inform staff and clients that some tobacco products are wrapped in tobacco-containing papers so ingestion of the paper alone may be toxic.
- Remind owners that nicotine products can be flavored, making them more appealing to pets. This warning applies to nicotine gums as well, which may also contain xylitol (see chapter 62, "Xylitol").
- Advise owners to not leave ashtrays/cigarette butts, packs of cigarettes, smoking-cessation drugs (e.g., gums, patches), or other nicotine-containing products in reach of pets.
- Many pets get exposed to nicotine after "purse-digging."

Patient Monitoring

- Regular monitoring of heart rate, blood pressure, ECG, and CNS status while hospitalized
- Once the animal is asymptomatic and stable without intervention, the pet may be discharged.

Expected Course and Prognosis

- Prognosis for low-dose ingestions is excellent.
- Prognosis for high-dose exposures is poor unless treatment is initiated early and the animal can be stabilized within the first 4 hours after ingestion.

Abbreviations

CNS = central nervous system
ECG = electrocardiogram
GIT = gastrointestinal tract
IM = intramuscular
IV = intravenous
LD_{50} = median lethal dose
q   = every
SQ = subcutaneous

See Also

Amphetamines
Chocolate and Caffeine
Cocaine
Ephedra/Ma Huang

Foreign Bodies
Imidazoline Decongestants
Metaldehyde Snail and Slug Bait
Methamphetamine
Mycotoxins—Tremorgenic
Organophosphate and Carbamate Insecticides
Phenylpropanolamine
Pyrethrins and Pyrethroids
Strychnine

Suggested Reading

Brutlag AG. Topical toxins. In: Ettinger SJ and Feldman EC, ed. Textbook of Veterinary Internal Medicine, 7th ed. St. Louis: Elsevier 2010; pp. 565–568.

Malson JL, Sims K, Murty R, Pickworth WB. Comparison of the nicotine content used in bidis and conventional cigarettes. Tob Control 2001; 10(2):181–183.

National Cancer Institute/National Institutes of Health. Questions and Answers About Cigar Smoking and Cancer. 2000. Available at http://www.cancer.gov/cancertopics/factsheet/Tobacco/cigars

Plumlee KH. Nicotine. In: Peterson ME, Talcott PA, eds. Small Animal Toxicology, 2nd ed. St Louis: Saunders, 2006; p 898.

Author Names: Carey L. Renken, MD; Ahna G. Brutlag, DVM
Consulting Editors: Ahna G. Brutlag, DVM; Justine A. Lee, DVM, DACVECC

chapter 39

Vitamins and Minerals

 ## DEFINITION/OVERVIEW

- Vitamins, in the form of single nutrient formulations, multivitamins, and pre-natal vitamins, are readily available in many homes. However, there is a paucity of veterinary literature describing toxicosis resulting from vitamin and mineral ingestion in small animals.
- In the United States, a multivitamin/mineral supplement is defined as a supplement containing three or more vitamins and minerals but does not include herbs, hormones, or drugs. Each nutrient is at a dose below the tolerable upper level determined for humans by the Food and Drug Board and the maximum daily intake to not cause a risk for adverse health effects.
- Among the common vitamins and minerals found within readily available multivitamin, prenatal, and single nutrient formulations, the most dangerous ingredients resulting in toxicosis following acute ingestion are vitamin A, vitamin D_3, and iron.
- Management of patients who have ingested any vitamin or mineral containing medication entails calculation of amount consumed, emesis, specific antidote therapy if indicated, monitoring, and supportive care.
- Prognosis following vitamin and/or mineral toxicosis depends on ingested ingredient(s), health status of the pet, prompt and appropriate care, and response to treatment.

 ## ETIOLOGY/PATHOPHYSIOLOGY

Mechanism of Action

- Common ingredients found within commercially available multivitamins in the United States may include the following items, though in variable amounts depending on the manufacturer and formulation.
  - Vitamin A
  - Vitamin B_1 (thiamine)
  - Vitamin B_2 (riboflavin)
  - Vitamin B_3 (niacin)
  - Vitamin B_6 (pyridoxine)

- • Vitamin B_{12} (cobalamin)
- • Vitamin C (ascorbic acid)
- • Vitamin D_3 (cholecalciferol)
- • Vitamin E
- • Biotin
- • Calcium
- • Copper
- • Folic acid
- • Iodine
- • Iron
- • Magnesium
- • Pantothenic acid
- • Phosphorus
- • Zinc

■ Many formulations are available in order to appeal to the vast array of consumer demands (e.g., adult, children, men, women), health needs, desired dosing regimen, and preferred formulation type (e.g., tablets, capsules, powders, liquids, and chewables; fig. 39.1). Vitamin and mineral supplements labeled "high potency" are required to have 100% of the recommended daily value for at least two-thirds of the ingredients contained within the supplement, as dictated by the Food and Drug Administration.

■ Prenatal vitamins, which are recommended for women of childbearing age who are attempting to become pregnant or are known to be pregnant, may contain many of the same ingredients found in multivitamins but tend to have higher

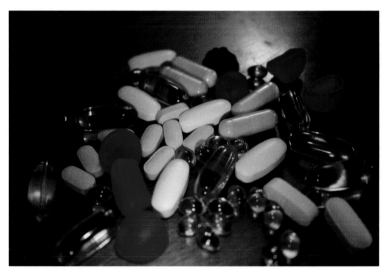

■ **Fig. 39.1.** An assortment of vitamin and mineral supplements in different shapes, sizes, and formulations. (Photo courtesy of Dana L. Clarke)

compositions of folic acid, calcium, and iron. However, as with multivitamins, the composition and nutrient amount varies greatly by manufacturer.

- All commercial pet foods contain added vitamins and minerals, in amounts to provide necessary nutrients and withstand manufacturing and storage impacts. Pet foods that have been certified by the Association of American Feed Control Officials (AAFCO) are guaranteed to meet minimal nutrient requirements for given stages of life. Therefore, additional supplementation of vitamins and minerals for pets being fed a high-quality balanced diet is not necessary.

Pharmacokinetics/Absorption, Distribution, Metabolism, and Excretion

- Vitamin absorption depends mostly on the solubility of the vitamin: fat-soluble vitamins require bile salts and fat in order to be passively absorbed in the duodenum and ileum, whereas water-soluble vitamins require active transport for uptake from the GIT.
- Mineral absorption depends on solubility, density, and mineral-mineral interactions in both the GIT and tissue storage level.
- Please see supplement 39.1 at the end of the chapter for further information on distribution, metabolism, and excretion of vitamins and minerals.

Toxicity

- Of the common vitamins and minerals contained within single nutrient supplements, multivitamin/multimineral supplements, and prenatal supplements, **vitamins A, D$_3$,** and **iron** are the most likely to cause significant clinical signs.
- The remaining vitamins and minerals are likely to cause mild GIT signs, such as vomiting, diarrhea, and anorexia, when ingested in large quantities. Specific vitamin or mineral toxicity is otherwise uncommon.
- **Vitamins E, K, B$_2$, B$_3$,** and **B$_6$** are considered to be minimally toxic. No toxicosis has been associated with supplements containing **vitamin C, pantothenic acid, folic acid, biotin,** and **zinc.**
- **Calcium, phosphorus, iodine,** and **magnesium** may be associated with specific clinical signs or end-organ damage (see Systems Affected).
- Massive ingestion of capsules or tablets can result in bezoar formation and may require gastric lavage for removal.
- **Vitamin A**—For acute vitamin A toxicosis, clinical signs are usually associated with ingested amounts that exceed 10 to 1000 x the daily requirement.
- **Vitamin D$_3$**—The reported LD$_{50}$ for vitamin D$_3$ is 88 mg/kg in dogs; however, ingested doses of less than 0.1 mg/kg can cause mild GIT signs, whereas doses of greater than 0.1 mg/kg can lead to hypercalcemia and ARF. To calculate the amount of vitamin D$_3$ ingested, it is important to note that 1 IU of vitamin D$_3$ equals 0.025 µg or 0.000025 mg of vitamin D$_3$. See chapter 100 on vitamin D$_3$/cholecalciferol.

■ **Iron**—In dogs ingesting less than 20 mg/kg of elemental iron, no clinical signs have been reported. When amounts between 20 and 60 mg/kg of elemental iron are consumed, mild clinical signs may be seen. Doses above 60 mg/kg may cause severe clinical sings, and death may result from doses between 100 to 200 mg/kg. See chapter 84 on iron toxicosis.

Systems Affected

■ Gastrointestinal
  • Vomiting—may be seen with ingestion of any vitamin or mineral
  • Diarrhea—may be seen with ingestion of any vitamin or mineral
  • Anorexia—may be seen with ingestion of any vitamin or mineral
  • Gastrointestinal bleeding—seen with iron toxicosis
  • Gastrointestinal strictures—late complication seen with iron toxicosis
  • Hematochezia—associated with vitamin B_3 (niacin) toxicosis
■ Nervous
  • Flaccid paralysis—associated with magnesium toxicosis
  • Tremors/convulsions—associated with vitamin A and B_3 toxicosis
  • Paralysis—seen with vitamin A toxicosis
  • Ataxia—seen with vitamin B_6 (pyridoxine) toxicosis
  • Abnormal reflexes—associated with vitamin B_{12} (cobalamin) toxicosis
■ Musculoskeletal
  • Lameness—associated with calcium and vitamin D_3 toxicosis
  • Soft tissue calcifications—associated with phosphorus toxicosis
  • Cervical spondylosis—seen with vitamin A toxicosis
  • Long bone fractures—seen with vitamin A toxicosis
■ Renal/urologic
  • ARF—seen with vitamin D_3 toxicity
  • Uroliths—seen with calcium, phosphorus, and magnesium toxicosis
■ Endocrine/metabolic
  • Hypercalcemia—seen with calcium and vitamin D_3 toxicosis
  • Secondary hyperparathyroidism—seen with phosphorus toxicosis
■ Hemic/lymphatic/immune
  • Coagulopathy—associated with vitamin A and E toxicosis
  • Anemia—seen with vitamin A toxicosis
■ Hepatobiliary
  • Hepatitis/increased liver enzymes/decreased hepatic function—seen with vitamin A and copper toxicosis
■ Cardiovascular
  • Hypotension and bradycardia—associated with vitamin B_1 (thiamine) toxicosis
■ Skin/exocrine
  • Rough haircoat—associated with chronic iodine toxicosis

SIGNALMENT/HISTORY

- There are no breed, sex, or age predilections for nutritional supplement toxicosis.
- While no mean age has been reported, it is likely that younger animals are more frequently affected given their increased incidence of ingesting foreign objects.

Risk Factors

- Animals living in homes or areas where vitamin or mineral supplements are stored
- Animals with renal disease could be at increased risk of more severe consequences after vitamin D_3 or calcium ingestion.

Historical Findings

- Ingestion of vitamin or mineral supplements may be witnessed by the owners, or suspected based on damaged packaging or spilled supplements.
- Owners may witness vomiting (which may or may not contain supplements), diarrhea, and neurologic changes.

Location and Circumstances of Poisoning

- Ingestion often occurs when plastic baggies are used to temporarily store medications.
- Ingestion often occurs when dogs chew on weekly plastic pill holders, which are not pet-proof.

 CLINICAL FEATURES

- Gastrointestinal—vomiting, diarrhea, anorexia, GIT bleeding, hematochezia
- Nervous—abnormal reflexes, ataxia, tremors, convulsions, flaccid paralysis, paralysis
- Musculoskeletal—lameness, soft tissue calcification, cervical spondylosis, long bone fractures
- Renal/urologic—pain on abdominal (specifically, kidney or bladder) palpation
- Cardiovascular—bradycardia, poor pulse quality
- Skin/exocrine—rough hair coat

 DIFFERENTIAL DIAGNOSIS

- Vomiting, diarrhea, anorexia, and GIT bleeding due to other primary or secondary GIT disease

- ARF
- Liver dysfunction or failure
- Ataxia, tremors, and paralysis due to other primary or secondary neurologic disease

 DIAGNOSTICS

- A baseline CBC and serum chemistry should be considered in any animal where **multivitamin/multimineral/prenatal supplement** ingestion is suspected, especially when the ingested amount is unknown.
- In animals known to have ingested near-toxic or toxic amounts of **vitamin D_3** and calcium, total calcium, ionized calcium, BUN, creatinine, and urinalysis (including urine specific gravity) should be measured.
- For patients ingesting near-toxic or toxic amounts of **vitamin A** and **copper**, special attention should be directed toward liver enzymes and measures of liver function (e.g., BUN, glucose, albumin, and cholesterol).
- For animals ingesting toxic or near-toxic doses of **vitamin A**, a complete coagulation panel (e.g., PT, PTT, platelets, and d-dimers) should be measured.
- For patients with severe tremors from **multivitamin** ingestion, serum AST and CK, as well as blood lactate, should be monitored.
- For any patient ingesting elemental **iron** at toxic or near-toxic doses, serum iron concentration and total iron binding capacity should be measured. See chapter 84 for more information about iron toxicity.

Pathological Findings

- Gross or histopathologic lesions seen in animals that have ingested multivitamins/multiminerals/prenatal supplements will depend on the ingested dose of a particular vitamin or mineral.
- Gross necropsy findings in pets that have ingested toxic amounts of vitamin or mineral supplements may include whole or partial tablets or capsules within the GIT, GIT bleeding (iron), GIT stricture formation (iron), soft tissue mineralization (calcium, phosphorus), long bone fracture (vitamin A), cervical spondylosis (vitamin A), nephroliths/uroliths (calcium, phosphorus), renomegaly due to ARF (vitamin D_3), and hepatomegaly associated with hepatitis (copper).
- Histopathologic lesions seen in pets ingesting toxic amounts of vitamin or mineral supplements include GIT ulceration (iron), fibrous tissue deposition within the GIT (iron), acute tubular necrosis (vitamin D_3), hepatitis (copper), and soft tissue calcification (phosphorus, calcium).
- For more detailed information on the gross and histopathologic lesions associated with iron toxicity, see chapter 84.

THERAPEUTICS

- If an animal is healthy and did not ingest a toxic or near-toxic amount of any vitamin or mineral, no further action aside from monitoring by the owner is needed.
- If an animal is found to have ingested a toxic or near-toxic dose of any vitamin or mineral, or if there is preexisting hepatic or renal dysfunction, emesis should be induced, and activated charcoal with a cathartic should be administered. For the most dangerous vitamin and mineral toxicoses (vitamins A and D_3), repeat doses of activated charcoal (without a cathartic) may be considered. Activated charcoal does not bind to iron well. See chapter 84 for more information on iron toxicosis.
- Intravenous fluids should be used to manage hydration and prevent hypovolemia in any patient showing clinical signs associated with vitamin or mineral toxicosis.
- Electrolytes, renal values, clotting times, and liver enzymes/measures of liver function should be monitored as indicated by the toxicosis and any underlying disease process.

Detoxification

- In patients presenting with recent, suspected, or confirmed multivitamin or multimineral toxicosis, emesis should be induced as quickly and safely as possible.
- For neurologically inappropriate patients who have ingested multivitamins, initial treatment should be aimed at managing neurologic signs, such as paralysis, tremors, or convulsions. Appropriate sedation, intubation (to protect the airway), and gastric lavage should be considered to facilitate decontamination if the supplements are still suspected to be within the stomach.
- As massive ingestion may result in a gastric bezoar, gastric lavage may be indicated for decontamination.

Appropriate Health Care

- In general, fluid therapy (either IV or SQ, depending on the severity of the toxicosis and clinical symptoms) should be used to manage hydration and prevent hypovolemia.
- Aggressive IV fluids and medications to increase calciuresis may be necessary for patients with vitamin D_3 toxicity; see chapter 100.
- With vitamin D_3 toxicosis, aggressive monitoring of renal values, electrolytes, and assessment for hydration (e.g., skin turgor, chemosis, peripheral edema, PCV/TS, weight, urine output) should be performed in all patients where there is concern for hypercalcemia-induced ARF, especially if furosemide has been given.

- Gastroprotectants and antiemetics may be necessary with multivitamin toxicity, including the following:
  - Famotidine 0.5–1.0 mg/kg IV q 12–24 hours
  - Pantoprazole 1 mg/kg IV q 24 hours
  - Sucralfate suspension 0.5–1 g PO q 8 hours, administered 30–60 minutes after any medication aimed at decreasing gastric acid production
  - Ondansetron 0.1–0.2 mg/kg IV q 8–12 hours
  - Maropitant 1 mg/kg SQ q 24 hours (for up to 5 days)
- For patients with tremors or convulsions, body temperature, patient comfort, hydration, and blood lactate should be closely monitored.
- For patients with severe tremors or convulsions secondary to vitamin or mineral supplement toxicosis, they should be controlled with diazepam (0.5–1 mg/kg IV) or midazolam (0.2–0.5 mg/kg IV). For patients with ongoing tremors or convulsions, a diazepam (0.25–1 mg/kg/hr) or midazolam (0.1–0.5 mg/kg/hr) CRI may be needed.

Drug(s) and Antidotes of Choice

- In patients at risk of iron toxicosis or those that are showing clinical signs, chelation therapy and gastroprotectants are indicated. See chapter 84 for more information on iron chelation and gastroprotection.

Follow-up

- The need for follow-up care will depend on extent of end organ damage or dysfunction and response to therapy.
- If there are derangements in liver or kidney values, patients will likely require follow-up blood work 5–10 days after discharge and may require more long-term monitoring if abnormalities persist.

Diet

- For patients with any neurologic compromise, vomiting, or regurgitation, oral food and water should be withheld until the patient is neurologically appropriate and GIT signs have resolved.

Prevention

- Proper storage of vitamin and mineral supplements in an area inaccessible to pets will help prevent toxicosis.
- Clients should be advised that pets being fed an AAFCO-approved, balanced commercial diet do not require additional vitamin or mineral supplementation; therefore, they should not administer any nutritional supplements unless specifically instructed by a veterinarian.

COMMENTS

Client Education

- Clients should be educated on the mechanism of action of the specific vitamin or mineral toxicosis, as well as given recommendations for safe storage.
- Clients should also be informed that children are also at risk of vitamin or mineral toxicosis if large doses are ingested.
- Information about the gradual reintroduction of a bland diet, monitoring for ongoing GIT and neurologic signs, and general observation instructions should be provided.
- For patients with persistent renal, hematologic, or hepatic derangements, clients should be given clear instructions about frequency of follow-up monitoring, possibility of permanent end organ injury, and dietary or medication adjustments that are required based on organ dysfunction.

Patient Monitoring

- For patients with hypercalcemia, serum total and ionized calcium should be monitored every 12–24 hours, and more frequently if therapy to treat hypercalcemia is being used. Electrolytes (e.g., sodium, potassium, and chloride) should be monitored every 12–24 hours if furosemide therapy is used.
- For patients at risk for or those with ARF, renal values and PCV/TS should also be measured at least every 12–24 hours. Urine output should be measured every 2–4 hours. Patients should be weighed every 6–8 hours to help assess fluid balance.
- For coagulopathic patients, clotting times should be measured at least every 24 hours and more frequently if being treated with FFP to assess success of therapy.
- In patients with hepatic failure, blood glucose should be monitored every 2–4 hours and supplemented as needed.
- In patients with elevations in liver enzymes, after baseline values are obtained, reassessment should be performed every 3–7 days depending on clinical course.
- Neurologic status should be monitored every 2–4 hours, as well as body temperature, gag reflex, and blood lactate in any patient with tremors, paralysis, or other neurologic impairment.
- For patients with iron toxicosis, serum iron concentration and total iron binding capacity should be measured at presentation and during chelation therapy. See chapter 84 for monitoring the patient with iron toxicosis.

Prevention/Avoidance

- Education about proper storage and handling of vitamin and mineral supplements will help prevent re-exposure.

Possible Complications

- ARF
- Chronic renal failure after resolution of ARF
- Liver failure/hepatitis
- GIT hemorrhage
- GIT stricture
- Paralysis, tremors

Expected Course and Prognosis

- For patients that do not consume a toxic amount of any vitamin or mineral, owners can expect self-limiting GIT signs that should resolve on their own within 12–48 hours.
- There are four stages associated with iron toxicosis: the first stage starts within 6 hours of iron ingestion, and the fourth stage may not be seen for 2–6 weeks after ingestion. Without aggressive supportive care, monitoring, and chelation therapy, acute iron poisoning is potentially lethal in animals. For more specific information about the prognosis and clinical course expected with iron toxicosis, please see chapter 84.
- For patients with hypercalcemia secondary to vitamin D_3 toxicity, prognosis and clinical course will depend on how soon treatment for hypercalcemia is initiated and response to therapy. For patients that develop ARF secondary to hypercalcemia, even though aggressive care is absolutely warranted, a guarded prognosis must be given.
- The prognosis for vitamin A toxicosis is likely favorable with appropriate treatment and supportive care.

Synonyms

multivitamin toxicosis, multimineral toxicosis, prenatal vitamin/mineral toxicosis, vitamin or mineral supplement toxicosis

Abbreviations

AAFCO = Association of American Feed Control Officials
ARF   = acute renal failure
AST   = aspartate aminotransferase
BUN   = blood urea nitrogen
CBC   = complete blood count
CK   = creatine kinase
FFP   = fresh frozen plasma
GIT   = gastrointestinal tract
IV   = intravenous
PCV   = packed cell volume

PO   = *per os* (by mouth)
PT   = prothrombin time
PTT   = partial thromboplastin time
q   = every
SQ   = subcutaneous
TS   = total solids

See Also

Calcium Supplements
Cholecalciferol
Iron

Suggested Reading

Albretsen A. The toxicity of iron, an essential element. Vet Med 2006; 82–90.
Gross KL, Wedekind KJ, Cowell CS, et al. Nutrients. In: Hand MS, Thatcher CD, Remillard RL, et al. Small Animal Clinical Nutrition, 4th ed. Marceline, MO: Walsworth, 2000.
McKnight KL. Ingestion of over-the-counter calcium supplements. Vet Tech 2006; 446–447, 451.
Murphy LA. Toxicities from over the counter drugs. In: Kahn CM, ed. Merck Veterinary Manual, 9th ed. Whitehouse Station, NJ: Merck, 2005.

Authors: Dana L. Clarke, VMD; Justine A. Lee, DVM, DACVECC
Consulting editors: Ahna G. Brutlag, DVM; Justine A. Lee, DVM, DACVECC

SUPPLEMENT 39.1. Information on distribution, metabolism, and excretion of vitamins and minerals. For further detail, the reader is referred to a veterinary nutrition textbook.

- **Vitamin A** is stored in the liver and can undergo enterohepatic circulation. Cats require preformed vitamin A, since they lack an enzyme necessary for β-carotene cleavage.
- **Vitamin B$_1$ (thiamine)** is absorbed primarily in the jejunum after intestinal phosphatases hydrolyze thiamine to free thiamine. Active, carrier-mediated transport is the primary mechanism of absorption; however, passive diffusion is also utilized during periods of increased thiamine intake. It is transported in red blood cells and plasma to the tissues.
- **Vitamin B$_2$ (riboflavin)** requires hydrolysis prior to absorption in the GIT. Absorbed riboflavin is bound in approximately equal percentages to albumin and globulin. Excess riboflavin is renally excreted.
- **Vitamin B$_3$ (niacin)** is readily absorbed by the mucosa of the stomach and small intestine and it is taken up by tissues, where it is often required for cofactor synthesis. Excessive amounts are excreted by the kidneys following methylation.
- **Vitamin B$_6$ (pyridoxine)** is absorbed via passive diffusion in the small intestine, but only small quantities are stored. Products of vitamin B$_6$ metabolism are renally excreted.
- **Vitamin B$_{12}$ (cobalamin)** absorption depends on both intake and GIT function, as it undergoes several transformations (hydrolysis, intrinsic factor binding, ileal absorption, protein bound transport, and cell surface receptor mediated uptake) in order to be utilized.

(Continued)

- **Vitamin C (ascorbic acid)**, though not technically a vitamin, can be synthesized from glucose by cats and dogs. Additional vitamin C is absorbed by passive diffusion. It is transported by albumin, distributed throughout the body, and excreted via urine, feces, and sweat.
- **Vitamin D (D$_3$, cholecalciferol)** can be synthesized by the skin after exposure to UV light. It is also absorbed in the small intestine, using bile salts, and subsequently transported with vitamin D binding protein to tissues where it is contained within lipid deposits.
- **Vitamin E** is absorbed in the small intestine by passive diffusion; however, it is absorbed with poor efficacy. Absorption can be increased by consuming fats at the same time. Transport to circulation is facilitated by the lymphatics. There is minimal metabolism of vitamin E, and the majority of it is fecally excreted.
- **Biotin** is released via protein hydrolysis in order to permit intestinal absorption and subsequent transfer from the blood to the tissues. In addition, intestinal microbes synthesize approximately half of the biotin requirements. Excessive biotin is excreted by the kidneys.
- **Calcium** absorption is variable in the GIT and can be achieved using three possible mechanisms. In the duodenum and jejunum, there is an active, transcellular method using a vitamin D–dependent, calcium-binding protein. The other two methods are passive and facilitated absorption, which are primarily localized to the distal GIT. Most calcium in dietary supplements is in the form of calcium salts, which are poorly absorbed by the GIT.
- **Copper** can be absorbed along the entire length of the GIT, though most is absorbed within the small intestine, by both active and passive mechanisms. The liver is the main site of copper metabolism, and excretion is via feces and bile.
- **Folic acid (folate)** is hydrolyzed in the intestine before enterocyte absorption. There are no folate reserves in the body; therefore, it must be ingested daily in the diet.
- **Iodine** within the plasma is trapped by the thyroid glands to ensure adequate supplies of thyroid hormone.
- **Iron** must be ionized in order to be absorbed. It is absorbed into mucosal cells lining the intestinal lumen, particularly in the duodenum and jejunum. The absorbed iron is then transferred to ferritin or transferrin. No distinct mechanism for iron excretion exists, which contributes to toxicosis with iron ingestion.
- **Magnesium** is absorbed is either actively or passively from the intestines, depending on the intraluminal concentration. The kidney is essential for magnesium homeostasis and is responsible for filtration, excretion, and reabsorption of this mineral.
- **Pantothenic acid** is released via protein hydrolysis within the intestinal lumen. Most of the vitamin is contained within erythrocytes.
- **Phosphorus** is well absorbed in the intestines, particularly when found in animal-based ingredients. Calcium and phosphorus absorption, metabolism, and hemostasis are under the delicate and intricate control of hormonal and renal influences.
- **Zinc** absorption is not completely understood, though the majority of absorption occurs in the duodenum, jejunum, and ileum. The liver is responsible for zinc metabolism, and excretion of excess zinc occurs via the feces.

Drugs: Veterinary Prescription

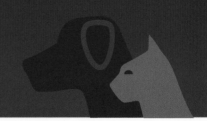

Alpha₂-Adrenergic Agonists (Detomidine, Dexmedetomidine, Romifidine, Xylazine)

chapter **40**

DEFINITION/OVERVIEW

- Alpha$_2$-adrenergic agonists are a widely used class of sedatives in veterinary medicine. They produce dose-dependent sedation, analgesia, and muscle relaxation.
- The four agents commonly used are xylazine, detomidine, romifidine, and dexmedetomidine.
- Toxicity is most often due to iatrogenic administration of an improper dose.
- All drugs in this class are can be rapidly and completely reversed with alpha$_2$ antagonists.

ETIOLOGY/PATHOPHYSIOLOGY

Mechanism of Action

- These agents have agonist actions on the alpha adrenergic receptor.
  - Alpha$_1$ receptors produce arousal, excitement, and increased locomotor activity.
  - Alpha$_{2A}$ receptors mediate sedation, supraspinal analgesia, centrally mediated bradycardia, and hypotension.
  - Alpha$_{2B}$ receptors mediate the initial increase in vascular resistance and reflex bradycardia.
  - Alpha$_{2C}$ receptors mediate hypothermia.
- Receptor selectivity ratios, alpha$_2$/alpha$_1$ are the following:
  - Xylazine 160:1
  - Detomidine 260:1
  - Romifidine 340:1
  - Dexmedetomidine 1620:1
- There is inhibition of norepinephrine and dopamine storage and release.

Pharmacokinetics/Absorption, Distribution, Metabolism, and Excretion

- Alpha agonists are well absorbed across the oral mucosa or sublingually.
- There is rapid absorption following IM administration and rapid onset with IV administration.

- The agents are highly water soluble.
- The volume of distribution of dexmedetomidine is 0.9 L/kg.
- Elimination is via biotransformation in the liver to inactive metabolites excreted, primarily, in the urine.
- The half-life of dexmedetomidine 40–50 minutes in dogs and 1 hour in cats.

Toxicity

- Toxicosis from these agents has been seen with 2 to 5 times the normal IV dose and 10 times the normal IM dose.
- Intensity and duration of effect is dose dependent

Systems Affected

- Cardiovascular—brief period of hypertension caused by activation of peripheral postsynaptic alpha$_2$ receptors. This leads to vascular smooth muscle contraction and vasoconstriction, with reflex bradycardia. Cardiac output can decrease by 30% to 50%.
  Sinus bradycardia and atrioventricular (AV) block can be seen following administration of alpha$_2$ agonists.
- Nervous—CNS depression as evidenced by sedation and anxiolysis. Analgesia (somatic and visceral) and muscle relaxation. Hypothermia may occur as a result of depression to the thermoregulatory center, muscle relaxation, and decreased shivering.
- Gastrointestinal—Vomiting is common immediately following administration. There may be decreased GI secretions as well as varying effects on intestinal muscle tone.
- Urinary—increased urine output due to action of antidiuretic hormone on the renal tubules and collecting ducts producing dilute urine
- Endocrine—transient hypoinsulinemia and hyperglycemia due to receptor mediated inhibition of insulin release from the pancreatic beta cells
- Respiratory—depression, decreased respiratory rate, and possible apnea

 # SIGNALMENT/HISTORY

- Any age or breed of dog or cat
- Overdose most commonly occurs due to iatrogenic administration of an improper dose.
- Xylazine comes in two concentrations, 20 mg/mL and 100 mg/mL, and overdose can occur when the 100 mg/mL is mistakenly used in place of 20 mg/mL.

 # CLINICAL FEATURES

- The onset of clinical signs is rapid (seconds to minutes).

- The duration of signs depends on the drug. However, as all drugs are easily reversible, signs typically only last until the reversal agent is administered.
- CNS—CNS depression, ataxia, sedation and hypothermia. May see muscle twitching
- Cardiac—bradycardia, AV block, decreased myocardial contractility and cardiac output, initial hypertension followed by hypotension. Pale (or cyanotic) oral mucus membranes may also be seen.
- Respiratory—decreased respiratory rate with possible apnea
- GI—vomiting
- May have death from circulatory failure and severe pulmonary congestion

 ## DIFFERENTIAL DIAGNOSIS

- Bradycardia and cardiac arrhythmias: beta-adrenergic blocking drugs, calcium channel blocking drugs, and opioids
- Respiratory depression: opioids

 ## DIAGNOSTICS

- ECG: sinus bradycardia and second degree AV block
- Blood glucose: hyperglycemia due to decreased insulin
- Blood pressure: hypertension followed by hypotension

 ## THERAPEUTICS

- All drugs can be rapidly reversed with alpha$_2$ antagonists.
- Overall, treatment consists of general supportive care, protection of the airway, and potentially, mechanical ventilation.
- Monitor heart rate and rhythm, blood pressure, body temperature, urine output, and glucose levels.

Detoxification

- All drugs are rapidly and completely reversible. See Drug(s) and Antidotes of Choice.

Appropriate Health Care

- Reversal with IM atipamezole
- IV crystalloid fluids to treat hypotension and increased urination
- IV anticholinergic therapy such as atropine or glycopyrrolate to treat severe bradycardia and hypotension

Drug(s) and Antidotes of Choice

- The alpha$_2$ agonists can be rapidly and completely antagonized by alpha$_2$ antagonists.
  - There are three available antagonists, atipamezole (Antisedan), yohimbine, and tolazoline.
  - Atipamezole is highly selective for the alpha$_2$ receptors and does not create significant hypotension.
    - ☐ It is recommended to give atipamezole IM due to the potential to create excitement and tachycardia. It can be given IV in emergency situations.
    - ☐ Reversal should take into consideration the amount of agonist given and the time duration since the agonist was administered.
    - ☐ Dose: Typically, give the same amount of atipamazole as was given of detomidine or dexmeditomidine.
  - Yohimbine (0.1 mg/kg IV for dogs) and tolazoline (4 mg/kg IV slow for dogs) produce variable effects and also antagonize alpha$_1$ receptors. This may lead to hypotension.
- Antagonism results in sympathetic outflow becoming enhanced.
- It is better to underdose the antagonist, as side effects from an overdose of the antagonist include excitement, muscle tremors, hypotension, tachycardia, salivation, and diarrhea. Large doses of antagonists will also reverse analgesia.
- Atipamezole is marketed to be paired as the reversal agent for dexmedetomidine but will also reverse all other alpha$_2$ agonist drugs.

Nursing Care

- Monitor the patient for bradycardia and hypotension.
- Monitor for respiratory depression and hypoventilation.
- Watch fluid balance due to increased urination.

Follow-up

- Make sure heart rate and blood pressure are within normal limits after reversal.

 COMMENTS

Patient Monitoring

- ECG and heart rate
- Blood pressure
- Blood glucose
- Urination

Prevention/Avoidance

- Be aware of proper dosing and drug concentration.

Expected Course and Prognosis

- The prognosis for alpha$_2$ agonist overdose is excellent with proper supportive care and prompt use of a reversal agent.

Suggested Reading

Lemke KA. Anticholinergics and sedatives. In: Tranquilli WJ, Thurmon JC, Grimm KA, eds. Lumb & Jones Veterinary Anesthesia and Analgesia, 4th ed. Ames, IA: Blackwell, 2007; pp. 203–239.

Author: Jane Quandt, DVM, MS, DACVA, DACVECC
Consulting Editor: Ahna G. Brutlag, DVM

chapter 41

Ivermectin/ Milbemycin/ Moxidectin

DEFINITION/OVERVIEW

- Ivermectin, milbemycin, and moxidectin are macrocyclic lactone derivatives used as anthelmintics and heartworm preventatives in veterinary medicine (see fig. 41.1).
- Toxicosis can occur when small animals ingest formulations intended for large animals and excessive amounts of products for small animals are consumed. In addition, when breeds of dogs that are sensitive to these drugs due to the MDR1 (multidrug resistance) gene mutation, now known as the ATP-binding cassette (ABCB-1Δ) polymorphism, are exposed to even therapeutic amounts of these drugs, toxicosis can be seen.
- Clinical signs of toxicosis include the following: lethargy, ataxia, hypersalivation, mydriasis, blindness, and seizures. Toxicosis can be fatal, especially in sensitive breeds.
- Treatment entails decontamination, activated charcoal administration, intensive monitoring, and supportive care. Novel use of intravenous lipid emulsion (ILE) therapy has also been explored.
- With appropriate supportive care, prognosis for recovery is often good. However, intensive respiratory, cardiovascular, and neurologic monitoring; mechanical ventilation; and prolonged hospitalization may be necessary.

ETIOLOGY/PATHOPHYSIOLOGY

Mechanism of Action

- Ivermectin is an antiparasitic drug that belongs to a class of compounds known as avermectins.
- Milbemycin and moxidectin, which is a derivative of milbemycin, belong to the milbemycin group of antiparasitics.
- The avermectins and milbemycins are similar in structure, mechanism of action, and effectiveness, and are collectively known as macrocyclic lactones.
- Macrocyclic lactones are fermentation products from *Streptomyces* species. They are also highly lipophilic and have excellent activity against nematodes and arthropods.

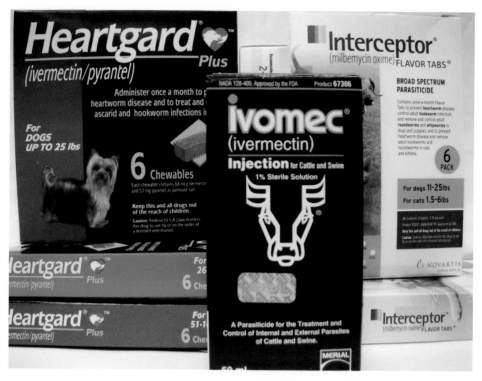

■ **Fig. 41.1.** An assortment of ivermectin- and milbemycin-containing products commonly used as small animal antiparasitic therapy and heartworm prevention. (Photo courtesy of Dana L. Clarke)

- Toxicosis in veterinary species is caused by drug binding to postsynaptic GABA-gated chloride channels in the CNS, which results in inhibition of neuronal impulse transmission. At therapeutic doses, toxicosis is prevented via the action of the BBB transmembrane transporter called p-glycoprotein.

Pharmacokinetics/Absorption, Distribution, Metabolism, and Excretion

- Absorption after oral administration is rapid. Peak plasma concentrations occur at 2 hours after moxidectin administration and 4 hours after ivermectin administration.
- Absorption after SQ drug administration is slower than orally. However, there is better bioavailability after SQ administration.
- They are highly lipophilic and extensively distributed to various tissues, especially fat. Moxidectin has a higher volume of distribution compared to ivermectin.
- The lipophilic nature of these drugs, combined with low plasma clearance, contributes to their long persistence in the body. Moxidectin has an approximately eight-fold longer elimination half-life than ivermectin.

- Canine ivermectin half-life: 3.3 days; moxidectin: 25.9 days.
- Ivermectin and moxidectin are primarily excreted in the feces, although small amounts of ivermectin are also excreted in urine. Also, a very small amount of ivermectin is oxidized in the liver.
- Though specific pharmacokinetic information about milbemycin in dogs and cats is not available, milbemycin's similar structure and mechanism of action to ivermectin and moxidectin likely indicate similar pharmacokinetics to these drugs.

Toxicity

- While there are dosage levels at which animals have been described to show clinical signs after ingestion, it is important to remember that each animal's reaction can be variable, especially if that animal is affected by the p-glycoprotein deletion (see Signalment/History).
- Ivermectin
    - For dogs not affected by the p-glycoprotein deletion, dosages up to 2.5 mg/kg can be tolerated without clinical signs. Doses ≥2.5 mg/kg may cause mydriasis.
    - Tremors can be seen at ≥5 mg/kg; severe tremors and ataxia at ≥10 mg/kg.
    - Reported fatalities at 40 mg/kg.
    - The reported LD_{50} in experimental beagle models is 80 mg/kg.
    - Dogs affected by the p-glycoprotein deletion can tolerate doses up to 0.1 mg/kg.
    - The LD_{50} in ivermectin-sensitive collies is 0.15–0.2 mg/kg.
    - Cats can tolerate oral doses of 0.75 mg/kg, though some reports indicate they are tolerant of higher doses.
    - Clinical signs of ivermectin toxicosis in cats and kittens has been reported at doses of 0.3–0.4 mg/kg.
- Moxidectin
    - No clinical signs at 0.9 mg/kg, which is 300x higher than the oral pharmacologic dose.
    - Clinical signs were observed in a collie after 0.09 mg/kg.
- Milbemycin
    - Beagles ingesting 100 mg/kg of milbemycin were reported to show no adverse clinical signs, which is 200x the monthly oral pharmacologic dose.
    - Hypersalivation, ataxia, mydriasis, and depression were observed in some collies at dosages of 5 mg/kg and all collies at the 10 mg/kg dose in one study.
    - Information about toxicosis of milbemycin in cats is not available.

Systems Affected

- Nervous

- Toxicosis primarily affects the CNS by binding to GABA-gated channels, which causes cell membrane hyperpolarization and subsequent inhibition of neuronal depolarization.
  - Severity of CNS signs increases with dose.
- Ophthalmic
  - Ophthalmic changes include mydriasis, central blindness, multifocal retinal edema, retinal folds, and changes in the ERG.
- Gastrointestinal
  - Hypersalivation, vomiting, anorexia, diarrhea
- Respiratory
  - Severe progression of neurologic impairment secondary to macrocyclic lactone ingestion can cause hypoventilation and respiratory failure.
  - In vomiting patients, or those with neurologic compromise that are unable to protect their airway, aspiration pneumonia is a possible complication of this toxicosis.
- Cardiovascular
  - In patients with a significant microfilaria burden, anaphylactic shock after sudden microfilaria death can cause severe hypotension and shock.

 SIGNALMENT/HISTORY

- Dogs and cats of any age, breed, or sex can be affected by this toxicosis.
- Toxicosis is more commonly reported in dogs.
- Pediatric animals are thought to be at higher risk for developing toxicosis due to incomplete development of the BBB.
- Many breeds of dogs, though most commonly collies, Shetland sheepdogs, border collies, Australian shepherds, and other herding breeds, carry a homozygous 4 base pair deletion of the MDR1 gene, now known as the ATP-binding cassette (ABCB-1Δ) polymorphism. This mutation causes the absence of p-glycoprotein in the BBB and increases the penetration and neurotoxic effects of macrocyclic lactones in the CNS.

Risk Factors

- Use of macrocyclic lactone antiparasitic therapies
- Access to large animal macrocyclic lactone formulation
- Ingestion of feces from large animals recently treated with macrocyclic lactones
- ABCB-1Δ polymorphism
- Concurrent administration of drugs that inhibit p-glycoprotein function, such as cyclosporine A and ketoconazole

Historical Findings

- If ingestion is witnessed by the owner or packaging material is found, the owner may report that their pet ingested a macrocyclic lactone medication.

Location and Circumstances of Poisoning

- Any area where the pet has access to the medication (e.g., home, garage, barn, farm, etc.)
- Inadvertent overdose by a veterinarian (home/farm call or in the veterinary hospital setting)
- Access to areas where large animals recently treated with these medications defecate (e.g., fields, paddocks, barn, etc.)

Interactions with Drugs, Nutrients, or Environment

- Concurrent administration of drugs that decrease or inhibit the function of p-glycoprotein:
  - Cyclosporine A
  - Ketoconazole
  - Verapamil
  - Tamoxifen
  - Loperamide

CLINICAL FEATURES

- Nervous—ataxia, weakness, disorientation, paddling, head pressing (seen in cats), tremors, seizures, coma
- Ophthalmic—mydriasis, central blindness, retinal edema (may be multifocal), retinal folds, attenuated or extinguished ERG wave amplitude (measure of retinal function)
- Gastrointestinal—hypersalivation, vomiting
- Respiratory—hypoventilation, poor chest excursions (e.g., intercostal breathing)
- Cardiovascular—hyperthermia, hypothermia, bradycardia, hypotension

DIFFERENTIAL DIAGNOSIS

- Anticholinesterase insecticide ingestion
- Tremorgenic mycotoxin ingestion
- Ethylene glycol ingestion
- Benzodiazepine ingestion
- Barbiturate ingestion
- Lead toxicosis
- Metabolic disease—hepatic encephalopathy, portosystemic shunt, etc.
- Primary ophthalmic disease

DIAGNOSTICS

- Depending on the patient's clinical status, diagnostics to assess the stability of the patient should take priority over confirmatory testing. Such emergency diagnostics may include the following:
    - Electrolytes, PCV/TS, blood glucose, BUN, creatinine
    - Blood pressure
    - Pulse oximetry
    - Arterial blood gas (to assess oxygenation and ventilation) or venous blood gas (to assess ventilation)
    - ECG
- Liquid chromatography mass spectroscopy to determine drug levels
    - Can be performed on serum, adipose tissue, and liver samples
    - Serum levels do correlate with clinical signs, as clinical signs are dependent on the concentration of the drug in the brain.
- PCR DNA test for MDR1 genotype
    - Should be considered in a susceptible breed or any canine patient whose clinical signs do not correlate with the amount of macrocyclic lactone ingested
    - Requires a cytology cheek brushing sample sent to the Veterinary Clinical Pathology Laboratory, College of Veterinary Medicine, Washington State University, Pullman, WA 99164–6610 (www.vetmed.wsu.edu/vcpl)
- Fundoscopy
    - Can be performed via direct or indirect ophthalmoscopy
- ERG
    - Allows for assessment of the neurosensory activity of the retina
    - Requires specialized equipment and training

Pathological Findings

- There are no characteristic gross or histopathologic lesions.

THERAPEUTICS

- Treatment entails decontamination, supportive care, and intensive monitoring.

Detoxification

- In neurologically appropriate patients, emesis should be induced as quickly and safely possible.
- For neurologically inappropriate, symptomatic patients, initial treatment should be aimed at managing neurologic signs, such as seizures. Sedation, intubation, and gastric lavage may also be considered.

- Due to enterohepatic recirculation, repeated doses of activated charcoal are indicated. Only the first dose should contain a cathartic. Administration of activated charcoal via a stomach tube for intubated patients may be necessary with an inflated ETT to prevent secondary aspiration pneumonia.

Appropriate Health Care

- Seizures must be aggressively controlled to prevent cerebral edema, noncardiogenic pulmonary edema, and aspiration of GIT contents. Intubation may be necessary.
- Serum electrolytes (e.g., sodium, potassium, glucose) should be monitored and treated if needed for patients receiving multiple doses of activated charcoal, large amounts of IV fluids, and those with seizures.
- Frequent lung auscultation as well as serial measurement of blood oxygenation (e.g., pulse oximetry, arterial blood gas) should be performed in patients where aspiration pneumonia is a concern. Mechanical ventilation is indicated for patients with severe hypoxemia unresponsive to supplemental oxygen therapy.
- Ventilation should be closely monitored in patients with severe neurologic impairment using venous or arterial (preferred) pCO_2 or end tidal capnography. Mechanical ventilation is indicated for patients with hypoventilation.
- Continuous ECG can be used in patients with concerning bradycardia.

Drug(s) and Antidotes of Choice

- There is no antidote.
- For control of tremors or seizures, patients can be loaded with phenobarbital (2–4 mg/kg IV as needed to control seizures, up to 16 mg/kg) or levetiracetam (Keppra, 20 mg/kg IV q 8 hours). The lowest effect dose should be used, due to the risks of severe sedation.
- The authors have experience with using intravenous lipid emulsion (ILE) to help treat a dog with ivermectin toxicosis. ILE is thought to create a lipid partition or "sink" within the intravascular space, which helps to contain the lipophilic macrocyclic lactone in the vasculature, and therefore prevent penetration into the brain. There is also a published case report describing the use of ILE to treat a puppy with suspected moxidectin toxicosis. The reader is encouraged to contact an established veterinary toxicology helpline or toxicologist if he or she wishes to consider this therapy, as it is still considered experimental in veterinary medicine.

Precautions/Interactions

- Benzodiazepines (e.g., midazolam, diazepam) should potentially be avoided for tremor or seizure management, as these drugs may potentiate the CNS toxicosis due to GABA binding and lead to prolonged recovery.

- Physostigmine is a cholinesterase inhibitor that has been used as it transiently improves clinical signs in affected patients. Since it causes lacrimation, salivation, defecation, urination, and seizures, its use is not currently recommended.
- Picrotoxin is a GABA antagonist that has been used to treat a case of ivermectin toxicosis. However, it can cause seizures and is therefore not recommended.

Alternative Drugs

- If tremors or seizures do not respond to phenobarbital or levetriacetam, propofol (1–2 mg/kg IV bolus, 0.1–0.2 mg/kg/min CRI) or etomidate (0.5–4 mg/kg IV) may be used. Etomidate should not be used as a sole agent.

Nursing Care

- Intensive neurologic monitoring (e.g., mentation, menace, visual ability, pupil size, PLR, ambulation, etc.) should be carried out every 2–4 hours, especially in patients with neurologic impairment at presentation.
- Care for recumbent patients, including frequent turning, passive range of motion, bladder and colon care, and eye and oral care should be provided.
- Special attention should be given to patients with central blindness to protect their corneas with frequent lubrication and prevent trauma to the eyes since patients may not blink as a protective mechanism.
- For patients with seizures and any concerns for cerebral edema, a board under the head and neck, positioned at a 15- to 30-degree angle, should be used to help decrease ICP. Compression of the jugular veins (especially for venipuncture) and hyperthermia should be avoided in such patients. If tolerated, supplemental oxygen via a mask should be considered for all recumbent, neurologic patients.
- Body temperature should be measured frequently. Heat support should be used for patients with hypothermia but should be discontinued when the body temperature has reached 99°F. In addition, gentle cooling measures, such as wetting of the fur and a fan, can be used for patients with hyperthermia. Cooling measures should be stopped once the patient's temperature has reached 103.5°F to prevent rebound hypothermia.

Follow-up

- Depending on the patient's clinical course, it is likely that follow-up care and monitoring will not be necessary after discharge.
- Patients that may require follow-up include those that develop aspiration pneumonia or severe seizures and neurologic impairment.

Diet

- For patients with any neurologic compromise, vomiting, regurgitation, or those that are sedated, oral food and water should be withheld until the patient is neurologically appropriate and any GIT signs have resolved.

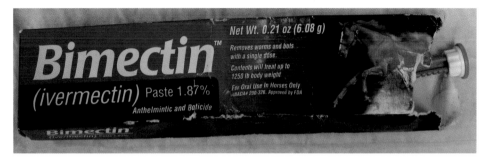

■ **Fig. 41.2.** A tube of equine ivermectin antihelminthic chewed by a dog. Ingestion of equine macrocyclic lactone antihelminthics is the most common cause of this toxicosis reported to Pet Poison Helpline. (Photo courtesy of Dana L. Clarke)

- In patients with prolonged neurologic compromise, recumbency, or those that require mechanical ventilation, parenteral nutrition may be necessary.

Activity

- Activity restriction is not necessary, as the patient's neurologic status will likely determine its activity level.
- Patients with any visual impairment should be assisted and monitored closely when navigating unfamiliar surroundings.

Prevention

- Proper storage of antiparasitic medications (see fig. 41.2)
- Ensuring correct dosage
- Preventing access to feces from large animals recently treated with these medications
- MDR1 genetic testing in all animals with toxicosis to rule out ABCB-1Δ polymorphism

 COMMENTS

Client Education

- Clients should be educated on the mechanism of action of toxicosis, as well as given recommendations for safe storage and use options.
- Information about the gradual reintroduction of a bland diet, monitoring for ongoing GIT and neurologic signs, and general observation instructions should be provided.
- For patients confirmed to be affected with the ABCB-1Δ polymorphism, recommendations on other medications that must be avoided should be made (e.g., loperamide).

Possible Complications

- Aspiration pneumonia
- Hypoventilation or hypoxemia requiring mechanical ventilation

Expected Course and Prognosis

- The prognosis for recovery ingestion is largely dependent on dose and ABCB-1Δ polymorphism status. Animals ingesting a larger dose, or those that lack p-glycoprotein in the BBB, are expected to require more intensive care and will likely have a more prolonged recovery.
- Duration to recovery can vary from days to weeks.
- Patients requiring more intensive care, especially mechanical ventilation, will also have increased costs associated with hospitalization, which may affect prognosis due to an owner's financial capabilities.
- Animals that recover often have no long-term complications secondary to this toxicosis.

Synonyms

ivermectin toxicosis/intoxication, milbemycin toxicosis/intoxication, moxidectin toxicosis/intoxication, macrolide toxicosis/intoxication

Abbreviations

ABCB-1Δ = ATP-binding cassette
BBB   = blood brain barrier
BUN   = blood urea nitrogen
CNS   = central nervous system
ECG   = electrocardiogram
ERG   = electroretinogram
ETT   = endotracheal tube
GABA   = gamma aminobutyric acid
GIT   = gastrointestinal tract
ICP   = intracranial pressure
ILE   = intravenous lipid emulsion
IV   = intravenous
MDR1   = multidrug resistance
pCO_2 = partial pressure of carbon dioxide
PCV   = packed cell volume
PCR   = polymerase chain reaction
PLR   = pupillary light reflex
q   = every
SQ   = subcutaneous
TS   = total solids

Suggested Reading

Al-Azzam SI, Fleckstein L, Cheng K, et al. Comparison of the pharmacokinetics of moxidectin and ivermectin after oral administration to beagle dogs. Biopharm Drug Disposition 2007; 28:431–438.

Beal MW, Poppenga RH, Birdsall WJ, et al. Respiratory failure attributable to moxidectin intoxication in a dog. J Am Vet Med Assoc 1999; 215(12):1813–1817.

Crandell DE, Weinberg GL. Moxidectin toxicosis in a puppy successfully treated with intravenous lipids. J Vet Emerg Crit Care 2009; 19(2):181–186.

Hopper K, Aldrich J, Haskins SC. Ivermectin toxicity in 17 collies. J Vet Int Med 2002; 16:89–94.

Kenny PJ, Vernau KM, Puschner B, et al. Retinopathy associated with ivermectin toxicosis in two dogs. J Am Vet Med Assoc 2008; 233(2):279–284.

Mealey KL. Ivermectin: macrolide antiparasitic agents. In: Peterson ME, Talcott PA, ed. Small Animal Toxicology, 2nd ed. St. Louis: Elsevier, 2006.

Authors: Dana L. Clarke, VMD; Justine A. Lee, DVM, DACVECC
Consulting Editor: Ahna G. Brutlag, DVM; Justine A. Lee, DVM, DACVECC

Phenylpropanolamine (PPA)

chapter 42

DEFINITION/OVERVIEW

- Phenylpropanolamine (PPA) is a sympathomimetic commonly used for the medical treatment of female urinary incontinence (urethral sphincter hypotonus).
- Overdoses are associated with tachycardia or reflex bradycardia, hypertension, agitation, excitability, tremors, and seizures.
- PPA is available primarily in veterinary preparations, often in chewable form. Proin and Proin Drops are some of the most common products, but multiple formulations are available through various manufacturers and compounding pharmacies.
- PPA was once commonly used in human OTC cold/flu preparations as a decongestant and also in OTC diet pills for appetite control. Due to the reported prevalence of strokes in female patients using the drug, it is rarely used in human medicine.
- Toxicity is often due to animals' ingesting large amounts of unsecured chewable medications.

ETIOLOGY/PATHOPHYSIOLOGY

Mechanism of Action

- PPA is a sympathomimetic agent that primarily works via alpha-adrenergic agonist stimulation.
  - The drug has some lesser effect on norepinephrine and beta-1 agonist receptors but has no effect on beta-2 receptors.
- PPA stimulates smooth muscle contraction in the urethra via its stimulation of alpha-adrenergic agonist receptors.

Pharmacokinetics/Absorption, Distribution, Metabolism, and Excretion

- Information on canine pharmacokinetics is sparse at best. Canines do, however, appear to follow human models closely.
- Orally, it is absorbed readily and almost completely.

- No enterohepatic recirculation
- The half-life is generally within 3–4 hours.
- Distributed widely throughout the body, including into the CNS
- Partially metabolized by the liver
- 80%–90% is excreted, unchanged, in urine within 24 hours.
- A small portion is metabolized into active metabolites.

Toxicity

- No known LD_{50} exists in veterinary medicine.
- The range of toxicity is not well documented in veterinary literature.
- In human literature, symptoms of toxicity have been recorded at 10 mg/kg in children, 3 mg/kg in infants.

Systems Affected

- Cardiovascular—hypertension, tachycardia/tachyarrhythmias, reflex bradycardia (rare)
- Nervous—agitation, hyperactivity, hyperesthesia, tremors and occasionally seizures or coma
- Ophthalmic—mydriasis (sympathomimetic stimulation), increased IOP
- Renal/urologic—urinary retention, myoglobinuria
- Musculoskeletal—rhabdomyolysis (sequela to prolonged seizure/tremors)
- Hemic—DIC (sequella to prolonged seizure activity and hyperthermia). There are rare reports of vascular accidents in human literature.
- Gastrointestinal—anorexia and vomiting
- Skin—piloerection in the absence of aggression/fear

 SIGNALMENT/HISTORY

- Although primarily prescribed for older spayed female dogs, any pet may ingest this medication.
- Dogs are the most common offenders.

Risk Factors

- Animals with preexisting cardiovascular disease (including hypertension), hyperthyroidism, or glaucoma may develop more severe clinical signs.
- Cats: PPA is rarely prescribed for cats as they may have symptoms of toxicity even at therapeutic doses.

Historical Findings

- History of accidental ingestion of medication (generally via dietary indiscretion but potentially through therapeutic error)

- Restlessness, CNS stimulation and tremors/seizures, excitability, irritability, tachycardia, or nonresponsive pet

Interactions with Drugs, Nutrients, or Environment

- Concurrent treatment with MAOIs, SSRIs, TCAs, potentially amitraz (if inadvertent oral exposure occurs), NSAIDs, and other sympathomimetic agents

 ## CLINICAL FEATURES

- Clinical signs generally develop within 1 hour of ingestion.
- The most common signs are agitation, hyperactivity, tremoring, hyperthermia, and mydriasis with decreased PLRs.
- Hypertension, tachycardia, and seizures may occur.
- Inappropriate piloerection or pets having their "hackles up" may be noted.

 ## DIFFERENTIAL DIAGNOSIS

- Other toxicities that may result in similar symptoms: 5-HTP, albuterol, amphetamines/methamphetamines, anticholinergics, antihistamines, antipsychotics, benzodiazepines (paradoxical response), cocaine, hops, imidazoline, methylxanthines (caffeine, chocolate, etc.), marijuana, metaldehyde, methionine, mycotoxins, nicotine, pseudoephedrine, SSRIs, TCAs, thyroid medication (generally very large overdoses)
- Pheochromocytoma
- Primary CNS lesion
- Hyperthyroidism

 ## DIAGNOSTICS

- ECG and blood pressure monitoring
- Baseline chemistry including renal values
- CBC
- UA to evaluate renal function and monitor for myoglobinuria
- CK to monitor for rhabdomyolosis
- Coagulation panel if DIC is suspected
- Cardiac troponin levels where available (normal range ≤0.07 ng/mL)
- CK myocardial band isoenzyme (not widely available) should be run to monitor for MI

Pathological Findings

- MI have been documented in humans, likely secondary to catecholamine-induced damage or ischemia.

- Acute renal failure
- Hemorrhagic stroke (most commonly documented in humans, notably females)

 THERAPEUTICS

Detoxification

- Induce emesis if within 30 minutes of ingestion if no CNS effects are present.
- May follow with one dose of activated charcoal/cathartic

Appropriate Health Care

- Observation for 8–12 hours or 24–36 hours if the product was a sustained-release formulation
- IV fluids at maintenance rate. High rates may exacerbate hypertension.
- Cooling measures for hyperthermia (alcohol on paw pads, wet towel, cooled IV fluids, fan on cage, etc.)
- Frequent TPRs

Drugs and Antidotes of Choice

- Tachycardia: propranolol 0.02–0.06 mg/kg IV slowly
- Hyperactivity: acepromazine 0.05–1.0 mg/kg IV, IM, SQ or chlorpromazine 0.5–1.0 mg/kg IV, IM as needed for sedation. Higher doses may be required. These drugs are preferred over other sedatives (see Precautions).
- Seizures/tremors: phenobarbitol 3 mg/kg IV to effect

Precautions/Interactions

- Benzodiazepines (diazepam) are not recommended in sympathomimetic overdoses as they may exacerbate clinical signs.
- Drugs used to treat bradycardia may exacerbate hypertension. Bradycardia is often reflexive and will resolve once hypertension is controlled.

Follow-up

- Uncomplicated cases do not require follow-up.
- Animals developing secondary complications such as rhabdomyolosis, DIC, or renal damage may require prolonged treatment.

Diet

- Normal diet unless significant kidney damage has occurred, requiring a renal diet.

Activity

■ Patient should be kept quiet and secure while symptomatic.

Surgical Considerations

■ Large amounts of ingested tablets can potentially cause a bezoar formation, which may require surgical removal if other decontamination processes (warm water gastric lavage) are unsuccessful.

Prevention

■ Secure all medications (especially chewable/flavored tablets) where they cannot be accessed by pets or children.

 # COMMENTS

Client Education

■ Educate clients about securing all medications, especially chewable/flavored tablets.
■ Due to the potential for drug interactions and PPA, instruct clients not to administer other medications without veterinary approval.
■ This medication is not intended for humans.

Patient Monitoring

■ ECG and blood pressure monitoring should be frequent, ideally every 2–4 hours. Continuous ECG monitoring in serious cases.
■ Patient should have constant seizure monitoring.

Possible Complications

■ Myglobinuric renal failure and DIC following prolonged seizures/tremors
■ Animals with preexisting renal insufficiency may have decreased rate of drug clearance. These animals may require a longer and more aggressive course of treatment.

Expected Course and Prognosis

■ Generally good if treated early
■ Animals exhibiting CNS symptoms or developing DIC or myoglobinuria have a poor prognosis.

Synonyms

PPA, Proin, Proin Drops, Cystolamine, Propalin, Propalin Syrup

Abbreviations

5-HTP = 5-hydroxytryptophan
CBC   = complete blood count
CK   = creatine kinase
CNS   = central nervous system
DIC   = disseminated intravascular coagulation
ECG   = electrocardiogram
IM   = intramuscular
IOP   = intraocular pressure
IV   = intravenous
MI   = myocardial infarction
MOAI   = monoamine oxidase inhibitor
NSAIDs = nonsteroidal anti-inflammatory drugs
OTC   = over-the-counter
PLR   = pupillary light reflex
PPA   = phenylpropanolamine
SQ   = subcutaneous
SSRI   = selective serotonin reuptake inhibitor
TCA   = tricyclic antidepressant
TPR   = temperature, pulse, respiration

See Also

Amphetamines
Decongestants (Pseudoephedrine, Phenylephrine)
Ephedra/Ma Huang
Methamphetamine

Suggested Reading

Bacon NJ, Oni O, White RAS. Treatment of the urethral sphincter mechanism incompetence in 11 bitches with a sustained-release formulation of phenylpropanolamine hydrochloride. Vet Rec 2002; 151:373–376.

Crandell JM, Ware WA. Cardiac toxicity from phenylpropanolamine overdose in a dog. J Am Anim Hosp Assoc 2005; 41:413–420.

Gupta RC. Veterinary Toxicology Basic and Clinical Principles. New York: Academic, 2007.

Phenylpropanolamine. Micromedex. Thomson Healthcare Evidence/Healthcare Series. Web. http://www.thomsonhc.com/hcs/librarian/ND_T/HCS/ND_PR/Main/CS/811810/DUPLICATIONSHIELDSYNC/FDACEF/ND_PG/PRIH/ND_B/HCS/ND_P/Main/PFActionId/hcs.ToxicSubstanceLists. Accessed September 2009.

Author: Nancy M. Gruber, DVM
Consulting Editor: Ahna G. Brutlag, DVM

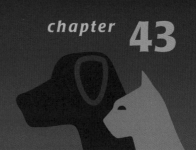

chapter 43

Pimobendan

DEFINITION/OVERVIEW

- Pimobendan is a drug used in management of canine congestive heart failure (CHF).
- The recommended dose is 0.2–0.3 mg/kg PO q 12 hours in dogs (0.5–0.6 mg/kg PO q 24 hours).
- Acute toxicosis has not been clinically reported in veterinary literature.

ETIOLOGY/PATHOPHYSIOLOGY

- Pimobendan is an inodilator, with both calcium-sensitizing properties and phosphodiesterase III inhibition.
  - Inodilators have both positive inotropic (increased contractility) and vasodilating effects.
- Pimobendan increases forward blood flow from the left ventricle by a combination of increased inotropy and arteriodilation.

Mechanism of Action

- Pimobendan alters sensitivity of troponin C to calcium, resulting in greater actin-myosin interaction (positive inotropy).
- Phosphodiesterase (PDE) III is expressed mainly in the heart and vascular smooth muscle. Inhibition of PDEIII causes increased contractility and vasodilation.

Pharmacokinetics/Absorption, Distribution, Metabolism, and Excretion

- Pimobendan is absorbed rapidly when given orally and has a bioavailability of 60%–65%.
- The onset of action is within 1 hour of administration.
- It is metabolized into its active form by the liver.
- The half-life of pimobendan in the blood is 0.4 hours and the half-life of its metabolite is 2 hours.
- Elimination is by excretion in the bile.
- Pimobendan is 90%–95% bound to plasma proteins in circulation.

Toxicity

- Acute toxicity has not been reported.
- Doses up to 8 mg/kg in experimental dogs have failed to produce acute clinical signs.
- No studies have demonstrated an increased risk of sudden death or arrhythmias in dogs.
- Long-term studies have shown development of mitral valve pathology in dogs.
- Dogs receiving 10–30x the recommended dose developed myxomatous changes after 4 weeks.
  - Oral administration of clinically relevant doses for 2 years resulted in development of similar lesions in research dogs.
- Dogs receiving supraphysiological doses had elevations in ALP without histological evidence of hepatotoxicity.
- One case study demonstrated a worsening of regurgitation in 2 dogs with mitral valve disease after pimobendan administration, which subsided upon withdrawal of the drug.
- In vitro evidence of platelet inhibition has failed to translate into clinical evidence of platelet inhibition or thrombocytopenia.
- Safety and efficacy have not been evaluated in cats. Anecdotal evidence suggests that the drug is well tolerated at doses similar to those in dogs.

Systems Affected

- Cardiovascular: possible hypotension, reflex tachycardia
- Hepatobiliary: increased ALP

 SIGNALMENT/HISTORY

Risk Factors

- Pimobendan is licensed for administration only to dogs with CHF secondary to mitral valve disease or DCM. Given the pathology of mitral and tricuspid valves with naturally occurring disease, administration of clinical doses of pimobendan is unlikely to cause additional valvular damage.
- Animals with HCM, aortic stenosis, other outflow obstructions or underlying arrhythmias may develop more severe clinical signs. However, studies of arrhythmogenesis with pimobendan have failed to demonstrate a significant proarrhythmic effect. No studies of the use of pimobendan in cats with HCM exist.
- Safety and efficacy have not been evaluated in cats. Anecdotal evidence suggests that the drug is well tolerated at doses similar to those in dogs.

Historical Findings

- Witness ingestion
- Discovery of a spilled/chewed pill canister

Location and Circumstances of Poisoning

▪ Usually unintended ingestion

Interactions with Drugs, Nutrients, or Environment

▪ There are no known interactions with other cardiac medications. Clinical experience of combination therapy with digoxin, sildenafil, diuretics, ACE inhibitors, and antiarrhythmic agents has failed to demonstrate significant drug interactions.

 # CLINICAL FEATURES

▪ Given pimobendan's wide margin of safety, clinical signs following most overdoses are unlikely. Should an animal present with clinical signs, strongly consider the animal's underlying health disorders (e.g., CHF) to be the primary cause.
▪ Following minor overdoses in healthy animals, clinical abnormalities are not expected.
  • Doses up to 8 mg/kg in experimental dogs have failed to produce acute clinical signs.
▪ Massive overdoses pose a theoretical risk for the following:
  • Hypotension
  • Arrhythmias (atrial fibrillation on increased ventricular ectopic beats), tachycardia, syncope, and weak or irregular pulses
  • Reflex tachycardia
  • Mild vomiting, diarrhea, anorexia
  • No cases of overdoses with significant toxic effects have been reported.
▪ Chronic high-dose administration could result in development of mitral valvulopathy. Several studies have demonstrated development of myxomatous mitral valvular lesions with high-dose (>2 mg/kg/day) pimobendan administration.

 # DIFFERENTIAL DIAGNOSIS

▪ Primary cardiac disease
▪ Primary respiratory disease

 # DIAGNOSTICS

▪ Given the wide margin of safety for this drug, the use of diagnostics is not anticipated.
▪ Should the animal develop clinical signs, consider underlying causes (CHF) and perform diagnostics accordingly.
▪ Monitor blood pressure on all tachycardic animals (reflex tachycardia).

Pathological Findings

■ Chronic high-dose administration results in development of myxomatous changes of the mitral valve, consistent with changes seen with other potent inotropes (milrinone).

 THERAPEUTICS

■ Pimobendan has a wide margin of safety, and studies have failed to demonstrate significant, acute toxicosis in overdose situations.
■ It is important to note that observed clinical signs are more likely to be directly related to the animal's underlying cardiac disease (CHF) than exposure to pimobendan.
■ Preexisting cardiac disease must be taken into account when considering therapeutic intervention.

Detoxification

■ With acute ingestion of large quantities of pimobendan, emesis is recommended.
■ Activated charcoal may reduce the amount of systemically absorbed drug.

Appropriate Health Care

■ Treatment is supportive and based on clinical signs.
■ Given the lack of clinical experience with acute intoxication, no specific or empirical therapy can be recommended.
■ Given the theoretical risk for hypotension/reflex tachycardia, blood pressure should be monitored on all symptomatic animals.
■ Fluid therapy must be used judiciously in patients with underlying cardiac disease.

Drug(s) and Antidotes of Choice

■ There is no antidote for pimobendan toxicosis treatment is supportive.

Precautions/Interactions

■ The effects of pimobendan may be attenuated by potent negative inotropes, vasoconstrictors, or calcium channel blockers.

Follow-up

■ Long-term adverse effects are not expected following acute toxicosis

Client Education

▪ Warn clients about the possible risks associated with long-term use.

Expected Course and Prognosis

▪ Prognosis for acute high-dose pimobendan ingestion is good.

Abbreviations

ACE = angiotensin converting enzyme
ALP = alkaline phosphatase
CBC = complete blood count
CHF = congestive heart failure
DCM = dilated cardiomyopathy
ECG = electrocardiogram
HCM = hypertrophic cardiomyopathy
PO   = *per os* (by mouth)
q   = every

See Also

Angiotensin-Converting Enzyme (ACE) Inhibitors
Beta-Blockers
Calcium Channel Blockers

Suggested Reading

Chetboul V, Lefebvre HP, Sampedrano CC, et al. Comparative adverse cardiac effects of pimo-bendan and benazepril monotherapy in dogs with mild degenerative mitral valve disease: a prospective, controlled, blinded, and randomized study. J Vet Intern Med 2007; 21(4):742–753.

FDA-CVM NADA 141–273 Pimobendan Freedom of Information Summary. Available at http://www.fda.gov/downloads/AnimalVeterinary/Products/ApprovedAnimalDrugProducts/FOIADrugSummaries/ucm062328.pdf. Accessed November 23, 2009.

Häggström J, Boswood A, O'Grady M, et al. Effect of pimobendan or benazepril hydrochloride on survival times in dogs with congestive heart failure caused by naturally occurring myxo-matous mitral valve disease: the QUEST study. J Vet Intern Med 2008; 22(5):1124–1135.

Smith PJ, French AT, Van Israël N, et al. Efficacy and safety of pimobendan in canine heart failure caused by myxomatous mitral valve disease. J Small Anim Pract 2005; 46(3):121–130.

Tissier R, Chetboul V, Moraillon R, et al. Increased mitral valve regurgitation and myocardial hypertrophy in two dogs with long-term pimobendan therapy. Cardiovasc Toxicol 2005; 5(1):43–51.

Author: Mark Rishniw, BVSc, MS, PhD, DACVIM
Contributing Editor: Ahna G. Brutlag, DVM

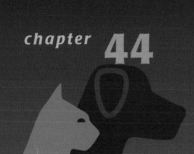

chapter 44

Veterinary NSAIDs (Carprofen, Deracoxib, Firocoxib, Ketoprofen, Meloxicam, Tepoxalin)

 DEFINITION/OVERVIEW

- NSAIDs are approved for use in small animals for the relief of pain and inflammation.
- They are inhibitors of COX-1, -2, and -3 as well as LOX enzymes, which decrease inflammation but can have adverse effects, most commonly on the GIT and kidneys and at higher doses on the liver and CNS.
- Veterinary NSAID drugs, formulations, and therapeutic doses:
  - Carprofen (Rimadyl) is available in 25-, 75-, and 100-mg caplet and chewable tablets and injectable at 50 mg/mL and is approved for dogs only. Therapeutic dose: 4.4 mg/kg/day PO, IM, or SQ, can divide into q 12 dosing.
  - Deracoxib (Deramaxx) is available in chewable tablets in 25-, 75-, 100-mg strength and is approved for dogs only. Therapeutic dose: 1–4 mg/kg PO q 24 hours.
  - Firocoxib (Previcox) is available in 57- and 227-mg chewable tablets and is approved for dogs only. Therapeutic dose: 5 mg/kg PO q 24 hours.
  - Ketoprofen (Ketofen) is available in 100 mg/mL injectable multidose vials. There are oral forms available in the UK and Canada. Therapeutic dose: 0.5–2 mg/kg PO, IM, SQ, IV q 24 hours.
  - Meloxicam (Metacam) is available in oral suspension in 1.5 mg/mL, 5 mg/mL injectable. Only the injectable is approved for use in cats. Dog therapeutic dose: 0.2 mg/kg PO, IV, or SQ once then 0.1 mg/kg PO q 24 hours. Cat therapeutic dose: 0.3 mg/kg SQ once.
  - Tepoxalin (Zubrin) is available in 30-, 50-, 100-, and 200-mg strength and approved for use in dogs. Therapeutic dose: 20 mg/kg PO once, then 10 mg/kg PO q 24 hours.

 ETIOLOGY/PATHOPHYSIOLOGY

Mechanism of Action

- Carprofen, deracoxib, firocoxib, and meloxicam are selective COX-2 inhibitors but may inhibit COX-1 at higher doses. Ketoprofen is a nonselective inhibitor of COX enzymes, and Tepoxalin inhibits COX-1 and -2 as well as LOX enzymes.

- These enzymes serve both inflammatory and constitutive functions in the body, which leads to the toxicity of these drugs at therapeutic doses and overdoses.

Pharmacokinetics/Absorption, Distribution, Metabolism, and Excretion

- All veterinary NSAIDs are well absorbed orally.
- They are highly protein bound and metabolized in the liver via glucuronidation and other hepatic metabolism.
- Enterohepatic recirculation: meloxicam (significant), carprofen (limited), keto-profen (suspected), deracoxib (none), tepoxalin (unknown). This will affect activated charcoal dosing during decontamination.
- Carprofen, deracoxib, firocoxib, meloxicam, and tepoxalin are mainly excreted in the feces. A small amount is excreted in the urine. Ketoprofen is excreted in the urine.

Toxicity

- Dogs
  - Acute: Doses greater than 5 times the therapeutic dose of most veterinary NSAIDs can result in clinical signs and require intervention.
  - Manufacturer safety data:
    - ☐ Carprofen: Acute doses of 22 mg/kg resulted in GI symptoms.
    - ☐ Deracoxib: Acute doses of >10 mg/kg resulted in GI ulceration. Doses up to 100 mg/kg did not show renal damage.
    - ☐ Firocoxib: Acute doses of 50 mg/kg resulted in GI symptoms.
    - ☐ Meloxicam: Acute doses up to 5 times therapeutic dose (0.1–0.5 mg/kg) resulted in some GI symptoms.
    - ☐ Tepoxalin: Acute doses from 100 to 300 mg/kg may result in GI symptoms.
    - ☐ No company reported renal damage in their safety studies.
  - Manufacturer safety data may differ from postmarked experience as it is not necessarily reflective of animals with underlying medical conditions.
  - Chronic: Therapeutic doses of all veterinary NSAIDs can result in clinical signs.
- Cats
  - Acute or chronic doses of any medication may cause toxicity in cats, especially off-label use.

Systems Affected

- Gastrointestinal: erosion, ulceration, perforation, gastroenteritis
- Renal: tubular damage, azotemia, oliguria to anuria
- Hemic/immune: blood loss anemia, platelet dysfunction, platelet loss/use
- Hepatobiliary: liver failure, hepatocellular necrosis
- Nervous: seizures, depression, agitation

SIGNALMENT/HISTORY

- Older animals or those with underlying kidney or liver disease may be more susceptible to adverse effects.
- Chewable tablets pose a greater risk of massive ingestion due to palatability, and younger animals may be more likely to chew on bottles or take them from the counter.
- Dogs
  - Labrador retrievers may develop idiosyncratic liver disease from carprofen use more often than other breeds.
  - No specific breed or sex predilection noted. Smaller breeds would require less ingested but larger breed dogs tend to chew more and may be able to ingest whole bottles.
- Cats
  - More sensitive due to decreased liver glucuronidation and longer half-life of certain NSAIDs (most notably carprofen).
  - Fewer products approved for use in cats and off-label use is common in this species.
  - No sex or breed predilection noted.

Risk Factors

- Animals with underlying GI, kidney, or liver disease, as well as animal with dehydration prior to use, are at greater risk.
- Concurrent steroids or NSAIDs may contribute to toxicity.
- Chronic use or off-label use (especially in cats) may increase likelihood of developing clinical signs.

Historical Findings

- The owners may report anorexia, vomiting ± hematemesis, melena or hematochezia, abdominal pain, polyuria, and polydipsia.

Location and Circumstances of Poisoning

- Most animals will ingest the medication at home, but some will have accidental overdose in the clinic.

Interactions with Drugs, Nutrients, or Environment

- Toxicity may be enhanced in animals taking or concurrently ingesting the following drugs:
  - ACE inhibitors, anticoagulants, aspirin, bisphosphonates, corticosteroids, cyclosporine, digoxin, fluconazole, furosemide, hepatic enzyme–inducing agents (e.g., phenobarbital), highly protein-bound drugs, methotrexate, nephrotoxic drugs, other NSAIDs, probenecid

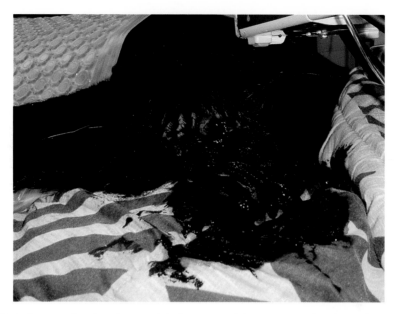

■ Fig. 44.1. Severe melena in a dog post-NSAID exposure. (Photo courtesy of Justine Lee)

 ## CLINICAL FEATURES

- Onset of clinical signs may occur within an hour after ingestion, but some symptoms such as renal failure or GI perforation may take 48–72 hours before clinical signs are evident.
- The most common signs will be GI and include vomiting, abdominal pain, melena, and diarrhea, which often cause secondary dehydration. See figure 44.1.
- Kidney damage will often manifest as increased drinking and urinating, anorexia, lethargy, and vomiting.
- Pale mucous membranes and tachycardia may occur after blood loss, hypovolemia, and poor perfusion develop.
- In severe ingestions, CNS symptoms can develop such as weakness, ataxia, and seizures; icterus may occur if liver damage is present.

 ## DIFFERENTIAL DIAGNOSIS

- Human NSAIDs may cause similar clinical signs but can result in a longer and more significant disease course due to prolonged half-life and differing metabolism in animals and should be ruled out. See Chapter 36 (Human NSAIDs).
- Gastrointestinal: gastroenteritis, IBD, HGE, metabolic disease, foreign body, pancreatitis
- Renal/urologic: chronic kidney disease, pyelonephritis, dehydration, ethylene glycol toxicity, ureteral obstruction, urethral obstruction

- • Cats: Asiatic/Easter lily toxicity
- Hepatic: xylitol or mushroom toxicity, hepatitis, pancreatitis, cholangiohepatitis
- Neurologic: epilepsy, other neurologic toxins (mushroom, antidepressants, xylitol)

 # DIAGNOSTICS

- CBC: blood loss anemia, thrombocytopenia noted with blood loss, high or low WBC with GI perforation and sepsis
- Serum chemistry profile: azotemia, liver enzyme/bilirubin elevations, elevated protein with dehydration, low albumin with liver failure or blood loss
- Urinalysis: inappropriate urine specific gravity, urinary casts with renal tubular damage
- Clotting profile: typically unaffected, platelet function tests can be prolonged
- Abdominocentesis or diagnostic peritoneal lavage: Intracellular bacteria, glucose <20 mg/dL in abdominal fluid versus peripheral glucose is consistent with GI tract perforation and a septic abdomen.
- Abdominal radiograph: loss of abdominal detail, free gas in the abdomen
- Abdominal ultrasound: complex free fluid, evidence of perforation

Pathologic Findings

- GI tract: erosions, ulceration and perforation of the stomach and small intestine
- Kidney: multifocal renal tubular necrosis, renal tubular regeneration, membranoproliferactive glomerulonephritis
- Liver: hepatocellular necrosis

 # THERAPEUTICS

- Treatment is aimed at prevention and palliation of gastric erosion, ulceration, and perforation as well as prevention of renal failure.

Detoxification

- Induce emesis within 1–2 hours after ingestion; may be difficult to identify chewable tablets in the emesis.
- Activated charcoal with a cathartic 1–4 g/kg. Give multidose charcoal (without a cathartic) for drugs that undergo enterohepatic recirculation.

Appropriate Health Care

- IV fluids as needed for dehydration and hypovolemia for 24–72 hours or as needed until clinical signs abate. Fluids will not enhance diuresis of the drugs but will support kidney perfusion.

- Exploratory laparotomy and repair of perforation as well as copious lavage of abdomen when a septic abdomen is identified. Standard postsurgical care as needed.
- Opioid pain medication to replace NSAID and for postoperative pain control or arthritis pain such as tramadol 1–4 mg/kg PO q 8–12 hours
- Hepato-protective medications and antioxidants can be used if liver damage is noted or prophylactically (silymarin/milk thistle, SAMe).
- A blood transfusion may be needed for significant blood loss.
- Nutritional supplementation may be required for anorectic animals.

Drug(s) and Antidotes of Choice

- GI protectants: Consider use of an H_2 blocker, proton pump inhibitor, or misoprostol, and sucralfate for 5–10 days after ingestion. Use multiple drugs if clinical signs are severe.
    - H_2 blocker: famotidine 0.5–1 mg/kg PO, IV, IM, SQ q 12–24 hours
    - Proton pump inhibitor: omeprazole 0.5–1 mg/kg PO q 24 hours
    - Misoprostol 1–5 mcg/kg PO q 8–12 hours
    - Sucralfate 0.25–1 g PO q 8 hours
- Antiemetic such as maropitant 1 mg/kg SQ or PO every 24 hours

Precautions/Interactions

- Discontinue use of other NSAIDs and steroids and use caution with drugs listed above that may have interactions with NSAIDs.

Nursing Care

- Keep animals clean and dry if having diarrhea.
- Soft, comfortable bedding is important for animals with arthritis.

Follow-up

- Recheck kidney values every 24 hours until normal or at a steady state.
- Patients should remain on GI protectants for 5–10 days or until GI symptoms resolve.
- Reinstate NSAIDs only after all clinical signs are resolved.

Prevention

- Owners should be educated on palatability of chewable medications and advised to keep this medication in a safe location.
- Owners should be advised to follow dosing instructions and only use if prescribed for the patient.

COMMENTS

Client Education

- Make sure owners are informed to discontinue use of all NSAIDs.
- Recommend keeping chewable medications out of reach.

Patient Monitoring

- Monitor hydration, kidney values, PCV/TP, CRT, urine output, heart rate, blood pressure, appetite, and stool quality.
- Animals can bleed into their GI tract without obvious melena or hematochezia. Monitor PCV/TP, CRT, and heart rate, where abnormalities can be early indicators of blood loss.

Prevention/Avoidance

- Discuss appropriate dosing of these medications and provide owners with symptoms to evaluate for at home, so that symptoms can be addressed early before significant morbidity develops.
- Discuss palatability of medication and keeping medications out of reach so that animals are not tempted to ingest large amounts of tablets. Animals will take these medications out of purses or bags if left unattended.

Possible Complications

- Oliguria or anuria may develop and these patients need aggressive therapy and monitoring.
- Chronic renal failure may occur after ingestion and requires lifelong therapy.
- GI perforation can occur and surgery is required for these cases. A septic abdomen and surgery will complicate recovery and carry a poor prognosis.

Expected Course and Prognosis

- Clinical signs generally resolve in 48–72 hours.
- Prognosis is fair to good with acute and chronic ingestion with appropriate decontamination and therapy. Surgery for GI perforation may complicate recovery and multiple surgeries may be required. Owners should be informed of the prolonged hospitalization and expense associated with these cases.
- Renal tubules may be able to regenerate with time, but full recovery may not be possible. Oliguria or anuria carries a guarded to poor prognosis.

Abbreviations

CBC = complete blood count
CNS = central nervous system

COX   = cyclooxygenase
CRT   = capillary refill time
GI   = gastrointestinal
HGE   = hemorrhagic gastroenteritis
IBD   = inflammatory bowel disease
IM   = intramuscular
IV   = intravenous
LOX   = lipoxygenase
NSAID = nonsteroidal anti-inflammatory drug
PCV   = packed cell volume
PO   = *per os* (by mouth)
q   = every
SQ   = subcutaneous
TP   = total protein
SAM-e = s-adenosyl methionine
WBC   = white blood cell

See Also

Aspirin
Human NSAIDs

Suggested Reading

Carroll GC, Simonson SM. Recent developments in nonsteroidal anti-inflammatory drugs in cats. JAAHA 2005; 41:347–354.
Enberg TB, Braun LD, Kuzme AB. Gastrointestinal perforation in five dogs associated with the administration of meloxicam. JVECC 2006; 16:34–43.
Lascelles BD, Blikslager AT, Fox SM, Reece D. Gastrointestinal tract perforation in dogs treated with a selective cyclooxygenase-2 inhibitor: 29 cases (2002–2003). Am Vet Med Assoc 2005; 7:1112–1117.
Matthews KA. Nonsteroidal anti-inflammatory analgesics. Vet Clin North Am Small Anim Pract 2000; 30(4):783–804.
Plumb DC. Plumb's Veterinary Drug Handbook, 6th ed. Ames, IA: Blackwell, 2008.

Author: Katherine L. Peterson, DVM
Consulting Editor: Ahna G. Brutlag, DVM

Envenomations

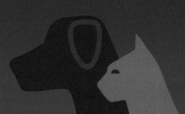

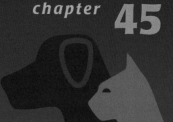

chapter 45

Black Widow Spiders

DEFINITION/OVERVIEW

- Black widow spider (*Lactrodectus* spp.) is a black, shiny spider about 2–2.5 cm in length with a red or orange hourglass mark on the ventral abdomen. The immature female is brown with red to orange stripes that change into the hourglass shape as she darkens with age (fig. 45.1). Males are brown, have no hourglass marks, and are generally thought to have fangs that are too small to penetrate the skin.
- Black widow spiders are found in every state except Alaska.

ETIOLOGY/PATHOPHYSIOLOGY

Mechanism of Action

- The venom contains a-latrotoxin, a potent neurotoxin that opens cation-selective channels at the presynaptic nerve terminal. This causes massive release and then depletion of acetylcholine and norepinephrine, resulting in sustained muscular spasms.
- Some proteolytic enzymes are also present, causing minimal localized tissue inflammation and pain.

Pharmacokinetics/Absorption, Distribution, Metabolism, and Excretion

- After the venom is injected, it is taken up by the lymphatics, entering the blood stream.
- In 30–120 minutes, muscle pain begins near the site of the bite.
- Within 2–3 hours, muscle pain and cramping spread to the muscles of the legs, abdomen, thorax, and back.
- Acute clinical signs generally resolve in 48–72 hours, but weakness and lethargy may continue for weeks to months.

Toxicity

- The neurotoxin is very potent.
  - LD_{50} in guinea pigs is 0.0075 mg/kg.
  - LD_{50} in mice is 0.9 mg/kg.

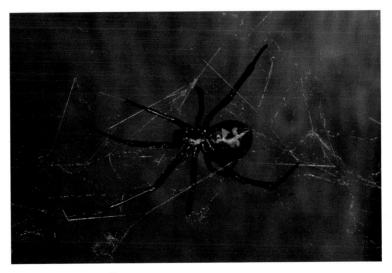

■ **Fig. 45.1.** Black widow spider (*Lactrodectus* spp.). (Photo courtesy of Richard Vetter, Dept. of Entomology, University of California–Riverside)

■ Cats are particularly sensitive to the venom, and many do not survive. The muscle pain and cramping can proceed to muscle tremors, ataxia, and paralysis.

Systems Affected

■ Musculoskeletal—severe muscle pain and cramping
■ Nervous—in cats especially, ataxia, tremors, and paralysis
■ Cardiovascular—mild tachycardia and hypertension
■ Gastrointestinal—vomiting, diarrhea, hypersalivation
■ Respiratory—Cheyne-Stokes pattern prior to death

 # SIGNALMENT/HISTORY

■ Diagnosis is based on history and clinical signs.

Risk Factors

■ Geriatric animals or animals with cardiac compromise may be at greater risk of complications.

Historical Findings

■ Owners have reported seeing the spider in the emesis of the animal.
■ Clinical onset is usually acute but may be delayed by several days with mild envenomation.

Location and Circumstances of Poisoning

■ Spiders are often found outside in leaf litter and debris or inside houses in dark areas under cabinets and in corners. Spiders are generally shy and will bite only if threatened by curious dogs and cats.

 # CLINICAL FEATURES

■ Clinical signs usually develop within 30 minutes to 2 hours postexposure, and the duration of clinical signs is generally 48–72 hours.
■ The most common signs are vomiting, diarrhea, vocalization, severe muscle spasms, pain and cramping, agitation, and restlessness.
■ Examination may show abdominal rigidity without tenderness, hypertension, tachycardia, regional tenderness, and lymph node tenderness.

 # DIFFERENTIAL DIAGNOSIS

■ Acute abdomen
■ Acute injury (hit by car, falling down stairs, etc.)
■ Back pain from disc disease

 # DIAGNOSTICS

■ CBC—leukocytosis
■ Serum chemistry—elevated CK

 # THERAPEUTICS

■ Therapeutic goals are to provide symptomatic and supportive therapy to minimize pain, muscle tremors, and agitation. If obtainable, antivenom can be used to rapidly shorten clinical signs.

Detoxification

■ None in particular

Appropriate Health Care

■ Monitor closely for signs of allergic reaction when giving antivenom.
■ Monitor for signs of tachycardia and hypertension and treat appropriately.

Drug(s) and Antidotes of Choice

- Antivenom is the definitive antidote. It should be reserved for high-risk patients (pediatric, geriatric, and metabolically compromised). In one case report, a cat was treated with antivenom 26 hours after becoming clinically compromised and quickly recovered neurologic function.
  - Lycovac Antivenin Black Widow Spider (Human Antivenin, equine origin); Merck, West Point, PA
    - One vial mixed with 100 mL crystalloid solution given IV slowly with monitoring of the inner ear pinna for evidence of hyperemia (an indicator of allergic response)
    - One dose is usually sufficient with a response occurring within 30 minutes.
    - With proper use, reactions are rare. If an adverse reaction occurs, stop antivenin and administer diphenhydramine (2–4 mg/kg IM, lower dose in cats). Wait 5 to 10 minutes and restart the antivenom at a slower rate.
  - New antivenin (Aracmyn; Instituto Biolclon, Mexico) has completed human phase three trials but is not yet approved for human use. This is an equine-origin Fab2 antivenin product and may be less likely to trigger an allergic reaction.
- Judicious use of IV fluids, especially if CK is elevated
- Muscle rigidity and anxiety
  - Methocarbamol 55–220 mg/kg/day slow IV. Do not exceed 330 mg/kg/day.
  - Diazepam 0.25–0.5 mg/kg IV as needed
- Opioids may be used at the lowest effective dose to control pain without compromising respiratory function.
  - Buprenorphine 0.005–0.02 mg/kg IM, IV or SQ q 6–12 hours
  - Tramadol 1–4 mg/kg PO q 8–12 hours for dogs (not yet labeled for use in cats)
- Antiemetics
  - Maropitant 1 mg/kg SQ q 24 hours, not labeled for cats
  - Ondansetron 0.1–0.2 mg/kg IV q 8–12 hours

Nursing Care

- Thermoregulation
- Frequent turning
- Monitor vitals closely
- Quiet environment

Follow-up

- Weakness, fatigue, and insomnia may persist for weeks to months. Pets should be monitored closely.

Expected Course and Prognosis

- Clinical signs generally resolve within 48–72 hours.
- Prognosis is uncertain for days; envenomation in cats is usually fatal without antivenom administration.

Abbreviations

CBC = complete blood count
CK   = creatine kinase
Fab = fragment antigen binding
IM   = intramuscular
IV   = intravenous
LD_{50} = median lethal dose
PO   = *per os* (by mouth)
q   = every
SQ   = subcutaneous

Suggested Reading

Gwaltney-Brant SM, Dunayer EK, Youssef HY. Terrestrial zootoxins. In: Gupta RC, ed. Veterinary Toxicology: Basic and Clinical Principles. New York: Elsevier, 2007; pp. 785–786.

Mebs D. Black widow spider. In: Mebs D, ed. Venomous and Poisonous Animals. Boca Raton: CRC Press, 2002; pp. 184–187.

Peterson ME. Spider envenomation: Black widow. In: Peterson ME, Talcott PA, eds. Small Animal Toxicology, 2nd ed. St. Louis: Saunders, 2006; pp. 1063–1069.

Twedt DC, Cuddon PA, Horn TW. Black widow spider envenomation in a cat. J Vet Int Med 2008; 13:613–616.

Authors: Michael E. Peterson, DVM, MS; Catherine M. Adams, DVM
Consulting Editor: Lynn R. Hovda, RPH, DVM, MS, DACVIM

chapter **46**

Brown Recluse Spiders

DEFINITION/OVERVIEW

- The brown recluse spider (*Loxosceles reclusa*) is a spider 8–13 mm in length with comparatively long legs of 20–30 mm in length. Its color ranges in shades of brown, and it has a violin shape on the dorsal cephalothorax (fig. 46.1).
- The spider is a hunter; the web is irregular and wispy.
- Various species of the *Loxosceles* spiders range over the temperate regions of Europe, Africa, and North and South America; however most are found in the Americas. In the United States, the range is primarily in the southern Midwest, with certain species being found in the southern western states. It is a common misconception that they are more widespread (see fig. 46.2).

ETIOLOGY/PATHOPHYSIOLOGY

Mechanism of Action

- The venom is a mixture of proteases and phospholipases, causing local and systemic clinical signs.
- Sphingomyelinase D, present in the venom, causes platelet aggregation, complement cascade, cellular lysis, apoptosis, and an immune response that leads to dermonecrosis.
- There appears to be tremendous variability between species regarding the extent of the response to the venom and the susceptibility to the venom.
  - Rabbits and humans had similar dermonecrotic lesions, but the rabbit's lesions healed more quickly.
  - Dogs had a milder version of the dermonecrotic lesion with the same injected dose of venom.

Pharmacokinetics/Absorption, Distribution, Metabolism, and Excretion

- After venom injection, little or no pain may be felt initially.
- Within 3–8 hours after envenomation, the area develops pruritus, pain, swelling, and a target lesion. The center may form a vesicle that later becomes a black scab (eschar).

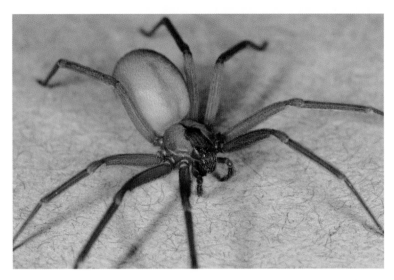

■ **Fig. 46.1.** Brown recluse spider (*Loxosceles reclusa*). Note the distinctive violin mark; it is often poorly demarcated in immature spiders or other species. (Photo courtesy of Richard Vetter, Dept. of Entomology, University of California–Riverside)

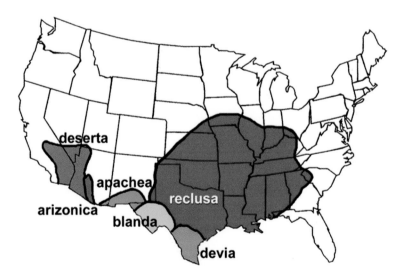

■ **Fig. 46.2.** North American distribution of the most widespread species of *Loxosceles* spiders. (Map courtesy of Richard Vetter, Dept. of Entomology, University of California–Riverside)

- Tissue around the lesion, along with the scab, may slough after 2–5 weeks, leaving a deep, slowly healing ulcer that usually spares muscle tissue.
- Less commonly, hemolytic anemia with hemoglobinuria may occur within the first 24 hours.
- Other systemic signs (tachycardia, fever, vomiting, dyspnea, renal failure, coma) may develop 6–72 hours after envenomation.

Toxicity

- Severity of signs varies with the amount of venom injected, but even minute amounts can cause severe clinical signs.
- Very little research has been done, and since the clinical signs mimic many other rule-outs, the concern is that misdiagnosis of spider venom may prevent correct diagnosis of another illness with more serious consequences such as Lyme disease, corrosive injury, dermal infection, and others.
- Little animal-related scientific data is available. There have been only two in vivo studies done in dogs to determine the effects of envenomation, and no studies in cats.

Systems Affected

- Skin/exocrine—localized pruritus, pain, swelling, classic target lesion, scabbing, ulceration
- Hemic/lymphatic/immune—leukocytosis, hemolytic anemia, thrombocytopenia, prolonged coagulation times
- Renal/urologic—renal failure
- Hepatobiliary—elevations in hepatic enzymes
- Endocrine/metabolic—fever, lethargy
- Gastrointestinal—vomiting

 SIGNALMENT/HISTORY

- Diagnosis is based on history, clinical signs, and appropriate geographic environment.
- No breed or sex predilection

Risk Factors

- Geriatric or pediatric patients may be at more risk of developing systemic effects.

Location and Circumstances of Poisoning

- The brown recluse spider is a shy, nocturnal creature that hides in dark areas under leaf litter, tree bark, or rocks. Inside houses, it hides in bedding, basements, under piles of clothes, and anywhere it will have protection.
- The spider will bite only if disturbed, attacking quickly and leaving immediately, making identification of the spider difficult.

 CLINICAL FEATURES

- There are two distinct forms as seen in human beings.

- Cutaneous. After an initial mild edema or erythema, the bite area becomes necrotic. An eschar forms over the area covering a deep ulcerating wound that heals very slowly. Secondary infection may occur.
- Viscerocutaneous. Rare systemic reactions are more likely in pediatric or geriatric patients. Severe hemolytic anemia, with hemoglobinuria, hematuria, and thrombocytopenia, may occur within 6–24 hours. Renal failure may be a sequela.

 # DIFFERENTIAL DIAGNOSIS

- Immune-mediated disease
- Injury
- Primary infections, including parasitic, fungal, bacterial, viral causes
- Neoplastic cutaneous disease
- Secondary cutaneous disease (diabetic ulcer, septic embolism)
- Vascular disease

 # DIAGNOSTICS

- There are no specific tests for the disease.
- Other tests should be used to rule out other diseases (Lyme test, autoimmune tests, coagulation tests, chemistry panel, CBC, UA) and to predict treatment in the case.
- Baseline CBC with platelet count and serum chemistry in those animals with evidence of systemic disease

Pathological Findings

- Pathological findings include dermal necrosis and ulceration with possible secondary infection.

 # THERAPEUTICS

- The treatment goals are to provide symptomatic and supportive care (rest, antibiotics if needed, IV, blood transfusion).
- There have been many suggested treatments, including surgical removal, dapsone, hyperbaric oxygen, anticoagulants, shock therapy, steroids, antihistamines, vitamin C, and meat tenderizer, but none have proven to be effective.

Detoxification

- None other than good wound care

Appropriate Healthcare

- Clean wound well with soap and water; prevent secondary infection.
- Cool compresses. Avoid application of heat.
- Elevation of area

Drug(s) and Antidotes of choice

- No specific antidote or antivenom is available.
- IV fluids as needed for dehydration and cardiovascular support
- Blood products as needed
- Broad-spectrum antibiotics if wound becomes infected
- Analgesics for pain
  - NSAIDs
    - Carprofen
      - Dogs: 2.2 mg/kg PO q 12–24 hours
      - Cats: 1–2 mg/kg SQ q 24 hours. Limit dosing to 2 days.
  - Opioids
    - Buprenorphine 0.005–0.02 mg/kg IM, IV or SQ q 6–12 hours
    - Tramadol 1–4 mg/kg PO q 8–12 hours for dogs (not yet evaluated in cats)
- Antiemetics
  - Maropitant 1 mg/kg SQ q 24 hours, not labeled for cats
  - Ondansetron 0.1–0.2 mg/kg IV q 8–12 hours
- Antihistamines for pruritus
  - Diphendyramine 2–4 mg/kg IM or PO as needed

Precautions/Interactions

- Heat treatment may exacerbate the condition.

Nursing Care

- Prolonged wound care may be necessary.

Surgical Considerations

- Wound debridement with Burrow's solution or dilute hydrogen peroxide followed by bandaging may be necessary.

Expected Course and Prognosis

- Full recovery may take weeks to months, but prognosis is good if systemic signs are not seen.

Abbreviations

CBC   = complete blood count
IM   = intramuscular
IV   = intravenous
PO   = *per os* (by mouth)
q   = every
SQ   = subcutaneous
NSAID = nonsteroidal anti-inflammatory
UA   = urinalysis

Suggested Reading

Gwaltney-Brant SM, Dunayer EK, Youssef HY. Terrestrial zootoxins. In: Gupta RC, ed. Veterinary Toxicology: Basic and Clinical Principles. New York: Elsevier, 2007; pp. 785–807.

Mebs D. Brown or fiddleback spiders. In: Mebs D, ed. Venomous and Poisonous Animals. Boca Raton: CRC Press, 2002; pp. 188–189.

Pace L, Vetter R. Brown recluse spider (*Loxosceles recluse*) envenomation in small animals. J Vet Emerg Crit Care 2009; 19(4):329–336.

Peterson ME. Spider envenomation: brown recluse. In: Peterson ME, Talcott PA, eds. Small Animal Toxicology, 2nd ed. St. Louis: Saunders, 2006; pp. 1071–1075.

Authors: Michael E. Peterson, DVM, MS; Catherine M. Adams, DVM
Consulting Editor: Lynn R. Hovda, RPH, DVM, MS, DACVIM

chapter 47

Bufo Toads

DEFINITION/OVERVIEW

- Two species of primary concern
    - Colorado River toad (*Bufo alvarius*). Found primarily in parts of California and along the Colorado River between Arizona and California.
    - Marine toad (*Bufo marinus*). Found primarily in Florida, Texas, Hawaii, and other tropical areas. Large toad that can grow up to 8 or 9 inches when mature (fig. 47.1).
- Marine toad is more toxic, and most exposed dogs will die if left untreated.
- Mouthing or ingestion of either can result in toxicity and death.
- Profuse salivation occurs within seconds of mouthing a toad.

ETIOLOGY/PATHOPHYSIOLOGY

Mechanism of Action

- Toxin produced by toad's parotid glands is rapidly absorbed across victim's mucous membranes.

Toxicity

- The toxin contains several major components, including bufotenines (pressor agents similar to oxytocin that may be hallucinogenic), bufagins (which act like digitalis cardiac glycosides), and noncardiac sterols.
- Limited information is available, but one rough estimate is that the contents of both parotid glands contain enough toxins to kill a 10–15 kg dog.
- Toads sitting in a water dish for several hours leave behind enough toxins to make an average-size dog ill after drinking the water.

Systems Affected

- Gastrointestinal—rapid onset of hypersalivation; occurs within seconds to minutes of mouthing or ingesting a toad
- Respiratory—increased respiratory rate and difficulty in breathing in 15 minutes

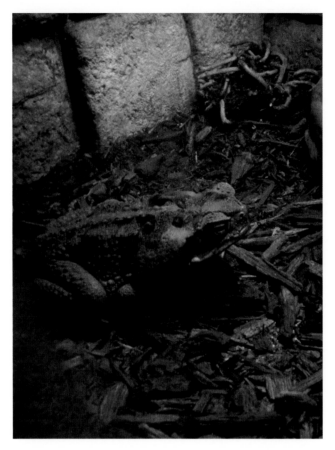

■ **Fig. 47.1.** Marine toad (*Bufo marinus*). (Photo courtesy of Tyne K. Hovda)

- Neurological—CNS stimulation ranging from ataxia to full seizures in 15–20 minutes
- Cardiovascular—Bradycardia or tachycardia with arrhythmias at any time

 ## SIGNALMENT/HISTORY

- Primarily dogs; rarely, ferrets and cats
- All ages can be affected.

Risk Factors

- Living in close proximity to toads. Toads are most active during periods of high humidity. Colorado River toads are especially active during the late summer monsoon season in the desert Southwest. Most encounters occur during the evening, night, or early morning hours.

CLINICAL FEATURES

- Onset is rapid, often occurring within a few minutes of exposure.
- Historical findings
    - Crying and pawing at the mouth
    - Ataxia or stiff gait
    - Seizures
- Physical examination findings
    - Profuse hypersalivation within seconds to minutes
    - Hyperexcitability with vocalization
    - Vomiting and diarrhea
    - Brick-red buccal mucous membranes
    - Hyperthermia
    - Recumbency, collapse
    - Marked cardiac ventricular arrhythmia—less common with Colorado River toad intoxication
    - Respiratory distress—dyspnea, tachypnea, cyanosis within 15 minutes
    - Neurological signs (ataxia, nystagmus, seizures) within 15–20 minutes

DIFFERENTIAL DIAGNOSIS

- Infectious diseases resulting in cardiovascular compromise
- Toxicants
    - Caustic agents and oral irritants
    - Cardiac glycoside plants
    - Calcium channel blockers and beta-blockers
    - Digoxin
    - Organophosphate and carbamate insecticides
    - Metaldehyde
- Underlying cardiac disease

DIAGNOSTICS

- CBC, serum chemistry, and urinalysis are generally unrewarding; may see hyperkalemia and acid/base imbalances
- Electrocardiogram may reveal ventricular arrhythmias.

THERAPEUTICS

- Marine toad intoxication is a medical emergency and death is common.
- Rinsing the mouth with water is a first line of therapy and should be instituted at home and again in the veterinary hospital.

Detoxification

- Emesis and activated charcoal are not recommended due to rapid onset of neurological signs.
- Emesis or endoscopic removal will be needed in those dogs that have swallowed an intact toad.
- Flush mouth with copious quantities of water for 10–15 minutes. Use a garden hose for larger dogs and put smaller ones in the sink. Be careful not to drown the animal while doing this.

Appropriate Health Care

- Rapid evaluation of cardiac activity is necessary, as is treatment of hyperthermia. Rectal temperatures can go as high as 105°F (40.6°C).
- Treat hyperthermia with a cool bath, cooling vest, or other measures. As temperature falls below 103°F (39.4C), stop measures. Do not overcool.

Drugs and Antidotes of Choice

- No specific antidote is available.
- IV fluids to treat hydration, electrolyte abnormalities, and hypotension
- Atropine
  - 0.04 mg/kg IM, SQ, IV as needed
  - Reduces the amount of salivation and helps prevent aspiration
  - Use with bradycardia, heart block, or other sinoatrial node alterations as a result of the digitalis-like effect of the toxin
  - Heart rate and secretions should guide redosing
  - Not recommended if severe tachycardia present
- Esmolol or propranolol for sinus tachycardia/tachyarrhythmias. Esmolol is very short acting and often used as a test dose. If the arrhythmia responds to treatment, propranolol should be used as the duration of action is much longer (hours).
  - Esmolol: 0.05–0.1 mg/kg IV every 5 minutes for a maximum dose of 0.5 mg/kg
  - Propranolol: 0.02 mg/kg IV slowly as needed up to a maximum dose of 1 mg/kg
- Lidocaine for ventricular tachycardia
  - 2 mg/kg IV slowly as a bolus; up to 8 mg/kg IV
  - If response is good, switch to CRI at 50–80 μg/kg/min.
- Antiemetics as needed
- Diazepam or phenobarbital for seizures
  - Diazepam 0.25–0.5 mg/kg IV
  - Phenobarbital 3–5 mg/kg IV PRN
- In severe cases, treatment with digoxin-specific Fab fragments may be indicated. Refer to chapter 3, "Antidotes and Other Useful Drugs," for specific information.

Precautions/Interactions

▪ Cardiac disease or bronchial asthma—patient may not tolerate the use of beta-blockers such as esmolol and propranolol. Use test dose of esmolol (very short duration of action) and monitor closely before using propranolol (much longer duration of action).

▪ Barbiturates may depress function of an already compromised myocardium; use with caution.

 # COMMENTS

Patient Monitoring

▪ Continuous electrocardiographic monitoring is recommended until the patient is fully recovered.

Expected Course and Prognosis

▪ Colorado River toad (*B. alvarius*) intoxication
  • Patients are usually normal within 30 minutes of onset of treatment.
  • Death is relatively uncommon if treated early.
  • Do not underestimate the risk of secondary heat stroke.
▪ Marine toad (*B. marinus*) intoxication is a true medical emergency and death is common.

Abbreviations

CBC = complete blood count
CRI = continuous rate infusion
Fab = fragment antigen binding
IM = intramuscular
IV = intravenous
SQ = subcutaneous

See Also

Beta-Blockers
Calcium Channel Blockers
Cardiac Glycosides

Suggested Reading

Otoni A, Palumbo N, Read G. Pharmacodynamics and treatment of animals poisoned by *Bufo marinus* toxin. Am J Vet Res 1969; 30:1865–1872.
Palumbo NE, Perri S, Read G. Experimental induction and treatment of toad poisoning in the dog. J Am Vet Med Assoc 1975; 167:1000–1005.

Peterson ME, Roberts BK. Toads. In: Peterson ME, Talcott PA, ed. Small Animal Toxicology, 2nd ed. St. Louis: Saunders, 2006; pp 1083–1093.

Reeves MP. A retrospective report of 90 dogs with suspected cane toad (*Bufo marinus*) toxicity. Aust Vet J 2008; 82(10):608–611.

Roberts BK, Aronsohn MG, Moses BL. *Bufo marinus* toxicity in dogs: 94 cases (1997–1998). J Am Vet Med Assoc 2000; 216:1941–1944.

Authors: Michael E. Peterson DVM, MS; Lynn Rolland Hovda, DVM, MS, ACVIM
Consulting Editors: Lynn R. Hovda, RPH, DVM, MS, DACVIM; Justine A. Lee, DVM, DACVECC

chapter 48

Crotalids (Pit Vipers)

DEFINITION/OVERVIEW

- Local and systemic venom-induced toxicity may both occur following bites by snakes in the subfamily Crotalinae (pit vipers), which comprises the genera *Agkistrodon* (cottonmouths [water moccasins] and copperheads) and *Crotalus* and *Sistrurus* (rattlesnakes) in North America (see figs. 48.1, 48.2, and 48.3).
- Identified by retractable fangs, heat-sensing pit between the nostril and eye, and a triangle-shaped head (see fig. 48.4)
- Venomous snakebite does not necessarily mean envenomation has occurred; in human beings, 20% of bites are "dry bites" with no venom injected.
- In some cases, the onset of clinical signs may be delayed up to 6 hours.
- Good emergent and supportive care coupled with antivenom therapy are key components for achieving an optimal outcome in cases of venomous snakebite.

ETIOLOGY/PATHOPHYSIOLOGY

- Inquisitive companion animals living in regions where venomous snakes are indigenous (particularly the southeastern and southwestern regions)
- Bites frequently are to the face and front legs due to the curious nature of dogs and cats when they encounter a snake.
- Fang punctures may be evident but can be missed due to hair.
- In cases where envenomation has occurred, swelling usually ensues.
  - Airway obstruction consistently occurs with bites to the tongue and rarely with bites to the face (fig. 48.5).
  - Neurotoxic venom may exhibit no local signs other than bite wounds.
- Further complications can result with development of coagulopathies.

Mechanism of Action

- Pit viper venoms are primarily composed of numerous proteins (both enzymatic and nonenzymatic) and small peptides. These typically will work in concert to produce insults on blood clotting and tissue integrity, alter fluid (blood and serum) distribution, and in some cases (depending on the species of snake) block central nervous system function.

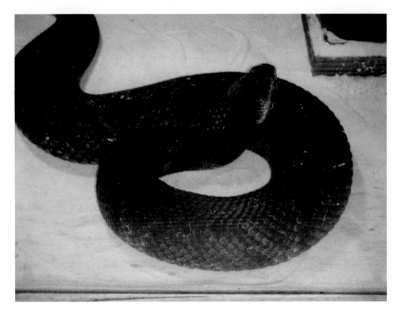

■ **Fig. 48.1.** Cottonmouth (*Agkistroton piscivorus*). (Photo courtesy of Tyne K. Hovda)

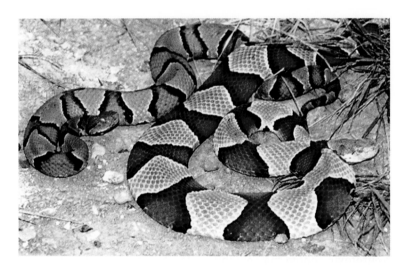

■ **Fig. 48.2.** Copperheads (*Agkistrodon contortrix*). (Photo courtesy of Dan Keyler)

- Most venom induces a drop in blood pressure, caused by pooling of blood within the splanchic (dogs) and pulmonary (cats) vessels, resulting in shock.
- Blood clotting factors can be inhibited, and the function of fibrinogen and platelets may be compromised, potentially producing significant coagulopathies.
- Red blood cells may be lost to the extravascular space or compromised, rendering them nonfunctional.

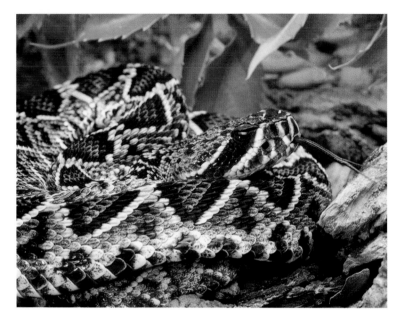

■ **Fig. 48.3.** Eastern diamondback rattlesnake (*Crotalus adamanteus*). (Photo courtesy of Barney Oldfield)

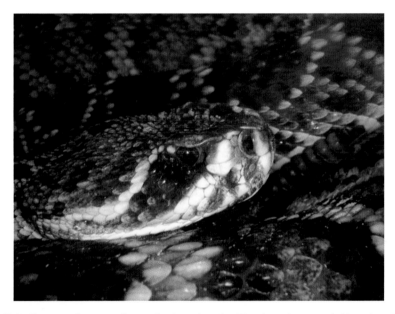

■ **Fig. 48.4.** Close-up of eastern diamondback rattlesnake (*Crotalus adamanteus*). Note the triangular-shaped head and heat-sensing pits between nostril and eye. (Photo courtesy of Tyne K. Hovda)

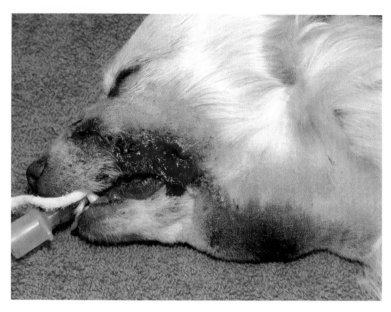

■ **Fig. 48.5.** Dog in respiratory distress and intubated secondary to prairie rattlesnake envenomation. (Photo courtesy of Barney Oldfield)

- Several species of rattlesnakes have subpopulations with venom containing a potent neurotoxin. It is possible for a snake to have both venom fractions. Strictly neurotoxic venoms produce no coagulopathies.

Pharmacokinetics/Absorption, Distribution, Metabolism, and Excretion

- The multiple toxins that compose snake venom all have their own individual kinetics but function collectively to enhance the distribution of specific toxins that are known to increase vascular permeability and alter clotting system functions.
- The rate of distribution of venom toxins can be quite rapid in the case of intravenous bites, slower with intramuscular bites, and slowest with subcutaneous bites (majority).
- Bites to the face and extremities generally have slower venom uptake than bites to the torso; peritoneal and tongue envenomations have rapid absorption.
- Metabolism and excretion kinetics are complex and, because of the multitoxin composition of venom, have not been well studied.
- Some toxins can form a repository or depot at a bite site, resulting in a slower sustained-release systemic absorption. Toxins that penetrate deeper tissues may redistribute with time back into the systemic circulation, resulting in recurrent toxicity. This process of redistribution can occur days after the bite.

Toxicity

- Although considered hematoxic, several species have subpopulations with lethal neurotoxic components (e.g., Mojave rattlesnake)
- General ranking of venom toxicity: (1) rattlesnakes, (2) water moccasins, (3) copperheads
- The route of administration of venom influences the time to effect of venom components and the level of systemic venom dosage (mg venom/kg BW).
- 85% of victims have altered laboratory values and clinically important swelling.
- Systemic toxic effects of venom occur greatest in highly perfused tissues with certain organ systems being more susceptible to thrombocytopenia, hypofibrinogemia (less commonly hyperfibrinogenemia), and the resultant coagulopathy.

Systems Affected

- Hemic/lymphatic/immune—coagulopathies and vascular hemorrhage
- Respiratory—fluid shifts to lungs, respiratory compromise secondary to neuromuscular complications
- Skin/exocrine—tissue destruction
- Cardiovascular—shock
- Renal/urologic—renal failure
- Gastrointestinal—vomiting and diarrhea
- Neuromuscular—generalized weakness

 SIGNALMENT/HISTORY

- Cats and dogs of any age may encounter venomous snakes that are indigenous to their region.
- The veterinarian should be aware of the venomous snake species in the geographic area in which they practice.

Risk Factors

- Smaller patients and older animals may be at greater risk of severe complications.
  - In smaller animals the venom dose (mg venom/kg BW of victim) may be quite large.
  - Geriatric animals lack resilience in their physiologic systems.
- Animals with cardiac, diabetic, renal, or other major physiologic system compromise are also at increased risk of medical complications. These factors may necessitate intensive supportive veterinary medical management in addition to treatment with antivenom.
- Animals receiving medications for existing medical problems

- NSAIDs may predispose to clotting anomalies.
- Corticosteroids may decrease natural defenses.
- Beta-blockers may mask the onset of anaphylaxis.
■ Aggressiveness and motivation of snake
  - Defensive strike—more likely to be "dry"
  - Feeding strike—more venom injected
  - Agonal bite—all available venom injected

Historical Findings

■ If the rattlesnake is not observed biting the animal, puncture wounds from fangs can frequently be observed; may require clipping hair in affected area.
■ Owners should be questioned as to whether antivenom has ever been given as prior exposure (may increase the chances of allergic reaction to antivenom).

Location and Circumstances of Poisoning

■ Copperheads account for the majority of venomous snakebites in areas where they are endemic. They are often found around human habitation.
■ In some cases owners may find their pet carrying around a snake that they have killed and chewed on. These patients should be checked carefully for multiple bite sites and are at high risk for agonal bites. If the snake has been killed, it is useful in correct identification.

Interactions with Drugs, Nutrients, or Environment

■ Because of the complex makeup of snake venom with numerous different toxins, there is the potential for interaction with many drugs. See Risk Factors.
■ Environmental factors such as excessive heat may be an additional burden beyond the effects of snake venom alone. Careful use of selective medications and the maintenance of euthermia and homeostasis are keys to an optimal outcome.

 CLINICAL FEATURES

■ Local signs may include the following:
  - Angioedema
  - Fang punctures—not always two punctures, may be multiple scratches, not always visible
  - Edema and swelling
  - Bleeding from the bite site
  - Erythema, ecchymosis
  - Lymphangitis

- Systemic signs may include the following:
  - Hypotension
  - Respiratory changes (dyspnea)
  - Weakness
  - Bleeding—epistaxis, gingival, hematuria, melena, retinal hemorrhage
  - Excessive salivation
  - Myokymia/fasciculations
  - Vomiting—hematemesis
  - Diarrhea
  - Oliguria

DIFFERENTIAL DIAGNOSIS

- Animal bites—nonsnake (e.g., rodents, shrews, etc.)
- Hymenoptera venom–induced angioedema. When touched, these swollen areas are generally not significantly painful in contrast to pit viper envenomation.
- Toxicants—brodifacoum or warfarin-based rodenticides
- Trauma-induced puncture wounds (e.g., nails, barbwire fence, etc.)
- Sepsis

DIAGNOSTICS

- If the snake is available, obtain proper identification. Determine species and if venomous or nonvenomous.
- Examine animal for fang marks, clip hair in affected area, examine for local tissue damage and ecchymosis.
- CBC, serum chemistry, UA, and coagulation profile—Initial bloodwork sets a baseline for monitoring progression of envenomation syndrome.
- CBC—If venom has been injected, 89% have echinocytosis (non-EDTA blood).
- Urinalysis—hemoglobinuria or myoglobinuria secondary to rhabdomyolysis
- Coagulation parameters (INR, Plts, PT, PTT, Fib)
  - International normalized ratio (INR)—prolonged
  - Prothrombin time (PT), partial thromboplastin time—prolonged
  - Platelets (Plts)—decreased
  - Fibrinogen (Fib)—decreased
- ECG—Ventricular arrhythmias may be detected in severely depressed patients.

Detoxification

- No particular detoxification at the site, best to transport to veterinary clinic immediately.

- Remove collars and other restrictive devices prior to transport.
- Clip and clean bite area.

Appropriate Healthcare

- Minimize exercise/movement.
- Observe closely for airway obstruction and be prepared to intubate.
- Monitor cardiovascular system closely.
- Blood pressure monitor.

Drug(s) and Antidotes of Choice

- Antivenom is the definitive antidote for venomous snakebite. In the United States, there are potentially four antivenom products available—one licensed for veterinary use, one licensed for human use in North America, and two for human use in Central America (usually maintained at zoos). In the absence of availability of the veterinary product, human antivenom products can be used. Availability and economic factors may determine whether antivenom therapy is an option.
  - The earlier antivenom is administered, the more effective it is; one vial early is equal to several later.
  - Specifics of use
    - Lyophilized antivenin should be reconstituted with diluent and gently agitated; the vial should be flushed as significantly more antivenin can be captured.
    - Dilute in 250 mL of crystalloids and administer IV slowly, looking for any sign of allergic reaction—pruritus, hyperemia of pinna, piloerection. If allergic-type reaction occurs, stop antivenin infusion.
    - Reaction is usually a complement-mediated anaphylactoid-type response to foreign proteins given too rapidly. Stop infusion, give diphenhydramine (2–4 mg/kg IM or PO), wait 5 minutes, and begin antivenin again at a slower rate. If problem persists, seek veterinary toxicology consult.
    - Anaphylactic reactions may also occur and the clinician should be prepared to respond.
  - Specific products
    - Antivenin (Crotalidae) Polyvalent (veterinary antivenin)—IgG (equine derived); Boehringer-Ingelheim, Ridgefield, CT
      - Dose varies from 1 to 5 vials IV depending on severity of symptoms.
      - 95% of cases controlled with a single vial
    - CroFab (human antivenin)—Crotalidae Polyvalent Immune—Fab1 (ovine derived); BTG, Brentwood, TN
      - Dose is not precisely determined for veterinary use.
      - Currently not licensed as specific veterinary product

- ○ Veterinary trial has been completed and is pending publication, average dose one vial (personal communication, Michael. E. Peterson).
  - □ Antivipmyn (human antivenin)—Polyvalent equine antiviper serum—Fab$_2$ (equine derived); Instituto Bioclon, S.A., Mexico
    - ○ Carried by many zoos in United States
    - ○ Currently in veterinary trials
  - □ Costa Rican pit viper antivenin (human antivenin)—Polyvalent Fab$_2$ (equine derived); Instituto Clodomino Picado, Costa Rica
    - ○ Not cross-reactive to all North American rattlesnakes
- ■ IV crystalloid fluids for volume resuscitation. The vast majority of cases are started on fluid therapy while antivenin is being prepared. Some envenomation syndromes can be controlled with IV fluids alone. Do not fluid overload.
- ■ Blood products may be needed for animals with marked hypoproteinemia. Coagulation defects can rarely be corrected with blood products alone, and persistent defects require additional antivenom.
- ■ Pain management
  - • Buprenorphine 0.005–0.02 mg/kg IM, IV or SQ q 6–12 hours
  - • Tramadol 1–4 mg/kg PO q 8–12 hours for dogs (not yet labeled for use in cats)
- ■ Antiemetics for persistent vomiting
  - • Maropitant 1 mg/kg SQ q 24 hours, not labeled for cats
  - • Ondansetron 0.1–0.2 mg/kg IV q 8–12 hours
- ■ Antibiotics are not routinely needed in cases of snakebite unless localized tissue damage is severe and infected. Fluoroquinolone antimicrobials improved survival in one study but wound infection was not assessed. No other antimicrobial agent had an effect on survival.

Precautions/Interactions

- ■ Antivenin reactions. The antibodies are foreign proteins and may precipitate allergic complications. This sometimes results from too-rapid administration; simply slowing/stopping the infusion rate may reduce the complication.
- ■ Other drugs
  - • Corticosteroids have no documented value in the treatment of venomous snakebite; evidence suggests they may worsen the condition.
  - • Colloids are avoided since they can alter coagulation and may pull fluids out of the intervascular space through damaged vessel walls.
  - • DMSO enhances uptake and spread of venom.
  - • Heparin should not be used as the coagulopathies induced by pit viper venoms work by a different mechanism. It has no clinical value and may worsen the condition.
  - • Morphine can cause reactions similar to early anaphylaxis.
- ■ Rattlesnake vaccine for dogs is currently marketed. The efficacy is unknown with only anecdotal evidence at this time.

COMMENTS

Patient Monitoring

- Baseline laboratory values should be obtained and repeated as necessary, particularly coagulation panel, packed cell volume, and total protein.
- Recurrence of clinical signs or coagulation abnormalities can occur with any antivenom. If patient has initial coagulopathy resolved with antivenom use, recurrence can occur usually within the next week (most commonly the next few days), although rarely as severe as initial defect. There have been no documented veterinary cases of clinical bleeding from subsequent coagulopathy; however, the clinician should be aware of the possibility.

Expected Course and Prognosis

- Animals may also suffer recurrent symptoms following an apparent recovery. These may be both local and systemic, and as such warrant that animals are closely monitored for up to several weeks following the snakebite and associated treatments.

Abbreviations

BW   = body weight
DMSO = dimethylsulfoxide
Fab   = fragment antigen binding
Fib   = fibrinogen
IgG   = immunoglobulin G
IM   = intramuscular
INR   = international normalized ratio; intravenous
IV   = intravenous
plt   = platelets
PO   = *per os* (by mouth)
PT   = prothrombin time
PTT   = partial thromboplastin time
q   = every
SQ   = subcutaneous
UA   = urinalysis

See Also

Elapids (Coral Snakes)

Suggested Reading

Boyer LV, Seifert SA, Cain, JS. Recurrence phenomena after immunoglobulin therapy for snake envenomations: part 2. Guidelines for clinical management with crotaline Fab antivenom. Ann Emerg Med 2001; 37:196–201.

Dart RC, McNally J. Efficacy, safety and use of snake antivenoms in the United States. Ann Emerg Med 2001; 37:181–188.

Gold BS, Barish RA, Dart RC. North American snake envenomation: diagnosis, treatment, and management. Emerg Med Clin North Am 2004; 22:423–443.

McCown JL, Cooke KL, Hanel R. Effect of antivenin dose on outcome from crotalid envenomation: 218 dogs (1988–2006). J Vet Emerg Crit Care 2009; 19(6):603–610.

Peterson ME. Snake bite: North American pit vipers. In: Peterson ME, Talcott PA, eds. Small Animal Toxicology. 2nd ed. St. Louis: Saunders, 2006; pp. 1017–1038.

Authors: Daniel E. Keyler Pharm D; Michael E. Peterson, DVM, MS
Consulting Editor: Lynn R. Hovda, RPH, DVM, MS, DACVIM

chapter 49

Elapids (Coral Snakes)

DEFINITION/OVERVIEW

- Members of Elapidae family
- Two clinically important species or subspecies in North America
  - *Micrurus fulvius fulvius*, eastern coral snake (North Carolina to the north; southern Florida to the south; west of the Mississippi River)
  - *Micrurus tenere* (formerly *Micrurus fulvius tenere*), Texas coral snake (west of Mississippi; in Arkansas, Louisiana, and Texas)
- Identification
  - Color pattern—red, yellow, and black bands (in this order) fully encircling the body (red and yellow colors touch each other; see fig. 49.1)
  - Relatively small head, black snout, round pupils

ETIOLOGY/PATHOPHYSIOLOGY

- Generally, coral snakes are timid and nonaggressive; bites to animals usually occur because the animal is harassing the snake.
- Fixed fangs and need to chew to inject venom
- Bites relatively uncommon due to snake's reclusive behavior and nocturnal habits

Mechanism of Action

- Bite wounds primarily to lips, tongue, mouth, and webbing of paws. May appear as scratches
- Envenomation usually associated with a prolonged contact bite and puncture of skin. Venom is a neurotoxin causing muscle paralysis and CNS depression.
- Primary site of action is at the neuromuscular junction. Both presynaptic and postsynaptic blockade actions occur, and on occasion cardiotoxin-like actions are observed.

Pharmacokinetics/Absorption, Distribution, Metabolism, and Excretion

- Onset of clinical signs may be delayed several hours (up to 18 hours) after envenomation.

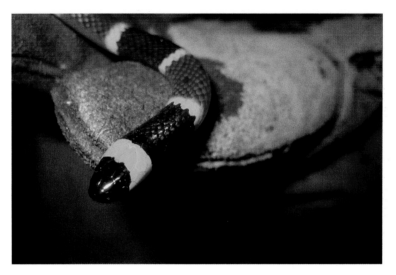

■ **Fig. 49.1.** Eastern coral snake (*Micrurus fulvius fulvius*); red and yellow bands touch each other; head is small with black snout. (Photo courtesy of David Seerveld, AAAnimal Control, Orlando, FL)

Toxicity

- Envenomations by *Micrurus tenere* seem to be less severe than *Micrurus fulvius fulvius.*

Systems Affected

- Neuromuscular—depolarization in muscle fibers
- Respiratory—respiratory depression
- Cardiovascular—antagonism of acetylcholine receptors

 SIGNALMENT/HISTORY

- Dogs and cats are equally affected.
- Cats may have a more difficult time surviving if prolonged respiratory support is needed.

Risk Factors

- Size of snake

 CLINICAL FEATURES

- Cats—primarily neurologic with respiratory depression, quadriplegia, CNS depression, hypotension, anisocoria, hypothermia

- Dogs—CNS depression, bulbar paralysis affecting cranial motor nerves, respiratory tract, and skeletal muscles; acute flaccid quadriplegia, dysphoria, dyspnea, respiratory depression, hypersalivation, hypotension, ventricular tachycardia
- Animals may be found staggering, salivating excessively, and may appear disoriented.

 ## DIFFERENTIAL DIAGNOSIS

- Botulism
- Myasthenia gravis
- Polyradiculoneuritis
- Tick bite paralysis

 ## DIAGNOSTICS

- CBC
  - Dogs—intravascular hemolysis, anemia, RBC burring
- Serum chemistry
  - Cats—increases in ALP and CK
- Urinalysis
  - Dogs—hematuria, hemoglobinuria
  - Cats—myoglobinuria
- If the snake is available, an accurate identification is useful in confirmation of coral snake envenomation.
- Often difficult to determine if a bite has actually occurred. Fangs are very small. Use of magnifying glass and good lighting can aid in determination of skin penetration.

Pathological Findings

- None specific

 ## THERAPEUTICS

Detoxification

- Avoid first aid measures; most effective treatment is rapid transport to a veterinary facility for antivenom administration.
- Australian technique for Elapidae bites is a pressure wrap of the bitten limb with ace-type bandage to decrease blood flow and venom uptake.

Appropriate Healthcare

- Do not wait for onset of clinical signs to initiate treatment.

- Hospitalize for a minimum of 48 hours.
- Clip and clean wound.
- Monitor respirations—be prepared to intubate.
- In the absence of antivenom, provide ventilatory support for several days in a critical care facility.
- ECG if tachycardia or abnormal rhythm
- Blood pressure monitoring for hypotension
- Treat signs as they develop. Aspiration pneumonia may occur secondary to loss of swallowing reflex.

Drug(s) and Antidotes of Choice

- Specific antivenom (*M. fulvius*) is no longer readily available in the United States; antivenom from other countries may sometimes be obtained from zoos. Follow manufacturer's guidelines for administration.
- Protective cross-reactivity does occur with the following antivenoms:
  - Coralmyn Instituto Bioclon, Mexico
  - Costa Rican coral snake antivenin; Instituto Clodomiro Picado, Costa Rica
  - Australian tiger snake (*Notechis scutatus*) antivenin; CSL Limited, Parkville, Victoria, Australia
  - Be prepared for a possible allergic reaction.
    - ☐ Anaphylaxis should be treated with fluids and epinephrine.
    - ☐ Anaphylactoid reactions should be treated by stopping the antivenin administration, administering diphenhydramine (2–4 mg/kg PO or IM, lower dose for cats), waiting 5 minutes, and resuming antivenin administration more slowly.
    - ☐ Serum sickness may occur 1–4 weeks after infusion and may be treated with corticosteroids and antihistamines.
- IV fluids to prevent dehydration and treat myoglobinuria and hematuria.
- Blood products if anemia is severe.
- Broad-spectrum antibiotics for 7–10 days may be needed if local tissue damage with infection has occurred.

Precautions/Interactions

- Corticosteroids use is controversial and not recommended. Reserve for true anaphylactic reaction to antivenom

Alternative Drugs

- Neostigmine—May be used if immediate restoration of neuromuscular transmission is needed until respiratory support can be implemented. This reversible cholinesterase inhibitor has been used successfully in human cases of coral snake envenomation.

Nursing Care

- Frequent vital signs
- Good wound care if enzymatic action of venom has resulted in local tissue damage

 COMMENTS

Expected Course and Prognosis

- Prognosis is fairly good with early intervention. Aspiration pneumonia worsens the prognosis.
- Marked clinical signs may last 1–1.5 weeks.
- Full recovery may take months as receptors regenerate.

Abbreviations

ALP = alkaline phosphatase
CBC = complete blood count
CK   = creatine kinase
CNS = central nervous system
ECG = electrocardiogram
Fab = fragment antigen binding
IM   = intramuscular
IV   = intravenous
PO   = *per os* (by mouth)

Suggested Reading

Brazil OV, Viera RJ. Neostigmine in the treatment of snake accidents caused by *Micrurus front-inalils*: report of two cases. Rev Inst Med Trop Sao Paulo 1996; 38:61–67.

Kitchens GS, Van Mierop LHS. Envenomation by the eastern coral snake (*Micrurus fulvius fulvius*). J Am Med Assoc 1987; 258:1615–1618.

Peterson ME. Snake bite: coral snakes. In: Peterson ME, Talcott PA, eds. Small Animal Toxicology 2nd ed. St. Louis: Saunders, 2006; pp. 1039–1048.

Sanchez EE, Lopez-Johnston JC, Rodriquez-Acosta, et al. Neutralization of two North American coral snake venoms with United States and Mexican antivenoms. Toxicon 2008; 51:297–303.

Wisniewski MS, Hill RE, Havey JM, et al. Australian tiger snake (*Notechis scutatus*) and Mexican coral snake (*Micrurus species*) antivenoms prevent death from United States coral snake (*Micrurus fulvius fulvius*) venom in a mouse model. J Clin Toxicol Clin Tox 2003; 41:7–10.

Authors: Michael E. Peterson, DVM, MS; Daniel E. Keyler, Pharm D
Consulting Editor: Lynn Rolland Hovda, RPH, DVM, MS, DACVIM

chapter 50

Scorpions

 DEFINITION/OVERVIEW

- There are over 1500 species of scorpions found in all parts of the world except Antarctica.
- Only one species in North America, found primarily in the Sonoran desert area, causes clinical signs after a venomous sting—the Arizona bark scorpion (*Centruroides exilicauda*, formerly *Centruroides sculpturatus*).
- This scorpion is light brown in color, nocturnal, ambushes its prey, and grows to about 8 cm (male) or 7 cm (female). See figure 50.1.
- It can be identified by the small tubercle under the stinger; magnification may be required to identify this. See figure 50.2.
- The majority of stings result only in localized pain or pruritus and usually resolve within 24 hours.

 ETIOLOGY/PATHOPHYSIOLOGY

Mechanism of Action

- The venom is a complex mixture of polypeptides, proteins, and neurotoxins. The neurotoxins of the bark scorpion block or delay the opening of the sodium channels of cell membranes, inhibiting neuromuscular transmission.
- Envenomation causes release of neurotransmitters, both sympathetic (causing tachycardia, hypertension, mydriasis) and parasympathetic (causing hypersalivation, bradycardia, hypotension).

Pharmacokinetics/Absorption, Distribution, Metabolism, and Excretion

- Animal studies involving other species of scorpions showed a distribution half-life of 4 to 7 minutes.
- Animal studies involving other species of scorpions showed an elimination half-life of 4.2 to 13.4 hours.

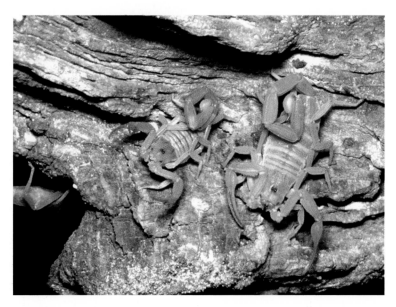

■ **Fig. 50.1.** Arizona bark scorpions (*Centruroides exilicaud*). (Photo courtesy of Arizona Poison and Drug Information Center, Tucson)

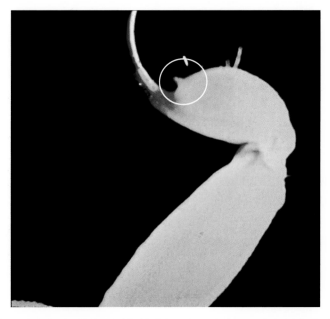

■ **Fig. 50.2.** The encircled tubercle located behind the stinger is characteristic of the bark scorpion. This tubercle may become less noticeable in some adults. (Photo courtesy of Arizona Poison and Drug Information Center, Tucson)

Toxicity

- There is very little data available in veterinary medicine. Anecdotal information documents pain and pruritus with the initial sting, followed by hypertension associated either with the toxins or secondary to the pain and distress.

Systems Affected

- Nervous—numbness at the site, paresthesia (human beings), tremors, ataxia
- Cardiovascular—hypertension, tachycardia; possible hypotension, bradycardia
- Endocrine/metabolic—hyperglycemia
- Respiratory—rarely, pulmonary edema secondary to cardiovascular compromise
- Ophthalmic—nystagmus
- Gastrointestinal—salivation

 SIGNALMENT/HISTORY

- No particular breed predilection
- Diagnosis is based on history, clinical signs, and appropriate geographic environment.
- No specific studies have been done on dogs and cats. Anecdotally, cats seem to be seldom, if ever, affected. They have been known to hunt the scorpions without consequence. There are, however, a few documented cases in Arizona where clinical signs in cats have occurred.

Risk Factors

- Geriatric or pediatric patients may be at higher risk of systemic involvement.

Location and Circumstances of Poisoning

- The bark scorpion is primarily nocturnal, hiding under rocks, clothes, or in shoes during the day. It will attack if threatened by an inquisitive animal or when crushed during movement of bedding, clothing, etc.

 CLINICAL FEATURES

- Immediate pain at the site following the sting. Edema and pruritus may follow.
- Hypertension may develop, especially in smaller animals. Whether this results from the venom itself or a pain response is unknown.
- Pulmonary edema may occur secondary to cardiovascular dysfunction.
- In human beings, paresthesia and numbness have been documented at the site of the sting. Tremors and neuromuscular dysfunction were also noted.

- Other clinical features in dogs and cats reported by owners to the Arizona Poison and Drug Information Center include respiratory changes, gastrointestinal distress, CNS changes (restlessness and lethargy), sneezing, and a pain response as evidenced by vocalizing, limping, licking, pawing, and head shaking. Signs usually persist for up to 24 hours, then resolve.

 # DIFFERENTIAL DIAGNOSIS

- Other venomous stings or bites (wasps, hornets, spiders) causing pain, allergic reaction

 # DIAGNOSTICS

- No specific diagnostics tests are recommended.
- Hyperglycemia due to decreased insulin production has been documented occasionally in human medicine.
- Identification of the scorpion, if possible, is the best diagnostic tool.

Pathological Findings

- Rarely, the skin at the site of the envenomation may slough.

 # THERAPEUTICS

- The goal is to provide symptomatic and supportive care. This includes the use of analgesics or opioids for pain control, appropriate treatment for CNS and CV changes, careful monitoring of the skin at the envenomation site, and medications for allergic reaction to the venom should it occur.

Detoxification

- Wash the sting area well and apply cool compresses as needed

Appropriate Healthcare

- Monitor the sting site for evidence of infection or skin sloughing.
- Frequent vital signs for first 24 hours to monitor for hypertension.
- Observe for onset of pulmonary edema and be prepared to intubate and provide oxygen as needed
- Watch closely for local and systemic signs associated with a rare allergic reaction to venom.

Drug(s) and Antidotes of Choice

- The use of antivenom is controversial. There are some locally prepared antivenoms available, but they are difficult to obtain and have not been approved by the FDA.
- IV fluids as needed to replace losses and prevent hypotension from hypovolemia
- Analgesics
  - Carprofen
    - Dogs: 2.2 mg/kg PO q 12–24 hours
    - Cats: 1–2 mg/kg SQ q 24 hours. Limit dosing to 2 days.
  - Deracoxib 1–2 mg/kg PO q 24 hours (dogs)
  - Buprenorphine 0.005–0.02 mg/kg IM, IV or SQ q 6–12 hours (dogs, cats)
  - Tramadol 1–4 mg/kg PO q 8–12 hours for dogs (not evaluated in cats yet)
- Antihistamine
  - Diphenhydramine 2–4 mg/kg IM or PO q 8–12 hours (dogs, cats)
- Hypertension—Acepromazine 0.05 mg/kg IV, IM, SQ (dogs, cats)

Nursing Care

- Cool compresses or ice may alleviate some of the local pain and swelling.
- Nonstimulating environment

Follow-up

- Monitor until clinical signs resolve.

 COMMENTS

Patient Monitoring

- Monitor hydration, pain level, blood pressure, heart rate, temperature, and development of hyperglycemia as needed based on degree of clinical signs being experienced.

Prevention/Avoidance

- Keep clothes picked up, shake out shoes and blankets prior to use; monitor pets' activities and keep them away from suspicious areas.

Possible Complications

- Allergic reactions, pulmonary edema, CV collapse, coma, and death are rare complications.

Expected Course and Prognosis

- Clinical signs generally resolve within 24 hours with no sequelae.

Abbreviations

CNS = central nervous system
CV   = cardiovascular
FDA = Food and Drug Administration
IM   = intramuscular
IV   = intravenous
PO   = *per os* (by mouth)
q   = every
SQ   = subcutaneous

Suggested Reading

Gwaltney-Brant SM, Dunayer EK, Youssef HY. Terrestrial zootoxins. In: Gupta RC, ed. Veterinary Toxicology: Basic and Clinical Principles. New York: Elsevier, 2007; pp. 785–786.

Mebs D. Scorpions. In: Mebs, D, ed. Venomous and Poisonous Animals. Boca Raton: CRC Press, 2002; pp. 172–178.

Peterson ME. Scorpion antivenom. In: Peterson ME, Talcott PA, eds. Small Animal Toxicology, 2nd ed. St. Louis: Saunders, 2006; p. 472.

Author: Catherine M. Adams, DVM
Consulting Editors: Lynn R. Hovda, RPH, DVM, MS, DACVIM; Ahna G. Brutlag, DVM

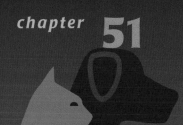

chapter **51**

Wasps, Hornets, Bees

DEFINITION/OVERVIEW

- Vespids (wasps and hornets) and apids (honeybees and African killer bees) are winged insects marked in yellows, blacks, and rarely white or red.
- With the exception of killer bees, they are found worldwide.
  - Wasps and hornets are in the Vespidae family and generally referred to as vespids.
  - Honeybees and African killer bees are in the Apidae family and generally referred to as apids.
- Venom is injected through an adapted ovipositor.
  - Vespids do not have barbs on the stinger and sting multiple times.
  - Apids have a barbed stinger that stays in the victim, continuing to pump toxin. Thus, a single sting by an apid causes the bee to die shortly after the sting.

ETIOLOGY/PATHOPHYSIOLOGY

Mechanism of Action

- Venom of the vespids and apids is a mixture of proteins, vasoactive amines and peptides, mastoparans, acetylcholine, kinins, serotonin, hyaluronidase, mellitin (apids only), and phospholipase A.
- The venom also promotes histamine release from mast cells and basophils (especially in sensitized individuals), which under the right circumstances can lead to vasodilation and loss of blood pressure.
- Together, all these components are responsible for the immediate pain, localized and regional reactions, and potential anaphylaxis experienced by animals.

Pharmacokinetics/Absorption, Distribution, Metabolism, and Excretion

- Absorption of the venom is immediate, causing intense pain.
- Onset of anaphylaxis occurs swiftly, usually within minutes of the sting.
- Delayed-type hypersensitivity reactions occur within 3–14 days.

Toxicity

- An estimated lethal dose in mammals is about 20 stings/kg BW.
- Each vespid sting contains about 17 µg of venom.
- African killer bee stings contain 94 µg of venom.
- European honeybee stings contain 147 µg venom.
- A single sting can be toxic to a susceptible animal, but the multiple stings delivered by the hornets and wasps and by many killer bees will result in far more serious consequences.

Systems Affected

- Skin/exocrine—wheals, erythema, edema, pruritus, pain
- Cardiovascular—collapse secondary to anaphylaxis
- Hemic/lymphatic/immune—DIC secondary to anaphylaxis
- Renal/urologic—acute renal failure secondary to anaphylaxis and DIC

 SIGNALMENT/HISTORY

- Diagnosis is based on history and clinical signs.
- Certain terrier breeds (bull, Staffordshire) and boxers appear to have a higher rate of reaction to the venom.

Risk Factors

- Geriatric, pediatric, and other individuals sensitive to the venom are at greater risk of serious clinical signs.

Location and Circumstances of Poisoning

- Honeybees are generally passive and only sting when aggravated.
- African killer bees travel in swarms but tend to mind their own business; when angry or provoked, a much more aggressive and deadly response occurs.
- Hornets and wasps resemble the approach of the killer bees, causing more injury because of the multiple stings each individual can produce and the large numbers of insects providing the attack.
- Animals that are confined in kennels or on tie-outs are at more risk if they cannot escape an attack.

 CLINICAL FEATURES

- There are four separate physiological responses to a sting.
  - Localized pain, erythema, and edema that occur within seconds to minutes; usually self-limiting within about 24 hours

- Regional edema and erythema sometimes affecting an entire limb.
- Anaphylaxis, usually within minutes
  - □ Anaphylaxis in dogs is characterized by urticaria, pruritus, angio-edema, vomiting, urination, weakness, respiratory and cardiovascular compromise, and seizures. Local upper airway edema can result in respiratory obstruction. Most deaths occur from respiratory compromise.
  - □ Anaphylaxis in cats is characterized by pruritus, vocalization, hyper-salivation, ataxia, and collapse.
- Delayed-type hypersensitivity reactions including serum sickness, DIC, arthritis, vasculitis, neuropathy, and renal compromise may occur within 3–14 days.

DIFFERENTIAL DIAGNOSIS

- Other venomous stings or bites (scorpions, fire ants) causing pain, allergic reaction
- Other causes of anaphylaxis

DIAGNOSTICS

Pathological Findings

- Consistent with anaphylaxis and DIC

THERAPEUTICS

- Most envenomations resolve without major intervention.

Detoxification

- Immediate removal of the bee stinger to limit further envenomation
- Careful removal of all wasps/hornets/bees from the hair to limit further stinging
- Cold compresses and basic wound care

Appropriate Healthcare

- Monitor closely for anaphylaxis and treat accordingly.
- Observe for respiratory compromise and be prepared to intubate and provide oxygen if needed.

Drug(s) and Antidotes of Choice

- No specific antidote is available.

- IV fluids as needed for hypotension secondary to cardiovascular compromise and hypovolemia. If hypotension persists after vigorous use of fluids (including colloids), and if the animal is well hydrated, consider adding the following:
  - Dopamine: 5–20 µg/kg/min IV CRI
  - Norepinephrine: 0.1–1.0 µg/kg/min IV CRI
  - Epinephrine: 0.1–0.4 µg/kg/min IV CRI
- Anaphylaxis
  - Diphenhydramine 1–4 mg/kg IM or SQ; can be given IV but must be given very slowly, and should be diluted.
  - Dexamethasone sodium phosphate 0.1–0.2 mg/kg IV q 12 hours
  - Epinephrine 0.01–0.02 mg/kg IV, IM, SQ
- Antiemetics if vomiting is severe or persists.
  - Maropitant 1 mg/kg SQ q 24 hours, not labeled for cats
  - Ondansetron 0.1–0.2 mg/kg IV q 8–12 hours
- Seizures
  - Diazepam 0.25–0.5 mg/kg IV PRN
  - Phenobarbital 3–5 mg/kg IV PRN
- Analgesics
  - Carprofen
    - Dogs: 2.2 mg/kg PO q 12–24 hours
    - Cats: 1–2 mg/kg SQ q 24 hours. Limit dosing to 2 days.
  - Deracoxib 1–2 mg/kg PO q 24 hours (dogs)
  - Buprenorphine 0.005–0.02 mg/kg IM, IV or SQ q 6–12 hours (dogs, cats)
  - Tramadol 1–4 mg/kg PO q 8–12 hours for dogs (not evaluated in cats yet)

Precautions/Interactions

- Since there is a potential for anaphylaxis, all animals should be monitored carefully for at least 30–90 minutes following envenomation.

Public Health

- Vespid and apid envenomation poses a risk to pet owners and clinic staff members. Use caution when removing attached wasps and hornets from the animal's hair coat.

 COMMENTS

Client Education

- Owners with dogs at risk for reactions to stings should keep diphenhydramine close at hand. Those with known reactions should have epinephrine readily available.

Patient Monitoring

▪ Monitor closely for signs of anaphylaxis following a sting.

Expected Course and Prognosis

▪ Prognosis is excellent for a localized reaction and fair to good for other reactions as long as prompt and aggressive treatment is provided. The total number of stings is more important than the species stinging in determining prognosis.

Abbreviations

BW = body weight
CRI = constant rate infusion
CV = cardiovascular
DIC = disseminated intravascular coagulation
IM   = intramuscular
IV   = intravenous
PO = *per os* (by mouth)
q   = every
SQ = subcutaneous

Suggested Reading

Fitzgerald K, Vera R. Insects: hymenoptera. In: Peterson ME, Talcott PA, eds. Small Animal Toxicology, 2nd ed. St. Louis: Saunders, 2006; pp. 744–756.

Gwaltney-Brant SM, Dunayer EK, Youssef HY. Terrestrial zootoxins. In: Gupta RC, ed. Veterinary Toxicology: Basic and Clinical Principles. New York: Elsevier, 2007; pp. 785–807.

Mebs D. Bees and bumblebees; Wasps and hornets. In: Mebs D, ed. Venomous and Poisonous Animals. Boca Raton: CRC Press, 2002; pp. 210–218.

Waddell L, Drobatz K. Massive envenomation by *Vespula* spp. in two dogs. J Vet Emerg Crit Care 1999; 9(2):67–71.

Author: Catherine M. Adams, DVM
Consulting Editor: Lynn R. Hovda, RPH, DVM, MS, DACVIM

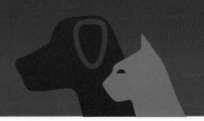

Foods

chapter 52

Bread Dough

DEFINITION/OVERVIEW

- Bread dough toxicosis occurs when uncooked or unbaked bread, pizza dough, bun, or roll products (including sourdough or "starters") that contain yeast are ingested during the process of rising.
- Although bread dough toxicosis can occur any time, the most commonly reported cases occur during the Easter and Christmas season, when many people bake their own bread.
- Although owners may be cognizant that the bread dough is missing and was ingested by their pet, most are not aware of the potential severe clinical signs that can develop due to the ingestion of rising dough. Because of this, most patients present once clinical signs have already become apparent.

ETIOLOGY/PATHOPHYSIOLOGY

Mechanism of Action

- During the process of rising, yeast within the dough produces ethanol gas. The fermentation rate increases once the dough is within the stomach due to the presence of a moist, warm environment and the internal body temperature (which acts as an "oven").
- The presence of a large amount of rising dough, coupled with the production of ethanol gas, can result in gastric bloat and, in severe cases, a life-threatening GDV.
- Ethanol is rapidly absorbed from the stomach and small intestines. It is metabolized in the liver by the enzyme alcohol dehydrogenase to form acetaldehyde and acetic acid.
- Acid production from the metabolism of ethanol can result in a severe metabolic acidosis.

Toxicology

- No known LD_{50} exists in dogs or cats.

Systems Affected

- Gastrointestinal—vomiting, distended abdomen, retching, bloat, GDV

- Cardiovascular—tachycardia, hypertension, tachyarrhythmias, hypovolemic shock; may also see bradycardia from severe ethanol toxicity and sedation; injected mucous membranes
- Nervous—behavior changes, vocalization, CNS depression, blindness, ataxia, weakness, recumbency, coma due to ethanol toxicity
- Respiratory—tachypnea, hypoxemia secondary to aspiration pneumonia, respiratory depression, and resultant cyanosis
- Endocrine/metabolic—hypoglycemia

 # SIGALMENT/HISTORY

- All reported cases of bread dough toxicosis have been in dogs.
- Dogs that are greedy or "garbage can" dogs are more likely to be affected (e.g., Labrador retrievers, beagles).
- Often, there is a history of dough ingestion prior to the onset of clinical signs.
- The presence of bread dough in emesis

 # CLINICAL FEATURES

- Dogs may present with gastric bloat, abdominal discomfort, vomiting, or unproductive retching.
- Ethanol toxicosis from the fermenting yeast will result in neurologic signs such as ataxia, weakness, and blindness. Severely affected dogs may present in semi-comatose to comatose states and require assisted mechanical ventilation.
- Hypoglycemia may occur due to depletion of glucose stores and depression of gluconeogenesis.

 # DIFFERENTIAL DIAGNOSES

- GDV or gastric dilatation
- Food bloat
- Foreign body obstruction
- Toxicities
  - Ethylene glycol toxicity
  - Salicylate toxicity
- Other diseases affecting the neurologic system, such as primary CNS disease, other neurogenic toxins, hepatic encephalopathy, drug overdose, other

 # DIAGNOSTICS

- Baseline blood work consisting of CBC, chemistry profile, and urinalysis should be performed.

- Quick assessment tests should be promptly performed, including blood glucose levels; electrolytes; blood gas analysis to assess acid-base status, oxygenation, and ventilation; blood lactate; and PCV/TP.
- Abdominal radiographs should be performed to assess the amount of gastric distension present and to verify correct positioning of the stomach. If GDV is diagnosed, emergency surgery is warranted following cardiovascular stabilization.
- Blood ethanol levels should be obtained if possible, to help verify the diagnosis and direct further therapy. Human hospitals have the ability to perform this analysis. Blood alcohol levels at 2–4 mg/mL in adult dogs have produced signs ranging from ataxia to coma.

Pathologic Findings

- The presence of bread dough in the stomach
- Evidence of gastric rupture, GDV, gastric necrosis, or septic peritonitis
- Splenic congestion
- Histopathologic findings consistent with GDV

 # THERAPEUTICS

- Goals of treatment include decontamination, gastric lavage to remove the presence of ethanol gas and bread dough, stabilization of cardiovascular collapse, prevention of further absorption of toxic compounds, and supportive/symptomatic care for cardiac, gastric, and neurologic symptoms.

Detoxification

- If recent ingestion with no clinical signs, immediate emesis with hydrogen peroxide or apomorphine can be performed, provided a GDV has been ruled out on history, physical exam, clinical signs, and/or radiographs.
- If emesis induction is unproductive and the presence of gastric material is evident (on physical examination or radiographs), gastric lavage with a large-bore stomach tube is indicated to remove the dough from the stomach and relieve the excess gas.
- Cold water lavage is very effective at decreasing further yeast fermentation by dropping the gastric temperature.
- Activated charcoal with cathartic should be administered via stomach tube 1x, once gastric evacuation and lavage have been performed.

Appropriate Health Care

- Severe gastric bloat or GDV can induce cardiovascular shock. Dogs should be initially triaged and fluid resuscitated if cardiovascular shock is diagnosed.

Intravenous crystalloid fluids should be administered at an initial dose of 30 mL/kg over 20 minutes and then readministered as further boluses if clinically indicated.

- Blood glucose levels should be maintained in the normal range. Hypoglycemic patients should be treated with a bolus of 50% dextrose (1 mL/kg, diluted) and followed with a CRI of dextrose supplementation in the IV fluids.
- Mild neurologic abnormalities should be treated with supportive care and are usually self-limiting.
- If severe neurologic signs are evident, direct therapy may include the administration of yohimbine. Ethanol has been demonstrated to affect specific receptors in the brain, including alpha$_2$-adrenergic receptors. Yohimbine is an alpha$_2$ receptor antagonist and therefore may block the effects of ethanol at these sites. One experimental study in ethanol-affected mice showed that yohimbine actually caused more sleepiness; however, it has been shown to arouse dogs in an ethanol-induced coma, increasing respirations and helping alleviate clinical signs of severe respiratory depression. Yohimbine should only be used in severely affected dogs, where respirations are affected and a mechanical ventilator is not available or an option.

Drug(s) and Antidotes of Choice

- There is no known antidote for bread dough toxicosis.

Nursing Care

- Patients that are nonambulatory due to severe ataxia from ethanol toxicosis should receive appropriate nursing care for a recumbent patient. Urinary catheterization may be necessary as part of nursing care.

 COMMENTS/PROGNOSIS

- Based on over 100 cases reported to Pet Poison Helpline and ASPCA Animal Poison Control Center combined, if dogs with this toxicosis are treated quickly and aggressively, they have an excellent prognosis for full recovery.

Abbreviations

CBC = complete blood count
CRI = continuous rate infusion
CNS = central nervous system
GDV = gastric dilatation volvulus
IV = intravenous
LD$_{50}$ = median lethal dose
PCV/TP = packed cell volume/total protein

Suggested Reading

Means C. Bread dough toxicosis in dogs. JVECC 2003; 13(1):39–41.

Suter RJ. Presumed ethanol intoxication in sheep dogs fed uncooked pizza dough. Aust Vet J 1992; 69(1):20.

Thrall MA, Freemyer FG, Hamar DW, et al. Ethanol toxicosis secondary to sourdough ingestion in a dog. JAVMA 1984; 184(12):1513–1514.

Author: Lisa L. Powell, DVM, DACVECC
Consulting Editor: Justine A. Lee, DVM, DACVECC

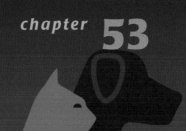

chapter **53**

Calcium Supplements

DEFINITION/OVERVIEW

- Calcium supplements range in dosage between OTC and prescription strength. Almost all contain vitamin D_3 to help increase the absorption of calcium from the GIT. Calcium salts are available as calcium carbonate, calcium chloride, calcium gluconate, and others.

ETIOLOGY/PATHOPHYSIOLOGY

- Through tightly controlled feedback mechanisms of parathyroid hormone (calcitonin and calcitriol), the body maintains its functional concentration of ionized calcium, the active component of total calcium.

Mechanism of Action

- Calcium is necessary for the normal functioning of the renal, musculoskeletal, nervous, respiratory, and coagulation systems.

Pharmacokinetics/Absorption, Distribution, Metabolism, and Excretion

- Calcium alone is poorly absorbed from the GIT.
- Activated vitamin D_3 is necessary for calcium absorption (see chapter 100, "Cholecalciferol").
- A small portion of calcium is distributed to the intracellular and extracellular fluid. The majority of calcium is taken up by bone.
- Calcium is excreted in the feces, with a very small amount excreted by the kidneys.

Toxicity

- Acute ingestions of most calcium supplements do not typically result in clinical signs of toxicosis in healthy animals.
- If enough vitamin D_3 is present in the ingestion, hypercalcemia can cause calcium deposits in the kidneys, in cardiac vessels, and in the GIT.
- Hypercalcemia can increase the excitation threshold of nerve and muscle cells, causing weakness and lethargy.

- Hypercalcemia decreases the GFR in the kidneys. Calcification occurs, further impairing the excretion of calcium.
- Calcium carbonate can produce alkalosis by mechanisms causing sodium to be excreted by the kidney. Volume depletion occurs, stimulating bicarbonate reabsorption.
- Increased calcium carbonate suppresses parathyroid hormone release, leading to further impairment of bicarbonate excretion.
- Hypercalcemia affects the GIT system by decreasing contractility of smooth muscle (potentially causing constipation) and increasing gastrin secretion (leading to increased hydrochloric acid secretion, which in turn causes GI irritation).
- Hypercalcemia inhibits ADH receptors in the renal tubules, leading to PU with compensatory PD (secondary nephrogenic diabetes insipidus).
- Deposition of calcium in the renal tubules causes mineralization and renal failure.

Systems Affected

- Gastrointestinal—vomiting, diarrhea, anorexia, nausea, constipation
- Urinary/renal—PU/PD, azotemia, oliguria, decreased GFR, renal mineralization, nephroliths, cystic calculi
- CNS—depression
- Endocrine/metabolic—transient hypercalcemia
- Musculoskeletal—weakness

 # SIGNALMENT/HISTORY

- All breeds and species are susceptible to GI irritation from ingestion of calcium supplements or to hypercalcemia from overdose of calcium supplements containing enough vitamin D_3 to allow calcium absorption.

Risk Factors

- Young animals or individuals with renal impairment are at increased risk of complications associated with hypercalcemia.

Historical Findings

- Owners often report PU/PD, lethargy, and anorexia when severe toxicosis has resulted in hypercalcemia.

Interactions with Drugs, Nutrients, or Environment

- Vitamin D enhances calcium absorption.
- Oral calcium may decrease the GI absorption of tetracyclines or phenytoin.

- The use of thiazide diuretics, vitamin A, or oral magnesium during calcium overdose may result in hypercalcemia.

 # CLINICAL FEATURES

- Mild and self-limiting GI distress (vomiting, diarrhea) are the most likely clinical signs following an acute ingestion of calcium supplements.
- Though transient hypercalcemia may occur following ingestion, it is rarely clinically significant (due to inadequate Vitamin D_3 levels found in calcium supplements).
- If enough Vitamin D has been ingested in conjunction with the calcium ingestion, clinical signs of hypercalcemia could be expected (PU/PD, weakness, lethargy, nausea, vomiting, diarrhea, constipation). Milk-alkali syndrome (back and loin pain related to kidney stones, polyuria) can also develop if the patient has concurrent renal compromise.

 # DIFFERENTIAL DIAGNOSIS

- Gastrointestinal disease—pancreatitis, foreign body, dietary indiscretion, gastroenteritis
- Renal disease
- Diabetes mellitus
- Diabetes insipidus
- Hypercalcemia of malignancy
- Feline idiopathic hypercalcemia
- Hypoadrenocorticism

 # DIAGNOSTICS

- Acute ingestions of calcium supplements alone are generally unlikely to result in significant changes in blood work.
- Acute ingestions of calcium supplements with concurrent large ingestions of vitamin D may result in signs of hypercalcemia (see chapter 100, Cholecalciferol).

Pathological Findings

- With acute ingestion of calcium supplements, GI irritation may be seen.
- With hypercalcemia, calcification in the kidneys, GIT walls, and cardiac vessels may be found.

 # THERAPEUTICS

- The objectives of therapeutics are decontamination, evaluation for the presence of hypercalcemia, and treatment of the hypercalcemia if present.

Detoxification

- If calcium supplements have been consumed, timely emesis may help remove tablets/chews/syrup, as well as the wrappers of the product.
- In most cases, no further intervention will be required.
- Unless toxic amounts of vitamin D have been consumed along with the calcium supplement, no activated charcoal is required.

Appropriate Health Care

- Monitoring at home for prolonged GI distress, then symptomatic and supportive care if necessary (fluids, antiemetics, antidiarrheals) should be all that is necessary for ingestion of calcium supplements without adequate vitamin D ingestion.

Drug(s) and Antidotes of Choice

- There is no specific antidote for ingestion of calcium supplements.

 COMMENTS

- The concomitant ingestion of vitamin D along with calcium is the key to the degree of toxicity. If enough vitamin D has been consumed along with the calcium supplement, calcium will be absorbed more easily and may cause hypercalcemia.
- 40,000 IU of vitamin D_3 = 1 mg vitamin D_3
- 1 IU vitamin D_3 = 0.000025 mg vitamin D_3
- Doses of vitamin D_3 <0.1 mg/kg BW may cause mild GI irritation.
- Doses of vitamin D_3 >0.1 g/kg BW may result in hypercalcemia.

Expected Course and Prognosis

- Clinical signs of ingestion of calcium supplements without enough vitamin D ingestion to cause hypercalcemia should be mild and self-limiting in the otherwise healthy patient, and prognosis is good. If there is previous renal compromise, the prognosis will depend on the amount of the ingestion, the timing of intervention, and the degree of previous compromise.

Abbreviations

ADH = antidiuretic hormone
BW   = body weight
CNS = central nervous system
GFR = glomerular filtration rate
GI   = gastrointestinal
GIT   = gastrointestinal tract
IU   = international unit

OTC   = over-the-counter
PU/PD = polyuria/polydipsia

See Also

Cholecalciferol

Suggested Reading

Plumb DC. Calcium salts. In: Plumb's Veterinary Drug Handbook, 6th ed. Ames, IA: Blackwell, 2008.

Feldman E, Nelson R. Hypercalcemia and primary hyperparathyroidism. In: Canine and Feline Endocrinology and Reproduction, 2nd ed. Philadelphia: Saunders, 1996; pp. 455–496.

Lucas P, et al. Treating paraneoplastic hypercalcemia in dogs and cats. Vet Med 2007; 5:314–331.

McKnight, K. Ingestion of over-the-counter calcium supplements. Vet Tech 2006; 7:446–448.

Author: Catherine M. Adams, DVM
Consulting Editor: Justine A. Lee, DVM, DACVECC

chapter 54

Chocolate and Caffeine

DEFINITION/OVERVIEW

- Theobromine and caffeine are methylated xanthine alkaloids (methylxanthines) that cause a variety of clinical signs when ingested by veterinary species.
- Clinical signs can include vomiting, diarrhea, PU/PD, ataxia, cardiac arrhythmias, CNS stimulation (including seizure activity and hyperexcitability), and potentially death.
- Dogs are the most frequently intoxicated species (due to their indiscriminate eating habits), having been poisoned through the ingestion of chocolate, over-the-counter caffeine tablets, or cacao bean mulch.

ETIOLOGY/PATHOPHYSIOLOGY

Mechanism of Action

- Methylxanthines exhibit four main mechanisms of action:
  - Inhibition of cellular phosphodiesterase, causing an increase in cAMP
  - Stimulation of the release of catecholamines from the adrenal medulla
  - Competitive inhibition of adenosine
  - Inhibition of calcium sequestration within the sarcoplasmic reticulum and an increase of calcium entry into cardiac and skeletal muscle cells

Pharmacokinetics/Absorption, Distribution, Metabolism, and Excretion

- Caffeine is rapidly absorbed and reaches peak plasma levels within 30 to 60 minutes. It is metabolized mainly in the liver, with excretion through the bile. Enterohepatic recirculation is thought to occur. The half-life of caffeine is estimated to be 4 hours in the dog. Approximately 10% of caffeine is excreted unchanged via the kidney.
- Caffeine crosses the blood-brain barrier and the placental barrier and is absorbed into the mammary gland as well.
- Theobromine is more slowly absorbed, reaching peak plasma levels in approximately 10 hours. It is also metabolized within the liver and undergoes

enterohepatic recirculation. The half-life of theobromine is approximately 17 hours in the dog.

■ Methylxanthines are thought to be reabsorbed intact through the bladder wall.

Toxicity

■ The LD_{50} of caffeine in dogs is 140 mg/kg and is 80–150 mg/kg in cats.
■ The LD_{50} of theobromine in dogs is 250–500 mg/kg and is 200 mg/kg in cats.
■ Clinical signs are dose dependent.
■ It should be noted that chocolate products often contain both theobromine and caffeine together.
■ Cacao bean shells are frequently used in horticulture as mulch; clinical signs have been reported from dogs ingesting this mulch, although death is rare.
■ Tables 54.1 and 54.2 provide the typical amounts of caffeine and theobromine found in common food products.

Table 54.1. Caffeine content of common products.

Source	Caffeine Content
Vivarin tablets	200 mg/tablet
Tea	4–18 mg/oz
Chocolate-containing products	2–40 mg/oz, depending on type
Coffee beans	280–570 mg/oz
Regular coffee	6–18 mg/oz
Decaffeinated coffee	0.4–0.8 mg/oz
Cola beverages	5–7.5 mg/oz

Table 54.2. Theobromine content of common chocolate products.

Source	Theobromine Content
Cacao beans	300–1500 mg/oz
Unsweetened baking chocolate	390–450 mg/oz
Dark chocolate	135 mg/oz
Milk chocolate	44–60 mg/oz
White chocolate	0.25 mg/oz
Cocoa powder	400–737 mg/oz
Cacao bean mulch	56–900 mg/oz

Systems Affected

- Cardiovascular—tachycardia, hypertension, VPCs, other tachyarrhythmias, bradycardia (rare)
- Nervous—hyperreactivity, ataxia, general CNS excitability, generalized tonic-clonic seizures (rare)
- Gastrointestinal—vomiting, diarrhea
- Musculoskeletal—muscle tremors
- Renal/urologic—PU/PD, often reported by owners as urinary incontinence
- Respiratory—tachypnea, hypoxemia secondary to aspiration pneumonia, respiratory failure, and resultant cyanosis (seen with high doses)
- Endocrine/metabolic—hypokalemia

 # SIGNALMENT/HISTORY

- Any age or breed of dog can be affected.
- A similar clinical course would be predicted in the cat but is infrequently reported due to discriminating eating habits.
- Toxicity has also been noted in pigs, calves, chickens, ducks, and horses when cacao bean shells were added to feedstuffs.

Risk Factors

- Preexisting liver disease may slow metabolism of methylxanthines.
- Preexisting heart disease may predispose to complications due to cardiac effects of methylxanthines.

Historical Findings

- Witnessed ingestion of chocolate or caffeine-containing products is often, but not always, noted.
- Discovery of chewed packages or wrappings of chocolate or caffeine-containing products is common.
- Owners should be questioned about access to or witnessed ingestion of cocao bean mulch.

Location and Circumstances of Poisoning

- Availability of chocolate or caffeine-containing products in the environment should be assessed in dogs presenting with clinical signs of toxicity.

 # CLINICAL FEATURES

- Initial clinical signs of restlessness, hyperactivity, PU/PD, urinary incontinence, and vomiting are generally noted within 1 to 2 hours for caffeine toxicity, and 2 to 4 hours for theobromine toxicity.

- As intoxication progresses, tachycardia, hypertension, weakness, ataxia, diarrhea, cardiac arrhythmias, and seizures may occur.
- Hyperthermia is frequently evident.
- Death may occur due to respiratory failure, cardiac arrhythmias, or terminal seizure activity.
- Bradycardia and hematuria are infrequent clinical features.
- Signs of toxicity generally last for 12 to 72 hours, depending on dose ingested.

DIFFERENTIAL DIAGNOSIS

- Toxicities
  - Strychnine, nicotine, or amphetamine intoxication
  - Metaldehyde toxicosis
  - Cardiac medication ingestion
  - Serotonin syndrome
- Primary cardiac disease
- Primary CNS disease

DIAGNOSTICS

- If the patient presents soon after exposure (<1–2 hours), physical examination may be within normal limits.
- If the patient is symptomatic at the time of presentation, restlessness, hyperactivity, dehydration, ataxia, weakness, tachycardia, cardiac arrhythmias, or seizure activity may be noted on physical examination. Evidence of chocolate may be seen or smelled from the vomitus or diarrhea.
- CBC, serum chemistry profile, and urinalysis are generally within normal limits with the exception of mild hypokalemia.
- Imaging studies are generally within normal limits.
- Hematuria may occasionally be present.
- High-performance liquid chromatography can be used to measure the level of methylxanthines within the serum, plasma, tissue, urine, or stomach contents. These compounds are stable for 7 days at room temperature, 14 days if refrigerated, or 4 months if frozen.

Pathological Findings

- Gross examination at necropsy may reveal chocolate or caffeine-containing products within the GIT.
- There are no specific histopathologic findings associated with caffeine or theobromine toxicosis.
- Findings consistent with gastroenteritis may be evident as well as postmortem congestion of other organs (liver, kidneys, spleen, thymus).

THERAPEUTICS

■ Goals of treatment for caffeine and theobromine toxicosis are similar, and include early decontamination, prevention of further absorption of toxic compounds, promotion of excretion of previously absorbed toxins, and supportive/symptomatic care for cardiac and neurologic symptoms.

Detoxification

■ Decontamination
  • Induce emesis if ingestion has occurred within the previous 2–6 hours and there are no contraindications (e.g., symptomatic, unable to protect the airway, high risk for aspiration pneumonia, etc.).
  • If the patient is symptomatic but stable, passage of an endotracheal tube with the cuff inflated followed by gastric lavage may be helpful if ingestion was fairly recent or if material is noted within the stomach on survey radiography.
  • Rarely, massive amounts of chocolate ingestion may congeal within the stomach, necessitating gastrotomy for removal.
  • Administration of activated charcoal is recommended to help prevent further absorption of toxic compounds. Repeated doses of activated charcoal have been shown to significantly decrease the half-life of caffeine and theobromine. Due to the enterohepatic recycling of these compounds, it has been recommended to continue activated charcoal treatments for up to 36–72 hours postingestion. Patients treated with repeated doses of activated charcoal should be adequately assessed for hydration and treated appropriately if needed, due to risks of hypernatremia. One way to prevent this occurrence would be to use activated charcoal free of cathartic for subsequent administrations.
  • Activated charcoal can be administered via stomach tube during the gastric lavage procedure if necessary.
  • The first dose of activated charcoal should ideally contain a cathartic, such as sorbitol.
  • Urinary catheterization or frequent voiding opportunities (q 2–4 hours) are recommended to prevent reabsorption of methylxanthines across the bladder wall.

Appropriate Health Care

■ Intravenous fluid therapy is recommended to combat dehydration and promote urinary excretion of caffeine and theobromine; electrolyte imbalances can also be addressed through fluid therapy.
■ Seizures, muscle tremors, and hyperreactivity should be treated symptomatically with diazepam at 0.5–2 mg/kg IV.

- If seizures are unresponsive to bolus dosing of diazepam, a diazepam CRI at 0.5–1 mg/kg/hour or treatment with barbituates or propofol may be necessary.
- The ECG should be monitored continuously. VPCs, if frequent or affecting cardiac output or perfusion, may be treated with lidocaine at an initial loading dose of 1–2 mg/kg IV followed by a CRI of 25–75 µg/kg/min.
- Persistent tachyarrhythmias (HR >180 bpm in dogs) or hypertension (systolic >200 mm Hg) should be treated with a beta-blocker such as metoprolol or propranolol. Metoprolol can be administered at 0.2–0.4 mg/kg PO q 12 hours. Alternatively, propranolol can be administered at a starting dose of 0.02–0.06 mg/kg IV q 6 hours.
- If bradycardia is present, atropine can be administered at a dose of 0.02–0.04 mg/kg IV, IM, or SQ.

Drug(s) and Antidotes of Choice

- There is no known antidote for caffeine or theobromine toxicity.

Nursing Care

- If urinary catheterization is not possible, the patient should have ample opportunities to void the bladder to help decrease the reabsorption of toxic compounds across the bladder wall.

 COMMENTS

Client Education

- While many pet owners may know anecdotally that chocolate is poisonous to dogs, they may not be aware of the variables that result in clinical toxicosis (e.g., milk vs. baking chocolate, or the amount that causes toxicity). In addition, clients may not know of other household items, such as chocolate-covered espresso beans, coffee, or tea, that may pose an additional danger to their pets. It is prudent to institute appropriate education regarding this common household toxin at well-pet and vaccination appointments.

Patient Monitoring

- Continuous ECG monitoring is recommended during hospitalization.
- Blood pressure, body temperature, and mental status monitoring every 4 to 6 hours for at least 24 hours postingestion is prudent.

Prevention/Avoidance

- Prevent access to theobromine- or caffeine-containing products in the home, particularly during seasonal events (e.g., Easter, Halloween, Christmas).

Expected Course and Prognosis

- Pet Poison Helpline had over 2500 cases of chocolate toxicity reported from 2004 to 2009. Overall, the prognosis for chocolate toxicity was fair with prompt aggressive medical treatment.
- For the patient that is presented within 1–6 hours following ingestion, if initial decontamination procedures are effective, the clinical prognosis is very good.
- For patients with clinical signs such as cardiac arrhythmias or seizure activity, the prognosis is guarded.

Abbreviations

bpm	=	beats per minute
cAMP	=	cyclic adenosine monophosphate
CBC	=	complete blood count
CNS	=	central nervous system
CRI	=	continuous rate infusion
ECG	=	electrocardiogram
GIT	=	gastrointestinal tract
HR	=	heart rate
IM	=	intramuscular
IV	=	intravenous
PD	=	polydipsia
PO	=	*per os* (by mouth)
PU	=	polyuria
q	=	every
SQ	=	subcutaneous

See Also

Metaldehyde Snail and Slug Bait
Strychnine
Ethylene Glycol
Amphetamines
Selective Serotonin Reuptake Inhibitors

Suggested Reading

Carson TL. Methylxanthines. In: Peterson ME, Talcott PA, eds. Small Animal Toxicology, 2nd ed. St. Louis: Saunders/Elsevier, 2006.

Glauberg A, Blumenthal HP. Chocolate poisoning in the dog. J Am Anim Hosp Assoc 1983; 19:246–248.

Hooser SB, Beasley VR. Methylxanthine poisoning (chocolate and caffeine toxicosis). In: Kirk RW, ed. Current Veterinary Therapy IX Small Animal Practice. Philadelphia: WB Saunders, 1986.

Sutton RH. Cocoa poisoning in a dog. Vet Rec 1981; 109:563–565.

Theobromine. http://www.hersheys.com/nutrition/theobromine.asp

Authors: Elise M. Craft, DVM; Lisa L. Powell, DVM, DACVECC
Consulting Editor: Justine A. Lee, DVM, DACVECC

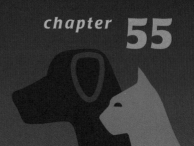
Grapes and Raisins

 ## DEFINITION/OVERVIEW

- Ingestion of grapes and raisins (*Vitis* spp.) by dogs has resulted in toxicosis characterized by lethargy, anorexia, vomiting, diarrhea, and ARF, possibly leading to death.
- Symptoms have also been noted after the ingestion of currants.
- The specific mechanism of toxicosis associated with grapes and raisins is unknown and currently is not definitely known to be dose related.
- Some dogs may show no adverse signs after ingestion of grapes or raisins due to the idiosyncratic nature of toxicosis.
- Anecdotal case reports of ARF in cats or ferrets have been reported.

 ## ETIOLOGY/PATHOPHYSIOLOGY

Mechanism of Action

- The mechanism of toxicosis associated with grapes and raisins is unknown.
- As not all dogs experience clinical signs following ingestion, proposed mechanisms for the development of ARF include the presence of mycotoxins or pesticide residues on the fruit itself, or an individual inability to metabolize a component of the fruit, such as tannins or the high monosaccharide content present within grapes or raisins. Organic grapes, homegrown grapes, seedless or seeded grapes have all been reported to be nephrotoxic.
- Grapeseed extract has not been associated with nephrotoxicty.
- Acute renal failure may result in oliguria, anuria, and death.

Pharmacokinetics/Absorption, Distribution, Metabolism, and Excretion

- Grapes and raisins are not rapidly broken down or absorbed and may be seen intact in vomitus or in feces several hours after ingestion (see fig. 55.1).
- Due to clinical signs associated with ingestion, metabolism and excretion are suspected to occur within the kidneys.

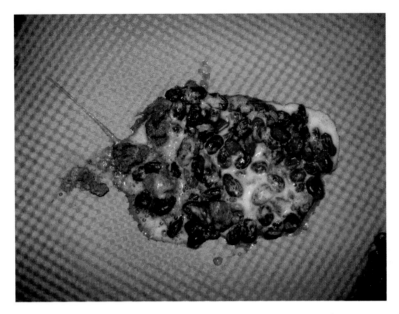

■ **Fig. 55.1.** Productive emesis induction post–raisin ingestion. (Photo courtesy of Justine A. Lee)

Toxicity

- Currently, clinical signs are not thought to be dose dependent.
- Up to 50% of dogs that ingest grapes or raisins may be unaffected. Nevertheless, due to the idiosyncratic toxicosis associated with grapes and raisins, appropriate decontamination and treatment should still be initiated.

Systems Affected

- Renal/urologic—acute renal tubular necrosis and subsequent ARF
- Gastrointestinal—vomiting, diarrhea, abdominal pain
- Hepatobiliary—mild elevations in liver enzymes possible
- Endocrine/metabolic—hypercalcemia and hyperphosphatemia noted in a majority of clinically affected cases; metabolic acidosis due to the presence of uremic acids
- Neuromuscular—weakness and ataxia noted in a small percentage of clinically affected cases

 SIGNALMENT/HISTORY

- Any age, sex, and breed of dog
- Anecdotally reported ARF in two cats and the death of one ferret after ingestion of *Vitis* spp.

Risk Factors

- Preexisting renal disease

Historical Findings

- Witnessed ingestion of grapes or raisins
- Suspected ingestion following discovery of chewed packages or trash that previously contained grapes or raisins (e.g., trail mix, granola, etc.)
- Emesis or stool/diarrhea containing intact grapes or raisins

Location and Circumstances of Poisoning

- Availability of grapes or raisins in the animal's environment

 CLINICAL FEATURES

- Physical examination may reveal dehydration, lethargy, uremic breath.
- Vomiting is consistently the initial clinical sign, generally within 24 hours following ingestion.
- Anorexia, lethargy, and possibly diarrhea follow within the next 12 to 24 hours.
- Serum creatinine and phosphorus begin to elevate soon after ingestion; BUN generally increases 24 hours postingestion.
- Hypercalcemia and hyperphosphatemia may be seen as early as 24 hours post-exposure, resulting in mineralization of soft tissues, possibly contributing to ongoing renal damage.
- Serum calcium levels begin to elevate at 48 to 72 hours following ingestion.
- Urine output generally begins to decline at 48 to 72 hours, eventually leading to oliguria or anuria.
- Oliguric or anuric renal failure leads to hyperkalemia, metabolic acidosis, and hypertension as the clinical course progresses.
- Severely affected dogs may require peritoneal dialysis or hemodialysis.

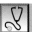 **DIFFERENTIAL DIAGNOSIS**

- Vomiting: dietary indiscretion, foreign body obstruction, intussusception, neoplasia, infectious disease, drug reaction, uremia, pancreatitis, hepatic disease, hypoadrenocorticism
- Acute renal failure:
    - Toxicities—NSAID ingestion, aminoglycoside administration, ethylene glycol, cardiac medication ingestion
    - Renal ischemia—hypovolemia, anesthetic/surgical procedures, trauma, heat stroke, sepsis/SIRS, pancreatitis

- Infectious and systemic disease—leptospirosis, pyelonephritis, myoglobinuria, hemoglobinuria, neoplasia
- Hypercalcemia: hyperparathyroidism, hyperadrenocorticism, hypervitaminosis D (e.g., psoriasis creams, vitamin D_3 rodenticide intoxication), idiopathic, neoplasia

 DIAGNOSTICS

- CBC—thrombocytopenia, mild anemia
- Chemistry—elevations of BUN and creatinine; elevations of liver enzymes (e.g., ALP, ALT); elevations of amylase/lipase, decreases in TCO_2, electrolyte derangements (e.g., hyponatremia, hyperkalemia, hypochloremia, hyperphosphatemia, hypercalcemia)
  - Monitor renal values at least every 24 hours.
  - Monitor potassium values at least every 8 hours, more frequently if patient is oliguric (<1 mL/kg/hr UOP) or anuric (<0.5 mL/kg/hr UOP).
- Urinalysis—isosthenuria/hyposthenuria, proteinuria, glucosuria, hyaline or granular casts
- Radiography—generally within normal limits, soft tissue mineralization may be evident
- Abdominal ultrasonography—renomegaly, hyperechoic renal cortices, or renal pelvic dilatation may be present.

Pathological Findings

- Moderate to severe renal tubular necrosis, with proximal tubules being more severely affected
- Proteinaceous debris present within damaged renal tubular lumen
- Intact basement membranes, and evidence of renal epithelial regeneration in a majority of histopathologic samples

 THERAPEUTICS

- Decontamination, supportive care, and monitoring are the objectives in the treatment of grape and raisin toxicosis. As it is unknown in which animals and at what dosage clinical signs will occur, treatment of all suspected intoxications is recommended. Serial monitoring of renal values is recommended every 24 hours for up to 72 hours.

Detoxification

- Decontamination

- Digestion and absorption of grapes and raisins is slow, and it may be beneficial to induce emesis even after several hours, provided there are no contraindications to the procedure (e.g., symptomatic, unable to protect the airway, high risk for aspiration pneumonia, etc.).
- As the toxic compound present in grapes and raisins is unknown, it is also unknown if the administration of activated charcoal is effective. Generally, it is believed that the benefits of activated charcoal administration outweigh the risks in an otherwise uncompromised patient. The benefit of repeated doses of activated charcoal is unknown and not currently recommended. Patients treated with activated charcoal should be adequately assessed for hydration, and treated appropriately if needed, due to rare reported risks for hypernatremia.

Appropriate Health Care

- Intravenous fluid therapy is indicated in the asymptomatic patient for 24 to 48 hours as it is unknown which patients will develop more serious renal disease. Preemptive fluid diuresis allows for preservation of renal blood flow, decreasing tubule obstruction from necrosis, and potentially increasing the excretion of a nephrotoxic agent.
- Serial monitoring of renal values, electrolytes, serum calcium levels, serum phosphorus levels, and urine sediment should be performed to allow for early detection of nephrotoxicity.
- If symptoms consistent with ARF occur, standard treatments and observations (e.g., aggressive intravenous fluid therapy, monitoring UOP, CVP, and blood pressure, etc.) should be instituted. Other possible interventions may include the use of CRI administration of dopamine, furosemide, and mannitol; antihypertensive therapy; and oral phosphate binder administration as indicated by the patient's clinical status.
- Critically ill patients (including those that are oliguric or anuric, volume overloaded, etc.) may require the use of aggressive peritoneal dialysis or hemodialysis.
- Gastric protectants and antiemetics should be administered to reduce the severity of uremic gastritis, gastric ulceration, and secondary aspiration pneumonia.
- Blood pressure monitoring and treatment for hypertension

Drug(s) and Antidotes of Choice

- There is no known antidote for grape and raisin toxicosis.

Follow-up

- Asymptomatic patients should have renal values, electrolytes, serum calcium, and serum phosphorus levels monitored for at least 48 to 72 hours postingestion.

Diet

- The patient should be encouraged to eat normally while hospitalized, provided GI symptoms allow it.
- Patients that are treated for ARF following ingestion of grapes or raisins may benefit from a low-protein, low-phosphorus prescription veterinary diet until normal renal function is obtained.

Prevention

- Prevent patient access to all *Vitis* spp. fruits.

 COMMENTS

Client Education

- Pet Poison Helpline had over 500 cases of grape and raisin toxicosis reported from 2004 to 2009. Overall, the prognosis was good with aggressive decontamination, IV fluid therapy, and supportive care.
- Many pet owners may not be aware of the danger that grapes and raisins pose to their pets. Appropriate education regarding this toxicosis at well-pet and vaccination appointments is encouraged.

Possible Complications

- Renal histopathology obtained from affected animals has revealed intact basement membranes and evidence of renal epithelial regeneration, indicative of renal healing. A majority of patients may be able to survive severe renal impairment caused by grapes and raisins, provided supportive care can be maintained until renal epithelial regeneration. The potential for long-term renal insufficiency following the ingestion of grapes and raisins is possible, and owners should be aware of the risks of CRF.

Expected Course and Prognosis

- The prognosis for grape and raisin toxicosis ranges from good to poor depending on the clinical signs the patient exhibits.
- For more than 50% of dogs that ingest grapes or raisins, there will be minimal to no clinical signs, making the prognosis quite good.
- For patients experiencing fulminant ARF, the prognosis may be poor to grave (particularly in anuric patients without access to peritoneal dialysis or hemodialysis).
- A majority of patients discharged from the hospital following treatment for ARF secondary to grape or raisin toxicosis will have no appreciable long-term renal insufficiency, although long-term follow-up in veterinary studies has not been evaluated.

Abbreviations

ALT   = alanine aminotransferase
ALP   = alkaline phosphatase
ARF   = acute renal failure
BUN   = blood urea nitrogen
CRF   = chronic renal failure
CRI   = continuous rate infusion
CVP   = central venous pressure
GI   = gastrointestinal
IV   = intravenous
NSAID = nonsteroidal anti-inflammatory drug
tCO_2 = total carbon dioxide
UOP   = urine output

See Also

Human NSAIDs
Cholecalciferol

Suggested Reading

Eubig PA, Brady MS, Gwaltney-Brant SM, et al. Acute renal failure in dogs after the ingestion of grapes or raisins: a retrospective evaluation of 43 dogs (1992–2002). J Vet Intern Med 2005; 19:663–674.
Gwaltney-Brant SM, Holding JK, Donaldson CW, et al. Renal failure associated with ingestion grapes or raisins in dogs. JAVMA 2001; 218:1555–1556.
Mazzaferro EM, Eubig PA, Hackett TB, et al. Acute renal failure associated with raisin or grape ingestion in 4 dogs. J Vet Emerg Crit Care 2004; 14:203–212.
Morrow CM, Valli VE, Volmer PA, et al. Canine renal pathology associated with grape or raisin ingestion: 10 cases. J Vet Diagn Invest 2005; 17:223–231.
Sutton NM, Bates N, Campbell A. Factors influencing outcome of *Vitis vinifera* (grapes, raisins, currants, and sultanas) intoxication in dogs. Vet Rec 2009; 164:430–431.

Author: Elise M. Craft, DVM; Justine A. Lee, DVM, DACVECC
Consulting Editor: Justine A. Lee, DVM, DACVECC

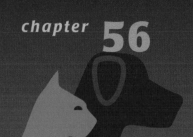

chapter **56**

Hops

DEFINITION/OVERVIEW

- Hops are the common name of the genus *Humulus* and are used for beer brewing to provide the bitter flavor and pungent aroma to beer.
- Hops should not be confused with wild hops (*Bryonia dioica*), which is a member of the gourd family.
- Hops originate from the female flower (or cone) and contain the following biologically active compounds: resins, essential oils, nitrogenous constituents, and phenolic compounds). These biologically active compounds are volatile and supposedly are not found in substantial amounts in boiled hops.
- Common clinical signs from hop ingestion include malignant hyperthermia-like reactions in susceptible dogs.
- Susceptible dogs include breeds such as the greyhound, Labrador retriever, Saint Bernard, pointer, Doberman, Border collie, English springer spaniel, and northern breed dog (e.g., Alaskan huskies, Siberian huskies, etc.).

ETIOLOGY/PATHOPHYSIOLOGY

Mechanism of Action

- The toxin and the mechanism of action are due to the biologically active compounds found within the hops, which may uncouple oxidative phosphorylation, resulting in malignant hyperthermia.
- Hops contain 0.5% to 2.5% essential oils, including hydrocarbons (including monoterpenes and sesquiterpenes), sulfur-containing components (including thiols, episulfides, sulfides, thioesters, and thiophenes), and oxygenated compounds (including humulene, myrcene, and farnesene). Essential oils are unstable and likely evaporate after 10 to 15 minutes of boiling.
- Hops contain 2% to 4% of phenolic compounds (including tannins such as coumaric acid, gallic acid, and caffeic acid). These compounds undergo rapid oxidation and disappear even with cold storage.
- Hops contain 2% to 3.5% nitrogenous constituents (including choline, adenine, hypoxanthine, betaine, and essential amino acids), with 0.5% being soluble.

436

Pharmacokinetics/Absorption, Distribution, Metabolism, and Excretion

- Clinical signs can be seen rapidly within hours; fatality has been seen within 6 hours of ingestion.
- The underlying absorption, distribution, metabolism, and excretion are currently unknown.

Toxicity

- No known LD_{50} exists in veterinary medicine.
- The toxin and the mechanism of action are due to the biologically active compounds found within the hops that may uncouple oxidative phosphorylation, resulting in malignant hyperthermia.
- A 28-g plug of hops can expand into approximately 900 mL of rehydrated plant material.

Systems Affected

- Endocrine/metabolic—electrolyte abnormalities, including hyperkalemia, hypermagnesemia, hyperphosphatemia, hypercalcemia; severe metabolic acidosis, elevated creatine kinase
- Cardiovascular—tachycardia
- Respiratory—panting, tachypnea
- Musculoskeletal—myoglobinuria from hyperthermia
- Nervous—hyperreactivity, pain, restlessness, death

 SIGNALMENT/HISTORY

- Any age and breed of dog can be affected.

Risk Factors

- Breeds predisposed to malignant hyperthermia are more at risk. These breeds include greyhounds, Labrador retrievers, Saint Bernards, pointers, Dobermans, Border collies, English springer spaniels, and northern breed dogs.

Historical Findings

- Witnessed ingestion of hops from a compost bin or brewing disposal area
- Emesis with hops present

Location and Circumstances of Poisoning

- Toxicity is typically seen in households with home brewers. Dogs may have access when composted or disposed hops are ingested when batches of beer are brewed.

CLINICAL FEATURES

- Initial clinical signs include hyperthermia, tachypnea, panting, tachycardia, pain, anxiety, and vomiting.
- Clinical signs can be seen quickly and can rapidly progress to death within 6 hours without treatment.

 DIFFERENTIAL DIAGNOSIS

- Malignant hyperthermia
- Hyperthermia—heat stroke, laryngeal paralysis, exogenous heat source
- Fever—infectious, immune-mediated, neoplasia, inflammatory
- Drug related—anesthetic agents, including amide local anesthetics, depolarizing skeletal muscle relaxants, and volatile inhalants

 DIAGNOSTICS

- CBC—mild elevation in WBC ($>18,000 \times 10^3/\mu L$)
- Chemistry—elevated CK, hyperkalemia, hypercalcemia, hyperphosphatemia, hypermagnesemia
- Venous blood gas analysis—metabolic acidosis, increased pCO_2, electrolyte imbalances
- Urinalysis—pigmenturia, myoglobinuria

 THERAPEUTICS

Detoxification

- Decontamination should be considered in cases when recent ingestion has occurred, especially if within 1–2 hours.
- Emesis induction in asymptomatic patients can be performed.
- In symptomatic patients, gastric lavage with an inflated endotracheal tube (to protect the airway) under sedation should be performed to remove the hops from the stomach.
- Administration of a single dose of activated charcoal with a cathartic may also delay further absorption and decrease the toxic effect of hops.
- Enemas may be performed to increase fecal expulsion.

Appropriate Health Care

- Treatment includes aggressive supportive care, cooling measures (including ice baths, cold IV fluids, the use of fans, alcohol on the paw pads, etc.) to the temperature of 103.5°F, and aggressive IV fluid therapy (to lower body temperature, prevent myoglobin-induced ARF, and maintain perfusion).

- The use of sodium bicarbonate can be used with severe cases of metabolic acidosis (pH <7.0, BE >−15 mmol/L, HCO_3 <11 mmol/L). Appropriate acid-base and electrolyte monitoring should be performed during hospitalization.
- Supportive care and monitoring as indicated.

Drug(s) and Antidotes of Choice

- Dantrolene sodium is a hydantoin derivative that is used for reversing malignant hyperthermia.
  - Dose: 2–3 mg/kg IV or 3.5 mg/kg PO immediately once following hops exposure. Repeated doses can be administered at 100 mg PO q 12 hours for 3 days thereafter.
- Supportive care
- Thermoregulation
- The use of dipyrone is not recommended as an antipyretic. Dipyrone works by inhibiting release of endogenous pyrogens, thereby lowering the hypothalamic thermostatic settings. As malignant hyperthermia secondary to hops ingestion is not due to endogenous pyrogens, dipyrone is not thought to be effective.

Nursing Care

- Patient monitoring for 24–72 hours until clinical signs subside.

Follow-up

- No long-term complications reported.

Activity

- Keep the pet quiet and confined until the clinical signs subside. Exercise should be limited for 3–5 days after discharge to prevent additional myoglobinuria.

 COMMENTS

Client Education

- Prevent any access of pets to hops, particularly with clients who are home brewers.

Patient Monitoring

- Supportive care, thermoregulation, ECG monitoring, acid-base and electrolyte monitoring, and maintaining hydration are imperative.

Prevention/Avoidance

- Prevent any access of pets to hops.

Possible Complications

- No long-term complications reported, although dogs should be tested for congenital malignant hyperthermia with erythrocyte osmotic fragility, caffeine muscle contracture tests, or halothane-succinylcholine challenge exposure test for confirmation of malignant hyperthermia.

Expected Course and Prognosis

- Clinical signs usually are self-limiting within 24–48 hours.

Abbreviations

ARF = acute renal failure
BE   = base excess
CBC = complete blood count
CK   = creatine kinase
DIC   = disseminated intravascular coagulation
ECG = electrocardiogram
HCO_3 = bicarbonate
IV   = intravenous
LD_{50} = median lethal dose
pCO_2 = partial pressure of carbon dioxide
PO   = *per os* (by mouth)
WBC = white blood cells

Suggested Reading

Duncan KL, Hare WR, Buck WB. Malignant hyperthermia-like reaction secondary to ingestion of hops in five dogs. J Am Vet Med Assoc 1997; 210(1):51–53.
Nelson TE. Malignant hyperthermia in dogs. J Am Vet Med Assoc 1991; 198:989–994.

Author: Justine A. Lee, DVM, DACVECC
Consulting Editor: Justine A. Lee, DVM, DACVECC

chapter 57

Macadamia Nuts

DEFINITION/OVERVIEW

- Processed or fresh macadamia nuts come from the trees of *Macadamia integrifolia* or *Macadamia tetraphylla*.
- Macadamia nuts contain up to 80% oil and 4% sugar.
- As little as 0.7 g/kg can cause clinical signs, although signs are typically seen at >2 g/kg.
- There are approximately 12 nuts per 1 ounce.
- Common clinical signs include weakness, depression, vomiting, ataxia, tremoring, joint pain, lameness, hind limb weakness, hyperthermia, recumbency, and mild abdominal pain.
- The onset of clinical signs is within 12 hours of ingestion. Clinical signs typically subside within 24–48 hours without treatment. No fatalities have been reported to date.

ETIOLOGY/PATHOPHYSIOLOGY

Mechanism of Action

- The exact toxin and the mechanism of action are unknown but may involve motor neurons, neuromuscular junctions, muscle fibers, or neurotransmitters.

Pharmacokinetics/Absorption, Distribution, Metabolism, and Excretion

- Unknown

Systems Affected

- Gastrointestinal—vomiting, mild abdominal pain
- Musculoskeletal—weakness (especially the hind limbs), lameness, joint pain
- Nervous—recumbency, ataxia, CNS depression, tremoring
- Endocrine/metabolic—hyperthermia
- Cardiovascular—pale mucous membranes

SIGNALMENT/HISTORY

- Any age and breed of dogs

Historical Findings

- Witnessed ingestion
- Chewed up, empty containers of macadamia nuts

 CLINICAL FEATURES

- The physical exam may be normal or any of the signs below may be seen within 12 hours after ingestion.
- Weakness (particularly hind limb weakness)
- CNS depression
- Vomiting
- Ataxia
- Tremor
- Hyperthermia
- Lameness
- Joint pain
- Pale mucous membranes
- Mild abdominal pain

 DIFFERENTIAL DIAGNOSIS

- Joint pain—tick-borne diseases (e.g., Lyme disease, ehrlichiosis, Rocky Mountain spotted fever); immune-mediated diseases (e.g., idiopathic, systemic lupus erythematosus); degenerative joint disease
- Musculoskeletal weakness (especially affecting the hind limbs)—spinal cord lesion (e.g., intervertebral disc disease, FCE, trauma, neoplasia, other myelopathy); tick paralysis; coonhound paralysis; botulism; protozoal polyradiculoneuritis (e.g., *Toxoplasma, Neospora*); cholinesterase inhibitor toxicity (e.g., organophosphate, carbamate)

 DIAGNOSTICS

- With a known history of macadamia nut ingestion in a previously healthy patient, usually no advanced diagnostics are indicated.
- Chemistry: mild elevation of serum triglycerides, alkaline phosphatase, and lipase

■ CBC: mild elevation in WBC (>18,000)

 THERAPEUTICS

■ Treatment is supportive and may be potentially done at home until clinical signs subside; resolution of clinical signs typically occurs within 24–48 hours.
■ In older patients and patients with other concurrent illness, hospitalization and supportive care (e.g., SQ fluids, nursing care, thermoregulation, etc.) should be given consideration as indicated.
■ Decontamination should be considered in cases when recent ingestion has occurred, especially if >1 g/kg is ingested.
■ Patients that ingest other concurrent toxins such as methylxanthine (e.g., chocolate-coated macadamia nut) should be treated accordingly (see chap. 54, "Chocolate and Caffeine," for further information).

Detoxification

■ Emesis induction in an asymptomatic patient within 1 hour of ingestion
■ Activated charcoal with sorbitol may decrease the toxic effect of macadamia nuts.

Appropriate Health Care

■ Supportive care and monitoring as indicated

Drug(s) and Antidotes of Choice

■ No antidote

Nursing Care

■ Patient monitoring for 24–48 hours until clinical signs subside

Follow-up

■ No long-term complications reported

Activity

■ Keep the pet quiet and confined until the clinical signs subside.

 COMMENTS

Client Education

■ Prevent any access of pets to macadamia nuts.

Patient Monitoring

▪ Nursing care, antiemetic therapy, and maintaining hydration are imperative.

Prevention/Avoidance

▪ Prevent any access of pets to macadamia nuts.

Possible Complications

▪ No long-term complications have been reported.

Expected Course and Prognosis

▪ Clinical signs usually are self-limiting within 24–48 hours.

Abbreviations

CBC = complete blood count
CNS = central nervous system
FCE = fibrocartilaginous embolism
SQ   = subcutaneous
WBC = white blood cells

See Also

Chocolate and Caffeine

Suggested Reading

Allen C. Treacherous treats: macadamia nuts. Vet Tech 2001;559: 572.
Cope RB. Four new small animal toxicoses. Aust Vet Pract 2004; 34:121–123.
Hansen SR. Macadamia nut toxicosis in dogs. Vet Med 2002; 97:274–276.
Hansen SR, Buck WB, Meerdink G, et al. Weakness, tremors, and depression associated with macadamia nuts in dogs. Vet Hum Toxicol 2000; 42:18–21.
McKenzie RA, Purvis-Smith GR, Czerwonka-Ledez BJ, et al. Macadamia nut poisoning of dogs. Aust Vet Pract 2000; 30:6–10.

Authors: Debra Liu, DVM; Justine A. Lee, DVM, DACVECC
Consulting Editor: Justine A. Lee, DVM, DACVECC

chapter 58

Mycotoxins–Aflatoxin

DEFINITION/OVERVIEW

- Aflatoxin is produced by some strains of various species of *Aspergillus* (*A. flavus*, *A. paraciticus*, and *A. nomius*).
- Contamination of food may occur prior to harvest (e.g., corn, cottonseed, peanuts, walnuts, pecans, potatoes), or in improperly stored foods after harvest and processing.
- Ingestion of other moldy foods (e.g., bread, garbage) has also caused toxicosis.

ETIOLOGY/PATHOPHYSIOLOGY

Mechanism of Action

- The active epoxide metabolite damages hepatocytes, resulting in cell necrosis, decreased liver function, fibrosis, and biliary hyperplasia.

Pharmacokinetics/Absorption, Distribution, Metabolism, and Excretion

- Intestinal absorption after ingestion
- Hepatic cytochrome P450 metabolism to an active epoxide: the epoxide then binds to DNA, RNA, and proteins in hepatocytes, interfering with cellular metabolism and protein synthesis.
- Activation to epoxide can also occur in the proximal renal tubular epithelial cells.
- Minimal accumulation in the liver (primarily), kidney, bone marrow, lungs, brain, muscle, and fat.
- Metabolites present in milk and eggs
- Excretion through bile, feces, and urine
- Variable rate of elimination, but usually within 24–72 hours postingestion.

Toxicity

- 60 ppb of aflatoxin in dog food has been associated with canine aflatoxicosis.
- 6.7–15 ppm aflatoxin in moldy bread has been reported toxic to dogs.

- Cats are reported to be as sensitive in dogs based on research animals; however, no natural cases of aflatoxicosis in cats have been reported.

Systems Affected

- Gastrointestinal—anorexia, vomiting, diarrhea
- Metabolic/endocrine—fever, jaundice, increased ALT, increased ALP
- Musculoskeletal—weakness
- Hemic/immune/lymphatic—anemia, thrombocytopenia, neutrophilia, hyperbilirubinemia, hypofibrinogenemia, elevated FDP, prolonged PT/PTT, decreased serum cholesterol and protein C
- Nervous—weakness, collapse, coma
- Renal—bilirubinuria, PU/PD

 # SIGNALMENT/HISTORY

- Toxicosis is rarely reported in small animals but has occurred sporadically in large outbreaks associated with contaminated pet foods.
- Diagnosis is based on history and clinical signs.
- More than one pet in the household is likely to be affected when pet food contamination is the cause.

Risk Factors

- Pediatric patients, intact males, and pregnant females are believed more susceptible.
- Field and storage conditions predispose grain to aflatoxin contamination.
  - Hot, dry weather
  - Insect damage to grain

Historical Findings

- Acute lethal exposure is not as common as chronic exposure.
- Grain-based contaminated pet foods have been associated with outbreaks.
- The amount ingested and the duration of exposure is difficult to determine, complicating diagnosis.
- Clinical signs may be delayed for 3 or more weeks postexposure.

 # CLINICAL FEATURES

- Acute clinical signs include anorexia, depression, dyspnea, vomiting, diarrhea (often with GI hemorrhage), fever, seizures, coagulopathy, epistaxis, icterus, DIC, and death.

- Laboratory findings associated with acute toxicosis include neutrophilia; elevated BUN, bilirubin, ALT; hypoalbuminemia; thrombocytopenia; bilirubinuria; anemia; and variable elevations in GGT, AST, ALP.
- Clinical signs of chronic ingestion are those of hepatic failure—weight loss, rough hair coat, anemia, icterus, hypoglycemia, hypocholesterolemia, hypoalbuminemia, melena, coagulopathy, anorexia, depression, ascites, and PU/PD.
- Laboratory results of chronic toxicosis may include thrombocytopenia; hypofibrinogenemia; elevated FDP; prolonged PT/PTT; decreased serum protein C, antithrombin, and cholesterol.

 DIFFERENTIAL DIAGNOSIS

- Other causes of hepatic disease
  - Inflammatory—hepatitis (chronic, active), copper storage disease
  - Infectious—bacterial disease (leptospirosis), viral disease (parvovirus)
  - Neoplastic disease
  - Other toxins—cyanobacteria, mushrooms
  - Drug-induced—acetaminophen
  - Congenital disease
- Other causes of hemorrhage, especially intestinal
  - Long-acting anticoagulant rodenticide toxicosis
  - Parvoviral enteritis

 DIAGNOSTICS

- CBC, chemistry, coagulation panel, UA (results within normal limits do not rule out possible aflatoxicosis)
- Abdominal ultrasound, liver aspirate/biopsy, and histopathology—characteristic lesions (see Pathologic Findings)
- Antithrombin and protein C activity
- Assay of the suspected aflatoxin source, if available
  - Available at many state veterinary diagnostic laboratories
  - See www.aavld.org for a list of accredited laboratories.
  - Aflatoxin assay is also available at many commercial analytical laboratories.
  - Assay of affected food may be difficult if the whole bag has already been consumed by the time clinical signs have developed (which may be delayed for up to 3 weeks).
- Aflatoxin residues can be found in urine, liver, and kidney of recently exposed animals.
  - Due to relatively rapid aflatoxin excretion, absence of tissue residues does not rule out aflatoxicosis.

Pathological Findings

- Hepatomegaly with lipidosis
- Icterus
- Ascites
- GI hemorrhage
- Subserosal edema of the gallbladder
- Multifocal petechia, ecchymosis, and hemorrhage
- Microvesicular fatty change in hepatocytes
- Centrilobular hepatocellular necrosis, with evidence of regeneration possible
- Canalicular cholestasis
- Bridging portal fibrosis with proliferation of bile ducts
- Possible renal proximal tubular necrosis

 THERAPEUTICS

- The goal of therapeutics is symptomatic and supportive care to limit hepatic and other organ damage.

Detoxification

- Early emesis followed by one dose of activated charcoal with a cathartic may be beneficial for recent ingestion of moldy food.

Appropriate Health Care

- Monitor vitals, blood pressure, and urine output.

Drug(s) and Antidotes of Choice

- No specific antidote is available for aflatoxicosis.
- Treatment is symptomatic and supportive.
- IV fluid therapy with B vitamins and dextrose (if hypoglycemic) to correct fluid and electrolyte imbalances
- Antiemetics as needed for persistent vomiting or prior to oral N-acetylcysteine
  - Maropitant 1 mg/kg, SQ q 24 hours, not labeled for cats
  - Ondansetron 0.1–0.2 mg/kg, IV q 8–12 hours
- GI protectants
  - H₂ blockers
    - Famotidine 0.5–1 mg/kg, PO, SQ, IM, IV q 12 hours
    - Ranitidine 1–2 mg/kg, PO, SQ, IM, IV q 8–12 hours
    - Cimetidine 5–10 mg/kg, PO, SQ, IM, IV q 6–8 hours
  - Omeprazole 0.5–1 mg/kg, PO q 24 hours
  - Sucralfate 0.25–1 g PO, q 8 hours

- Vitamin K$_1$ 3–5 mg/kg PO, divided twice daily
- Hepatic support
  - SAMe 17–20 mg/kg or higher, PO per day given on an empty stomach
    - Cats at 200 mg/day on an empty stomach
- Parenteral N-acetylcysteine in severely affected dogs or cats—refer to *Plumb's Veterinary Drug Handbook* for dosing
- Replace suspect diet with appropriate hepatic diet.

Precautions/Interactions

- Avoid drugs metabolized by the liver.
- Avoid pyrethroid insecticides, which may potentiate aflatoxicosis experimentally.

Alternative Drugs

- Silymarin (Marin) can be used alternatively to SAMe as a hepatoprotectant (SAMe with milk thistle).
- Oral N-acetylcysteine may be used instead of parenteral—refer to *Plumb's Veterinary Drug Handbook* for dosing.

Prevention

- Recognize that a major source is contaminated grain in commercial diets.
- Report suspected cases associated with pet food to the manufacturer, FDA, and state regulatory agencies.
- Ask pet food manufacturers about aflatoxin quality control measures.
- Keep all food in clean containers in a cool, dry storage area.
- Keep garbage out of reach of pets.

 COMMENTS

Patient Monitoring

- Monitor hydration, electrolytes, heart rate, blood pressure, heart rhythm (ECG), and body temperature.
- Frequency of monitoring will vary with severity of clinical syndrome.

Possible Complications

- None reported in surviving dogs and cats
- Cirrhosis is possible from prolonged toxicosis.

Expected Course and Prognosis

- Prognosis is guarded to poor, even with treatment, once clinical signs are evident.

Abbreviations

ALT = alanine aminotransferase
ALP = alkaline phosphatase
AST = aspartate transaminase
BUN = blood urea nitrogen
CBC = complete blood count
DIC = disseminated intravascular coagulation
DNA = deoxyribonucleic acid
ECG = electrocardiogram
FDP = fibrin degradation products
GI = gastrointestinal
GIT = gastrointestinal tract
IM = intramuscular
IV = intravenous
PO = *per os* (by mouth)
ppb = parts per billion
ppm = parts per million
PT = prothrombin time
PTT = partial thromboplastin time
PU/PD = polyuria, polydipsia
q = every
RNA = ribonucleic acid
SAMe = S-adenosyl-methionine
SQ = subcutaneous
UA = urinalysis

Suggested Reading

Bischoff K, Garland T. Aflatoxicosis in dogs. In: Bonagura JD, Twedt DC, eds. Kirk's Current Veterinary Therapy XIV. St. Louis: Saunders, 2009; pp. 156–159.

Hooser SB, Talcott PA. Mycotoxins. In: Peterson ME, Talcott PA, eds. Small Animal Toxicology, 2nd ed. Philadelphia: Saunders, 2006; pp. 888–897.

Meerdink GL. Aflatoxin. In: Plumlee KH, ed. Clinical Veterinary Toxicology. St. Louis: Mosby, 2004; pp. 231–235.

Plumb DC. Plumb's Veterinary Drug Handbook, 6th ed. Ames, IA: Wiley-Blackwell, 2008.

Stenske KA, Smith JR, Newman SJ, et al. Aflatoxicosis in dogs and dealing with suspected contaminated commercial foods. JAVMA 2006; 228(11):1686–1689.

Authors: Catherine M. Adams, DVM; Karyn Bischoff DVM, MS, DABVT
Consulting Editors: Gary D. Osweiler, DVM, PhD, DABVT; Justine A. Lee, DVM, DACVECC

chapter 59

Mycotoxins–
Tremorgenic

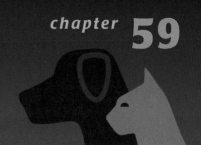

DEFINITION/OVERVIEW

- Toxicosis is caused by ingestion of toxins penitrem A and roquefortine, typically found in moldy food or decomposing organic matter such as compost.
- The degree of illness is dependent upon the quantity of toxin ingested.
- Food most often containing these toxins include moldy dairy foods, moldy walnuts or peanuts, moldy spaghetti, and stored grains.
- The most common effects from exposure are neurologic and GI signs.
- Death can occur if decontamination and treatment are not performed in a timely manner.

ETIOLOGY/PATHOPHYSIOLOGY

Mechanism of Action

- The exact mechanism is unknown, but the toxins are thought to interfere with the normal release of neurotransmitter amino acids.
- Varies depending on the specific mycotoxin ingested
- Roquefortine
  - Toxin produced by *Penicillium roqueforti*
  - Very little is known about the mechanism of action.
- Penitrem A
  - Toxin produced by *Penicillium crustosum*
  - May induce tremors by acting as a glycine antagonist in the brain, or by influencing presynaptic neurotransmitter release
  - Other mechanisms have also been proposed.

Pharmacokinetics/Absorption, Distribution, Metabolism, and Excretion

- Depends on type of toxin
- Many are absorbed through the GIT and metabolized by the liver.
- Excreted primarily through the bile

Toxicity

- Due to the toxins penitrem A and roquefortine
- Specific clinically significant toxic doses have not been described but seem to vary among species.
- A dose of 0.5 mg/kg of purified penitrem A, when given intraperitoneally, resulted in acute onset of tremors in dogs.
- There is one reported case of a small-breed dog developing tremors after ingesting one moldy piece of bread.

Systems Affected

- Nervous—muscle tremors, hyperresponsiveness to external stimuli, seizures, agitation, ataxia, stiff gait, secondary hyperthermia from tremor activity
- Gastrointestinal—hypersalivation, vomiting of ingested material can occur
- Heme/lymphatic/immune—metabolic acidosis, DIC secondary to severe hyperthermia
- Respiratory—panting, respiratory depression
- Cardiovascular—tachycardia
- Muscular—rhabdomyolysis (rare)

 SIGNALMENT/HISTORY

- Dogs are most commonly affected by this toxicosis due to their indiscriminate eating habits.
- Rarely occurs in cats
- No breed, sex, or age predilection
- Patients may present with the following clinical signs—hypersalivation, agitation, hypersensitivity to external stimuli (e.g., noise, touch), panting, ataxia, muscle tremors, seizures, vomiting of "brown" material (compost), hyperthermia, and tachycardia.

Risk Factors

- Exposure to moldy foods in garbage or compost piles
- Animals left outside unattended and having access to garbage or compost
- Roaming dogs that have access to dead, decaying matter while wandering unsupervised

Historical Findings

- History of exposure to or ingestion of compost piles or moldy food in garbage
- Owners may report, upon further inquiry, that their compost bin is improperly secured (e.g., inadequate fencing, etc.)

Location and Circumstances of Poisoning

- Cases occur throughout North America.

 CLINICAL FEATURES

- The onset of clinical signs ranges from minutes to hours, with most clinical signs occurring within 2 to 4 hours of exposure.
- The duration of clinical signs ranges from hours to days (typically 24–48 hours, although excessive exposures may result in prolonged clinical signs for 4–5 days).
- Systems most commonly affected include the following:
  - Nervous—agitation, muscle tremors, ataxia, seizures, stiff gait, secondary hyperthermia from tremor activity
  - Gastrointestinal—hypersalivation, vomiting, possible diarrhea from secondary gastroenteritis
  - Hemic/lymphatic/immune—metabolic acidosis, DIC secondary to severe hyperthermia
  - Cardiovascular—tachycardia
  - Respiratory—panting, respiratory depression
  - Muscular—rhabdomyolysis, dark pigmenturia secondary to tremors (rare)

 DIFFERENTIAL DIAGNOSIS

- Toxicities resulting in seizures—strychnine, insecticides (e.g., organophosphate, carbamate, organochlorine, nicotine, pyrethroid), metaldehyde, zinc phosphide, bromethalin rodenticides, methylxanthines, amphetamines, cocaine, and concentrated DEET
- Primary neurologic disease—inflammation, congenital disease, tumor, idiopathic, cerebellar disorders, tremor syndrome of white dogs, infection
- Primary metabolic conditions—hepatic, renal, hypoglycemia, secondary hepatic encephalopathy

 DIAGNOSTICS

- CBC, serum chemistry profile, and urinalysis to assess the status of the patient and rule out other causes of tremors and seizures
- Venous blood gas to evaluate severity of metabolic acidosis
- Thin-layer chromatography (TLC) or high-pressure liquid chromatography analysis of vomitus, stomach contents, and gastric lavage washings for penitrem A or roquefortine.
- Roquefortine C in vomit or stomach contents serves as a biomarker for penitrem A intoxication.

Pathological Findings

- No specific lesions associated

 THERAPEUTICS

- The objectives of treatment are decontamination to prevent further toxin absorption and supportive care.

Detoxification

- Induce emesis if animal is not at risk of aspiration. This is especially important if large amounts of garbage, compost, or decaying matter have been ingested.
- Gastric lavage if emesis ineffective or patient cannot tolerate emesis (i.e., has clinical signs that would put it at risk of aspiration pneumonia such as tremors, seizures, sedation, etc.). Gastric lavage should be performed with the patient sedated and the airway protected with an inflated endotracheal tube.
- Administer activated charcoal and a cathartic once to limit absorption of the toxin.

Appropriate Health Care

- Monitor for hyperthermia. Patients with a temperature >105.5°F should be treated with cooling measures (e.g., IV fluids, cool water bath, etc.). Cooling measures should be discontinued when temperature reaches 103.5°F.
- IV fluids to assist in hydration, perfusion, cooling, and to prevent ARF from secondary myoglobinuria from severe tremors or seizures. Hydration status should be measured frequently based on physical examination, PCV/TS, weight, and urine output.
- Monitor for hypoglycemia—hypoglycemic patients should be treated appropriately with dextrose supplementation and frequent monitoring.
- Monitor tachycardia and treat appropriately with IV fluids, muscle relaxants, sedation, and analgesics if needed.
- Monitor the need for ventilation support and intubate if necessary.
- If patients are tachypneic, dyspneic, or hypoxemic, chest radiographs should be performed to rule out secondary aspiration pneumonia.

Drug(s) and Antidotes of Choice

- No specific antidote is available.
- Muscle tremors should be treated aggressively.
  - Methocarbamol 55–220 mg/kg, IV for control of muscle tremors, PRN to effect; not to exceed 330 mg/kg/day.

- Seizures should be treated aggressively with anticonvulsant therapy.
  - Diazepam for control of seizures—mycotoxin-induced seizures often do not clinically respond well to diazepam, and higher dosages may be necessary in conjunction with methocarbamol and phenobarbital.
    - Diazepam 0.25–1 mg/kg, IV to effect
  - Barbiturates can be used if seizures cannot be controlled with diazepam.
    - Phenobarbital 4–16 mg/kg IV, PRN to effect
    - Pentobarbital 3–15 mg/kg, IV, PRN to effect
- Anti-emetic therapy as needed
  - Maropitant 1 mg/kg SQ, q 24 hours
  - Ondansetron 0.1–0.2 mg/kg SQ, IV q 8–12 hours
  - Metoclopramide 0.2–0.5 mg/kg SQ q 8 hours
- Tachycardia
  - Propranolol 0.02–0.06 mg/kg IV, slowly to effect

Precautions/Interactions

- Electrolytes should be monitored while the patient is hospitalized.

Diet

- Oral intake should be avoided until vomiting and neurological signs cease.

Prevention

- Prevent animals from eating moldy food items, garbage, or compost.
- Appropriate fencing of compost area (e.g., with chicken wire fencing, etc.) so animals and wildlife do not have access

 COMMENTS

Client Education

- Educate the client on the toxicity of moldy foods.
- Stress the necessity to eliminate the animal's access to garbage and compost piles.

Patient Monitoring

- Patients should be monitored for occurrence of tremors or seizures, hyperthermia, dehydration, acid-base imbalances, liver damage, rhabdomyolysis, and respiratory difficulties.

Possible Complications

- Seizures are generally nonresponsive to diazepam, and additional anticonvulsant therapy may be necessary.

- Hepatic damage and rhabdomyolysis may occur with severe toxicosis.
- Aspiration pneumonia has been reported as a sequela to vomiting and/or gastric lavage.

Expected Course and Prognosis

- Very good if aggressive therapy is instituted, the toxin is removed from the GIT, and seizures are well controlled
- Recovery in most clinical cases is complete within 24–48 hours with no residual signs.
- In a few reported cases, signs of weakness, muscle rigidity, and incoordination were persistent and slowly resolved over 1–2 weeks.
- Exposure can be fatal if lethal doses are consumed and are absorbed before GI decontamination and therapy are instituted.

Abbreviations

ARF   = acute renal failure
CBC   = complete blood count
DEET = diethyltoluamide
DIC   = disseminated intravascular coagulation
GI   = gastrointestinal
GIT   = gastrointestinal tract
IV   = intravenous
PCV   = packed cell volume
PRN   = *pro re nata* (as needed)
q   = every
SQ   = subcutaneous
TS   = total solids

Suggested Reading

Boysen SR, Rozanski EA, Chan DL, et al. Tremorgenic mycotoxicosis in four dogs from a single household. J Am Vet Med Assoc 2002; 221(10):1441–1444.
Schell MM. Tremorgenic mycotoxin intoxication. Vet Med 2000; April: 283,286.
Young KL, Villar D, Carson TL, Imerman, et al. Tremorgenic mycotoxin intoxication with penitrem A and roquefortine in two dogs. J Am Vet Med Assoc 2003; 222(1) 52–53.
Tiwary AK, Puschner B, Poppenga RH. Using roquefortine C as a biomarker for penitrem A intoxication. J Vet Diagn Invest 2009; 21:237–239.

Authors: Christy A. Klatt, DVM; Stephen B. Hooser, DVM, PhD, DABVT
Consulting Editor: Justine A. Lee, DVM, DACVECC

chapter 60

Onions and Garlic

DEFINITION/OVERVIEW

- The *Allium* species of plants belongs to the Alliaceae family and includes onions, garlic, chives, and leeks. These plants contain propyl disulfides and can cause Heinz body anemia when ingested by companion animals.

ETIOLOGY/PATHOPHYSIOLOGY

Mechanism of Action

- Toxic compounds are disulfides and thiosulfates.
- Metabolism of these compounds causes oxygen free radicals, which can result in eccentrocytes (erythrocytes that have a pale crescent space in the middle of the cell due to direct oxidative damage), denatured hemoglobin (Heinz bodies), and methemoglobin, which forms when the iron in the heme protein is oxidized.

Pharmacokinetics/Absorption, Distribution, Metabolism, and Excretion

- Onions and garlic are readily absorbed by the GIT system.
- Chewing the plant converts organosulfoxides to the compounds responsible for the distinctive odors and pharmacologic effects.
- Cooking, drying, processing, and spoiling do not negate the toxic effect.
- Metabolism occurs via several oxidase pathways in the liver and the RBC, which ultimately result in eccentrocytes, Heinz bodies, decreased blood oxygen transportation ability, impaired delivery of oxygen to tissues, intravascular and extravascular hemolysis, and scavenging of damaged red blood cells by the reticuloendothelial system.
- Excretion is thought to occur through the GIT, the kidneys, and the lungs.

Toxicity

- *Allium* species can be toxic in varying amounts depending on status (e.g., cooked, fresh, dried, juiced, powdered, added to other ingredients and foods or supplements), species of plant, time of year, species of companion animal, and acute or chronic exposure.

- Decontamination and treatment are recommended if ingestion is ≥ 0.5% of the animal's body weight.
- Toxicity occurs when the oxidant concentration overwhelms the antioxidative pathways in the RBC.
- Onions and garlic also contain compounds that are antithrombotic agents, cardiac and smooth muscle relaxants, vasodilators, and hypotensives, exacerbating the effects of the anemia.
- Un-aged garlic compounds can cause gastric and ileal mucosal damage, resulting in diarrhea and discomfort.
- Garlic can have a dose-dependent, hypoglycemic effect.

Systems Affected

- Hematologic—Heinz body anemia, anemia, methemoglobinemia
- Gastrointestinal—vomiting, diarrhea
- Respiratory—hypoxemia from methemoglobinemia

 # SIGNALMENT/HISTORY

- Pets on homemade diets with *Allium* supplementation (e.g., onion powder) may be chronically poisoned.
- Cats are more susceptible to the effects of oxidative damage because of differences in their hemoglobin (as cats have 8 sulfhydryl groups on hemoglobin, while dogs have 4).
- Dogs have low catalase antioxidant activity in their RBC, which can make them more susceptible to oxidative damage from *Allium* toxicity.
- Reduced glutathione and potassium concentrations in certain breeds of dogs (e.g., Akita, Shiba, and Jindo) and certain individuals may predispose them to higher susceptibility to oxidative damage.

 # CLINICAL FEATURES

- Clinical signs may not present for several days following ingestion.
- May take up to 2 weeks for the PCV to normalize, and anemia may persist for 3 weeks.
- Heinz body anemia
- Eccentrocytosis
- Hemoglobinemia
- Hemoglobinuria
- Methemoglobinemia
- Bilirubinemia
- Lethargy

- Tachycardia
- Oral, esophageal, and gastric irritation and pain
- GI signs (e.g., vomiting, diarrhea, anorexia)

DIFFERENTIAL DIAGNOSIS

- Medications (e.g., acetaminophen, benzocaine, zinc-containing compounds)
- Foods (e.g., cauliflower, broccoli, cabbage, turnip, mustard, cress, watercress, horseradish)
- Long-acting anticoagulants
- Naphthalene-containing mothballs
- Heavy metals (e.g., pennies with zinc, copper)
- Diabetic ketoacidosis
- Neoplasia
- dl-methionine
- Hepatic lipidosis

DIAGNOSTICS

- CBC—Heinz body anemia, eccentrocytosis, regenerative anemia, methemoglobinemia, leukocytosis
- Chemistry—hyperbilirubinemia due to hemolysis, renal and hepatic damage secondary to anemia
- Urinalysis—hemoglobinuria, pigmenturia

Pathological Findings

- Postmortem findings: pale or jaundiced mucous membranes, hepatic necrosis, renal necrosis, and hemosiderosis in the liver, spleen, and renal tubules.

THERAPEUTICS

Detoxification

- Emesis within 2 hours if acute ingestion, and if patient is asymptomatic
- Activated charcoal once (for acute ingestion only)

Appropriate Health Care

- Monitor CBC, renal values, blood glucose, blood pressure, urine output, venous blood gases
- Symptomatic and supportive care

- Intravenous crystalloid and/or colloid fluid therapy
- Dextrose supplementation if hypoglycemic
- GI support (e.g., gastric protectants, antiemetics)
- Whole blood transfusion if indicated

Drug(s) and Antidotes of Choice

- No antidote
- Supportive care

 COMMENTS

Expected Course and Prognosis

- Prognosis is good with appropriate care and timely intervention.

Abbreviations

CBC = complete blood count
GI   = gastrointestinal
GIT = gastrointestinal tract
PCV = packed cell volume
RBC = red blood cell

Suggested Reading

Caruso K. Applied cytology case study of the month presentation. NAVC Clinician's Brief 2003; 2:42–43.
Cope RB. *Allium* species poisoning in dogs and cats. Vet Med 2005; 100:562–566.
Plumlee, P. Propyl disulfide. In Clinical Veterinary Toxicology. Philadelphia: Mosby, 2004; pp 408–410.
Poppenga RH. Hazards associated with the use of herbal and other natural products. In: Peterson ME, Talcott PA, eds. Small Animal Toxicology, 2nd ed. St. Louis, Elsevier Saunders, 2006, p 323.
Yamato O, et al. Heinz body hemolytic anemia with eccentrocytosis from ingestion of Chinese chive (*Allium tuberosum*) and garlic (*Allium sativum*) in a dog. J Am Anim Hosp Assoc 2005; 41(1):68–73.

Author: Catherine M. Adams, DVM
Consulting Editor: Justine A. Lee, DVM, DACVECC

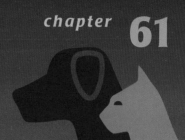
Salt

DEFINITION/OVERVIEW

- Hypernatremia can be caused by either solute gain or from water losses (hypotonic or free water loss). This chapter will focus on the patient's abnormalities that result from solute gain (e.g., sodium intake or salt poisoning).
- Sodium sources include homemade play dough (fig. 61.1), table salt, rock salt used to de-ice roads, salt emetics, sodium phosphate enemas, paintballs, sea water, iatrogenic administration of sodium-containing fluids such as sodium bicarbonate and hypertonic saline, and ingestion of improperly mixed or formulated feeds (typically for large animals).
- Common clinical signs include GI and neurologic signs, including vomiting, diarrhea, depression, lethargy, tremors, seizures, and coma.

ETIOLOGY/PATHOPHYSIOLOGY

- The GIT signs are due to a direct irritant effect on the gastric mucosa.
- Neurological signs are due to rapid fluid shifts within the CNS, resulting in initial cell shrinkage, hyperosmolality, and hemorrhage. Cerebral edema may then occur secondary to treatment with crystalloid fluid therapy or due to unlimited access to oral water.
- The amount of salt ingested, water availability, duration of time since ingestion, and underlying health conditions of the patient all influence the clinical course and toxicity.

Mechanism of Action

- Sodium is rapidly absorbed following oral ingestion or through parenteral administration of hypertonic saline and results in hypernatremia (serum sodium levels >155 mEq/L in the dog or >158 mEq/L in the cat).
- The brain is affected by sodium by two main mechanisms:
  - Sudden increases in osmolality result in fluid shifts and cellular dehydration. Cerebral tissue dehydration then results in secondary hemorrhage of fine meningeal vessels.

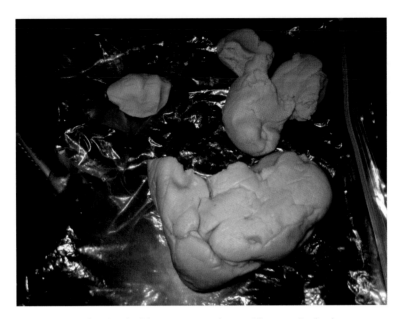

■ **Fig. 61.1.** Homemade play dough. (Photo courtesy of Anne Okerman Gardner)

- Once treatment with IV fluids begins, or if the animal has free access to oral water, acute fluid shifts can result in cerebral edema. Cerebral edema occurs as a result of two theories:
  - □ Rapid, inappropriate IV administration of free water (D5W) causes water to move from the vasculature into the CNS, resulting in cerebral edema.
  - □ Sodium passes from plasma to the CSF passively, but transfer of sodium back into plasma requires energy. As the sodium load increases, the CSF sodium increases. The higher CSF sodium levels (>145–185 mEq/L) result in decreased energy production, preventing the CSF from being able to transport sodium back into plasma. This then results in CSF hypernatremia. When water is taken in (orally) or given intravenously (D5W), it may result in inappropriate movement of water into the CNS, resulting in edema formation.

Pharmacokinetics/Absorption, Distribution, Metabolism, and Excretion

- Sodium is an important osmotic molecule.
- Rapid increases in sodium serum levels will cause fluid shifts from the ICF compartment into the vasculature, resulting in hypervolemia.
- If hypernatremia is chronic (or slow in onset), the CNS will protect itself from cell shrinkage via the production of idiogenic osmoles.

- Idiogenic osmoles typically form with chronic dehydration (i.e., water deprivation, starvation, DKA), and take 4–7 days to form.
- Examples of these osmoles include the following:
  - Inositol
  - Glutamate
  - Glutamine
  - Taurine
  - β-aminosulfonic acid
  - Phosphocreatine
- Sodium correction should occur no faster than 0.5 mEq/L/hr or no more than 10–12 mEq/L per day. With chronic hypernatremia, the sodium correction should be done even more slowly (over 48–72 hours), as this will allow for elimination of idiogenic osmoles; too rapid a correction will result in cerebral edema formation.

Toxicity

- Signs of toxicosis are generally seen with serum sodium concentrations ≥170 mEq/L; more severe signs are seen at a serum sodium level of ≥180 mEq/L.
- 4 g/kg of sodium is reported to be a lethal dose in the dog, and dogs ingesting 2–3 g/kg of sodium have shown signs of toxicity.
- Clinical signs of salt toxicosis have been reported to occur within 3 hours.
- One tablespoon of table salt contains approximately 17.85 g of sodium chloride, or one cup of table salt contains 285.6 g of sodium chloride.
- Ingestion of 1.9 g/kg of homemade play dough can be toxic. Homemade play dough can contain 8 g of sodium per tablespoonful of dough.
- Sodium bicarbonate or baking soda contains about 1/20th the sodium content of sodium chloride or table salt. It takes about 10 to 20 g/kg to produce signs of toxicity in the majority of animals. This is roughly 2–4 teaspoonfuls/kg.

Systems Affected

- Gastrointestinal—vomiting, diarrhea, anorexia
- Nervous—lethargy, depression, ataxia, tremors, seizures, coma
- Respiratory—pulmonary edema
- Cardiovascular—tachycardia, arrhythmias
- Respiratory—pulmonary edema or pleural effusion may develop from hypervolemia
- Renal/urologic—azotemia, acute tubular necrosis
- Endocrine/metabolic—metabolic acidosis, PU/PD, hyperthermia, hyperosmolality
- Musculoskeletal—muscular rigidity, myoclonus, ataxia

SIGNALMENT/HISTORY

- There is no known breed or sex predilection.
- Vomiting has been the most common initial clinical sign reported. Signs may occur in as short as 30 minutes to as long as 4 hours following ingestion. Diarrhea may also be present.
- Neurological progression often follows the initial GI signs and includes ataxia, disorientation, tremors, seizures, and coma.

Risk Factors

- Lack of access to fresh water (e.g., water deprivation from a frozen water bowl) or unlimited access to water (after salt exposure) both may predispose to clinical signs.

Historical Findings

- A thorough history should be obtained. The sodium source may have been iatrogenic (e.g., administered by the owners to induce emesis). Likewise, with patients presenting with hypernatremia, one should inquire regarding other sources of potential salt ingestion (e.g., from the animal's hair during the winter from de-icers or ingestion of homemade play dough ornaments from a Christmas tree).
- Acute onset of vomiting followed by tremors or seizures with documented hypernatremia is suspicious for possible increased solute intake.

Location and Circumstances of Poisoning

- The animal's history should help to guide if hypernatremia is due to gain of solute versus loss of water.
- The finding of hypernatremia on an electrolyte panel may be due to two primary causes:
  - Gain of a solute (e.g., salt toxicity)
  - Loss of water (e.g., free water losses [frozen water bowl for an outdoor dog] or hypotonic fluid losses [profound vomiting and diarrhea])
    - When hypernatremia is due to hypotonic fluid losses, these patients may also be clinically dehydrated and the administration of volume replacement fluids (e.g., 0.9% saline, LRS, Norm-R, etc.) may be needed first to correct dehydration before the addition of D5W is administered as adjuvant therapy.
- In either circumstance, the hypernatremia should be corrected slowly.

CLINICAL FEATURES

- The most common initial clinical signs are vomiting, diarrhea, and anorexia occurring within 3 hours.
- This may be followed by the development of neurological signs such as ataxia, tremors, seizures, and coma.
- On physical exam, the animal may appear dehydrated despite the presence of hypervolemia. They may be hyperthermic, tachypneic, tachycardic, or have the presence of arrhythmias. The neurological assessment will vary depending on the degree of CNS effects.

 DIFFERENTIAL DIAGNOSIS

- Hypernatremia can be due to increased solute load or due to water losses.
- Pure water losses:
  - Heat stroke
  - Diabetes insipidus (central or nephrogenic)
  - Fever
  - Inadequate access to water (e.g., frozen water bowl in the winter in an outdoor dog)
  - Severe burns
- Hypotonic fluid losses:
  - Vomiting
  - Diarrhea
  - Chronic or acute renal failure
  - Diabetes mellitus
  - Diuretic administration

 DIAGNOSTICS

- Measurement of the serum sodium level will confirm the presence of hypernatremia but not the inciting cause.
- Other confirmatory testing includes evaluation of CSF sodium levels; values >160 mEq/L are supportive. Postmortem cerebral tissue levels >1800 ppm is supportive of salt toxicity, but this is rarely performed.

Pathological

- Gross pathologic findings: hemorrhage to the GIT (stomach, small intestines, and colon), retraction of the brain from the calvarium, trauma to meningeal vessels, and hematoma formation

- Microscopic changes: diffuse cerebral edema with widened extracellular spaces, blood vessel congestion, necrosis of vessel walls with extravasation of RBC and protein, renal necrosis, and hepatic necrosis

 THERAPEUTICS

- The goal of therapy is to lower the serum sodium concentration safely. This should be done over 48 hours or no faster than 0.5 mEq/L/hr.
- The water deficit can be calculated to help safely guide therapy.
- Intensive electrolyte monitoring is needed every 2–3 hours.
- Any animal that has worsening neurological signs after the initiation of treatment is likely suffering from cerebral edema resulting from rapid correction of the sodium. Careful fluid management, head elevation, nursing care, and mannitol with furosemide may be needed.

Detoxification

- Depending of the source of solute and timing since ingestion, emesis or gastric lavage may be helpful.

Appropriate Health Care

- Aggressive supportive care to decrease sodium levels is imperative.
- Carefully monitor for clinical signs of cerebral edema.
- Sodium levels should be monitored frequently to ensure that levels do not change too rapidly.

Drugs and Antidotes

- Hospitalization for appropriate electrolyte monitoring and IV fluid therapy (using both balanced crystalloids and D5W) are indicated.
- Free water replacement in the form of slow oral water administration (via a nasoesophageal feeding tube) or IV D5W.
- Water deficit = [(0.6) × (BW in kg)] × [(current serum sodium/desired serum sodium) − 1]. This should be replaced over 48 hours or no faster than 0.5 mEq/L/hr.
- Once the patient is euhydrated, the administration of 3.7 mL/kg/hr of D5W is estimated to lower the serum sodium level by 1 mEq/L/hour.
- Furosemide (2.2–4.4 mg/kg, IV q 12–24 hours) may help with sodium excretion, especially in those animals that have underlying cardiac or renal disease, as they may not tolerate the additional volume in an already hypervolemic state.
- Antiemetics should be used due to the irritant effects of salt on the GI mucosa:
  - Maropitant 1 mg/kg, SQ q 24 hours, not labeled for cats

- Ondansetron 0.1–0.2 mg/kg, IV q 6–12 hours
- Metoclopramide 0.2–0.5 mg/kg, SQ, IM q 8 hours
■ Anticonvulsants:
  - Diazepam 0.5 mg/kg, IV to effect, followed by CRI at 0.5–1 mg/kg/hr, IV, to effect if needed
  - Phenobarbital 4–16 mg/kg, IV to effect
  - Propofol 1–8 mg/kg, IV to effect, followed by CRI dose of 0.1–0.6 mg/kg/min if uncontrolled seizures
■ If signs worsen after treatment begins, this may be due to the development of cerebral edema.
  - D5W should be slowed or stopped.
  - Treatment for cerebral edema:
    □ Head elevation at 15–30 degrees to decrease ICP (if the patient is laterally recumbent)
    □ Minimize jugular restraint to prevent increased ICP
    □ Mannitol 0.5–2 g/kg, IV slow over 20–30 minutes to effect
    □ Furosemide 2.2–4.4 mg/kg, IV, to effect

Precautions/Interactions

■ Do not lower the serum sodium level faster than 0.5–1 mEq/L/hr.
■ Patients with underlying renal or cardiac disease will need to monitored closely for the development of pulmonary edema, as they may be less tolerant of the hypervolemic state caused by hypernatremia.

Nursing Care

■ Intensive care may be needed depending on the patient's neurological status.

Diet

■ Due to the GI effects, a bland diet and soft foods may be indicated for 5–7 days.

Prevention

■ Decrease potential exposure to salt sources.
■ Always ensure that outdoor dogs have access to water (e.g., frozen water bowl).

 COMMENTS

■ Clinical signs in salt toxicosis are related to fluid shifts.
■ Use caution when correcting the sodium level even in patients that have had rapid onset of hypernatremia.

Client Education

- Make owners aware of possible sources of sodium, including paintballs, home-made play dough, and de-icing salts.
- Avoid the use of salt for emesis induction.

Patient Monitoring

- Monitoring of the serum sodium level every 2–3 hours during fluid correction is indicated. The fluid rate and type of fluid should be titrated based on the sodium level.
- Evaluation of the liver and kidney function should be repeated to evaluate for delayed injury.

Prevention/Avoidance

- Preventing ingestion of salt sources, including homemade play dough, paint-balls, table salt, and cold weather de-icing salt are imperative. Wiping a pet's feet after walking on ice is an easy way of avoiding accidental ingestion.

Possible Complications

- Treatment can result in cerebral edema if the serum sodium is dropped too quickly.
- There are reports of renal and hepatic necrosis; monitoring a chemistry panel may be indicated, depending on the patient's progression.

Expected Course and Prognosis

- Symptomatic patients should have their sodium corrected over a 48–72 hour period.
- Prognosis has been linked to the patient's sodium level and clinical signs on presentation. In human reports, age also played a role in prognosis; younger patients had a better survival.

Abbreviations

CNS = central nervous system
CRI = continous rate infusion
CSF = cerebral spinal fluid
D5W = 5% dextrose in water
DKA = diabetic ketoacidosis
ECF = extracellular fluid
GI   = gastrointestinal
GIT = gastrointestinal tract
ICF = intracellular fluid

ICP   = intracranial pressure
IM   = intramuscular
IV   = intravenous
PD   = polydipsia
PU   = polyuria
q   = every
RBC   = red blood cells
SQ   = subcutaneous

See also

Paintballs

Suggested Reading

Ajito T, Suzuki K, Iwabuchi, S. Effect of intravenous infusion of a 7.2% hypertonic saline solution on serum electrolytes and osmotic pressure in healthy beagles. J Vet Med Sci 1999; 61:637–641.

Barr JM, Safdar AK, McCullough, SM, et al. Hypernatremia secondary to homemade play dough ingestion in dogs: a review of 14 cases from 1998 to 2001. J Vet Emerg Crit Care 2004; 14:196–202.

DiBartola SP. Disorders of sodium and water: hypernatremia and hyponatremia. In: DiBartola SP, ed. Fluid, Electrolyte, and Acid-Base Disorders in Small Animal Practice, 3rd ed. St. Louis: Elsevier Saunders, 2006.

Pouzot C, Descone-Junot C, Loup J, et al. Successful treatment of severe salt intoxication in a dog. J Vet Emerg Crit Care 2007; 17:294–298.

Tegzes JH. Sodium. In: Peterson ME, Talcott PA, ed. Small Animal Toxicology, 2nd ed. St. Louis: Elsevier Saunders, 2006.

Authors: Sarah L. Gray, DVM; Justine A. Lee, DVM, DACVECC
Consulting Editor: Justine A. Lee, DVM, DACVECC; Lynn R. Hovda, DVM, MS, DACVIM

chapter *62*

Xylitol

DEFINITION/OVERVIEW

- Xylitol is a five-carbon sugar alcohol commonly used as a sugar substitute in chewing gums, candies, nicotine gums, toothpastes, and baked goods.
- Xylitol exists naturally in low levels in fruits and vegetables.
- Ingestion of xylitol can cause hypoglycemia and acute hepatic necrosis, leading to vomiting, depression, diarrhea, weakness, ataxia, seizures, coagulopathy, and potentially death.
- Other sugar-free products (aspartame, acesulfame, malitol, sorbitol) are generally considered nontoxic.

ETIOLOGY/PATHOPHYSIOLOGY

Mechanism of Action

- Xylitol is a potent stimulator for insulin secretion from the pancreas in dogs.
- The mechanism of hepatic necrosis is unknown. There are two proposed mechanisms: depletion of hepatic cellular ADP, ATP, and inorganic phosphorus molecules or production of reactive oxygen species during the metabolism of xylitol in the liver.
- Severe hepatic necrosis results in secondary impaired clotting factor production and DIC.
- Profound hypokalemia can be seen secondary to endogenous insulin secretion, contributing to signs of muscle weakness and lethargy.

Pharmacokinetics/Absorption, Distribution, Metabolism, and Excretion

- Rapidly absorbed after oral ingestion, with hypoglycemia seen within 10–15 minutes.
- Peak plasma concentration: 30 minutes to 1 hour.
- The liver is the major organ of metabolism.

Toxicity

- Hypoglycemia—a dose >0.1 g/kg may cause hypoglycemia.

470

- Hepatic failure—a dose >0.5 g/kg may cause hepatic toxicity. However, it is unclear if it is truly dose dependent or an idiosyncratic reaction.

Systems Affected

- Endocrine/metabolic—hypoglycemia
- Hepatobiliary—acute hepatic necrosis, elevated liver enzymes, icterus, hypoglycemia, melena, hepatic encephalopathy
- Gastrointestinal—vomiting, diarrhea, melena
- Nervous—weakness, ataxia

 # SIGNALMENT/HISTORY

- Any age and breed of dogs

Risk Factors

- Preexisting liver diseases
- Preexisting conditions predisposing to hypoglycemia (e.g., insulinoma, hepatoma, hepatocellular carcinoma, hunting dog hypoglycemia, diabetes mellitus with insulin administration)
- Availability of xylitol in the environment

Historical Findings

- Witnessed ingestion
- Discovery of chewed up packages of xylitol products or baked goods. The owner may note the smell of gum from the pet's mouth.

Location and Circumstances of Poisoning

- Availability of xylitol in the environment (commonly ingested from "purse digging")

 # CLINICAL FEATURES

- Vomiting is usually the initial sign.
- Clinical signs of hypoglycemia (including weakness, depression, collapse, ataxia, tremoring, or seizures) may occur within 10–60 minutes postingestion.
- Hepatic damage may occur as early as 9–12 hours post-ingestion, or may be delayed up to 72 hours post-ingestion. The patient may experience hepatic necrosis in the absence of initial hypoglycemia at presentation.
- Hepatic necrosis may lead to exacerbation of hypoglycemia and secondary DIC. Depression, vomiting, icterus, melena, diarrhea, petechiae/ecchymosis, and hepatic encephalopathy may be seen as the clinical condition progresses.

DIFFERENTIAL DIAGNOSIS

- Hypoglycemia—insulinoma, juvenile hypoglycemia, hunting dog hypoglycia, sepsis, drug administration or toxicosis (insulin overdose, glipizide)
- Liver failure:
  - Toxicities—Sago palm (*Cycas revoluta*), acetaminophen, hepatotoxic mushrooms (*Amanita phalloides*), iron, aflatoxin, blue green algae, metaldehyde
  - Infectious diseases—leptospirosis, mycoses, toxoplasmosis, infectious canine hepatitis
  - Metabolic—cirrhosis, portosystemic shunt, microvascular dysplasia
  - Neoplasia

 DIAGNOSTICS

- Blood glucose—hypoglycemia
  - Monitor BG every 1–2 hours for the first 6–8 hours. Adjust frequency subsequently based on the patient's clinical progression and degree of glucose supplementation.
- CBC—mild neutrophilic leukocytosis, thrombocytopenia, hemoconcentration from dehydration
- Chemistry—elevations of ALT, AST, ALP; hyperbilirubinemia; electrolyte derangements (e.g., hypokalemia, hypophosphatemia or hyperphosphatemia, and hypercalcemia)
- Clotting profile—prolonged coagulation tests (e.g., ACT, PTT, PT), thrombocytopenia, increased D-dimer or FDP
- Abdominal ultrasound—With acute hepatic necrosis, the liver may be normal to increased in size. Echogenicity of the liver may be normal to hypoechoic or mottled. Cytology of the liver by fine needle aspirate may show degenerative changes such as nonlipid vacuolar changes, increased nuclear to cytoplasmic ratio, anisokaryosis, and lysed cellular debris.

Pathological Findings

- Diffuse hepatic cell necrosis and organizational collapse may be seen as with other hepatotoxins.
- Widespread hemorrhage from DIC and icterus are common with acute hepatic necrosis.

 THERAPEUTICS

- Early decontamination, supportive care, and monitoring are the mainstay of xylitol toxicity treatment. Severe hepatic failure and coagulopathy may have a delayed onset (up to 72 hours reported) in the absence of hypoglycemia. Serial liver value monitoring is recommended.

Detoxification

- Decontamination
  - Emesis induction for an asymptomatic patient if the ingestion is within 1–6 hours. Do not induce emesis if the patient has signs of hypoglycemia to avoid the risk of aspiration pneumonia.
  - With large ingestions (e.g., bulk packages containing 200 pieces of gum), delayed emesis may still be beneficial, provided the patient's hypoglycemia has been treated appropriately, as xylitol may conglomerate in the stomach, delaying gastric emptying.
  - Activated charcoal is not recommended due to poor and unreliable binding to xylitol.

Appropriate Health Care

- Intravenous crystalloid fluids with 2.5% to 5% dextrose supplementation to maintain hydration and blood glucose. Dextrose supplement is recommended to prevent hypoglycemia even if initial BG at presentation is normal. Additional dextrose boluses may be given if the patient develops hypoglycemia.
- In hypoglycemic patients (BG <60 mg/dL), 0.5–1.5 mL/kg of 50% dextrose (diluted with saline) should be bolused IV over 1–2 minutes, followed by a CRI of 2.5%–5% dextrose supplementation in IV fluids.
- If the patient is not vomiting, small frequent meals should be fed to help prevent hypoglycemia.
- Preemptive hepatic function supportive medications are recommended, especially in cases of large dose ingestion.
  - S-adenosylmethionine (SAM-e)
  - Silymarin (milk thistle)
  - Vitamins C and E
  - N-acetylcystine
  - Vitamin K_1
- Fresh frozen plasma in the presence of DIC or coagulopathy
- Antiemetics and GI protectants as indicated for the patient's GI signs

Drug(s) and Antidotes of Choice

- There is no known antidote for xylitol.

Nursing Care

- Close patient monitoring for signs of hypoglycemia, liver failure, and DIC.

Follow-up

- Serial evaluation of the patient's clinical signs and liver values until at least 72 hours postingestion is prudent.

COMMENTS

Client Education

- Early aggressive medical treatment for xylitol toxicity is imperative to avoid possible life-threatening consequences. Pet owners should be made aware of this toxicity on wellness visits or via client education handouts on pet safety.

Patient Monitoring

- BG
- Liver values
- Electrolytes
- Hematological profile
- Coagulation profile

Prevention/Avoidance

- Prevent any access of pet to xylitol-containing products.
- Prevent any "purse digging."

Possible Complications

- For severely affected patients, data evaluating long-term liver function is lacking.

Expected Course and Prognosis

- The prognosis for xylitol toxicity is fair to guarded with prompt aggressive medical treatment. For patients affected by transient hypoglycemia only, the long-term prognosis is good after discharge from the hospital. For patients affected with liver failure, the prognosis is guarded.

Abbreviations

ACT = activated coagulation time
ADP = adenosine diphosphate
ALT = alanine transaminase
ALP = alkaline phosphatase
AST = aspartate transaminase
ATP = adenosine triphosphate
BG   = blood glucose

CBC = complete blood count
CRI = continuous rate infusion
DIC = disseminated intravascular coagulation
FDP = fibrin degradation products
GI   = gastrointestinal
IV   = intravenous
PT   = prothrombin time
PTT = activated partial thromboplastin time

See Also

Acetaminophen
Blue-green Algae (Cyanobacteria)
Iron
Metaldehyde Snail and Slug Bait
Mushrooms
Sago Palm

Suggested Reading

Dunayer EK. Hypoglycemia following canine ingestion of xylitol-containing gum. Vet Human Toxicol 2004; 46(2):87–88.

Dunayer EK. New findings on the effects of xylitol ingestion in dogs. Vet Med 2006; 101:791–798.

Dunayer EK, Gwaltney-Brant SM. Acute hepatic failure and coagulopathy associated with xylitol ingestion in eight dogs. JAVMA 2006; 229:1113–1117.

Kuzuya T, Kanazawa Y, Kosaka K. Stimulation of insulin secretion by xylitol in dogs. Endocrinol 1969; 84:200–207.

Todd JM, Powell LL. Xylitol intoxication associated with fulminant hepatic failure in a dog. J Vet Emerg Crit Care 2007; 17:286–289.

Authors: Ta-Ying Debra Liu, DVM; Justine A. Lee, DVM, DACVECC
Consulting Editor: Justine A. Lee, DVM, DACVECC

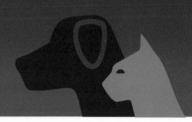

Foreign Objects

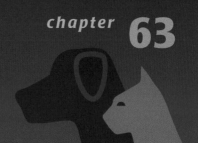

chapter 63

Foreign Bodies

DEFINITION/OVERVIEW

- A foreign body is an object located in any part of the body in which it does not belong. In this chapter, we will discuss foreign bodies specifically related to the GIT tract.
- Common GIT foreign bodies in the dog include corn cobs, cloth, carpet, rubber objects, toys, string, and bones.
- Common GIT foreign bodies in the cat include string, thread, yarn, and hairballs.

ETIOLOGY/PATHOPHYSIOLOGY

- GI obstruction can be seen in both dogs and cats. The degree of clinical signs and illness will be based on many factors, including the duration of obstruction, location of the obstruction, if the obstruction is partial or complete, and the severity of the intestinal injury (e.g., perforation, necrosis).
- Clinical signs of GIT obstruction may include loss of appetite, dehydration, vomiting, abdominal pain, and lethargy. Clinicopathologic abnormalities may also be present, including electrolyte derangements, hemoconcentration, and acid-base abnormalities.

Mechanism of Action

- **Gastric foreign body obstructions (FBOs)** may result in chronic irritation of the stomach, with secondary anorexia, nausea, and vomiting.
- **Small intestinal (SI) FBOs** may result in decreased outflow of intestinal contents, proximal intestinal dilation, vomiting, diarrhea, electrolyte losses, abdominal pain from distension, profound fluid losses, and dehydration.
- **Pyloric FBOs** may result in a profound hypochloremic metabolic alkalosis, projectile vomition, secondary electrolyte losses, and dehydration.

Systems Affected

- Gastrointestinal—anorexia, nausea, retching, regurgitation, vomiting, diarrhea, colic, "prayer" position, abdominal distension, absence of bowel sounds, borborgymi, absence of defecation, painful defecation, dehydration

- Endocrine/metabolic—hypochloremia, hypokalemia, metabolic alkalosis
- Cardiovascular—tachycardia, hypotension
- CNS—lethargy, generalized malaise

 SIGNALMENT/HISTORY

- Young animals are more likely to present with a GIT foreign body as they tend to be more curious and mischievous. The Labrador and golden retriever breeds, along with mixed breed dogs, tend to be the most common dogs to present with GIT foreign bodies.

Risk Factors

- Young dogs that are not crated are predisposed to FBO, particularly if adequate pet proofing has not occurred in the house or if the environment contains material at risk for FBO.

Historical Findings

- Pet owners may find evidence of foreign bodies chewed up in the environment or may find remnants of wrappers, part of boxes, pill vials, etc.
- The presence of foreign material may be seen in emesis or in stool.

Interactions with Drugs, Nutrients, or Environment

- Patients with underlying metabolic disease (such as renal disease, hypoadrenocorticism, IBD, etc.) may be more difficult to diagnose with a FBO due to chronic vomition.
- Underlying disease may predispose these patients to more profound dehydration or electrolyte imbalances, and rapid diagnosis and treatment is imperative.

 CLINICAL FEATURES

- Dogs and cats with GIT foreign bodies may present with a wide array of clinical signs, ranging from a mild decrease in appetite to hypovolemic shock and septic peritonitis.
- Common presenting clinical signs may include vomiting, loss of appetite, lethargy, abdominal pain, borborgymi, decreased bowel movements, diarrhea, hypersalivation, and nausea. Other signs and symptoms may include weight loss and dehydration.
- Clinical signs will vary based on the foreign body causing the obstruction, duration of obstruction, location of the obstruction, if the obstruction is partial or complete, and the severity of the intestinal injury (e.g., perforation, necrosis).

- **Esophageal FBOs**—hypersalivation, dysphagia, transient pawing at the mouth, regurgitation, and even signs of respiratory distress due to compression of the trachea
- **Gastric FBOs**—inappetence, vomiting. Depending on the duration of the presence of the gastric foreign body, either chronic, intermittent, or acute projectile vomiting may be seen.
- **Proximal SI obstructions**—acute, protracted vomiting
- **Distal SI obstructions**—more gradual onset of vomiting, weight loss, and anorexia
- **Large intestinal obstructions**—dyschezia, constipation, vomiting, loss of appetite, and weight loss

 # DIFFERENTIAL DIAGNOSIS

- Gastrointestinal disease—IBD, pancreatitis, gastritis, gastroenteritis, mesenteric torsion, GDV, intestinal infarction/ischemia, neoplasia
- Abdominal—peritonitis, splenic torsion, intraabdominal testicular torsion, acute abdomen
- Metabolic disease—renal disease, liver disease
- Endocrine disease—hypoadrenocorticism, hyperthyroidism

 # DIAGNOSTICS

- Thorough history, specifically the following:
  - Past medical history
  - Clinical signs (e.g., loss of appetite, vomiting, diarrhea, lethargy)
  - Foreign material ingested
  - Time ingested
  - Amount ingested
- Thorough physical exam, paying special attention to:
  - Oral cavity (specifically under the tongue to evaluate for linear FBO, particularly in cats)
  - Abdominal palpation
  - Rectal exam
- CBC, serum chemistry, UA, venous blood gas analysis
  - Evaluate for severity of dehydration/hemoconcentration (elevated PCV/TS).
  - Evaluate for elevated WBC count ± left shift (due to peritonitis from intestinal perforation).
  - Monitor acid-base and electrolyte imbalances (e.g., hypokalemia, metabolic alkalosis, etc.).
- Chest radiographs:
  - Evaluate for esophageal FBO or evidence of aspiration pneumonia.

- Abdominal radiographs:
  - Evaluate for SI diameter:
    - Dog: SI diameter is not normally uniform, but on the lateral radiographic projection, the ratio of the maximal SI diameter to the height of the vertebral body of L$_5$ at its narrowest point should be less than 1.6.
    - Cat: SI diameter is normally more uniform, and >12 mm diameter of SI on lateral or VD radiographic projection suggests FBO.
  - Evaluate for the following:
    - Peritonitis—loss of abdominal detail
    - Pneumoperitoneum—free gas in the abdominal cavity seen as gas bubbles not contained in a viscous. This is typically found at the highest point of the peritoneal cavity on radiographs and is often superimposed on abdominal organs such as the liver or the GIT. Recent abdominal surgery, artifical insemination, and other benign causes for pneumoperitoneum should be ruled out.
  - Additional diagnostics:
    - Repeat radiographs
    - Upper GI (barium) contrast study ± fluoroscopy
    - Abdominal ultrasound

Foreign Body Evaluation

Cat Litter—Clumping
- Although inert and nontoxic, cat litter ingestion is not an uncommon problem in a multipet and multispecies household.
- With small ingestions, GIT signs may include loss of appetite, vomiting, and diarrhea.
- With large ingestions, there is an increased risk of pyloric outflow obstruction, SI obstruction, or large intestinal obstruction.
- Radiographic description: stippled, mineralized, foreign material
- Generally, treatment is not necessary unless a massive ingestion has occurred. Radiographs should be performed and emesis induction initiated if gastric foreign material is still present. See the general treatment recommendations under "Treatment."

Charcoal/Barbeque Briquettes
- Charcoal or barbeque briquettes are generally considered nontoxic but carry a risk of FBO.
- Barbeque briquettes may contain charcoal and a combination of petroleum distillates, limestone, and sawdust. Used barbeque briquettes may have grill grease drippings dried on, resulting in increased palatability and secondary gastroenteritis/pancreatitis.
- Ingestion may result in loss of appetite, vomiting, diarrhea, and the potential for FBO.

- Radiographic evidence—stippled material within the GIT, possible FBO
- See the general treatment recommendations under "Treatment."

Crayons

- Most crayons are manufactured for children and are generally nontoxic. It is important to check the package/label to verify this.
- Small ingestions typically do not result in clinical signs.
- Large ingestions can cause clinical signs and illness, including loss of appetite, vomiting, diarrhea, and/or FBO.
- Radiographic evidence—foreign material within the GIT, generally not radiopaque and may be difficult to identify radiographically.
- Generally, treatment is not necessary unless a massive ingestion has occurred. Radiographs should be performed and emesis induction initiated if gastric foreign material is still present. See the general treatment recommendations under "Treatment."

Silica Gel Packets/Oxygen Absorbers

- Commonly found with newly purchased clothing, shoes, and other retail items
- This is an inert substance and is not toxic.
- Although inert, ingestion can lead to expansion of the silica gel as it absorbs water, leading to GI signs such as diarrhea, vomiting, or even a gastric or intestinal FBO with massive ingestion (rare).
- Radiographic evidence—not radiopaque, difficult to see on radiographs
- Generally, treatment is not necessary unless a massive ingestion has occurred.

Firestarter Logs (e.g., Duraflame logs composed of wax and sawdust)

- Constructed from sawdust, agricultural fibers, and nonpetroleum renewable waxes and oils
- Toxicity is not expected if the product is ingested, but there is an increased risk of FBO with a large amount ingested.
- FBO may be due to indigestible wood fibers within the product. Rarely, a gastroenteritis, pyloric outflow obstruction, SI obstruction, or even large intestinal obstruction may occur with massive ingestions.
- Radiographic evidence—may see evidence of foreign material or matter within the stomach or GIT
- Generally, with small ingestions, treatment is not necessary. When a large amount of firestarter is ingested, radiographs should be performed and emesis induction initiated if gastric foreign material is still present. See the general treatment recommendations under "Treatment."

Wood Glues (Diphenylmethane diisocyanate)

- Diphenylmethane diisocyanate is an active ingredient in many industrial-strength wood glues as well as polyurethane foams, various industrial paints, and other adhesives.

- When ingested, an exothermic reaction occurs, leading to expansion of the glue within the stomach.
- Following ingestion, even a small amount of liquid glue can quickly develop into a large, firm foreign body resulting in a FBO.
- Radiographic evidence—may see a large amount of material within the stomach, often confused for kibble. Additional diagnostics such as contrast studies, abdominal ultrasound, or fluoroscopy may be needed to rule out a FBO.
- Decontamination should be rapidly performed if immediate ingestion has occurred; otherwise, surgical intervention may be necessary. Emesis is not typically recommended due to the concern for the material to become an esophageal foreign body as the liquid becomes a more solid form following the exothermic reaction. In general, immediate decontamination with gastric lavage with a large-bore cuffed tube may be performed; however, FBO often occurs quickly due to the rapid exothermic reaction. See the general treatment recommendations under "Treatment."

Medication Bezoars
- Certain medications, when ingested in large quantities, can form bezoars, specifically a pharmacobezoar.
- Medications reported to cause bezoars include aluminum hydroxide gel, enteric-coated aspirin, sucralfate, guar gum, cholestyramine, enteral feeding formulas, psyllium preparations, nifedipine XL, chewable iron supplements, and meprobamate.
- Pharmacobezoars can result from excessive administration or ingestion of the medication, altered motility (due to dehydration, the ingested drug's effect on gastric emptying, concomitant use of anticholinergics and narcotics, ileus, etc.), or abnormal anatomy of the GIT tract.
- Medications that are hygroscopic (absorb water) may also have an increased propensity to form pharmacobezoars.
- Radiographic evidence—may see a large amount of material within the stomach, often confused for kibble. If present, aggressive decontamination (e.g., emesis induction, gastric lavage) should be performed, followed by repeat radiographs to verify removal of all product. See the general treatment recommendations under "Treatment."

 # THERAPEUTICS

- Dehydration, hypovolemia, and electrolyte abnormalities should be corrected with appropriate IV fluid therapy. Options for fluid therapy include crystalloid or colloid solutions. Crystalloid solutions are classified as replacement or maintenance solutions. Replacement solutions are most often used in veterinary medicine, including lactated Ringer's solution, Normosol-R, Plasmalyte 148, and

0.9% NaCl. These solutions have electrolyte concentrations similar to the patient's serum concentrations and can be given rapidly. With illness as a result of GIT disease, electrolytes and osmolarity may be altered, emphasizing the importance of acid-base and electrolyte testing in these patients.

- Colloid solutions are indicated when the patient's colloid osmotic pressure (COP) is decreased. This can be determined using a colloid osmometer, or estimated to be decreased when the patient's albumin drops below 2.0 g/dL or the TS is less than 3.5 g/dL. When the COP is low, the patient is at risk for developing interstitial edema. As compared to crystalloid solutions, larger molecules found in colloid solutions remain in the vascular space and increase the oncotic pressure. Examples of colloid solutions include whole blood, plasma, dextrans, hetastarch, and Oxyglobin.
- If diagnostics (e.g., x-rays, contrast studies, or an ultrasound) show an abnormality that would indicate the need for surgical intervention, including intestinal dilation (criteria above), peritonitis, abdominal effusion consistent with a septic peritonitis, or pneumoperitoneum, the patient should be stabilized with fluid therapy prior to surgery, but definitive correction will then require surgical removal of the inciting cause.
- Treatment for GI exposure:
  - If a small amount was ingested, and the patient is asymptomatic, no treatment is necessary.
  - Radiographs may help to confirm ingestion and aid in additional treatment options (e.g., fluid therapy, antinausea/antiemetics). See figure 63.1.
  - With large ingestions, or if the patient is symptomatic, radiographs should be considered to confirm and identify the FBO within the GIT.
  - If present within the stomach, options for decontamination may initially include either emesis or gastric lavage to resolve a pyloric outflow obstruction or decrease the likelihood of a subsequent SI obstruction. While emesis is often safe and effective, emesis induction is contraindicated following ingestion of caustic or corrosive substances (e.g., battery ingestion) or sharp objects (e.g., glass, sharp bones) as they can lead to esophageal damage such as strictures, perforation, or further irritation.
  - With large ingestions, surgical removal may be necessary if decontamination is inadequate, if the patient does not respond to medical management, or if there is evidence of a pyloric outflow obstruction or SI obstruction.
  - If present within the stomach and gastric lavage was not successful, treatment options may include either endoscopy or surgical removal (gastrotomy).
  - If present within the SI and the radiographs are suspicious for an SI obstruction, an exploratory laparotomy should be performed.
  - If present within the colon/large intestine and the patient presents with signs of constipation, fluid therapy to correct dehydration should be performed and enema therapy can be considered.

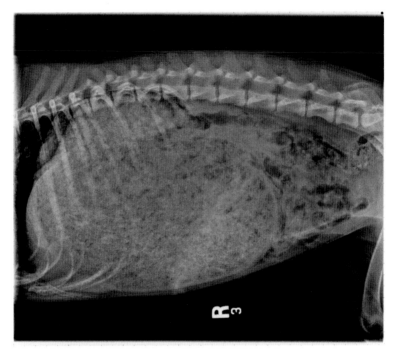

■ **Fig. 63.1.** Lateral radiograph of a dog with the presence of a large amount of gastric foreign material. (Radiograph courtesy of Garret E. Pachtinger)

 COMMENTS

Client Education

■ Pet owners should be taught how to pet proof their home to prevent accidental foreign body ingestion.

Patient Monitoring

■ The use of radiographs, ultrasonography, contrast radiography (e.g., barium series), or even fluoroscopy may be necessary to aid in diagnosis of a FBO.

Prevention/Avoidance

■ Dogs should be appropriately crate trained to prevent foreign body ingestion or FBO.

Possible Complications

■ Risks of complications include dehiscence, septic peritonitis, stricture, and adhesions postsurgical exploratory.

Expected Course and Prognosis

- Overall, the prognosis for surgical removal of a gastric or intestinal FBO is fair to good, depending on the viability and integrity of the tissue.

Abbreviations

CBC = complete blood count
CNS = central nervous system
COP = colloid osmotic pressure
FBO = foreign body obstruction
GDV = gastric dilatation volvulus
GI   = gastrointestinal
GIT   = gastrointestinal tract
IBD   = inflammatory bowel disease
IV   = intravenous
PCV = packed cell volume
SI   = small intestine
TS   = total solids
UA   = urinalysis
WBC = white blood cell
XL   = extended release

Suggested Reading

Beal MW. Approach to the acute abdomen. Vet Clin North Am Small Anim Pract 2005; 35(2):375–396.

Bebchuk TN. Feline gastrointestinal foreign bodies. Vet Clin North Am Small Anim Pract 2002; 32(4):861–880.

Graham JP, Lord PF, Harrison JM. Quantitative estimation of intestinal dilation as a predictor of obstruction in the dog. J Small Anim Pract 1998; 39:521.

Morgan JP: The upper gastrointestinal examination in the cat: normal radiographic appearance using positive-contrast medium. Vet Radiol 1981; 22:159.

Taylor JR, Streetman DS, Castle SS. Medication bezoars: a literature review and report of a case. Ann Pharmacother 1998; 32(9):940–946.

Authors: Garret E. Pachtinger, VMD; Kenneth J. Drobatz, DVM, MSCE, DACVIM, DACVECC
Consulting Editor: Justine A. Lee, DVM, DACVECC

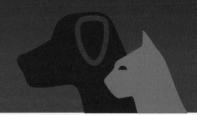

Garden, Yard, and Farm Chemicals

chapter 64

Bone and Blood Meal

DEFINITION/OVERVIEW

- Bone meal and blood meal are by-products from the meatpacking industry that are widely utilized as soil amendment products, fertilizer components, or as deer, rabbit, and wildlife repellants.
- Bone meal may also be a component in calcium and phosphorus mineral supplements.
- In general, these meals are considered a low-level toxicity; however, they can result in GIT irritation, foreign body obstruction (FBO), and severe pancreatitis when ingested.
- Iron may be added to bone meal or blood meal, resulting in additional toxicity. (See chap. 84 on iron toxicity for more information.)

ETIOLOGY/PATHOPHYSIOLOGY

- Bone meal and blood meal are highly palatable to dogs and can result in unintentional, large ingestions.
- Tulip, daffodil, and hyacinth bulbs may be dusted in bone meal when planted to fertilize bulbs and aid in repelling squirrels. The scent of bone meal may entice dogs to dig up newly planted bulbs and subsequently ingest both the potentially toxic bulb and bone meal.
- Increased use of organic products that contain blood meal and bone meal in lawn and gardening have increased exposure opportunities for animals.

Pharmacokinetics/Absorption, Distribution, Metabolism, and Excretion

- Bone meal and blood meal are poorly absorbed through GIT and dermal routes and are primarily GIT irritants.

Toxicity

- Bone meal and blood meal are generally considered low-level toxins.
- Bone meal may be added to fertilizers, herbicides, or insecticides (organophosphates), which can result in toxicity and in larger ingestions of other amendment

products due to increased palatability (see appropriate chapters for more information).

- Bone meal or blood meal may be iron fortified and can increase toxicity risk if the iron content is ≥1%.
- Large ingestions of bone meal can congeal into a solid ball in the stomach, resulting in an FBO.
- Large ingestions of blood meal can congeal into a gelatinous FBO.
- Decontamination is recommended with recent large ingestions or for dogs with a prior history of pancreatitis.

Systems Affected

- Gastrointestinal

 # CLINICAL FEATURES

- GIT signs (e.g., persistent foul-smelling vomiting and/or diarrhea, anorexia, bloating, and abdominal discomfort)

 # DIFFERENTIAL DIAGNOSIS

- Toxicity of other GI irritants
- Foreign body obstruction
- Pancreatitis
- Inflammatory bowel disease
- Metabolic disease—liver or renal disease

 # DIAGNOSTICS

- CBC with PCV/TS to monitor for dehydration, particularly if vomiting is persistent
- Pancreatitis blood tests (e.g., amylase, lipase, canine pancreas–specific lipase [cPL], pancreatitis lipase immunoreactivity) or abdominal ultrasound
- Radiographic evaluation for FBO

Pathological Findings

- Evidence of foreign material or FBO
- Evidence of aspiration pneumonia if secondary aspiration of vomitus has occurred

THERAPEUTICS

Detoxification

- Emesis within 2 hours if (1) spontaneous emesis has not occurred and (2) ingestion was a significant amount that could result in FBO or pancreatitis, or (3) the patient had a prior history of pancreatitis.
- Unsuccessful emesis may result in the need for aggressive gastric lavage (with an inflated endotracheal tube to prevent aspiration) to remove contents from the stomach.
- If gastric lavage is unsuccessful or time since ingestion is significantly delayed, surgical intervention may be necessary to remove the bone meal or blood meal if there is evidence of FBO (e.g., based on radiographic appearance).

Appropriate Health Care

- Antiemetics if vomiting is severe or persists
  - Maropitant 1 mg/kg SQ q 24 hours, not labeled for cats
  - Ondansetron 0.1–0.2 mg/kg IV q 8–12 hours
- GI protectants as needed
  - H_2 blockers
    - Famotidine 0.5 mg–1 mg/kg PO, SQ, IM, IV q 12 hours
    - Ranitidine 1–2 mg/kg PO, SQ, IM, IV q 8–12 hours
    - Cimetidine 5–10 mg/kg PO, SQ, IM, IV q 6 hours
  - Omeprazole 0.5–1 mg/kg PO q 24 hours
  - Sucralfate 0.25–1 g PO q 8 hours × 5–7 days if evidence of active ulcer disease

Drug(s) and Antidotes of Choice

- No antidote
- Supportive care

Nursing Care

- Symptomatic and supportive care (e.g., SQ or IV fluid therapy, antiemetic therapy, bland or low-fat diet, etc.)

 # COMMENTS

Expected Course and Prognosis

- Prognosis is good with timely intervention involving decontamination and supportive care.

Abbreviations

CBC = complete blood count
cPL = canine pancreas-specific lipase
FBO = foreign body obstruction
GI   = gastrointestinal
GIT = gastrointestinal
IM   = intramuscular
IV   = intravenous
PCV = packed cell volume
PO   = *per os* (by mouth)
q   = every
SQ   = subcutaneous
TS   = total solids

See Also

Iron

Suggested Reading

Plumlee, K. Clinical Veterinary Toxicology. Philadelphia: Mosby, 2004; pp. 408–409.

Authors: Josephine L. Marshall, CVT; Justine A. Lee, DVM, DACVECC
Consulting Editor: Gary D. Osweiler, DVM, PhD, DABVT

chapter 65

Fertilizers

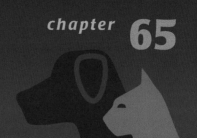

DEFINITION/OVERVIEW

- Fertilizers are soil amendment products used in agriculture, lawn and garden care, and indoor plant applications.
- Fertilizers contain varying percentages of nitrogen, phosphorus, and potassium (potash) as indicated by the three numbers on the packaging (e.g., 30-10-10).
- Fertilizer may also contain the following minerals: iron, copper, zinc, cobalt, boron, manganese, and molybdenum.
- In general, fertilizer ingestions are a low-level toxicity and symptoms are primarily limited to GIT irritation.

ETIOLOGY/PATHOPHYSIOLOGY

- Accidental ingestion of fertilizer may be increased with the addition of palatable soil amendments like blood meal and/or bone meal. (See Chapter 64)
- Appropriately diluted fertilizers (e.g., "ready-to-use" or "RTU") and fertilizers applied according to labeled directions rarely result in toxicity.
- The widespread use of lawn and garden fertilizers results in frequent exposure opportunities for animals.

Mechanism of Action

- Generally result in low level of toxicity
- With high nitrate concentrations in some fertilizers, methemoglobinemia may be seen if nitrates convert to nitrates in the intestine or colon.
- Some fertilizers may also contain other additives like fungicides, insecticides, and herbicides, which may produce an additive, synergistic, or even antagonist toxic effect.

Pharmacokinetics/Absorption, Distribution, Metabolism, and Excretion

- Fertilizers generally have poor GIT and dermal absorption.

Toxicity

- The primary toxic components of fertilizers are nitrogen, phosphorus, and potassium.

- Toxicity from ingestion of fertilizer is rare due to low concentrations of nitrogen, phosphorus, and potassium, combined with poor GIT absorption of the fertilizer.
- Additional ingredients (such as iron, herbicides, pesticides, and fungicides) may be added to fertilizers, increasing the risk of toxicity (see appropriate chapters for more information).
- Fertilizers containing iron in concentrations of ≥1% can result in iron toxicity.
- Stored, concentrated products present greater risk of toxicity due to higher concentration of fertilizer.
- Once appropriate fertilizer applications have dried, there is little concern with ingestion or dermal exposure.
- Ingestion of crops, plants, or grass that have recently been fertilized are not anticipated to result in fertilizer toxicity, although mild GIT signs may occasionally be seen.
- Decontamination is recommended if recent ingestion of a concentrated product occurred, or when ingestion of >0.5 g/kg of body weight is ingested.

Systems Affected

- Gastrointestinal

 # CLINICAL FEATURES

- Clinical signs usually occur within 2 to 10 hours of ingestion.
- GIT signs (e.g., salivation, vomiting, diarrhea, abdominal discomfort, anorexia)
- GIT symptoms generally resolve in 12 to 24 hours.
- LD_{50} in rats: 5 g/kg

 # DIFFERENTIAL DIAGNOSIS

- Toxicosis from other GI irritants
- Foreign body obstruction
- Pancreatitis
- Inflammatory bowel disease
- Metabolic disease—liver or renal disease

 # DIAGNOSTICS

- No specific or diagnostic features
- Evaluation of hydration (based on PCV/TS) should be assessed.
- Abdominal radiographs and other advanced diagnostics may need to be performed to rule out other differential diagnoses.

Pathological Findings

■ Evidence of GIT lesions. No other specific lesions are found with fertilizer ingestions alone.

 # THERAPEUTICS

Detoxification

■ Emesis within 2 hours if spontaneous emesis has not occurred and ingestion is
significant (e.g., of stored, concentrated product)
■ Single dose of activated charcoal and cathartic

Appropriate Health Care

■ Antiemetics if vomiting is severe or persists
  • Maropitant 1 mg/kg SQ q 24 hours, not labeled for cats
  • Ondansetron 0.1–0.2 mg/kg IV q 8–12 hours
■ GI protectants as needed
  • H$_2$ blockers
    □ Famotidine 0.5–1 mg/kg PO, SQ, IM, IV q 12 hours
    □ Ranitidine 1–2 mg/kg PO, SQ, IM, IV q 8–12 hours
    □ Cimetidine 5–10 mg/kg PO, SQ, IM, IV q 6 hours
  • Omeprazole 0.5–1 mg/kg PO q 24 hours
  • Sucralfate 0.25–1 g PO q 8 hours × 5–7 days if evidence of active ulcer
    disease

Drug(s) and Antidotes of Choice

■ No antidote
■ Supportive care

Nursing Care

■ Symptomatic and supportive care (e.g., SQ or IV fluid therapy, anti-emetics,
bland diet)

 # COMMENTS

Expected Course and Prognosis

■ Prognosis is good with minimal treatment (e.g., supportive care) or no
treatment.

Abbreviations

GI   = gastrointestinal
GIT = gastrointestinal

IM   = intramuscular
IV   = intravenous
PCV = packed cell volume
PO   = *per os* (by mouth)
q   = every
RTU = ready-to-use
SQ   = subcutaneous
TS   = total solids

Suggested Reading

Albretsen JC. Fertilizers. In: Plumlee KH. Clinical Veterinary Toxicology. St Louis: Mosby, 2004; pp. 154–155.

Campbell A, Chapman M. Handbook of Poisoning in Dogs and Cats. Ames, IA: Blackwell Science, 2000; pp. 133–134.

Gerken DF. Lawn care products. In: Bonuagura JD, ed. Kirk's Current Veterinary Therapy XII, Philadelphia: WB Saunders, 1995; pp. 248–249.

Levengood JM, Beasley VR. Principles of ecotoxicology: environmental contaminants. In: Gutpa RC, ed. Veterinary Toxicology: Basics and Clinical Principles. New York: Elsevier, 2007; pp. 693–694.

Yeary RA. Oral intubation of dogs with combinations of fertilizers, herbicide and insecticide chemicals commonly used on lawns. Am J Vet Res 1984; 45:288–290.

Authors: Josephine L. Marshall, CVT; Justine A. Lee, DVM, DACVECC
Consulting Editor: Gary D. Osweiler, DVM, PhD, DABVT

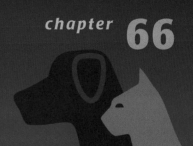

chapter 66

Herbicides

 DEFINITION/OVERVIEW

- Herbicides are plant control chemicals that may also have varying effects on animals under high exposure conditions.
- Selected herbicides with frequent use in urban and suburban locations include the following:
    - Phenoxy acid herbicides and their derivatives (2,4-D, MCPA, MCPP)
    - Benzoic acids (dicamba)
    - Dinitroanilines (trifluralin, pendimethalin, prodiamine)
    - Phosphonomethyl amino acids (glyphosate)
- The term *herbicide* includes a range of chemical structures. Modern herbicides are largely designed to affect plant biochemistry rather than animal systems.
- Herbicides are among the most heavily and widely used pesticide category, but poisonings are a very limited portion of small animal toxicosis.
    - Pet owners/guardians often consider herbicides as equivalent in risk to insecticides, rodenticides, and other pet control chemicals. Veterinarians must carefully evaluate exposure and toxicity of specific herbicides and explain relative risk to their clients.
    - A combination of low acute toxicity and low application rates reduces dosage and risk to animals that consume or have contact with treated plants (lawn grasses, garden weeds).
    - Most illness from herbicide exposure is by accidental exposure to concentrates or mixed sprays before application or improper disposal of containers or unused spray.
- Accurate information about application rate, potential contact with concentrates, and time since exposure is essential to accurate evaluation of risk.
- Simple examples can be used to illustrate herbicide risk:
    - One pound of herbicide per acre of lawn delivers approximately 150 ppm of herbicide to the grass (see table 66.1).
    - Expected concentrations of herbicides to lawns range from 150 to 1000 ppm
- Older herbicides (arsenicals, dinitrophenols, chlorates) and paraquat are generally more toxic to animals than contemporary lawn and garden herbicides. See chapter 68 for paraquat toxicosis.

TABLE 66.1. Calculation and comparison of risk to small animals from grass treated with example herbicides.

Herbicide	Typical Grass Concentration (ppm)	Canine No-Effect Dietary Concentration (ppm)	Ratio of Dietary No-Effect Concentration to Grass Concentration (column 3 divided by column 2)
2,4-D	150	500	3.3
Dicamba	15–40	50	1.25–3.3
MCPA, MCPP	300–450	160	0.53–0.36[a]
Paraquat	75–150	34	0.45–0.23
Pendimethalin	80–120	500	6.25–4.2

a. Ratio <1.0 suggests high risk. MCPA or MCPP and paraquat are available above the "no effect" concentration.

- Antidotes are not available for herbicides. Prompt detoxification and systemic supportive therapy can prevent poisoning and mitigate effects.
- Common responses to the most available herbicides include dermal or ocular irritation, or vomiting and nausea from consumption of concentrates or spray mixes.
- For many products, effects may be a combination of the herbicide in addition to effects from solvents or adjuvants added to improve herbicide performance.
- Response is usually shortly after direct exposure, and often the signs subside within 24–48 hours.
- Prolonged or excessive exposure may cause renal damage by some products.
- Since the majority of useful toxicology information is for the phenoxy acid herbicides, this chapter will cover primarily that group of herbicides.

 ETIOLOGY/PATHOPHYSIOLOGY

Mechanism of Action

- Phenoxy acid herbicides include 2,4-D, MCPA, and MCPP.
- Depress ribonuclease synthesis, uncouple oxidative phosphrylation and increase hepatic peroxisomes. Relationship of these effects to animal poisoning is uncertain.
- Prolonged exposure is associated with mild to moderate reversible renal damage.
- In dogs, phenoxy acid herbicides affect muscle membranes and cause myotonia. The reported potential mechanism is increased paranitrophenyl phosphatase with increased potassium and compensatory chloride conductance at muscle membranes.

Pharmacokinetics/Absorption, Distribution, Metabolism, and Excretion

- 2,4-D is absorbed almost completely from GIT, skin, and lungs.
- Peak concentrations appear within 6 hours in blood, liver, kidney, lungs, and spleen.
- Renal anion transport in dogs may be less effective than in other animals.
- Excretion is rapid with >80% unchanged 2,4-D in urine and a T½ of 10–20 hours.
- Peak serum concentration is >100 ppm at a dosage of 100 mg/kg BW, and serum values are >700 ppm when dosage is >175 mg/kg BW.
- At high dosages, serum and kidney 2,4-D concentrations are approximately equal.
- MCPA and MCPP kinetics are believed similar to 2,4-D but less well described.

Toxicity

- Residues on turf range from 35 to 75 ppm and may persist 1–3 days. This is approximately equivalent to 1.4–3.0 mg/kg BW.
- Oral LD$_{50}$ in dogs is 100 mg/kg, but dogs have survived up to 200 mg/kg.
- Multiple oral dosage toxicity studies in dogs produced fatalities at 20 mg/kg for 3 weeks or 25 mg/kg for 6 days.
- Vomiting and myotonia occur at dosages >175 mg/kg and electromyograph changes occur at ≥8.8 mg/kg.
- Dogs exposed to 4 times the recommended application on turfgrass and held there for 7 days displayed no observed adverse effects and had no abnormal clinical chemistry or hematology changes.
- Toxicity is reduced when herbicide is delivered in food.
  - Dogs fed 25 mg/kg 2,4-D in their diet for 2 years had no detectable adverse effects.
- MCPA canine no-effect dosage is 1 mg/kg. Dosages ≥20 mg/kg for 4 weeks caused only dry hair coat and mild changes in liver and kidney function.
  - A nonlethal chronic toxic dosage is 4.0 mg/kg BW, resulting in retarded growth and altered kidney function.
- MCPP canine oral dosage of 64 mg/kg BW for 13 weeks caused decreased weight gains and anemia. Dosages of ≤16 mg/kg caused no effect.

Systems Affected

- Gastrointestinal
  - Initial response is vomiting; may be followed by diarrhea and bloody feces.
  - Solvents, adjuvants, or other inert ingredients may also cause nausea and vomiting when dogs access freshly treated lawns.
- Musculoskeletal
  - Reluctance to move followed by myotonia, including muscle rigidity, ataxia, and posterior weakness.

- Spastic movements, opisthotonus, and mild seizures can occur.
  - Musculoskeletal effects do not appear to be caused by other common herbicides.
- Ophthalmic and skin
  - Some but not all herbicide concentrate and spray solutions may cause ocular or skin irritation.
- Renal
  - Renal function may be mildly affected with congestion, enlargement of kidneys, and tubular degeneration.

 SIGNALMENT/HISTORY

Risk Factors

- Combination products, especially containing herbicides, insecticides, and/or fertilizers can raise risk of chemical poisoning from one or more ingredients.

Historical Findings

- Observations or events
  - Recent mixing, spraying, or other use of granular lawn or garden chemicals; pet owners/guardians may generalize any lawn care chemical use as including or implicating herbicides.
  - History of pet gaining access to sprayed or treated areas
  - Spray drift or chemical odor from adjacent or nearby properties
  - Spilled container of chemicals on property, in garage, or elsewhere
  - Recent history of cleaning garages, basements, or garden sheds
- Clinical signs
  - Acute and unexpected onset of signs
  - Prominent signs of vomiting, nausea, depression, or skin or eye irritation.

Location and Circumstances of Poisoning

- Often reported after lawn treatment, especially when commercial applicator used or nearby properties use chemical products
- Most incidents or suspected poisoning is in the growing season, or during spring or fall treatments of lawns or gardens. Exception is subtropical/tropical regions where applications occur year round (e.g., Florida, California, Hawaii)

Interactions with Drugs, Nutrients, or Environment

- Known interactions with other drugs or chemicals are rarely reported.
- Herbicides that are metabolized by hepatic mixed function oxidases could interact with other chemicals metabolized in the same way.

CLINICAL FEATURES

- Anorexia, vomiting, diarrhea, melena
- Lethargy, depression, hesitant to move
- Myotonia, muscle rigidity (reported only in dogs)
- Ataxia
- Posterior weakness
- Clonic seizures (rare)
- Oral ulcers (occasional)

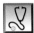 **DIFFERENTIAL DIAGNOSIS**

- Anionic/cationic detergent exposure
- Arsenical poisoning
- Coenuriasis, cystercosis, cestodiasis
- Eclampsia, hypocalcemia
- Granulomatous meningoencephalomyelitis
- Cholecalciferol (vitamin D_3) toxicosis
- Ionophore feed additive toxicosis
- Myotonia congenital (chow chow, miniature schnauzers, several other breeds less prevalent) if no gastrointestinal signs
- Nicotine toxicosis (2,4-D and dicamba group only)

 DIAGNOSTICS

- **Clinical laboratory**: Increased ALP, LDH, and CK reflect mild to moderate damage to renal tubules and skeletal muscle
- **Serum/tissue assay**: 2,4-D or other phenoxy herbicides in serum or renal tissue at 100–700 ppm confirm recent exposure to potentially toxic dosage.
- **Electromyographic changes**: Increased insertional activity (harmonic change when electrode is inserted) at dosages lower than clinical toxicosis.
- **Pathological findings**: oral ulcers, gastritis, renal congestion and/or mild tubular necrosis, friable liver, hyperemia of lymph nodes

 THERAPEUTICS

Treatment Objectives

- All categories discussed have no specific effective antidote.
- Treatment should emphasize decontamination.
- Carriers and adjuvants in herbicides may be a risk to attending personnel. Protect involved persons with aprons, gloves, and goggles.

Detoxification

- Bathe exposed animals in warm water with soap or mild detergent.
- Flush eyes with isotonic saline or water for 10–15 minutes.
- Consider emesis or gastric lavage in asymptomatic animals with recent (<2 hours) ingestion.
  - Use caution with emesis since carriers and adjuvants can promote GI tract irritation.
  - Avoid emesis if signs of oral/pharyngeal irritation are present, gag reflex is depressed, or CNS excitation or depression are evident.
  - Emesis is NOT recommended for glyphosate exposure (tissue irritant).
- Administer activated charcoal with a cathartic (2–5 g/kg BW) within 2 hours of ingestion.

Appropriate Health Care

- Supportive care is indicated if clinical signs are seen. This may include fluids (oral, SQ, or IV) to maintain hydration and generalized GI support. (See Precautions/Interactions and Diet.)

Drug(s) and Antidotes of Choice

- No specific antidotes or drugs for herbicide exposure.
- Clinical supportive care must be judged according to physical and laboratory evaluation.

Precautions/Interactions

- IV fluids should be saline only or amended with bicarbonate or lactate. Avoid acidification of urine, which will retard excretion of acidic agents such as phenoxy herbicides.

Nursing Care

- Nursing care is important for most patients with true herbicide toxicosis.
- Maintain hydration as needed to replenish fluids or electrolytes and maintain urine flow.

Diet

- Bland low-protein diet is recommended for 2–5 days postrelease.

Activity

- Limit physical exertion for 2–3 days postrecovery.

Prevention

- Instruct owner/guardian in proper use of home chemicals.
- Keep pets off treated lawns and gardens for 24–48 hours.
- Package and dispose of lawn chemicals to avoid exposure to leftover concentrates.
- Always follow label directions.
- If adverse postapplication effects appear on lawn or garden, keep pets away until cause is determined.

Public Health

- Limited reports suggest association of phenoxy herbicides with lymphoma and/or urinary bladder transitional cell carcinoma in Scottish terriers. Subsequent studies have not confirmed early reports.
- Similar associations have been made for Hodgkins lymphoma in humans exposed repeatedly to phenoxy herbicides.
- Although causal relationships have not been confirmed for these associations, pet owners/guardians should be aware of the issue and avoid unnecessary exposure.

Environmental Issues

- Herbicides are generally substantially more toxic to fish than to mammals.
- Disposal should be done in a manner to avoid contamination of landscaping ponds or water features that may contain aquatic species.
- Follow label directions for application to minimize chemical runoff that could reach ponds, rivers, or lakes.

 # COMMENTS

Client Education

- See comments under Prevention above.
- Remember that herbicides used as directed have a very good safety record with companion animals.
- Most often the veterinarian will need to actively explain the risk factors and why herbicide toxicosis may not be an appropriate diagnosis.

Patient Monitoring

- Monitor kidney and liver function for 2–5 days.

Possible Complications

- Lasting or recurring health issues are not expected in recovered animals.

Expected Course and Prognosis

■ Expected course and prognosis are good with early detoxification and supportive therapy.

Abbreviations

2,4-D = 2,4 dichlorophenoxyacetic acid
BW   = body weight
GI   = gastrointestinal
IV   = intravenous
MCPA = 2-methyl-4-chlorophenoxyacetic acid
MCPP = 2-(4 chloro-methylphenoxy) propionic acid
SQ   = subcutaneous

Suggested Reading

Arnold EK, Lovell RA, Beasley VR, et al. 2,4-D toxicosis. III: an attempt to produce 2,4-D toxicosis in dogs on treated grass plots. Vet Hum Toxicol 1991; 33(5):457–461.

Beasley VR, Arnold EK, Lovell RA et al. 2,4-D toxicosis. I: a pilot study of 2,4-dichlorphenoxyacetic acid and dicamba-induced myotonia in experimental dogs. Vet Hum Toxicol 1991; 33(5):435–440.

Burgat V, Keck G, Guerre P. Glyphosate toxicosis in domestic animals: a survey from the data of the Centre National d'Informations Toxicologiques Veterinaries (CNITV). Vet Hum Toxicol 1998; 40:363–376.

Gupta PK. Toxicity of herbicides. In: Gupta RC, ed. Veterinary Toxicology: Basic and Clinical Principles. New York: Elsevier, 2007; pp. 567–586.

Yeary YA. Miscellaneous herbicides, fungicides, and nematocides. In: Peterson ME, and Talcott PA, eds. Small Animal Toxicology, 2nd ed. St. Louis: Elsevier-Saunders, 2006; pp. 732–743.

Author: Gary D. Osweiler, DVM, PhD, DABVT
Consulting Editor: Ahna G. Brutlag, DVM

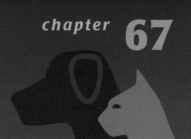

chapter 67

Methionine

DEFINITION/OVERVIEW

- Essential amino acid that is a glutathione and sulfate precursor; supplies both methyl and sulfhydryl groups to the liver
- Used in veterinary medicine as a urine acidifier and feed additive
- Given orally to dogs (tablets, chews, crunchies) to decrease brown spots in lawns associated with dog urine
- Clinical signs in dogs and cats—GI, CNS, metabolic acidosis; Heinz body anemia and methemoglobinemia in cats

ETIOLOGY/PATHOPHYSIOLOGY

Mechanism of Action

- Exact mechanism unknown but may be related to one of the following:
  - Methionine metabolism leading to liver ATP depletion and hepatic encephalopathy
  - Increase in metabolites including mercaptan-like compounds, such as homocysteine, may act synergistically with ammonia
  - Underlying liver disease impairs methionine metabolism, which likely contributes to toxicity
- Metabolites likely cause oxidative injury, resulting in Heinz body formation and methemoglobinemia.

Pharmacokinetics/Absorption/Distribution/Metabolism/ Excretion

- Pharmacokinetic data in animals is very limited and is extrapolated from human information.
  - Absorption through GIT
  - Metabolized in the liver by transamination and transulfuration pathways
  - Sulfate excreted in the urine as sulfuric acid, which results in acidification
- Half-life is unknown.

Toxicity

- Dogs
  - Reported in healthy dogs—1.35 g/kg or >25 g/dog
    - Doses as low as 200 mg/kg have been associated with weakness and ataxia.
    - Doses as low as 400 mg/kg have been associated with the development of hepatic encephalopathy.
  - Hepatic/pancreatic disease—31.4 mg/kg has resulted in clinical signs.
  - GI distress can develop at normal doses.
- Cats
  - Can develop Heinz body anemia at normal doses.
  - Doses >0.5 g/kg or 2 g/cat (about 400 mg/kg for 5-kg cat) have resulted in severe clinical signs.

Systems Affected

- Dogs
  - Gastrointestinal—abdominal pain, salivation, vomiting
  - Nervous—somnolence, posterior ataxia, tremors, and seizures
- Cats
  - Hemic/lymphatic/immune—Heinz body anemia and methemoglobinemia
  - Endocrine/metabolic—metabolic acidosis, often even in small overdoses
  - Gastrointestinal—abdominal pain, salivation, vomiting
  - Nervous—tremors and seizures with high doses

 SIGNALMENT/HISTORY

- All breeds and species are equally affected.
- Dogs with documented liver or pancreatic issues are much more likely to develop toxicity at lower doses.
- Younger dogs may be more inclined to chew bottles and ingest large quantities of pills.
- Younger kittens may be more susceptible.

Risk Factors

- Concurrent acidifying diets

 CLINICAL FEATURES

- Dogs
  - Gastrointestinal signs are common including vomiting, drooling, and abdominal pain.

- Nervous signs including ataxia, seizures, agitation, disorientation, restlessness, hyperactivity, and pacing occur within 4 hours of dosing. Some patients present similar to a spinal cord trauma or injury.
- Cats
  - Heinz body formation and methemoglobinemia may cause pale mucous membranes and cyanosis.
  - Cardiovascular signs such as tachycardia and hypotension secondary to anemia may be seen.
  - Gastrointestinal signs including vomiting, secondary dehydration, abdominal pain, and anorexia can occur.

DIFFERENTIAL DIAGNOSIS

- Toxicities—onions/garlic, acetaminophen, zinc, skunk musk, benzocaine, mushrooms, antidepressants
- Primary neurologic disease (inflammatory, infectious, structural, trauma)
- Primary gastrointestinal disease (IBD, gastroenteritis, dietary indiscretion, pancreatitis)
- Primary metabolic disease (renal, hepatic)

DIAGNOSTICS

- CBC—Heinz body formation, methemoglobinemia, chocolate brown blood color, regenerative anemia
- Serum chemistry—increased liver enzymes, possible hepatic failure/insufficiency (e.g., low BUN, hypoglycemia, hypocholesterolemia), elevated amylase and lipase, azotemia
- Serum ammonia can be normal or elevated.
- Arterial or venous blood gas analysis—metabolic acidosis
- Urinalysis—acidic urine, hyposthenuria

THERAPEUTICS

Decontamination

- Emesis or gastric lavage, followed by one dose of activated charcoal with a cathartic
- Appropriate decontamination with large ingestions of chewable tablets to decrease the incidence of bezoar formation

Appropriate Health Care

- Address underlying disease processes.
- Monitor renal function and liver enzymes daily until animal is clinically normal.

Drugs and Antidotes of Choice

- No specific antidote is available.
- IV fluids as needed to maintain hydration and perfuse kidneys. Any balanced, isotonic, buffered crystalloid fluid (e.g., LRS, NormR) can be used.
- For severe metabolic acidosis (pH <7.0, BE <−15 mmol/L, or HCO_3 <10 mmol/L), sodium bicarbonate can be used at 0.5–1 mEq/kg, IV slowly over 30 minutes.
- Antiemetics as needed for vomiting
  - Maropitant 1 mg/kg SQ q 24 hours, not labeled for cats
  - Ondansetron 0.1–0.2 mg/kg IV every 8–12 hours
- GI protectants as needed
  - H_2 blockers
    - Famotidine 0.5–1 mg/kg PO, SQ, IM, IV q 12–24 hours
    - Ranitidine 1–2 mg/kg PO, SQ, IM, IV q 8–12 hours
    - Cimetidine 5–10 mg/kg PO, SQ, IM, IV q 6 hours
  - Omeprazole 0.5–1 mg/kg PO q 24 hours
  - Sucralfate 0.25–1 g PO q 8 hours × 5–7 days if evidence of active ulcer disease
- Control agitation.
  - Acepromazine 0.025–0.2 mg/kg IV, IM, SQ PRN to effect
  - Diazepam 0.25–0.5 mg/kg IV PRN to effect
- Control seizures.
  - Diazepam 0.25–0.5 mg/kg IV PRN to effect
  - Phenobarbital 3–5 mg/kg IV PRN to effect
- Hematologic support
  - In patients with signs of hemorrhagic shock (e.g., tachycardia, pallor, hypotension) that do not respond to IV fluids, colloids or blood transfusions may be needed.
  - Methylene blue for treatment of Heinz body anemia
    - Dogs: 1–4 mg/kg slow IV once. The use in cats is not currently recommended due to the potential for worsening Heinz body anemia.

Alternate Drugs

- S-adenysyl-methionine (SAMe) 20 mg/kg PO once daily as a hepatoprotectant

Diet

- Discontinue acidifying diet.
- Bland diet until GI distress has passed.

COMMENTS

Expected Course and Prognosis

- Prognosis is generally good with ingestion, but underlying disease processes may hinder recovery. Recovery is generally seen within 1–3 days.
- Seizures and acute renal failure complicate therapy and worsen the prognosis.

Abbreviations

ATP   = adenosine triphosphate
BUN   = blood urea nitrogen
CBC   = complete blood count
CNS   = central nervous system
GI   = gastrointestinal
GIT   = gastrointestinal tract
IBD   = inflammatory bowel disease
IM   = intramuscular
IV   = intravenous
PO   = *per os* (by mouth)
PRN   = *pro re nata* (as needed)
q   = every
SAMe = S-adenysyl-methionine
SQ   = subcutaneous

See Also

Mushrooms

Suggested Reading

Branam JE. Suspected methionine toxicosis associated with a portocaval shunt in a dog. J Am Vet Med Assoc 1982; 181:929–931.

Maede Y, Hoshino T, Inaba M, et al. Methionine toxicosis in cats. Am J Vet Res 1987; 48:289–292.

Plumb DC. Plumb's Veterinary Drug Handbook 6th ed. Ames, IA: Blackwell, 2008; pp. 589–591.

Villar D, Carson T, Osweiler G, et al. Overingestion of methionine tablets by a dog. Vet Hum Tox 2003; 45:311–312.

Author: Katherine L. Peterson, DVM
Consulting Editors: Gary D. Osweiler, DVM, PhD, DABVT; Justine A. Lee, DVM, DACVECC

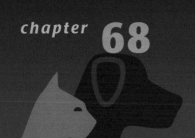

chapter **68**

Paraquat

DEFINITION/OVERVIEW

- Paraquat's chemical name is 1,1'-dimethyl-4,4'-bipyridyl, and it is one of the most selective pulmonary toxins known.
- Widely used nonselective contact herbicide, desiccant, and defoliant.
- Trade names include Cepupat, Dextron X, Dextrone, Gramoxone, Herbaxon, PP-148, and PP-910.
- Use is restricted to application by licensed applicators.
- In the USA, is often colored blue and has a noxious odor added to prevent accidental consumption and an emetic to induce vomiting if consumed.
- Available in pressurized spray formulations that contain less than or equal to 0.44% paraquat bis (methyl sulfate) and liquid fertilizer formulations that contain no more than 0.04% paraquat dichloride.
- Related dipyridyl compound (Diquat) available OTC may be confused with paraquat but is considerably less toxic than paraquat.

ETIOLOGY/PATHOPHYSIOLOGY

Mechanism of Action

- Cyclic reduction-oxidation reactions in lung generate oxygen, hydroxyl, and free radicals and deplete antioxidants such as superoxide dismutase and NADPH.
- Membrane damage, functional cellular incapacitation, and organ damage ensue.

Pharmacokinetics/Absorption, Distribution, Metabolism, and Excretion

- Absorption after oral ingestion is rapid but incomplete.
  - Peak plasma concentration in about 75 minutes
  - Roughly 25% absorbed and is dose dependent
  - Can be absorbed by inhalation or through skin, which is usually secondary to more chronic exposure and has a less severe reaction

Distribution

- Selectively accumulates in lung alveolar Type 1, Type 2, and Clara cells as well as renal proximal tubule epithelium

512

TABLE 68.1. Comparative toxicity of paraquat in selected species. The most susceptible animal shown is the dog.

	Dogs	Cats	Pigs, Sheep, Humans	Rats	Turkeys
LD_{50} (mg/kg)	25–50	40–50	25–75	100	290

- At 4 hours postexposure, concentration in lung is already 10x higher than at other selective sites; at 4–10 days after exposure, concentration in lung is 30–80x higher than plasma.

Metabolism and Excretion

- Paraquat undergoes extensive cyclic oxidation-reduction reactions in sequestering tissues but is excreted largely unchanged in the urine.
- Renal tubules actively excrete paraquat in higher concentrations than creatinine initially, but as kidney damage worsens, the T½ increases dramatically from <12 hours to >120 hours.

Toxicity

- LD_{50} varies by species (see table 68.1).
- In chronic or subacute exposure, symptoms may be seen by day 7 and progress to pulmonary fibrosis and progressive respiratory distress over several weeks.

Systems Affected

- Response secondary to ingestion is dose dependent and usually fatal (see fig. 68.1).
  - High-dose ingestion:
    - Rapid multisystem organ failure, massive pulmonary edema, ARF, liver damage, and death in 1–4 days
  - Moderate or sub-acute dose ingestion:
    - Slower onset of organ failure but eventual death from respiratory failure and pulmonary edema
  - Low and/or chronic exposure ingestion:
    - Death may not occur for several weeks and is usually secondary to pulmonary fibrosis and respiratory failure.
  - Chronic exposure through the skin or inhalation:
    - Usually a less severe clinical presentation

 SIGNALMENT/HISTORY

- There are no breed, sex, or age predilections, as paraquat is toxic to all mammals.
- Dogs are most likely to ingest paraquat.

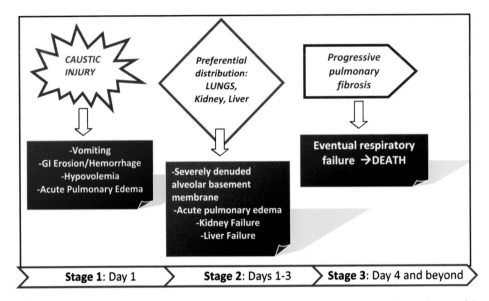

■ **Fig. 68.1.** Paraquat has a relatively unique pathogenesis, with early direct gastrointestinal injury, followed by preferential accumulation in lungs and less in liver and kidney. Oxidant and free radical damage to lungs results in progressive lung injury, which is typically fatal.

Historical Findings

■ Owners with high-risk jobs (pesticide industry)
■ Exposure to agricultural areas, where pesticides are used
■ Recent spraying activity
■ Observed ingestion or finding baits intended for dogs

Location and Circumstances of Poisoning

■ Primarily accidental, malicious, or intentional (by a human) oral ingestion
■ Skin absorption from concentrated or prolonged exposure
■ Animals near paraquat sources exposed to spray concentrates (agricultural centers, etc.)
■ Available since the 1960s and may still be stored in many places, including homes and garages

 CLINICAL FEATURES

Systems Affected

■ Gastrointestinal
  • Usually the first presenting signs due to caustic action of paraquat
  • Vomiting, diarrhea, aphagia, pain, possible esophageal or gastric ulceration, and GI hemorrhage may occur.

- GI dysfunction contributes to fluid loss, electrolyte imbalances, and hemo-dynamic instability.
- Respiratory
  - Acute toxicosis due to necrosis of type II pneumocytes, denuding alveolar basement membrane, secondary severe pulmonary edema, and clinical symptoms of acute respiratory distress syndrome (ARDS)
  - Chronic pulmonary effects with death over days to months from increasingly severe pulmonary fibrosis
  - Respiratory exposure possible from spray formulations
- Cardiovascular
  - Cor pulmonale and cardiovascular collapse may occur after large doses and secondary to acute pulmonary and renal damage.
- Renal
  - Acute tubular necrosis (ATN) 1–3 days postingestion.
  - If survival is past the acute phase, may see signs of renal tubular recovery
  - Hypovolemic prerenal azotemia combined with ATN often followed by oliguric renal failure
- Neurological (occasional)
  - While rare, neurologic clinical signs may occur, including hyperexcitability, depression, ataxia, and seizures.
- Skin (usually from dermal exposure) leading to irritation
  - Paraquat is a desiccant, so ulceration, erythema, irritation, and blistering can be seen with large epidermal exposure.
  - Direct contact can cause a transverse white discoloration of the nail plate or discoloration of the nail.
  - Usually a more chronic and lower dose exposure

 DIFFERENTIAL DIAGNOSIS

- Gastrointestinal disease
  - Ingestion of strongly alkaline or acidic compounds, zinc or zinc phosphide, inorganic arsenic, mercury, or lead
  - Infectious agents/gastroenteritis
  - Pancreatitis
  - Parvovirus
- Primary cardiac disease
- Primary or secondary pulmonary disease
  - Canine distemper (especially puppies 3–6 months old)
  - Toxoplasmosis (especially young to middle-aged, indoor/outdoor male cats)
  - Asthma (e.g., Siamese cats)
  - *Pneumocystis carinii*
  - Pulmonary interstitial fibrosis in West Highland white terrier

DIAGNOSTICS

- Dithionate spot test may detect paraquat in tissues and is important for rapid diagnosis.
- Serum paraquat levels: This is most predictive of severity and prognosis but not readily available in veterinary laboratories, and levels are quickly undetectable.
- Spectrometry and quantitative analysis of urine up to 48 hours after ingestion
- Paraquat in stomach contents, vomitus, tissues, and organs
- Chest radiographs should be performed for the first 1–3 days postingestion, due to severity of pulmonary changes that can be observed.

Pathological Findings

- Gross pulmonary congestion, bullous emphysema, hemorrhage, bronchodilation, or atelectesis
- Microscopic: alveolar necrosis of type II pneumocytes denuding alveolar basement membrane with severe pulmonary edema and/or fibroplasias

THERAPEUTICS

Detoxification

- Traditional emesis or gastric lavage as early as possible (<1 hour postingestion)
  - *Caution:* further caustic injury may be created, and absorption is very rapid so must be done immediately to decrease absorption effectively.
  - Activated charcoal is preferred for GI decontamination.
  - Fuller's earth or even clay soil may provide some decrease in absorption.

Appropriate Health Care

- Standard emergency supportive measures should be implemented, including airway, respiratory, and cardiovascular support.
- Clients should be advised of the complexity and need for extended therapy that is often accompanied by a grave prognosis.
- *Early oxygen therapy is typically contraindicated because of oxidant damage.* However, oxygen therapy may be useful for patient comfort secondary to respiratory compromise and progressive lung failure. Progressive pulmonary fibrosis is typical and is usually eventually fatal with significant exposure.
- Fluid therapy should be titrated to appropriately treat hypovolemia and to increase perfusion. IV fluids may also enhance excretion of paraquat. Colloids should be avoided, due to the risks of pulmonary edema. Cautious IV crystalloid fluid therapy should be used but titrated to effect, again to prevent pulmonary edema.

- Supportive care, including analgesics, antibiotic therapy (for secondary infections), antiemetic therapy, and treatment of secondary complications should be implemented.
- Antioxidant therapy (e.g., vitamins E and C, N-acetylcysteine, superoxide dismutase analogs, etc.) may eventually provide an antidote to paraquat; however, this is still in development.
- Aggressive cardiac and blood oxygen monitoring
- Hemodialysis may be somewhat effective in decreasing plasma concentrations, but peritoneal dialysis is not useful.
- Hemoperfusion through charcoal may be the most effective treatment, decreasing plasma concentrations dramatically.

Drug(s) and Antidotes of Choice

- There is no proven treatment in animals other than early oral detoxification.
- There is no antidote and no post-onset treatment that has been clearly shown to be effective. Emergency detoxification and supportive therapy are crucial.

Precautions/Interactions

- Emesis and gastric lavage may further damage the esophagus or stomach if concentrated paraquat ingestion has caused erosions or ulcers.
- *Oxygen therapy early is typically contraindicated because of oxidant damage.*

Prevention

- Prevent access to the poison.
  - Clean out garages or sheds that may have outdated paraquat or other pesticides used as gardening herbicides.
  - Storage at licensed applicator locations
- Take measures during manufacturing to ensure safety of the product (i.e., distinctive coloring, bittering agents, emetic agents, etc.).

Public Health Issues

- Possible use as bioterrorism agent or malicious baiting of dogs
- Animal exposure may suggest potential human (pediatric) risk.

Environmental Issues

- Public education and possibly community toxin disposal events. When used as directed by the manufacturer, no adverse effects on groundwater, soil, earthworms, fish, wildlife, or birds have been reported.

Abbreviations

ARDS = acute respiratory distress syndrome
ARF   = acute respiratory failure
ATN   = acute tubular necrosis
IV   = intravenous
LD_{50} = median lethal dose
NADPH = Nicotinamide adenine dinucleotide phosphate
OTC   = over-the-counter

Suggested Reading

Cope RB. Toxicology brief: helping animals exposed to the herbicide paraquat. Vet Med 2004; pp. 755–762.

FAO Specifications and evaluations of agricultural pesticides. 2003. Available at http://www.fao.org/Ag/AGP/AGPP/Pesticid/Specs/docs/Pdf/new/paraquat.pdf. Accessed October 11, 2009.

Oehme FW, Mannala S. Paraquat. In: Peterson ME, Talcott PA, ed. Small Animal Toxicology, 2nd ed. St. Louis: Saunders, 2006.

Author: Carey L. Renken, MD
Consulting Editor: Gary D. Osweiler, DVM, PhD, DABVT

Herbals

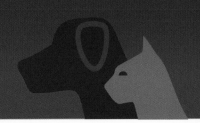

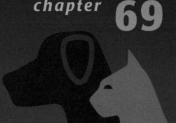

chapter 69

Ephedra/Ma Huang

DEFINITION/OVERVIEW

- *Ephedra sinica*, common name ma huang, is an herbal sympathomimetic used primarily as a weight loss aid, decongestant, and recreational drug known as herbal ecstasy.
- Overdoses cause hyperactivity, tachycardia, hypertension, tremors, seizures, hallucinations, and serotonin syndrome.

ETIOLOGY/PATHOPHYSIOLOGY

Mechanism of Action

- Ma huang contains ephedrine and pseudoephedrine. These alkaloids are structurally similar to amphetamines.
- Ma huang stimulates alpha- and beta-adrenergic receptors and releases endogenous catecholamines at synapses in the brain and heart. This results in peripheral vasoconstriction and cardiac stimulation.
- The clinical effects are increased blood pressure, tachycardia, mydriasis, ataxia, and restlessness. Central nervous systems effects include tremors, seizures, agitation, and serotonin syndrome.
- Serotonin syndrome is the overstimulation of serotonin receptors in the nervous system, gastrointestinal tract, cardiovascular and respiratory system. Clinical signs associated with serotonin syndrome seen in ma huang toxicity include tremors and seizures, hyperesthesia, hyperthermia, hypersalivation, and death.

Pharmacokinetics/Absorption, Distribution, Metabolism, and Excretion

- Ma huang is absorbed orally.
- It is metabolized in the liver and excreted in the urine.
- Ma huang excretion is enhanced if the urine is acidified.

Toxicity

- Clinical signs may be seen at 5–6 mg/kg.
- Death has been seen at 10–12 mg/kg.

Systems Affected

- Nervous: hyperactivity, hallucinations, tremors, seizures, head bobbing, serotonin syndrome
- Cardiovascular: tachycardia, hypertension
- Metabolic: hyperthermia
- Musculoskeletal: rhabdomyolysis (sequella to prolonged seizure activity and hyperthermia)
- Hemic: DIC (sequella to prolonged seizure activity and hyperthermia)
- Renal: myoglobinuria

 SIGNALMENT/HISTORY

- Dogs are the most common species to be affected by ma huang, although any species may develop toxicity if a sufficient dose of ma huang is ingested.
- Younger dogs may be more likely to "counter-surf" or get into purses and thus have exposure to a supplement.
- Diagnosis is based on history and clinical signs.

Risk Factors

- Animals with preexisting cardiovascular disease (including hypertension) or seizure disorders may develop more severe clinical signs.

Historical Findings

- Witnessed ingestion
- Access to herbal decongestants, diet products, and/or recreational drugs
- Owners frequently report restlessness, pacing, vocalizing, hyperactivity, panting, apparent hallucinations, head bobbing, and tremors or seizures.

Location and Circumstances of Poisoning

- Most animals will ingest supplements in a home or car.

Interactions with Drugs, Nutrients, or Environment

- If ingested with other sympathomimetic agents (pseudoephedrine, phenylpropanolamine), methylxanthines (chocolate or caffeine), MAO inhibitors (seligiline), or tricyclic antidepressants, toxicity may be enhanced.

 CLINICAL FEATURES

- Clinical signs can develop within 30 minutes to 8 hours postexposure.
- The duration of clinical signs is 24–72 hours.

- The most common signs are mydriasis, hyperactivity, panting, hyperthermia, nervousness, and tachycardia, followed by collapse.
- Hypertension, muscle tremors, and/or seizures may be noted on exam.
- Head bobbing has been associated with increased mortality.
- Death is usually due to cardiovascular collapse.

 # DIFFERENTIAL DIAGNOSIS

- Clinical signs are similar to the ingestion of pseudoephedrine found in cold and sinus medications, as well as amphetamine ingestion (attention deficit disorder drugs such as methylphenidate and dextroamphetamine) and illicit substances.

 # DIAGNOSTICS

- Clinical pathology: Hyperglycemia and hypokalemia may be noted.
- OTC drug tests will test positive for amphetamines if ma huang is ingested. Most OTC tests require urine.

Pathological Findings

- No specific gross or histopathologic findings have been reported.

 # THERAPEUTICS

- The treatment plan goals are to prevent further absorption, stabilize the cardiovascular system, control CNS signs, and provide supportive care.

Detoxification

- Induce emesis only in asymptomatic animals within 1 hour of ingestion.
- Activated charcoal may be given within 4 hours of ingestion in an asymptomatic animal.

Appropriate Health Care

- IV fluids as needed for supportive care in symptomatic animals

Drug(s) and Antidotes of Choice

- Acepromazine, 0.05–1.0 mg/kg IM or IV, to control restlessness and agitation. Start at low end of range and increase as needed.
- Propranolol, 0.02–0.06 mg/kg, slow IV to effect, for tachycardia. Propranolol also is a serotonin antagonist and may help reduce some clinical signs associated with serotonin syndrome.

- Cyproheptadine, 1.1 mg/kg q 6–12 hours for dogs, 2–4 mg/cat q 6–12 hours, for serotonin syndrome. Cyproheptadine is a specific serotonin antagonist.

Precautions/Interactions

- Diazepam can potentially cause increased CNS excitation resulting in crying, head bobbing, and death.

Alternative Drugs

- If propranolol is unavailable, or if an animal is hypertensive and tachycardic, a specific beta-1 antagonist may be preferred:
  - Esmolol 0.05–0.1 mg/kg IV boluses up to 0.5 mg/kg, or an infusion of 50–200 µg (0.05–0.2 mg)/kg/min in dogs. A loading dose of 200–500 µg/kg IV over 1 minute followed by a CRI of 10–200 µg/kg/min can be used in cats.
  - Atenolol 0.2–1 mg/kg PO q 12–24 hours for dogs, 2 mg/kg or 6.25–12.5 mg PO q 24 hours for cats
  - Metoprolol 0.2 mg/kg PO q 12 hours for dogs, 2–15 mg PO q 8 hours for cats
- If acid-base status can be monitored, administer ammonium chloride, 200 mg/kg/day, divided 4 times daily orally, or ascorbic acid/vitamin C, 20–30 mg/kg IM or IV q 8 hours, to acidify the urine.

Nursing Care

- Thermoregulation
- Minimize sensory stimulation.

Follow-up

- An animal should be monitored until clinical signs resolve, generally in 1–3 days.

Prevention

- Owners should be educated about keeping medications out of reach of pets.

 COMMENTS

Client Education

- Make sure the environment is safe for the pet before releasing to go home. Owners should check crates, blankets, under beds, etc. to make sure all pills or capsules have been removed.

Patient Monitoring

- Hydration
- Electrolytes
- Heart rate
- Blood pressure
- Heart rhythm (ECG)
- Body temperature
- Frequency of monitoring will vary with severity of clinical syndrome.

Prevention/Avoidance

- Discuss "counter-surfing," keeping purses, briefcases, etc. out of pet's reach. Discuss use of training aids like scat mats for pets constantly getting items off of counters.

Possible Complications

- DIC, rhabdomyolysis, and myoglobinuria (with subsequent renal failure) are possible if prolonged, untreated tremors/seizures or hyperthermia present.

Expected Course and Prognosis

- Clinical signs generally resolve within 24–72 hours.
- Prognosis is generally good.
- If head bobbing, myoglobinuria, or DIC present, prognosis is poor.

Synonyms

- Ma huang is also known as yellow horse or sea grape.
- There are several *Ephedra* species, but *Ephedra sinica* is the plant used in manufacturing of supplements.
- *Sida cordifolia*, also known as Indian common mallow, is another plant containing pseudoephedrine and ephedrine alkaloids sometimes used in herbal supplements.

Abbreviations

CNS = central nervous system
CRI   = constant rate infusion
DIC   = disseminated intravascular coagulation
ECG = electrocardiogram
IM   = intramuscular
IV   = intravenous
MAO = monamine oxidase
OTC = over the counter
PO   = *per os* (by mouth)
q   = every

See Also

Amphetamines
Decongestants (Pseudoephedrine, Phenylephrine)
Methamphetamine

Suggested Reading

DerMarderosian A, Beutler JA. The Review of Natural Products, 3rd ed. Saint Louis: Facts and Comparisons, 2002; 265–266.

Fugh-Berman A. The 5-minute Herb and Dietary Supplement Consult. Philadelphia: Lippincott Williams & Wilkins, 2003; 116–117.

Means C. Selected herbal toxicities. Vet Clin North Am Small Anim Pract 2002; 32:367–382.

Ooms TG, Khan SA, Means C. Suspected caffeine and ephedrine toxicosis resulting from ingestion of an herbal supplement containing guarana and ma huang in dogs: 47 cases (1997–1999). JAVMA 2001; 218:225–229.

Author: Charlotte Means, DVM, MLIS, ABVT, ABT
Contributing Editor: Ahna G. Brutlag, DVM

chapter 70

Essential Oils/ Liquid Potpourri

 ## DEFINITION/OVERVIEW

- Essential oils are the volatile, organic constituents of plants that contribute to plant fragrance and taste. They are extracted from plants via distillation or cold pressing.
- Essential oils are utilized in a variety of ways: insecticides, aromatherapies, personal care products (e.g., antibacterials), flavorings, herbal remedies, and liquid potpourri.
- A number of essential oils are not recommended for use on animals due to their potential for toxicity (e.g., pennyroyal oil, bitter almond, wormwood, concentrated melaleuca/tea tree oil).

 ## ETIOLOGY/PATHOPHYSIOLOGY

Mechanisms of Action

- There is limited data with regard to specific pathophysiologic mechanisms for many essential oils.

Pharmacokinetics/Absorption, Distribution, Metabolism, and Excretion

- Essential oils are lipophilic and are well absorbed through mucous membranes and the skin.
- Specific pharmacokinetic data for cats or dogs is generally lacking.
- Because of differences in detoxification pathways, some essential oil constituents are more toxic to cats than dogs (e.g., oil of wintergreen which, when hydrolyzed, releases methylsalicylate).
- Pulegone, the main constituent in pennyroyal oil, is bioactivated to a hepatotoxic metabolite called menthofuran.

Toxicity

- Toxicity varies considerably (reported LD_{50}s range from 1.90 g/kg for melaleuca/tea tree oil to 0.4 g/kg for pennyroyal oil).

- Toxicity data specific to cats and dogs is limited; most data are derived from laboratory animal studies.
- Liquid potpourri also contains cationic detergents, which can cause some of the reported clinical signs. Small ingestions (2–3 licks) and dermal exposures may result in corrosive injury.

Systems Affected

- Affected systems vary depending on the specific essential oil.
  - Pennyroyal oil—hepatobiliary
  - Citrus oil—gastrointestinal, musculoskeletal, nervous
  - Oil of wintergreen—gastrointestinal, hemic, hepatobiliary, respiratory
  - Melaleuca oil—nervous, musculoskeletal
- Many essential oils and cationic detergents in liquid potpourri are irritating (and potentially corrosive) to the skin and mucous membranes.

 # SIGNALMENT/HISTORY

Risk Factors

- Cats are more severely affected by liquid potpourri than dogs.
- Cats more likely to be exposed to liquid potpourri due to the placement of containers on countertops or tables.
- Animals with underlying liver disease may be more severely affected.

Historical Findings

- History of use on or in animals (especially for external parasite control)
- Access to essential oils or products containing essential oils (e.g., liquid potpourri)
- Discovery of spilled essential oils or disturbed liquid potpourri simmer pots
- Characteristic smell on hair coat, skin, breath, or in vomitus

Location and Circumstances of Poisoning

- Most typically in the household (e.g., liquid potpourri simmer pots or spills)
- Following direct application to skin or mucous membranes (e.g., using melaleuca/tea tree oil for external parasite control)

Interaction with Drugs, Nutrients, or Environment

- Limited data are available.
- Essential oils contain high concentrations of terpenes, which are metabolized by the liver. Thus, the coingestion of other chemicals undergoing significant hepatic metabolism can potentially cause interactions.

CLINICAL FEATURES

- Clinical features are variable depending on the essential oil.
  - Pennyroyal oil—dog (and presumably other species as well): acute hepatic failure
  - Citrus oil—cat: hypersalivation, muscle tremors, ataxia, lateral recumbency, coma, death
  - Melaleuca oil—dog: hind limb paralysis, ataxia, depression. Cat: hypothermia, ataxia, dehydration, nervousness, trembling, coma
  - Liquid potpourri—cat and dog: gastrointestinal, dermal, and mucosal irritation or caustic injury; CNS depression; ocular exposure can cause mild to severe corneal injury
    - Ingestion of cationic detergents (occasionally found in potpourri) can cause systemic effects such as emesis, dyspnea secondary to pulmonary edema, hypotension, metabolic acidosis, and CNS depression.

 DIFFERENTIAL DIAGNOSIS

- Pennyroyal oil—hepatotoxins such as microcystins, amanitins, aflatoxins, phenolic compounds (cats), acetaminophen, cycads, acute or chronic copper intoxication. Also, idiosyncratic drug reactions, leptospirosis, infectious canine hepatitis, toxoplasmosis, rickettsial disease, acute necrotizing pancreatitis
- Citrus oil—CNS-depressant drug overdose, hypoglycemia, hypotension, ethylene glycol, head trauma, and many etiologies associated with trembling, stupor, or coma
- Melaleuca/tea tree oil—CNS-depressant drug overdose, hypoglycemia, hypotension, ethylene glycol, head trauma, and many etiologies associated with trembling, stupor, or coma
- Liquid potpourri—many etiologies associated with gastrointestinal upset, other acid or alkaline corrosives, ethylene glycol, paraquat, and digoxin intoxications

 DIAGNOSTICS

- Pennyroyal oil—serum ALT, AST, ALP, CK, total bilirubin, coagulation profile, abdominal imaging, liver needle biopsy
- Liquid potpourri—Endoscopy will assist in determining the degree of damage to upper GI tract if exposure to cationic detergent-containing potpourri has occurred.
- Melaleuca/tea tree oil or citrus oils—no specific diagnostics

Pathological Findings

- Limited information is available.

- Pennyroyal oil—severe hepatic necrosis
- Other essential oils or liquid potpourri formulations—dermal, ocular, or mucosal irritation or caustic injury

 # THERAPEUTICS

Detoxification

- Bathe thoroughly if dermal exposure using a mild hand-dishwashing detergent or noninsecticidal pet shampoo.
- Irrigate eyes copiously with tepid tap water or physiologic saline if ocular exposure.
- Oral exposures:
  - For noncaustic exposures, induction of emesis within 1 to 2 hours might be useful followed by administration of activated charcoal.
  - For caustic exposures, dilution with milk or water is recommended. Do not induce emesis.

Appropriate Health Care

- Treatment is largely symptomatic and supportive (and empiric).
- For severe oral irritation or caustic damage, provide adequate hydration via IV fluids.
- If caustic damage:
  - Buprenorphine 0.005–0.03 mg/kg, IM, IV, SQ or PO (transmucosally) q 6–8 hours
  - Sucralfate 0.25–1 g, PO q 8 hours as a slurry, for oral, esophageal, gastric, or duodenal ulcers
  - Corticosteroids such as prednisone, 1–2 mg/kg IV, for one dose. Note, this is controversial. While one dose may be beneficial, there is limited evidence to support this.
- Antiemetics
  - Metoclopramide 1–2 mg/kg/day, IV as a CRI for mild or infrequent emesis
  - Maropitant 1 mg/kg, SQ q 24 hours, not labeled for cats
  - Ondansetron 0.1–0.2 mg/kg, IV q 8–12 hours
- Hepatoprotectants (consider use of one or all):
  - Silymarin (milk thistle):
    - Dose: 20–50 mg/kg PO q 24 hours
    - Silymarin is composed of three flavonoids (silybin, silydianin, and silychristin).
    - Serious adverse effects have not been observed.
  - N-acetylcysteine, loading dose at 140 mg/kg IV or PO; if using the oral formulation IV, dilute to a 5% solution in saline and administer via 0.2 μm nonpyrogenic filter, followed by 70 mg/kg q 6–12 hours.

▪ Corneal burns should be treated with ophthalmic lubricant ointments and anti-biotics such as gentamicin sulfate or tobramycin 4+ times per day.
▪ Fresh whole blood or fresh frozen plasma if needed for coagulopathies.

Drug(s) and Antidotes of Choice

▪ No antidotes are available for any essential oil or cationic detergent-containing liquid potpourri. See Appropriate Health Care.

Alternative Drugs

▪ S-adenosyl-methionine (SAM-e), 18–20 mg/kg PO q 24 hours. Consider loading at 40 mg/kg PO q 24 for the first 2–4 days of treatment.

Precautions/Interactions

▪ If significant liver damage is present, use drugs metabolized by the liver cautiously.

Nursing Care

▪ IV fluids to maintain hydration and tissue perfusion
▪ Maintain body temperature since hypothermia is reported with some essential oils.
▪ Provide pain control if caustic damage

Follow-Up

▪ If hepatic damage, monitor liver function every 2 to 3 days until improvement.

Diet

▪ Feed a soft or easily digestible diet if there is GI irritation or caustic damage.

Surgical Considerations

▪ For severe oral irritation or caustic damage, a gastrotomy tube might be necessary to provide adequate nutrition.
▪ For severe ocular exposure and corneal damage, conjunctival flaps might be warranted.

Prevention

▪ Owner should be educated about the risks associated with specific essential oils or use of liquid potpourri.
▪ Educate owners about the dangers of using concentrated melaleuca/tea tree oil for external parasite control.

COMMENTS

Patient Monitoring

- Pennyroyal oil—monitoring of hepatic function
- Caustic damage due to cationic detergent exposure—follow-up endoscopy to assess healing or residual damage (strictures due to scar tissue)

Possible Complications

- Pennyroyal oil—hypoglycemia, DIC, hepatic encephalopathy, chronic hepatic insufficiency
- Liquid potpourri—scarring and stricture formation if significant caustic damage to upper GI tract

Expected Course and Prognosis

- Variable depending on specific exposure
  - Pennyroyal oil—guarded to poor
  - Melaleuca/tea tree oil—good to guarded
  - Others—good to guarded

Abbreviations

ALP = alkaline phosphatase
ALT = alanine aminotransferase
AST = aspartate aminotransferase
CK = creatine kinase
CNS = central nervous system
CRI = constant rate infusion
IM = intramuscular
IV = intravenous
DIC = disseminated intravascular coagulation
LD = lethal dose
PO = per os (by mouth)
q   = every
SQ = subcutaneous

See Also

Phenols/Pine Oils
Soaps, Detergents, Fabric Softeners, Enzymatic Cleaners, and Deodorizers
Tea Tree Oil/Melaleuca Oil

Suggested Reading

Bischoff K, Guale F. Australian tea tree (*Melaleuca alternifolia*) oil poisoning in three purebred cats. J Vet Diagn Invest 1998; 10:208–210.

Hooser SB, Beasley VR, Everitt JI. Effects of an insecticidal dip containing D-limonene in the cat. J Am Vet Med Assoc 1986; 189:905–908.

Richardson JA. Potpourri hazards in cats. Available at http://www.aspcapro.org/animal-poison-control/documents/zh-toxbrief_1299.pdf. Accessed on September 30, 2009.

Sudekum M, Poppenga RH, Raju N, et al. Pennyroyal oil toxicosis in a dog. J Am Vet Med Assoc 1992; 200:817–818.

Villar D, Knight MJ, Hansen SR, et al. Toxicity of melaleuca oil and related essential oils applied topically on dogs and cats. Vet Hum Toxicol 1994; 36:139–142.

Author: Robert H. Poppenga, DVM, PhD, DABVT
Consulting Editor: Ahna G. Brutlag, DVM

chapter 71

Tree Oil/Melaleuca Oil

DEFINITION/OVERVIEW

- An essential oil produced from the Australian tea tree, *Melaleuca alternifolia*
- Tea tree oil is also known as melaleuca oil.
- It has known antibacterial and antifungal properties, and possible antipruritic and anti-inflammatory properties also.
- Found in gels and body lotions, shampoos, conditioners, toothpastes, balms, insect repellants, and other household cleaning products ranging from <1% to 100% oil
  - Marketed for use on dogs, cats, ferrets, and horses
- Toxicosis commonly results when 100% oil is applied as an external parasite repellant.
  - As little as 7 drops of 100% oil have caused clinical toxicity.
  - Toxicosis generally produces CNS dysfunction, muscle tremors, and hypothermia. May also result in hepatic injury.

ETIOLOGY/PATHOPHYSIOLOGY

- Toxicosis results from dermal application or ingestion.
- The prevalence of toxicosis may increase as pet owners' interest in "natural" therapies grows.
- The resulting toxicosis is similar to that of other essential oils, such as pine oil, eucalyptus, and d-limonene.
- Composed of 50%–60% terpenes, 6%–8% cineole, and other alcohols
- Terpinen-4-ol is the main antimicrobial and antifungal agent.
- Cineole produces irritation of mucous membranes and skin.

Mechanism of Action

- Exact mechanism of action is unknown; it is presumed to be similar to turpentine and other essential oils.

Pharmacokinetics/Absorption, Distribution, Metabolism, and Excretion

- Dermal and GI absorption is rapid due to its highly lipophilic nature.

- Terpene metabolism is largely hepatic.
- Phase I and phase II biotranformation via cytochrome P-450 enzymes
- Conjugated to glycine or glucuronide in the liver
- Undergoes enterohepatic recirculation
- Urinary excretion of metabolites takes 2–3 days; small amount via fecal elimination

Toxicity

- Exact toxic doses are not established.
- Oral LD_{50} (various species) = 1.9–5 g/kg or 1.9–2.6 mL/kg.
- Toxicosis is most often seen with direct application of 100% oil. Products with low concentrations (e.g., shampoos, face/body washes, toothpastes) are generally not considered toxic.
- Clinical toxicosis occurred following the application of 7–8 drops of 100% oil to the skin of a dog.
- Applications of approximately 10–20 mLs of 100% oil have resulted in toxicosis and death in both cats and dogs.

Systems Affected

- Nervous—target system of toxicity resulting in CNS depression/coma (similar to other terpenes)
- Hepatobiliary—elevated liver enzymes secondary to induction of microsomal P-450
- Skin—possible contact irritation, especially of the mucous membranes
- Musculoskeletal—generalized or rear limb weakness from a possible direct effect of toxic metabolites
- Cardiovascular—peripheral vasodilation following all routes of absorption
- Respiratory—primary or secondary effects due to CNS depression

 # SIGNALMENT/HISTORY

- There are no reported breed, sex, or age predilections.
- Cats may be more sensitive due to altered glucuronidation metabolism.

Risk Factors

- Animals with underlying CNS or hepatic disease may exhibit more severe clinical signs or develop toxicosis at lower doses.

Historical Findings

- Well-intentioned but misinformed owners may admit to administering tea tree oil directly to the pet.

- There may be a characteristic and strong odor (minty) associated with the pet.
- Oily/greasy fur on the neck/back from topical application
- Owners may report CNS depression, unresponsiveness, difficulty or inability to walk, shaking, or tremoring.
- Witnessed ingestions/discovery of chewed tea tree oil containers

Location and Circumstances of Poisoning

- Well-intentioned but misinformed owners use concentrated oil to treat external parasites.
- Given the heightened interest in "natural remedies," the incidence of misuse may increase.

 # CLINICAL FEATURES

- Onset of clinical signs is 1–2 hours after application (up to 8 hours).
- Signs slowly resolve over 2–4 days. Mild cases may resolve within hours.
- The most common clinical signs are mild to moderate hypothermia, weakness, CNS depression, ataxia, and generalized muscle tremors.
- Less common signs include skin/mucus membrane irritation, bradypnea, bradycardia, hypotension secondary to shock or CNS depression, unresponsive pupils, paralysis, and coma.

 # DIFFERENTIAL DIAGNOSIS

- Cardiovascular—shock, primary cardiac disease, other toxins (e.g., narcotics, benzodiazepine overdose)
- Neuromuscular—focal or diffuse primary CNS disease (e.g., neoplasia, distemper, other infectious disease), ethylene glycol, hypocalcemia, hepatic or uremic encephalopathy, IVDD, FCE, other neurotoxins
- Respiratory—primary respiratory disease (e.g., allergic and parasitic airway disease, fungal or bacterial pneumonia), congestive heart failure, pain, sedative/narcotic overdose
- Integument—Drug eruption/reaction, sunburn, thermal burn, vasculitis, contact dermatitis, pyoderma, insect/arthropod bite, parasitic, or other primary skin disease may be suspected based on location of lesion

 # DIAGNOSTICS

- Confirmation of terpinen-4-ol in urine by GC-MS (levels will decrease with IV fluid therapy, so pretreatment samples should be obtained)
- Chemistry profile—possible increase in AST and ALT (only reported in cats)

THERAPEUTICS

Detoxification

- Bathe with liquid dishwashing detergent to remove excess oil and reduce dermal absorption.
- Given the risk of oil aspiration, the induction of emesis is controversial. Induce emesis only if asymptomatic and the ingestion was within 15–30 minutes. Due to rapid GI absorption, emesis is unlikely to prevent toxicosis.
- Repeated doses of activated charcoal (PO q 4–6 hours over 24 hours) due to enterohepatic recirculation
- If mucous membrane/oral irritation is present, consider flushing the oral cavity.

Appropriate Health Care

- Supportive treatments:
  - IV fluid therapy to maintain hydration and tissue perfusion. The use of colloid therapy (e.g., Hetastarch) and vasopressors (e.g., dopamine 2–10 µg/kg/min IV CRI) may be necessary for persistent hypotension.
  - Body temperature regulation and heat support PRN, as hypothermia is common.
  - Atropine, 0.02–0.04 mg/kg IV, IM, or SQ as needed, for severe bradycardia.
  - Other supportive measures are largely dependent upon the CNS status of the patient (see Nursing Care).
  - With severe CNS depression, intubation and mechanical ventilation may be needed.

Drug(s) and Antidotes of Choice

- No antidote available
- Hepatoprotectants if indicated based on lab results (e.g., SAMe, loading dose 40 mg/kg q 24 hours × 2–4 days, maintenance dose 18–20 mg/kg PO q 24 hours × 2–3 weeks).

Precautions/Interactions

- Do not administer oral medications/activated charcoal to animals with CNS depression unless the airway is protected.

Nursing Care

- Monitor during use of warming therapies to prevent hyperthermia or burns.
- If severe CNS signs:
  - Monitor TPR every 5–15 minutes until stable.
  - Rotate body position to prevent atelectasis or thermal burns.
  - Monitor blood pressure closely until stable.

Follow-up

- With mild signs and no liver enzyme elevation, follow-up is generally not necessary (see Patient Monitoring).

Diet

- Typically, no changes are needed.
- With severe CNS depression, withhold feeding until stable.

Activity

- Restrict until neurological signs are minor or resolved.

Public Health

- Owners should be aware that concentrated tea tree oil is toxic to humans if ingested. Severe toxicosis has also been reported in children and adults.

 COMMENTS

- Specific and thorough history and PE are of utmost importance.

Client Education

- Provide appropriate client education regarding the use of herbal or "natural" remedies.
- Urge clients to consult with a veterinarian prior to use of any alternative therapies.
- Appropriate dilutions of tea tree oil can be used, but clients should consult with veterinarian prior to use; the use of 100% oil is never recommended.

Patient Monitoring

- Daily renal values should be evaluated while hospitalized.
- Hepatic values may not normalize immediately, and appropriate short-term monitoring is needed.
  - Recheck liver enzymes q 5–7 days until clinical signs and liver enzymes return to normal.
  - PRN monitoring of vital parameters until stabilized, then 3–4 times daily.

Prevention/Avoidance

- Veterinary consultation prior to administering alternative/home therapies (see Client Education)

Possible Complications

■ Severe and unresponsive CNS depression leading to bradycardia, hypoperfusion, and coma.

Expected Course and Prognosis

■ Good with appropriate treatment and no underlying health problems

Abbreviations

ALT   = alanine aminotransferase
AST   = aspartate aminotransferase
CNS   = central nervous system
CRI   = continuous rate infusion
FCE   = fibrocartilaginous emboli
GC-MS = gas chromatography–mass spectrometry
GI   = gastrointestinal
IM   = intramuscular
IV   = intravenous
IVDD   = intervertebral disc disease
LD   = lethal dose
PE   = physical exam
PO   = *per os* (by mouth)
PRN   = *pro re nata* (as needed)
SAMe   = s-adenosyl-methionine
SQ   = subcutaneous
TPR   = temperature, pulse, respiration

See Also

Essential Oils/Liquid Potpourri
Phenols/Pine Oils

Suggested Reading

Bischoff K, Fessessvork G. Australian tea tree (*Melaleuca alternifolia*) oil poisoning in three purebred cats. J Vet Diag Invest 1998; 10:208–210.
Carson CF, Riley TV. Toxicity of the essential oil of *Melaleuca alternifolia* or tea tree oil. Clin Toxicol 1995; 33:193–194.
Poppenga RH. Flora and fauna: Hazardous biotoxins for pets. CVC Proceedings Aug 1, 2008. Available at http://veterinarycalendar.dvm360.com/avhc/article/articleDetail.jsp?id=571086&sk=&date=&%0A%09%09%09&pageID=4. Accessed July 18, 2010.
Villar D et al. Toxicity of melaleuca oil and related essential oils applied topically on dogs and cats. Vet Hum Toxicol 1994; 36:139–142.

Wismer T. Toxicity of household products. International Veterinary Emergency and Critical Care Symposium 2006. Available at http://www.vin.com/Members/Proceedings/Proceedings.plx? CID=iveccs2006&PID=pr14142&O=VIN. Accessed July 30, 2009.

Authors: Seth L. Cohen, DVM; Ahna G. Brutlag, DVM
Consulting Editors: Ahna G. Brutlag, DVM; Justine A. Lee, DVM, DACVECC

Home Care and Recreational Products

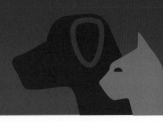

chapter 72

Acids

DEFINITION/OVERVIEW

- Acids have a pH <7, are proton donors, and have a sour taste.
- Tissue injury from acids depends on the pH, specific acid, concentration, volume, and duration of tissue contact time.
- Common household products containing acids:
  - Automobile battery fluid—sulfuric acid (25%–30%)
  - Drain cleaners—sulfuric acid (95%–99%)
  - Engraver's acid—nitric acid (63%)
  - Hair wave neutralizers—acetic acid (6%–40%)
  - Lemon juice—citric acid (2%–8%)
  - Metal cleaners and antirust compounds—phosphoric acid (5%–90%), oxalic acid (1%), hydrochloric acid (5%–25%), sulfamic acid (5%–10%), sulfuric acid (10%–20%), chromic acid (5%–20%)
  - Toilet bowl cleaners—hydrochloric acid (9%–25%), oxalic acid (2%), sodium bisulfate forms sulfuric acid upon contact with water (70%–100%), sulfuric acid (up to 80%)
  - Vinegar—acetic acid (4%–6%)
- Exposure to weak (pH 2–4) or dilute acids may cause mild tissue irritation.
- Exposure to strong (pH <2) or concentrated acids may cause corrosive injury (see Toxicology).
  - Products likely to cause corrosive injury include toilet bowl and drain cleaners, calcium/rust/lime-removing compounds, swimming pool sanitizers, automotive batteries, and gun barrel cleaners.
  - Many U.S. household products containing corrosive agents will display the signal word *Danger* clearly on the packaging.
- Treatment following exposure to acids is focused on the prevention/management of caustic injury, including analgesia and nutritional support.
- Serious complications include severe caustic injury followed by systemic infection, stricture formation, GIT perforation, and septic peritonitis.

ETIOLOGY/PATHOPHYSIOLOGY

- Exposure in animals generally occurs following accidental ingestion or dermal contact.

- Small ingestions/tastes of corrosive acids are unlikely to result in severe tissue damage.
- Strong acids have a sour/bitter taste and typically cause immediate pain upon tissue contact. Thus, large ingestions of strong acids are very rare.

Mechanism of Action

- Acids cause rapid, surface protein coagulation (leading to coagulation necrosis) followed by the formation of a thick eschar.
- Theoretically, the eschar may limit tissue penetration and damage.
- Significant tissue damage from caustic injury may result in stricture formation.

Pharmacokinetics/Absorption, Distribution, Metabolism, and Excretion

- Systemic absorption of acids is not typically a concern (except hydrofluoric acid).
- Rarely, acidemia may result from systemic absorption through injured tissue.
- Ions such as hydrogen, chloride (hydrochloric acid), or sulfate (sulfuric acid), if systemically absorbed, are well distributed and may disrupt normal metabolic function.

Toxicity

- Tissue damage of most acids is directly related to pH and concentration.
  - pH 2–4: Agents cause mild to moderate tissue irritation.
  - pH <2: Agents are extremely corrosive.
- Specific acids
  - Weak irritants
    - Acetic acid 5%–10%
    - Aluminum sulfate 5%–20%
    - Hydrochloric acid <5%
    - Phosphoric acid 15%–35%
  - Strong irritants
    - Acetic acid 10%–50%
    - Aluminum sulfate 20%
    - Glycolic acid 0.5%–10%
    - Hydrochloric acid 5%–10%
    - Oxalic acid <10%
    - Phosphoric acid 35%–60%
    - Sulfuric acid <10%
  - Corrosive
    - Acetic acid >50%
    - Aluminum sulfate >20%

☐ Glycolic acid >10%
☐ Hydrochloric acid >10%
☐ Oxalic acid >10%
☐ Phosphoric acid >60%
☐ Sulfamic acid >10%
☐ Sulfuric acid >10%

Systems Affected

- Organs having direct contact with acid (GIT, skin, eyes, and lungs) are most at risk.
- Gastrointestinal—ingestion causes mild tissue irritation to significant ulceration of the oral cavity, esophagus, stomach, and duodenum. The GIT is most often involved in life-threatening exposures.
- Skin—mild irritation to severe caustic injury of the superficial layers of the skin followed by eschar
- Ophthalmic—mild irritation to severe caustic injury of the cornea and conjunctiva with ocular exposure
- Respiratory—inhalation of powdered acids/fumes may cause irritation (common) or pulmonary edema, shock, or caustic injury (very rare).
- Hemic/lymphatic/immune—Sepsis may result following severe caustic injury.

 # SIGNALMENT/HISTORY

- There are no species, breed, or sex predilections.
- Animals with known dietary indiscretion may be at higher risk of accidental exposure.

Risk Factors

- Animals with preexisting dermal or upper GI disease may have an increased risk of developing tissue injury.

Historical Findings

- Witnessed ingestion or discovery of chewed acid-containing cleaners or products.
- If acid is ingested, owners may report excessive salivation, vomiting, oral lesions, stridor, and abnormal behavior (due to pain) such as pawing at the mouth or hiding, refusal of food/water, and vocalization.
- If animal is dermally exposed, owners may report red, irritated skin, excessive licking at the skin, "burned" or damaged hair, or open sores.

Location and Circumstances of Poisoning

■ Often in areas where acids are kept: bathroom, utility/hobby room, garage, workshop, etc.

 # CLINICAL FEATURES

■ Evidence of irritation or corrosive injury to the exposed tissues is often immediate.
■ In cases of severe caustic injury, ulcerations may persist for weeks to months.
■ Oral cavity—corrosive lesions typically progress from white/grey to black and wrinkled (eschar).
  • Up to 37% of patients with esophageal damage will NOT exhibit oral lesions (human beings).
■ Upper GI—ptyalism, dysphagia, vomiting/regurgitation, hematemesis, abdominal pain
■ Dermal—hyperemia, irritated or abraded skin, damaged hair
■ Ocular—conjunctivitis, blepharospasm, ± grossly visible corneal damage
■ Respiratory—stridor (laryngeal/epiglottic edema), tachypnea (pain), coughing

 # DIFFERENTIAL DIAGNOSIS

■ Toxicities
  • Tissue injury caused by alkalis or neutral caustic agents (e.g., phenol)
  • Oral injury secondary to chewing on electrical cords
  • GI erosion/ulceration secondary to NSAID or aspirin toxicity
■ Primary or secondary esophageal or GI disease resulting in esophagitis, esophageal stricture, gastric ulceration, or gastric outflow obstruction

 # DIAGNOSTICS

■ Endoscopy—cautious examination of the esophagus, stomach (especially pyloric region), and duodenum to determine the extent and severity of injury
  • Ideally, use a flexible endoscope with minimal insufflation.
  • Endoscopy is recommended in all cases involving the following:
    ▫ The ingestion of large volumes of acid
    ▫ The ingestion of a corrosive agent
    ▫ The ingestion of agents with a pH <4
    ▫ If clinical signs have not resolved in <12–24 hours
■ CBC or PCV/TS—blood loss anemia, WBC changes with GI perforation and sepsis
■ Chemistry panel—Monitor electrolytes, BUN, and creatinine in cases of caustic injury.

- Acid/base—monitor for acidemia in cases of severe caustic injury/large ingestions.
- Abdominocentesis—increased WBCs, protein, and fibrinogen levels, bacteria, and amorphous cellular debris are consistent with GI perforation and a septic abdomen.
- Radiographs of the neck, thorax, and abdomen for evidence of perforation
- Positive contrast barium esophagogram to look for strictures/evaluate motility
- Abdominal ultrasound—complex free fluid, evidence of perforation
- Fluoroscopy to evaluate esophageal motility/strictures

Pathological Findings

- Gross—evidence of partial- or full-thickness caustic injury (involving the mucosal, serosal, submucosal, and muscular layers)
- Histopathologic findings will be consistent with coagulation necrosis, including evidence of edema, acute inflammation (polymorphonuclear leukocyte infiltrate), and granulation tissue. Damage may extend through multiple tissue layers.

 # THERAPEUTICS

- Initial management following caustic ingestions involves rapidly evaluating the airway and obtaining vital signs.
- Once stable, treatment focuses on the prevention or management of caustic injury, including gastroprotection, analgesia, and nutritional supplementation.

Detoxification

- Flush exposed skin, eyes, or oral membranes with large volumes of water or saline for 20 minutes.
- Decontamination of the GIT is very limited (see Precautions/Interactions).
  - The induction of emesis is contraindicated.
  - Activated charcoal is contraindicated.
  - Neutralizing ingested acids with alkalis is not recommended.
  - Dilution with water can be attempted but has not been proven effective.

Appropriate Health Care

- Use injectable instead of oral drug formulations in the event of caustic injury.
- Manage caustic injury.
  - Gastroprotection (treat for weeks to months, depending on extent of injury)
    - Sucralfate liquid (0.25–1.0 g PO q 6–8 hours)
    - H_2 blockers (e.g., famotidine 0.5 mg/kg PO, IV, SQ q 12 hours)
    - Proton-pump inhibitors (e.g., omeprazole 0.7–1.4 mg/kg, PO q 12–24 hours)

- IV fluids—use a balanced electrolyte crystalloid to maintain euvolemia, hydration, and renal perfusion.
- Analgesia—powerful analgesics may be warranted.
- Nutritional support—patients with caustic injury become hypercatabolic and require substantial nutritional support, including total parenteral nutrition, gastrostomy, or jejunostomy. See Diet and Surgical Considerations.
- Corticosteroids—use remains controversial.
  - Unlikely to benefit in cases of minor injury
  - If significant injury and stricture formation is very likely, anti-inflammatory doses may be of slight benefit.
  - Must be accompanied by antibiotics due to the increased risk of infection
- Antibiotics—prophylactic use remains controversial.
  - In cases of known infection, parenteral use is advised.
  - Broad-spectrum coverage is recommended (e.g., enrofloxacin with ampicillin).
- If hypoproteinemia results, artificial colloid therapy (e.g., Hetastarch at 1–2 mL/kg/hr) should be considered to maintain colloid osmotic pressure.
- Blood transfusion with pRBCs as needed to maintain PCV $\geq$15%–20% if gastric hemorrhage noted.
- In cases of shock/loss of consciousness (very rare), intubation with mechanical ventilation if necessary

Drug(s) and Antidotes of Choice

- No antidote exists.
- Sucralfate liquid, 0.25–1 g PO immediately upon ingestion, may be beneficial.
- See Appropriate Health Care.

Precautions/Interactions

- Neutralization of the exposed tissue by adding an alkali is not recommended as exothermic reactions may result (thermal burns).
- The induction of emesis or gastric lavage is contraindicated due to the increased risk of aspiration, reexposure injury, and GIT perforation.
- Activated charcoal does not bind to caustic agents and is contraindicated.
- The use of oral NSAIDs is not typically recommended due to the compromised GIT.

Follow-up

- Esophageal and gastric ulcerations may persist for weeks to months.
- Esophageal strictures may not form until weeks to months after the initial injury.

Diet

- Depending on the extent and severity of injury, a soft or liquid diet or parenteral nutrition may be needed. See Surgical Considerations.

Surgical Considerations

- A feeding tube placed distal to GIT ulcerations may be needed to maintain nutritional support (e.g., gastrostomy or jejunostomy tubes).
- Strictures in the GIT may necessitate surgical attention (bougienage, balloon dilation, resection, etc.).

 COMMENTS

Client Education

- Inform clients that esophageal strictures may form until weeks to months after the initial injury.
- Alert clients to common household items that may cause caustic injury (toilet bowl, metal, drain, and metal cleaners; calcium/lime/rust removers; and pool sanitizers).

Prevention/Avoidance

- Potentially caustic cleaners and products should be stored in original containers and kept in pet/child-proof areas.

Possible Complications

- Esophageal strictures (may form weeks to months after the initial injury)
- Gastric stricture, pyloric stenosis, or GIT perforations with septic peritonitis
- Long-term esophageal dysmotility
- Esophageal carcinomas (humans)

Expected Course and Prognosis

- Most acid ingestions will be small and are unlikely to result in caustic injury. In such cases, the prognosis is excellent.
- In cases involving caustic injury, the prognosis is dependent on the extent and severity of injury. Prognosis is grave in cases of severe injury and no medical management and fair in cases of severe injury with aggressive management.

Abbreviations

BUN   = blood urea nitrogen
CBC   = complete blood count

GI   = gastrointestinal
GIT   = gastrointestinal tract
IV   = intravenous
NSAID = nonsteroidal anti-inflammatory drug
PCV   = packed cell volume
PO   = *per os* (by mouth)
pRBC = packed red blood cells
q   = every
SQ   = subcutaneous
TS   = total solids
WBC   = white blood cell

See Also

Alkalis
Aspirin
Batteries
Essential Oils/Liquid Potpourri
Hydrofluoric Acid
Phenols/Pine Oils
Soaps, Detergents, Fabric Softeners, Enzymatic Cleaners, and Deodorizers

Suggested Reading

Acids. In: POISINDEX® System [Internet database]. Greenwood Village, CO: Thompson Healthcare. Updated periodically. Available at: http://www.thomsonhc.com/hcs/librarian/ND_T/HCS/ND_CPR/ToxicSubstanceLists/ND_PR/Toxicology/CS/D711AC/DUPLICATIONSHIELDSYNC/FCFE8C/ND_PG/PRIH/ND_B/HCS/ND_P/Toxicology/PFActionId/hcs.common.RetrieveDocumentCommon/DocId/115/ContentSetId/51#TopOfPage. Accessed January 23, 2010.

Brutlag, AG. Chemical toxicities. In: Ettinger SJ, Feldman EC, eds. Textbook of Veterinary Internal Medicine, 7th ed. St. Louis: Elsevier, 2010; pp. 571–575.

Oehme FW, Kore AW. Miscellaneous indoor toxicants. In: Peterson ME, Talcott PA, eds. Small Animal Toxicology, 2nd ed. St. Louis: Elsevier, 2006; pp. 223–243.

Rella JG, Hoffman RS. Acids and bases. In: Brent J, Wallace KL, Burkhart KK, et al., eds. Critical Care Toxicology: Diagnosis and Management of the Critically Poisoned Patient. Philadelphia: Mosby, 2005; 1035–1043.

Tohda G, Sugawa C, Gayer C, et al. Clinical evaluation and management of caustic injury in the upper gastrointestinal tract in 95 adult patients in an urban medical center. Surg Endosc 2008; 22:1119–1125.

Author: Ahna G. Brutlag, DVM
Consulting Editor: Lynn R. Hovda, RPH, DVM, MS, DACVIM

chapter 73

Alkalis

DEFINITION/OVERVIEW

- Alkaline substances (also called bases) have a pH >7, produce hydroxide ions upon contact with water, and are proton acceptors.
- Tissue injury from alkaline agents depends on the pH, specific agent, concentration, volume, and duration of contact.
  - Exposure to weak (pH 10–11) or dilute alkalis may cause mild tissue irritation.
  - Exposure to strong (pH greater than 11–12) or concentrated alkalis may cause corrosive injury (see Toxicology).
  - Many U.S. household products containing corrosive agents will display the signal word *Danger* clearly on the packaging.
- The most common household alkaline agent is regular-strength chlorine bleach.
  - Sodium hypochlorite, 4–6%; typical pH = 11–12
  - Regular bleach is typically irritating to tissues, not corrosive (see Toxicology).
- Common household products containing potential alkaline corrosives:
  - Automatic dishwasher detergents
  - Batteries (dry cell such as AA, C, D)
  - Bleach—non-chlorine ("Color Safe," "Oxy," and "Ultra") formulations may be corrosive in large amounts or with prolonged tissue contact. They contain sodium percarbonate, sodium perborate, sodium carbonate, and sodium metasilicate.
  - Cement—when mixed with water, becomes corrosive (60% to 65% calcium oxide)
  - Dairy and industrial pipeline cleaners
  - Drain cleaners
  - Hair relaxers
  - Lye (sodium or potassium hydroxide)
  - Oven cleaners
- Treatment following exposure to alkaline agents is focused on the prevention/management of caustic injury, including analgesia and nutritional support.
- Serious complications include severe caustic injury followed by systemic infection, stricture formation, GIT perforation, and septic peritonitis.

ETIOLOGY/PATHOPHYSIOLOGY

- Exposure in animals generally occurs from accidental ingestion or dermal contact.
- Small ingestions/tastes of alkaline corrosives are unlikely to result in severe tissue damage.
- Alkaline products typically have little odor or taste; thus, larger ingestions may occur. Bittering agents may be added to deter ingestion.
- Pain, though common, is not always evident immediately upon contact.

Mechanism of Action

- Alkaline corrosives cause liquefaction necrosis with resulting edema and inflammation.
- They rapidly penetrate deeply into tissues, often involving multiple tissue layers (transmural necrosis).
- Fat and proteins become saponified; thrombosis occurs in arterioles and venules.
- Tissues release heat and gases upon contact with caustic alkalis.
- Significant tissue damage from caustic injury may result in stricture formation.

Pharmacokinetics/Absorption, Distribution, Metabolism, and Excretion

- Systemic absorption of alkalis is not typically concerning, and systemic alkalosis is not expected.
  - Exception: Large ingestions of chlorine bleach may cause hyperchloremic acidosis and hypernatremia.

Toxicology

- Corrosive injury occurs rapidly, within seconds of tissue contact.
- Exposures to large volumes and high concentrations cause more severe injury.
- For most alkaline agents, serious burns are less likely if the pH <11.5–12.
- Experimental cat model: 1 mL of 30% sodium hydroxide (lye) = transesophageal necrosis.
- Toxicity of household bleach (sodium hypochlorite, 4%–6%)
  - Typical pH = 11–12; corrosive if pH >12–12.5
  - Expect corrosive injury with ingestions >5 mL/kg or concentrations >10%.
  - When mixed with a strong acid, chlorine gas is released.
  - When mixed with ammonia, chloramine gas is released.
    - Gases irritate the nasal and oral mucosa, respiratory tract, eyes, etc.
    - In significant exposures, the gas may cause corrosive damage to mucosal membranes.

- Toxicity of specific alkaline chemicals
  - Irritants (mild-moderate)
    - Sodium hydroxide <2%
    - Sodium hypochlorite <10%
  - Corrosives
    - Sodium carbonate >15%
    - Sodium hydroxide >2%
    - Sodium hypochlorite >10%
    - Sodium metasilicate >0.5%
    - Sodium silicate >20%–40%
  - Sodium percarbonate, on contact with water, breaks down into hydrogen peroxide and sodium carbonate. Depending on concentration, may irritate or corrode tissue.

Systems Affected

- Organs having direct contact with acid (GIT, skin, eyes, and lungs) are most at risk.
- Gastrointestinal—ingestion causes mild tissue irritation to significant ulceration of the oral cavity, esophagus, stomach, and duodenum. The GIT is most often involved in life-threatening exposures.
- Skin—mild irritation to severe caustic injury of the superficial layers of the skin followed by an eschar.
- Ophthalmic—mild irritation to severe caustic injury of the cornea and conjunctiva with ocular exposure.
- Respiratory—inhalation or aspiration of powdered alkaline agents/gaseous by-products may cause irritation (common) or pulmonary edema, shock, or caustic injury (very rare).
- Hemic/lymphatic/immune—sepsis may result following severe caustic injury.
- Endocrine/metabolic—large ingestions of chlorine bleach may cause hyperchloremic acidosis and hypernatremia.

 SIGNALMENT/HISTORY

- There are no species, breed, or sex predilections.
- Animals with known dietary indiscretion or "chewers" may be at higher risk of accidental exposure.

Risk Factors

- Animals with preexisting dermal, upper GI, or respiratory disease may have an increased risk of developing tissue injury or clinical signs.

Historical Findings

- Witnessed ingestion or discovery of chewed alkaline-containing products
- If an alkaline is ingested, owners may report excessive salivation, vomiting, oral lesions, stridor, and abnormal behavior (due to pain) such as pawing at the mouth or hiding, refusal of food/water, and vocalization.
- If animal is dermally exposed, owners may report red, irritated skin, excessive licking at the skin, "burned" or damaged hair, or open sores.

Location and Circumstances of Poisoning

- Often in areas where alkaline agents are kept: bathroom, utility/hobby room, garage, workshop, etc.

Interactions with Drugs, Nutrients, or Environment

- Chlorine bleach, when mixed with strong acid or ammonia, produces chlorine and chloramines gases, respectively.
  - Gases irritate the nasal and oral mucosa, respiratory tract, eyes, etc.
  - In significant exposures, these gases may cause corrosive damage to mucosal membranes.

 CLINICAL FEATURES

- Evidence of irritation or corrosive injury is often immediate.
- In cases of severe caustic injury, ulcerations may persist for weeks to months.
- Oral cavity—corrosive lesions typically progress from white/grey to black and wrinkled (eschar).
  - Up to 37% of patients with esophageal damage will NOT exhibit oral lesions (human beings).
- GI—ptyalism, dysphagia, vomiting/regurgitation, hematemesis, abdominal pain, diarrhea
- Dermal—hyperemia, irritated or abraded skin, damaged hair
- Ocular—conjunctivitis/edema, blepharospasm, lacrimation, photophobia, corneal edema, ± grossly visible corneal damage
- Respiratory—stridor (laryngeal/epiglottic edema), tachypnea (pain), coughing

 DIFFERENTIAL DIAGNOSIS

- Toxicities
  - Tissue injury caused by acids or neutral caustic agents (e.g., phenols or quaternary ammonium cationic surfactants)
  - Oral injury secondary to chewing on electrical cords
  - GI erosion/ulceration secondary to NSAID or aspirin toxicosis

- Primary or secondary esophageal or GI disease resulting in esophagitis, esophageal stricture, gastric ulceration, or gastric outflow obstruction

DIAGNOSTICS

- Endoscopy—cautious examination of the esophagus, stomach and duodenum to determine the extent and severity of injury
  - Ideally, use a flexible endoscope with minimal insufflation.
  - Endoscopy is recommended in all cases involving the following:
    - □ The ingestion of large volumes of any alkaline agent (>5 mL/kg)
    - □ Ingestion of a corrosive agent
    - □ Ingestion of agents with a pH >11.5
    - □ If clinical signs have not resolved in <12–24 hours
  - Endoscopic evaluation of lesions aids in prediction of stricture formation.
- CBC or PCV/TS—blood loss anemia, WBC changes with GI perforation and sepsis
- Chemistry panel—monitor electrolytes, BUN, and creatinine in cases of caustic injury. Large ingestion of chlorine bleach may cause hyperchloremic acidosis and hypernatremia.
- Acid/base—monitor for acidosis if a large volume of chlorine bleach was ingested.
- Abdominocentesis—increased WBCs, protein and fibrinogen levels, intracellular bacteria, and amorphous cellular debris are consistent with GI perforation and a septic abdomen.
- Radiographs of the neck, thorax, and abdomen for evidence of perforation. Positive contrast barium esophagogram to look for strictures/evaluate motility.
- Abdominal ultrasound—complex free fluid, evidence of perforation
- Fluoroscopy to evaluate esophageal motility/strictures (if available)

Pathological Findings

- Gross—evidence of partial- or full-thickness caustic injury (involving the mucosal, serosal, submucosal, and muscular layers)
- Histopathologic findings will be consistent with liquefaction necrosis, including evidence of edema, acute inflammation, and granulation tissue. Damage may extend through multiple tissue layers.

THERAPEUTICS

- Initial management following caustic ingestions involves rapidly evaluating the airway and obtaining vital signs.
- Once stable, treatment focuses on the prevention or management of caustic injury, including gastroprotection, analgesia, and nutritional supplementation.

Detoxification

- Flush exposed skin, eyes, or oral membranes with large volumes of water or saline for 20 minutes.
- Decontamination of the GIT is very limited (see Precautions/Interactions).
    - The induction of emesis is contraindicated.
    - Activated charcoal is contraindicated.
    - Neutralizing ingested alkaline agents with acids is not recommended.
    - Dilution with water can be attempted but is often ineffective.

Appropriate Health Care

- Use injectable drug formulations (when possible) in the event of caustic injury.
- Manage caustic injury.
    - Gastroprotection (treat for weeks to months, depending on extent of injury)
        - Sucralfate liquid (0.25–1.0 g PO q 6–8 hours) binds to damaged tissue.
        - H_2 blockers (e.g., famotidine 0.5 mg/kg PO, IV, SC q 12 hours)
        - Proton-pump inhibitors (e.g., omeprazole 0.7–1.4 mg/kg, PO q 12–24 hours)
    - IV fluids—use a balanced electrolyte crystalloid to maintain euvolemia, hydration, and renal perfusion.
    - Analgesia—powerful analgesics may be warranted (see Precautions/ Interactions).
    - Nutritional support—patients with caustic injury become hypercatabolic and require substantial nutritional support, including total parenteral nutrition, a gastrostomy, or jejunostomy. See Diet and Surgical Considerations.
    - Corticosteroids—use remains controversial.
        - Unlikely to benefit in cases of minor injury.
        - If significant injury and stricture formation is very likely, anti-inflammatory doses may be of slight benefit.
        - Must be accompanied by antibiotics due to the increased risk of infection.
    - Antibiotics—prophylactic use remains controversial.
        - In cases of known infection, parenteral use is advised.
        - Broad-spectrum coverage is recommended.
    - If hypoproteinemia results, artificial colloid therapy (e.g., Hetastarch at 1–2 mL/kg/hr) should be considered to maintain colloid osmotic pressure.
    - Blood transfusion with pRBCs as needed to maintain PCV ≥15%–20% if gastric hemorrhage is noted.
    - In cases of shock/loss of consciousness (very rare), intubation ± mechanical ventilation if necessary.

Drug(s) and Antidotes of Choice

- No antidote exists.
- See Appropriate Health Care.

Precautions/Interactions

- Neutralization of the exposed tissue by adding an acid is not recommended as exothermic reactions may result (thermal burns).
- The induction of emesis or gastric lavage is contraindicated due to the increased risk of aspiration, reexposure injury, and GIT perforation.
- Activated charcoal does not bind to caustic agents and is contraindicated.
- The use of oral NSAIDs is not typically recommended due to the compromised GIT.

Follow-up

- Esophageal and gastric ulcerations may persist for weeks to months.
- Esophageal strictures may not form until weeks to months after the initial injury.

Diet

- Depending on the extent and severity of injury, a soft or liquid diet or parenteral nutrition may be needed. See Surgical Considerations.

Surgical Considerations

- A feeding tube placed distal to GIT ulcerations may be needed to maintain nutritional support (e.g., gastrostomy or jejunostomy tubes).
- Strictures in the GIT may necessitate surgical attention (bougienage, balloon dilation, resection, etc.).

 COMMENTS

Client Education

- Inform clients that esophageal strictures may form weeks to months after the initial injury.
- Alert clients to common household items that may cause caustic injury (drain and toilet bowl cleaners, dry cell batteries, concentrated bleach, lye, hair relaxers, wet cement).

Prevention/Avoidance

- Caustic cleaners and products should be stored in original containers and kept in pet/child-proof areas.

Possible Complications

- Esophageal strictures (may form weeks to months after the initial injury)
- Gastric stricture, pyloric stenosis, or GIT perforations with septic peritonitis
- Long-term esophageal dysmotility
- Esophageal carcinomas (humans)

Expected Course and Prognosis

- Most ingestions will be small and are unlikely to result in caustic injury. In such cases, the prognosis is excellent.
- In cases involving caustic injury, the prognosis is dependent on the extent and severity of injury. Prognosis is grave in cases of severe injury and no medical management and fair in cases of severe injury with aggressive management.

Abbreviations

CBC   = complete blood count
GI   = gastrointestinal
GIT   = gastrointestinal tract
IV   = intravenous
NSAID = nonsteroidal anti-inflammatory drug
PCV   = packed cell volume
PO   = *per os* (by mouth)
pRBC = packed red blood cells
q   = every
SC   = subcutaneous
TS   = total solids

See Also

Acids
Batteries
Essential Oils/Liquid Potpourri
Hydrofluoric Acid
Phenols/Pine Oils
Soaps, Detergents, Fabric Softeners, Enzymatic Cleaners, and Deodorizers

Suggested Reading

Brutlag AG. Chemical toxicities. In: Ettinger SJ, Feldman EC, eds. Textbook of Veterinary Internal Medicine, 7th ed. St. Louis: Elsevier, 2010; pp. 571–575.
Corrosives: Alkaline. In: POISINDEX® System [Internet database]. Greenwood Village, CO: Thompson Healthcare. Updated periodically. Available at: http://www.thomsonhc.com/hcs/librarian/ND_T/HCS/ND_CPR/ToxicSubstanceLists/ND_PR/Toxicology/CS/DB5F92/DUPLICATIONSHIELDSYNC/C733DE/ND_PG/PRIH/ND_B/HCS/ND_P/Toxicology/

PFActionId/hcs.common.RetrieveDocumentCommon/DocId/11/ContentSetId/51.   Accessed January 23, 2010.

Oehme FW, Kore AW. Miscellaneous indoor toxicants. In: Peterson ME, Talcott PA, eds. Small Animal Toxicology, 2nd ed. St. Louis: Elsevier, 2006; pp. 223–243.

Rella JG, Hoffman RS. Acids and bases. In: Brent J, Wallace KL, Burkhart KK, et al, eds. Critical Care Toxicology: Diagnosis and Management of the Critically Poisoned Patient. Philadelphia: Mosby, 2005; pp. 1035–1043.

Tohda G, Sugawa C, Gayer C, et al. Clinical evaluation and management of caustic injury in the upper gastrointestinal tract in 95 adult patients in an urban medical center. Surg Endosc 2008; 22:1119–1125.

Author: Ahna G. Brutlag, DVM

Consulting Editor: Lynn R. Hovda, RPH, DVM, MS, DACVIM

chapter 74

Batteries

DEFINITION/OVERVIEW

- When the casing of a battery is ruptured, alkaline or acidic material can leak from the battery and ulcerate exposed tissues.
- The design of button- or disc-shaped batteries allows an electric current to be passed to the tissues of the GIT. This current causes necrosis and possible GIT perforation, tracheoesophageal fistulas, fistulization into major vessels, and massive hemorrhage/exsanguination.
- The greatest damage occurs from lithium disc/button batteries. One 3-volt battery can cause esophageal necrosis with 15 minutes of contact.
  - In children, the most serious outcomes and greatest number of deaths have been reported with larger-diameter lithium cell batteries (≥20 mm). Death is often due to exsanguination after fistulization into major vessels (following esophageal entrapment).
- Batteries may also contain the metals lead, mercury, zinc, cobalt, nickel, or cadmium. Heavy metal toxicosis may occur if batteries are retained in the GIT for more than 2–3 days.

ETIOLOGY/PATHOPHYSIOLOGY

Mechanism of Action

- **Lithium disc/button batteries:** Contain no corrosive compounds, but the esophagus becomes increasingly alkalinic on the cathode side and acidic on the anode side as the current passes through the battery. This results in severe tissue damage/possible perforation.
- **Dry cell batteries:**
  - Acid dry cells usually contain ammonium chloride or manganese dioxide. When either component comes in contact with mucosa it causes coagulation necrosis.
  - Alkaline dry cells (the majority of household batteries) contain potassium hydroxide or sodium hydroxide. When the compounds come in contact with tissue, liquefaction necrosis occurs resulting in deeply penetrating ulcers.

Pharmacokinetics/Absorption, Distribution, Metabolism, and Excretion

- **Lithium disc/button batteries:** Significant systemic absorption of lithium rarely occurs occurs. Stomach acid does not significantly alter the battery casing. The battery is passed unchanged in the feces.
- **Dry cell batteries:** The alkaline or acidic component can leak if the casing is ruptured. This may occur before ingestion or within the stomach as the casing is further degraded. As the acid or alkaline contents react with local tissues, the contents become nonreactive and systemic absorption does not typically occur. If the battery remains lodged in the gastrointestinal tract for a prolonged period, the heavy metals in the casing (lead, mercury, zinc, cobalt, cadmium) may cause toxicity.

Systems Affected

- Gastrointestinal—ulcerations in the oral cavity, esophagus, stomach, and small intestine are possible. Ulceration may lead to GIT perforation, secondary peritonitis, and tracheoesophageal fistulas.
- Skin—ulceration and irritation if exposed to battery contents
- Respiratory—stridor from pharyngeal or esophageal ulceration. Dyspnea from obstruction of the airway. Pleuritis, dyspnea, or fever if esophageal perforation occurs and ingesta leaks into pleural cavity. Chemical pneumonitis if corrosive material inhaled.
- Hemic—ulceration of the GIT may lead to fistulization into major vessels, and massive hemorrhage/exsanguination. Intravascular hemolysis may occur secondary to heavy metal toxicosis if batteries are retained in the GIT (see Metallic Toxicants).
- Hepatobiliary—hepatic damage may occur secondary to heavy metal toxicosis if batteries are retained in the GIT (see Metallic Toxicants).
- Nervous—CNS abnormalities may occur secondary to heavy metal toxicosis if batteries are retained in the GIT (see Metallic Toxicants).

 SIGNALMENT/HISTORY

- There are no breed, age or sex predilections.

Risk Factors

- Use of toys or bedding with batteries in them; chewing on remote controls, hearing aids, or other battery operated devices

Historical Findings

- Owner often reports having witnessed the ingestion or finding the partially ingested battery or battery-containing device. With an unwitnessed ingestion, owners may report hypersalivation, pawing at the mouth, anorexia, or vomiting. Signs typically begin 2–12 hours after ingestion.

Location and Circumstances of Poisoning

- Ingestion usually occurs within the home. The holiday season has been anecdotally associated with a greater number of ingestions (battery-containing gifts).

 # CLINICAL FEATURES

- Physical examination should begin with a good evaluation of the oral cavity. Look for erythema and ulceration of the gums, tongue, and laryngeal/pharyngeal area. Teeth may be discolored (black or grey) from exposure to battery contents.
- Signs of nausea such as hypersalivation and frequent swallowing
- Abdominal palpation may reveal pain, free abdominal fluid, or distention.
- Other clinical signs (e.g., evidence of hemolysis) may develop if sufficient time has passed for heavy metal toxicosis to develop (see Metallic Toxicants).
- In children, serious outcomes and death from tracheoesophageal fistulas, fistulization into major vessels, and massive hemorrhage/exsanguination have been reported.

 # DIFFERENTIAL DIAGNOSIS

- There are multiple other conditions that can cause acute gastroenteritis with ulceration and possible perforation. NSAID toxicity, foreign body ingestion, pancreatitis, corrosive chemical ingestion, and endotoxemia ("garbage gut") can all present with very similar clinical signs.

 # DIAGNOSTICS

- Radiograph the GIT to look for a retained battery. This should include the back of the mouth, the esophagus, stomach, and small and large intestine.
- PCV/TS or CBC—to assess blood loss, hydration, inflammation or infection
- Endoscopy to characterize ulcerations and potentially removed lodged batteries from the esophagus or stomach.

Pathological Findings

- Ulceration, necrosis, and perforation anywhere along the GIT with hemorrhage and adjacent tissue injury; edema and ulceration of the larynx, trachea, and lower airways from inhalation of caustic battery components

 # THERAPEUTICS

- Do not induce vomiting. See Detoxification.

■ Initial therapy should include dilution of caustic components, removal of retained batteries, treatment for corrosive injury, pain management, and infection control.

Detoxification

■ The induction of emesis is not often advised due to the potential for corrosive injury or esophageal entrapment of the battery.
■ Activated charcoal is not recommended as it will not bind to battery contents and increases the risk of vomiting.
■ Dilution:
  • Give small amounts of tepid tap water every 10–15 minutes until evaluation can be completed. Rinse the oral cavity and any exposed skin for 10–15 minutes with water to remove or dilute any remaining caustic material.
■ Battery removal:
  • Once radiographs have revealed the location of the battery, an appropriate method of removal should be selected.
  • Esophagus—Immediate endoscopic removal is ideal as it is minimally invasive and quick. If the battery is known to be leaking, passage of the battery through the esophagus may create further damage. Thus, leaking/ruptured batteries should be surgically removed.
  • Stomach—Surgical removal is appropriate to protect the esophagus as endoscopic removal of a punctured battery may cause further ulcerations. Small, unpunctured disc and dry cell batteries *may* pass through the GIT without causing further damage. Repeated GI radiographs are needed to ensure passage of the battery/casing. Retention may lead to heavy metal toxicity and leakage of caustic contents.
  • Small intestine—Immediate surgical removal if the battery is punctured/leaking. Monitor (radiographs, examination of stool) for GI passage if the battery is not leaking.

Appropriate Health Care

■ Depending on the extent of corrosive injury, these patients may have significant discomfort when eating and drinking. Placement of a gastrostomy (PEG) tube may be necessary to ensure adequate nutrition, reduce the likelihood of infection, allow earlier release from the hospital, and improve patient comfort. PEG tubes may be placed at the time of battery removal.

Drug(s) and Antidotes of Choice

■ GI protectants and antacids to allow ulceration to heal rapidly with less discomfort.
  • H_2 blockers (e.g., famotidine 0.5 mg/kg IV, IM, or PO q 12 hours)
  • Proton pump inhibitors (e.g., omeprazole 0.5–1 mg/kg PO q 24 hours)
  • Sucralfate 0.25–1 g PO q 8 hours, on an empty stomach

- Antimicrobials if necessary
  - Cefazolin 10–30 mg/kg IV q 8 hours and enrofloxacin 5–20 mg/kg IV q 12–24 hours
  - Metronidazole 15 mg/kg PO q 12 hours
- Analgesics (see Precautions/Interactions)
  - Buprenorphine 0.005–0.01 mg/kg IV, IM, SQ or sublingual q 8 h
  - Tramadol 1–4 mg/kg PO q 8 hours

Precautions/Interactions

- Avoid early use of NSAIDs as prostaglandin inhibition will reduce the protective lining of the stomach.

Alternative Drugs

- H$_2$ blockers: Cimetidine and ranitidine are also excellent choices.
- Analgesics: Other opioid analgesics can be used, such as hydromorphone, morphine, oxymorphone, or butorphanol.
- Antimicrobials: Any broad-spectrum antibiotic can be used to prevent infection.

Follow-up

- Follow-up endoscopy may be needed to evaluate the esophagus for stricture formation. Consider balloon therapy to relieve a stricture.

Diet

- Keep pet NPO for 12–24 hours after exposure if any tissue damage is suspected.
- Consider placing a feeding tube to bypass the most severely affected areas (see Appropriate Health Care).

Surgical Considerations

- Standard anesthetic protocols are appropriate as long as the patient has no underlying medical conditions.
- Surgical versus endoscopic removal of battery material should be carefully considered (see Detoxification).
- Efforts need to be focused around preventing esophageal damage and rapid removal of the material.

Prevention

- Do not give pets toys or bedding containing batteries. Prevent access to batteries by removing old batteries from the environment.

Public Health

- Owner can sustain injuries from touching a ruptured battery and should use protection to prevent damage to their skin.
- In children, the most serious outcomes and greatest number of deaths have been reported with larger-diameter lithium cell batteries (≥20 mm). Death is often due to exsanguination after fistulization into major vessels (following esophageal entrapment).

Environmental Issues

- Consult your local recycling service before disposing of used batteries.

 COMMENTS

Client Education

- The owner will need to monitor closely for evidence of esophageal strictures, including anorexia, hypersalivation, and regurgitation.

Patient Monitoring

- Patients who initially have mild lesions can be monitored based on resolution of clinical signs. Those with more severe lesions should have an endoscopy performed in 7–14 days to determine progression and look for esophageal stricture or diverticulum.

Possible Complications

- Long-term esophagitis, esophageal stricture, or esophageal diverticulum

Expected Course and Prognosis

- Lithium disc battery in the esophagus:
  - With rapid removal, expect short-term esophagitis with complete recovery. Risk for stricture is low.
  - With delayed removal or no removal, expect extensive tissue damage. Risk for esophageal perforation is high. Long-term esophageal malformation is likely.
- Lithium disc battery in the stomach:
  - With rapid surgical removal, expect mild to moderate gastritis with possible stomach ulceration. Complete recovery expected in 7–10 days (with appropriate care).
  - With delayed or no removal, expect extensive tissue damage. The risk of perforation is high. If perforation is prevented, long-term affects are unlikely. If perforation occurs, septic peritonitis will likely result and immediate surgical intervention is needed to correct the perforation.

- Dry cell battery that is intact:
  - No ulcerations in the oral cavity or esophagus are expected. If the battery is removed from the stomach, recovery is expected to be uneventful.
  - If the battery is not removed from the stomach, it may pass uneventfully or it may become trapped in the stomach causing symptoms of a pyloric obstruction. Over time, the casing will corrode, leading to content leakage, stomach ulceration, and heavy metal toxicity.
- Dry cell battery that is ruptured/leaking:
  - Mild to severe ulcerations of the oral cavity, esophagus, and stomach are expected. Esophageal damage may result in long-term esophageal malformation or may heal normally.
  - With delayed or no removal, expect extensive tissue damage. The risk of perforation is high. If perforation is prevented, long-term effects are unlikely. If perforation occurs, septic peritonitis will likely result and immediate surgical intervention is needed to correct the perforation.

Synonyms

dry cell battery, lithium ion battery, button battery, disc battery, alkaline battery, acid battery, nickel-cadmium battery

Abbreviations

CBC	= complete blood count
CNS	= central nervous system
GI	= gastrointestinal
GIT	= gastrointestinal tract
IM	= intramuscular
IV	= intravenous
NPO	= *nil per os* (nothing by mouth)
NSAID	= nonsteroidal anti-inflammatory drug
PCV	= packed cell volume
PEG	= percutaneous endoscopic gastrostomy
PO	= *per os* (by mouth)
q	= every
SQ	= subcutaneous
TS	= total solids

See Also

Acids
Alkalis
Metallic Toxicants

Suggested Reading

Litovitz, T, Whitaker N, Clark L, White NC and Marsolek M. Preventing battery ingestion: An analysis of 8648 cases. Pediatrics 2010; 125:1178–1183.

Rebdandl W, Steffan I, Schramel P, Puig S, Paya K, Schwanzer E, Strobl B, Horcher E. Release of toxic metals from button batteries retained in the stomac: an in vitro study. J Pediatr Surg 2002; 37:87–92.

Tanaka J, Yamashita M, Yamashita Ma, et al. Effects of tap water on esophageal burns in dogs from button lithium batteries. Vet Hum Tox 1999; 41:279–282.

Wormald PJ, Wilson DAB. Battery acid burns of the upper gastro-intestinal tract. Clin Otolaryngol Allied Sci 2007; 18:112–114.

Yoshikawa T, Asai S, Takekaway, Kida A, Ishikawa K. Experimental investigation of battery-induced esophageal burn injury in rabbits. Crit Care Med 1997; 25:2039–2044.

Author: Catherine Angle, DVM, MPH
Consulting Editor: Ahna G. Brutlag, DVM

chapter 75

Matches and Fireworks

 ## DEFINITION/OVERVIEW

- Most match ingestions only cause GI signs, while serious toxicosis can result with firework ingestions.
- Poisoning by matches and fireworks is not common.
- Matches contain potassium chlorate and possibly phosphorus sesquisulfide. The chlorates are the biggest concern for toxicosis. Animals exposed to chlorates can develop methemoglobinemia.
- In fireworks, chlorates and barium appear to be the toxins of most concern. They can cause methemoglobinemia, cardiovascular effects, and renal failure. (See table 75.1 for other possible ingredients.) Used fireworks can have a different composition from unused, and the kinetics and toxicity can vary (increased or decreased bioavailability).

 ## ETIOLOGY/PATHOPHYSIOLOGY

Mechanism of Action

- Barium: causes severe hypokalemia by blocking the exit channel for potassium in skeletal muscle cells. Barium also stimulates skeletal, smooth, and cardiac muscle, causing violent peristalsis, arterial hypertension, and arrhythmias.
- Chlorates: locally irritating and potent oxidizing agents. The irritation leads to vomiting and diarrhea while the oxidation of the red blood cells causes hemolysis and methemoglobin formation. Chlorates are directly toxic to the proximal renal tubules, producing necrosis and renal vasoconstriction. Hemoglobinemia and methemoglobin catalysis also contribute to the renal effects.

Pharmacokinetics/Absorption, Distribution, Metabolism, and Excretion

- **Barium:** Oral absorption of barium is generally rapid but depends on the solubility of the particular barium salt. Peak serum concentrations are reached within 2 hours after ingestion. Barium is distributed into the bone, with an estimated half-life of 50 days. The main route of excretion of barium is fecal (less than 3% is excreted renally).

TABLE 75.1. Toxicologic information on the ingredients commonly found in fireworks.

Ingredient	Fireworks Usage/Toxicity Information
Aluminum	Silver and white flames and sparks (common in sparklers)
	Poor oral absorption; little risk of toxicity
Antimony (antimony sulfide)	Glitter effects
	Poor oral absorption; poisoning is very rare
Barium (barium chlorate, barium nitrate)	Green colors and can help stabilize other volatile elements
Beryllium	White sparks
	Poor oral absorption; inhalation can cause lung cancer
Calcium (calcium chlorate)	Orange coloring and used to deepen other colors
Cesium (cesium nitrate)	Indigo colors
	Toxicity is of minor importance
Chlorine	Component of many oxidizers in fireworks
Copper (copper chloride, copper halides)	Blue colors
	Copper salts are locally corrosive
Iron	Gold sparks
	(see chap. 84, "Iron")
Lithium (lithium carbonate)	Red color
Magnesium	White sparks and improves brilliance
Phosphorus	Glow-in-the-dark effects and may be a component of the fuel
	Red phosphorus (safety matches) is an insoluble substance that is nontoxic in oral ingestions. White phosphorus (fireworks) can cause severe gastroenteritis and cardiotoxic effects.
Potassium (potassium nitrate, potassium perchlorate)	Violet color, black powder explosive and used to oxidize firework mixtures
	Animals with normal renal function have minimal toxicity consisting of GI signs
Rubidium (rubidium nitrate)	Violet color
Sodium (sodium nitrate)	Gold or yellow colors
Strontium (strontium carbonate)	Red color and used to stabilize firework mixtures
Sulfur (sulfur dioxide)	Component of black powder
	Vomiting and diarrhea are common following sulfur ingestion
Titanium	Silver sparks
	Poor oral absorption; heavy dust exposures can cause coughing and dyspnea
Zinc	Smoke effects

■ Chlorates: Chlorates are well absorbed orally and are slowly excreted unchanged by the kidney.

Toxicity

■ Barium: LD_{LO} (oral) human = 11 mg/kg; LD_{50} (oral) human = 1 g
■ Barium chloride: LD_{50} (oral) rat = 220 mg/kg
■ Chlorates: LD_{50} (oral) dog = 1000 mg/kg
■ Potassium chlorate: LD_{50} (oral) rat = 1870 mg/kg
■ Sodium chlorate: LD_{50} (oral) mouse = 596 mg/kg; rat = 1200 mg/kg

Systems Affected

■ Gastrointestinal—vomiting (possibly bloody), diarrhea, hypersalivation
■ Skin—dermal burns
■ Nervous—lethargy
■ Hemic—hemolysis, methemoglobinemia
■ Cardiovascular—arrhythmias, hypertension
■ Respiratory—tachypnea, dyspnea
■ Endocrine/metabolic—hyperkalemia (chlorates), hypokalemia (barium)
■ Renal—renal failure (rare, chlorates)
■ Musculoskeletal—weakness, paresis (rare, barium)

 # SIGNALMENT/HISTORY

Risk Factors

■ Animals that ingest wooden matches are at risk for developing a GI foreign body.

Historical Findings

■ Vomiting, lethargy, diarrhea, bloody diarrhea
■ Owners may report matches or fireworks in vomitus

 # CLINICAL FEATURES

■ Overall, vomiting, lethargy, diarrhea, hypersalivation, and bloody vomiting are most common.
■ Tachycardia, hemolysis, hyperkalemia, methemoglobinemia and nephropathy have also been reported.
■ Barium: Ingestion can cause vomiting, diarrhea, salivation, cyanosis, bradycardia, and dyspnea within 10–60 minutes after exposure. Later signs (2–3 hours) include tremors, seizures, paralysis, mydriasis, severe hypokalemia, hypertension, arrhythmias, tachypnea, respiratory failure, and cardiac shock. If no signs within 6–8 hours, none are expected to develop.

- Chlorates: Vomiting, tachycardia, hemolysis, hyperkalemia, methemoglobinemia, and nephropathy can be seen in sodium chlorate toxicosis. Methemoglobinemia may not develop for 1–10 hours after exposure.

DIFFERENTIAL DIAGNOSIS

- Methemoglobinemia—acetaminophen, 3-chloro-p-toluidine hydrochloride (Starlicide), phenols (cats), garlic, onions, aniline dyes, naphthalene, phenazopyridine
- Hemorrhagic gastroenteritis—arsenic, parvoviral enteritis

DIAGNOSTICS

- CBC: methemoglobin level (chlorates), hematocrit (chlorates)
- Chemistry panel and electrolytes:
  - Renal panel (chlorates)
  - Potassium (barium, chlorates)
- Urinalysis: hemoglobinuria (chlorates)
- Blood gases (barium)
- ECG: QRS or QTc interval changes (barium)
- Special tests: contact lab for most appropriate sample and volume required.
  - Chlorate levels: blood or urine

Pathological Findings

- Chocolate-colored blood and tissues (methemoglobinemia), dark kidneys, renal tubular necrosis (chlorates)
- Oral, esophageal, GI ulcers (corrosive salts)

THERAPEUTICS

- Objectives of treatment include decontamination if asymptomatic, administration of an antidote (if appropriate), and supportive care.
- With firework ingestion, it is common that the exact composition is unknown and treatment is tailored to the clinical signs.

Detoxification

- Emesis if asymptomatic and only if noncorrosive agents were ingested
- Dilution with milk or water with corrosive agents
- Gastric lavage: only if noncorrosive agents ingested and large amount of material
- Barium: Magnesium sulfate will precipitate barium in the GI tract and prevent further absorption.

- Chlorates: Mineral oil gastric lavage may prevent further GI absorption of chlorates and help speed unabsorbed chlorate through the intestinal tract. It may be mixed with 1% sodium thiosulfate for increased efficacy.

Appropriate Health Care

- Intravenous fluids to maintain normal blood pressure and urine production
- See Drugs and Antidotes of Choice

Drug(s) and Antidotes of Choice

- Oxygen if cyanotic
- Saline diuresis to increase excretion (barium)
- Silver sulfadiazine topically for burns
- Sucralfate (0.25–1 g PO q 6–8 hours) for gastric irritation (corrosive salts)
- Famotidine (0.5–1 mg/kg PO, SQ, IM, IV q 12–24 hours) or other H_2 blocker for gastric irritation (corrosive salts)
- Sodium bicarbonate (1–2 mEq/kg IV, titrate up as needed) to shift potassium intracellularly (chlorates)
- Potassium chloride (do not exceed 0.5 mEq/kg/hr IV) to correct hypokalemia, cardiac arrhythmias and diarrhea (barium)
- Methylene blue (10 mg/kg IV, as a 2–4% solution) to convert methemoglobin to hemoglobin (chlorates)
- Sodium thiosulfate (2–5 g in 200 mL of 5% sodium bicarbonate, PO or IV) to inactivate chlorate ions

Precautions/Interactions

- Charcoal does not bind to chlorate or heavy metals and, with the risk of aspiration, it should be avoided. Charcoal should also not be given if corrosive agents were ingested.

Alternative Drugs

- Ascorbic acid (10–20 mg/kg IV, SQ, PO q 4 hours to aid in the conversion of methemoglobin to hemoglobin (chlorates)

Diet

- NPO while symptomatic, may need an esophagostomy or gastrostomy tube if severe oral or esophageal burns are evident.

Activity

- Cage rest while symptomatic

COMMENTS

Patient Monitoring

- Monitor SPO_2 to evaluate oxygenation (initially, monitor continuously)
- Liver and renal function—baseline, 24, 48, and 72 hours
- Urine output—daily

Expected Course and Prognosis

- Most animals will recover within 24 to 72 hours with supportive care. Barium and chlorate ingestion carries a more guarded prognosis.

See Also

Metallic Toxicants
Iron
Smoke Inhalation
Zinc

Abbreviations

CBC = complete blood count
ECG = electrocardiogram
GI = gastrointestinal
IM = intramuscular
IV = intravenous
LD_{50} = median lethal dose
LD_{LO} = lowest lethal dose
NPO = *nil per os* (nothing by mouth)
PO = *per os* (by mouth)
q = every
SQ = subcutaneous

Suggested Reading

DiBartola SP. Fluid Therapy in Small Animal Practice, 2nd ed. New York: W.B. Saunders, 2000.
Sheahan BJ, Pugh DM, Winstanley EW. Experimental sodium chlorate poisoning in dogs. Res Vet Sci 1971; 12:387–389.
Smith EA, Oehme FW. A review of selected herbicides and their toxicities. Vet Hum Toxicol 1991; 33:596–608.

Author: Tina Wismer DVM, DABVT, DABT
Consulting Editor: Ahna G. Brutlag, DVM

chapter 76

Mothballs

DEFINITION/OVERVIEW

- Moth repellants are composed of two major toxic ingredients: naphthalene or paradichlorobenzene (PDB). Camphor is also used in some countries.
- Moth repellants are sold as flakes, crystals, cakes, scales, powder, cubes, and spheres ("mothballs").
- Naphthalene is a dry, white, solid crystalline material with a classic "mothball odor."
  - Historically, naphthalene has been used as an antiseptic, expectorant, anthelmintic and insecticide (in dusting powders), and as a treatment for intestinal and dermal diseases.
- PDB is an organochlorine insecticide.
  - Found in deodorizers for diaper pails, urinals, and bathrooms
  - PDB is considered less toxic than naphthalene.
- Routes of exposure include inhalation, ingestion, and transdermal absorption.
- Mothballs may take several days to completely dissolve in the GIT.
- GI signs are most common.
- Hepatic, renal, neurological signs have also been reported.

ETIOLOGY/PATHOPHYSIOLOGY

- Ingestion, inhalation, and dermal contact with mothballs can lead to toxicosis.
- The majority of toxicoses are due to ingestion.

Mechanism of Action

- Depletes cellular glutathione, impeding the ability to counteract oxidative damage
- GI, dermal, and ocular effects are likely secondary to irritant properties.

Pharmacokinetics/Absorption, Distribution, Metabolism, and Excretion

- Absorption
  - Readily soluble in oils and fats. Dermal absorption is increased if oils/lotions have been applied. Oral absorption is increased if ingested with fatty meals.
  - Rapid uptake by the lungs with inhalational exposure

- GI absorption can be delayed as mothballs may be slow to dissolve in the GIT.
- Distribution
  - Greatest affinity for adipose tissue. High concentrations are also found in the lungs, kidneys, and liver.
  - Can enter placental blood supply and affect the fetus
- Metabolism
  - Naphthalene is metabolized in the liver by microsomal P450 enzymes and conjugated to glutathione, glucuronide, sulfate, or mercapturate.
  - PDB's major metabolite is 2,5-dichlorophenol, which can cause oxidative damage to the liver, kidneys, lungs, and CNS. PDB is oxidized to phenolic compounds prior to conjugation with sulfate and glucuronide.
  - Detoxification depends on glucuronide conjugation in the liver.
  - Glutathione depletion may result secondary to oxidative damage.
  - Metabolite oxidation of Hb to MetHb results in Heinz body formation and erythrolysis.
- Excretion
  - Excreted almost exclusively via the kidneys (91%–97%). PDB is eliminated via the urine in 5 days.
  - Small amounts may be eliminated in bile, feces, and breast milk.
  - Half-life of naphthalene in guinea pig blood is 10.4 hours; the decay is biphasic in other tissues.

Toxicity

- PDB is less toxic than naphthalene (by approximately one-half).
- PDB
  - Rat oral LD_{50} = 3.8 g/kg
  - Dogs ingesting 1.5 g/kg developed no clinical signs.
  - Rats receiving 770–1200 mg/kg for 5 days showed CNS signs.
- Naphthalene
  - Rat oral LD_{50} = 1.8 g/kg
  - Hemolytic anemia was reported in 1 dog from a single 1.525 g/kg dose.
  - Hemolytic anemia was reported in 1 dog from 263 mg/kg/day over 7 days.
  - Lowest reported canine oral lethal dose = 400 mg/kg
- Mothballs typically weigh 2.7–4g; rarely 5 g/mothball

Systems Affected

- Gastrointestinal—vomiting, diarrhea due to irritant properties
- Neuromuscular—CNS stimulation followed by depression (with PDB)
- Hemic/lymphatic/immune—oxidation of Hb to MetHb; depletion of glutathione
- Hepatobiliary—direct injury via oxidative damage; secondary to hemolysis or metabolism of toxin

- Respiratory—cellular damage via direct inhalation or secondary to anemia
- Skin—local irritation if absorbed/contacted
- Renal—primary or secondary damage, likely secondary to hemolysis. With chronic toxicity of PDB, kidney is primary organ injured.
- Ophthalmic—metabolized in the lens, causing free radical damage
- Cardiovascular—secondary to hematological effects/hemorrhagic shock

 # SIGNALMENT/HISTORY

Risk Factors

- Cats may be more sensitive to toxic effects based on metabolism (glucuronidation).
- There is no known breed, age, or sex predilection.

Historical Findings

- Witnessed ingestion, inhalation, or contact with substance
- Discovery of ingested material in the emesis
- Mothball-scented breath
- Owner may notice signs of toxicity from mothballs, including vomiting, lethargy, trembling, depression, weakness, anorexia, and seizures.

Location and Circumstances of Poisoning

- Exposure often occurs in the home.
- Not confined to mothballs—active ingredients are found in cake deodorizers used in diaper pails, urinals, and bathrooms
- Pet owner may find cat playing with mothballs.

Interactions with Drugs, Nutrients, or Environment

- GI and dermal absorption is enhanced by fat, oil, or lotion.

 # CLINICAL FEATURES

- Clinical signs typically begin within minutes to hours of exposure.
- Duration of signs is based on effect and dose (may last for days).
- GI—dehydration, nausea/hypersalivation, anorexia, vomiting, lethargy, abdominal pain
- CNS—depression, trembling, tremors, ataxia, seizures
- Cardiovascular—mucous membrane pallor/icterus/brown discoloration, tachypnea, tachycardia, weakness, hypotension
- Respiratory—tachypnea, dyspnea, hypoxemia
- Integument—dermal abrasions/irritation if contact exposure, jaundice

DIFFERENTIAL DIAGNOSIS

- Gastrointestinal signs:
    - Primary GI disease
    - Secondary GI disease
    - Toxicities—NSAIDs, aspirin, iron, soaps/detergents, etc.
- Neurologic signs:
    - Primary CNS disease—inflammatory, infectious, neoplasia, epilepsy
- Anemia:
    - Blood loss—melena, neoplasia, coagulopathy, DIC, cavital bleed, antico-agulant rodenticide toxicity
    - Lack of production—bone marrow disease, aplastic anemia, drug/toxin
    - Destruction—immune- and non-immune-mediated disease/causes for hemolysis, zinc toxicosis, toxins such as zinc, onions, chives, garlic, acetaminophen, etc. that result in Heinz body anemia anemia
- Primary metabolic disease—renal, hepatic, hypoadrenocorticism, hypoglyce-mia; other hepatic toxicities: *Amanita* mushroom, xylitol, blue-green algae (cyanobacteria)
- Dermatologic signs:
    - Infectious—pyoderma, insect/arthropod bite, parasitic
    - Inflammatory—drug eruption/reaction, vasculitis
- Other—sunburn, thermal burn, contact dermatitis

DIAGNOSTICS

- To help differentiate naphthalene from PBD mothballs, float mothballs in both plain water and a saturated salt solution.
    - To make a saturated salt solution, mix 4 ounces of tepid water with 3 heaping tablespoons of table salt. Stir vigorously until the salt will not dissolve any further.
    - Naphthalene mothballs sink in water and float in salt solution.
    - PDB mothballs sink in both.
- CBC—anemia, Heinz bodies, evidence of hemolysis
- Chemistry—azotemia, liver enzyme elevation, hyperbilirubinemia
- Venous blood gas analysis—metabolic acidosis, electrolyte abnormalities from vomiting
- Urinalysis—pigmenturia, hemoglobinuria, isosthenuria if underlying renal injury
    - Urine can be submitted to a laboratory for isolation of naphthalene and metabolites using TLC or HPLC and identification using GC-MS.
- Radiographs—PDB mothballs are densely radiopaque; naphthalene mothballs are radiolucent or faintly radiopaque.

THERAPEUTICS

Detoxification

- Stabilize symptomatic animals prior to decontamination.
- Induce emesis in asymptomatic patients (due to slow dissolution, emesis may be effective many hours after ingestion).
- Emesis is contraindicated in animals exhibiting CNS signs (e.g., depression, ataxia, tremors, seizures).
- Gastric lavage if emesis is nonproductive or in cases of massive ingestions
- Activated charcoal with a cathartic may be given once within 24 hours of ingestion.
- Decontaminate dermal exposures by bathing the area (see chap. 1, "Decontamination and Detoxification of the Poisoned Patient").
- Irrigate exposed eyes with isotonic saline or water for 10–15 minutes.
- Animals exposed to naphthalene fumes should be removed from the source of exposure.

Appropriate Health Care

- Immediate patient assessment and stabilization are extremely important.
- Treatments are supportive and symptomatic, based upon the clinical signs of the patient.
- Dyspneic patients should receive supplemental oxygen if needed.
- Patients with signs of hemorrhagic shock (e.g., hypotension, tachycardia, anemia, severe hemolysis, or MetHb) should be volume resuscitated and transfused if needed.

Drug(s) and Antidotes of Choice

- IV fluid therapy with a balanced, isotonic crystalloid should be used for all symptomatic animals.
- GI signs may be treated with the following:
    - Antiemetic (e.g., metoclopramide 0.2–0.5 mg/kg, PO, IM, SQ q 8 hours; 1–2 mg/kg/day CRI IV).
    - Sucralfate 0.25–1 g, PO q 8 hours
    - H_2 antagonist (e.g., famotidine 0.5–1.0 mg/kg, PO, SQ, or IV q 12–24 hours)
    - Proton pump inhibitor (e.g., omeprazole, 0.5–1.0 mg/kg PO q 24 hours in dogs and 0.7 mg/kg PO q 24 hours in cats)
- Anticonvulsant therapy:
    - Diazepam, 0.5–1 mg/kg, IV to effect
    - Phenobarbital 4 mg/kg, IV q 4–6 hours × 4 doses. Use higher doses if needed. If refractory, may add to diazepam CRI IV at 0.25–0.5 mg/kg/hour.
- MetHb can be treated with ascorbic acid and/or methylene blue.
    - Ascorbic acid reduces MetHb to Hb but is a slow conversion.

□   20 mg/kg, PO, IM, SQ q 6 hours
- Methylene blue converts to leucomethylene blue to rapidly reduce MetHb to Hb.
    □   Dogs: 1–4 mg/kg IV, slow infusion given once
    □   Cats: 1–1.5 mg/kg IV, slow infusion given once

Precautions/Interactions

- Methylene blue can induce further MetHb.
- Cats are at greater risk for adverse effects from methylene blue.

Alternative Drugs

- N–acetylcysteine (NAC) may be useful to replenish glutathione stores and provide a substrate for sulfation.
    - Initial loading dose of 140 mg/kg PO, then 70 mg/kg PO every 4–6 hours for 7–17 treatments (consider premedicating with an antiemetic)
    - Oral formation may be given IV (off label) slowly over 15–20 minutes through a 0.2-micron bacteriostatic filter. Loading dose of 140 mg/kg IV
    - 10% or 20% solutions should be diluted to a 3–4% solution prior to IV administration.
- The IV preparation (Acetadote) is preferred if the drug is to be given IV. Dilute to 3–5%. Loading dose of 150 mg/kg over 15 minutes; then 50 mg/kg over 4 hours; then 100 mg/kg over 16 hours.
- S–adenosylmethionine (SAMe), 18–20 mg/kg, PO q 24 hours on an empty stomach, may help with glutathione production and maintenance.

Nursing Care

- Proper monitoring and nursing care should be provided accordingly as it pertains to symptoms of each patient (e.g., TPR, oxygenation).
- Patients with CNS depression and/or who are heavily sedated from anticonvulsants should have appropriate nursing care and be monitored carefully.

Follow-up

- CBC and chemistry values should be monitored to ensure a return to normal.

Client Education

- Clients should be made aware of potential toxicants and locations in/around the home.

Patient Monitoring

- PCV should be assessed at least twice daily in anemic patients.
- Hepatic and/or renal values should be monitored daily in affected patients.
- Visual assessment of drawn blood/blood smears for resolving MetHb or presence of hemolysis as needed

Expected Course and Prognosis

- Good, provided treatment is initiated early and there is no underlying hepatic or renal impairment

Abbreviations

CBC	= complete blood count
CNS	= central nervous system
CRI	= continuous rate infusion
CRT	= capillary refill time
DIC	= disseminated intravascular coagulopathy
GC-MS	= gas chromatography–mass spectrometry
GI	= gastrointestinal
GIT	= gastrointestinal tract
Hb	= hemoglobin
HPLC	= high-performance lipid chromatography
IM	= intramuscular
IV	= intravenous
LD_{50}	= median lethal dose
MetHb	= methemoglobin
NAC	= N–acetylcysteine
NSAID	= nonsteroidal anti-inflammatory drug
PCV	= packed cell volume
PDB	= paradichlorobenzene
PO	= *per os* (by mouth)
q	= every
RR	= respiratory rate
SQ	= subcutaneous
TLC	= thin-layer chromatography
TPR	= temperature, pulse rate, respiratory rate

See Also

Essential Oils/Liquid Potpourri
Phenols/Pine Oils

Suggested Reading

Bischoff K. Naphthalene. In: Plumlee KH, ed. Clinical Veterinary Toxicology. St. Louis: Mosby, 2004; pp. 163–164.

DeClementi C. Moth repellant toxicosis. Vet Med 2005; 100:24.

Desnoyers M, Hebert P. Heinz body anemia in a dog following naphthalene ingestion. Vet Clin Path 1995; 24(4):124–125.

Oehme FW, Kore AM. Miscellaneous indoor toxicants. In: Peterson ME, Talcott PA, eds. Small Animal Toxicology, 2nd ed. St. Louis: Elsevier, 2006; p. 223.

Authors: Seth L. Cohen, DVM; Ahna G. Brutlag, DVM
Consulting Editor: Justine A. Lee, DVM, DACVECC

chapter 77

Paintballs

DEFINITION/OVERVIEW

- Paintball toxicosis in dogs and, rarely, cats and ferrets is an uncommon toxicity presented to veterinarians. While the ingredients within paintballs are nontoxic, the components are osmotically active and can pull free water into the GIT. (See figs. 77.1 a and b.)
- Common components of paintballs include glycerol, glycerin, polyethylene glycol (PEG), sorbitol, gelatin, propylene glycol, wax, mineral oil, and dye. The exact ingredients within a given paintball vary by manufacturer.
- Common clinical signs include vomiting, diarrhea, ataxia, and tremors.
- Treatment includes decontamination of the GIT, management of hypernatremia and neurologic complications, and supportive care.
- Though clinical reports detailing paintball toxicosis are very limited in veterinary medicine, the prognosis appears to be good with appropriate supportive care.

ETIOLOGY/PATHOPHYSIOLOGY

Mechanism of Action

- The ingredients in paintballs are nontoxic (see Definition/Overview).
- After the paintballs are ingested, the osmotically active ingredients (e.g., sorbitol, glycerol, propylene glycol, and PEG) pull water from the body tissues into the GIT resulting in an increase in plasma osmolality and hypernatremia. Neurologic effects are often secondary changes in osmolality and serum sodium concentrations.
- Large volumes of free water within the GIT, in addition to the osmotically active ingredients of the paintballs themselves, can cause vomiting and diarrhea.

Pharmacokinetics/Absorption, Distribution, Metabolism, and Excretion

- The osmotically active ingredients within paintballs remain in the GIT until the patient vomits or they are excreted through the feces. They are not absorbed from the GIT or metabolized by other organs.

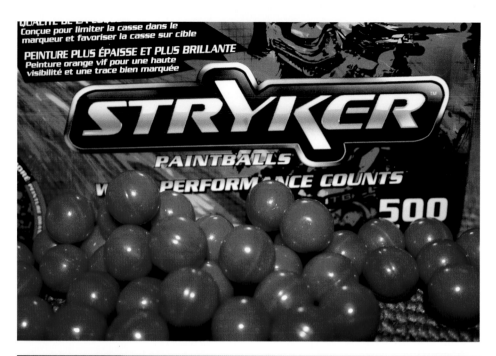

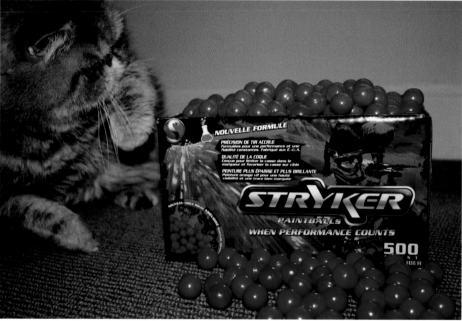

■ **Fig. 77.1.** Commercially available paintballs and their packaging. Figure 77.1a shows paintball size and appearance, as well as the original packaging materials. Figure 77.1b shows the author's own cat, which was instantly very interested in playing with the paintballs being photographed. (Photo courtesy of Dana L. Clarke)

Toxicity

- None of the commonly used components of paintballs are toxic. Toxicosis results from the fluid and electrolyte shifts secondary to the osmotically active nature of many of the ingredients used.
- As few as 5–10 paintballs have caused symptoms in a 30-kg dog.

Systems Affected

- Gastrointestinal
  - Direct irritation of the esophageal or gastric mucosa by ingredients may cause vomiting.
  - Free water movement into the stomach (with secondary fluid distension of the stomach) and intestines may result in vomiting and diarrhea.
  - Polydipsia may occur as a consequence of hypernatremia.
- Nervous
  - Movement of free water into the GIT leads to increased serum osmolality via hypernatremia and hyperchloremia.
  - Acute increases in serum sodium results in increased serum osmolality, which causes dehydration, free water shifts, and eventually leads to cerebral cellular dehydration and cell shrinkage. Cerebral and meningeal vessels may tear with cellular shrinkage and lead to cerebral and subarachnoid hemorrhage, resulting in acute neurologic signs.
- Renal/urologic
  - Prerenal azotemia, secondary to dehydration, may result.
- Endocrine/metabolic
  - Antidiuretic hormone (ADH) may be released secondary to significant free water shifts/loss.
  - A metabolic acidosis can result from hyperchloremia secondary to free water loss, bicarbonate loss through diarrhea, prerenal azotemia, and lactic acidosis if perfusion is compromised.
- Cardiovascular
  - Hypovolemia may occur secondary to significant fluid losses, resulting in tachycardia (compensatory) and hypotension.
- Neuromuscular
  - Weakness may occur secondary to electrolyte imbalances, dehydration, and hypovolemia.
- Ophthalmic
  - Cerebral cellular shrinkage may cause central blindness.

 SIGNALMENT/HISTORY

- There are no breed, sex, or age predilections.
- Paintball toxicosis has been reported in dogs, cats, and ferrets; however, dogs represent the majority of animals affected.

- No mean age has been reported. Younger animals are more frequently affected, given their increased incidence of ingesting foreign objects.

Risk Factors

- Animals living in homes or areas where paintballs are stored
- Animals that have access to outdoor areas where paintballs are fired
- Animals with diseases that cause increased water loss (such as renal, metabolic, or gastrointestinal disease) could be at increased risk of more severe consequences.

Historical Findings

- Witnessed ingestion
- Discovery of damaged/chewed packaging or spilled paintballs
- Owners may see paint on the pet's coat or face and may witness vomiting (which may or may not contain paint), diarrhea, and CNS changes.

Location and Circumstances of Poisoning

- Pets with access to paintballs, either indoors or outdoors, are those that could ingest these objects.

 CLINICAL FEATURES

- The onset of clinical signs can occur quickly (within 1 hour) due to rapid shifting of free water into the GIT.
- The severity of clinical signs is dependent upon the number of paintballs consumed. Given that packages may contain up to 1000 paintballs, and the exact amount ingested is often unknown, it can be difficult to predict the severity of signs that will result.
  - Gastrointestinal—vomiting, diarrhea
  - Renal/urologic—polydipsia, polyuria
  - Nervous—depression, ataxia, stupor, coma, hyperexcitability, seizures
  - Cardiovascular—tachycardia, hypotension
  - Neuromuscular—weakness
  - Ophthalmic—central blindness
  - Skin/exocrine—paint on the skin or hair coat

 DIFFERENTIAL DIAGNOSIS

- Diabetes insipidus
- Salt toxicosis (e.g., sea water, homemade play dough, salt emetic)
- Ethanol ingestion

- Ethylene glycol toxicosis
  - The early clinical signs of ethylene glycol toxicosis are similar to those seen with paintball toxicosis. In addition, several common paintball components, including sorbitol, glycerol, and propylene glycol, can react with the chemicals used in blood ethylene glycol tests to produce false positive results. For more information on ethylene glycol toxicosis, see chapter 6.

DIAGNOSTICS

- There are no specific diagnostic tests.
- Serum sodium concentration and other electrolytes should be determined at presentation and monitored frequently during treatment (q 2–4 hours during hospitalization).
- To distinguish true ethylene glycol toxicosis from other chemicals that cross-react with ethylene glycol tests, high-performance liquid chromatography is needed.

Pathological Findings

- There are no characteristic gross or histopathologic lesions.
- Gross necropsy findings may include paintball paint and remnants within the alimentary tract, edema of the intestinal wall, and increased fluid content within the GIT. If hypernatremic patients have a necropsy performed prior to fluid therapy, there may be gross signs of brain shrinkage and retraction from the meninges and attachments to the calvarium. If necropsy is performed after aggressive fluid therapy for hypernatremia, there may be signs of cerebral edema such as herniation of the cerebellum or brainstem.
- Histopathology may reveal edema of the mucosa and submucosa of the GIT, cerebral cellular shrinkage, torn meninges and meningeal vessels, or cerebral cellular swelling.

THERAPEUTICS

- Treatment includes aggressive decontamination if the patient is presented soon after ingestion, electrolyte and neurologic monitoring, fluid therapy, and supportive care.
- The use of activated charcoal is contraindicated.

Detoxification

- In asymptomatic animals, emesis should be induced as quickly and as safely as possible.
- The use of activated charcoal is contraindicated (see Precautions/Interactions).

▪ For neurologically inappropriate patients, initial treatment should be aimed at managing neurologic signs, such as seizure control. Appropriate sedation, intubation (to protect the airway), and gastric lavage should be considered.

▪ Warm water enemas (2–4 mL/kg) may be considered to help evacuate the osmotically active paintball remnants from the large intestine and to help decrease free water loss into the GIT. In addition, given the large absorptive capacity of the colon for water, the enemas may provide an additional source of free water. The frequency will depend on the patient's serum sodium concentration and clinical signs.

Appropriate Health Care

▪ Acute hypernatremia (<18 hours) may be treated aggressively to normalize the sodium level, and sodium levels can be dropped relatively quickly with IV fluids with *acute* toxicosis.

▪ Chronic hypernatremia (>18 hours) must be treated slowly and sodium should not be altered more than 0.5 mEq/L per hour.

▪ Serum electrolytes (e.g., sodium, potassium, glucose), PCV/TS, and blood glucose should be obtained at presentation and monitored at least every 2–4 hours initially, depending on the extent of electrolyte derangements. Once electrolyte derangements have stabilized, monitor every 4–6 hours.

▪ Aggressive fluid therapy may be necessary, given the large volumes of free water that may be lost into the GIT. Careful monitoring of hydration parameters (e.g., patient weight, physical exam, UOP, urine specific gravity, PCV/TS) should be done.

▪ When managing hypernatremia, the chronicity or duration of time for which the electrolyte was increased is imperative information. If this information cannot be ascertained from the patient's history and clinical course, hypernatremia must be assumed to be chronic and therefore treated as such (slowly).

  • For patients with both acute and chronic hypernatremia that require fluid boluses, 0.9% NaCl should be used, as this isotonic crystalloid will have the least impact on serum sodium concentration when compared with other crystalloids. Hypertonic saline (7.5%) should be avoided for the management of hypovolemia, as this will perpetuate interstitial dehydration and hypernatremia. Hypovolemia should be treated prior to attempting to safely manage dehydration and hypernatremia.

  • For patients with **chronic** (>18 hour) duration of hypernatremia, serum sodium should be decreased by no more then 0.5 mEq/L/hr, due to the presence of idiogenic osmoles and their ability to osmotically pull fluid into cerebral cells. The isotonic crystalloid's sodium content should be selected so that it is closest to the patient's current serum sodium concentration.

  • Once hydration is restored, D5W (5% dextrose in sterile water) or 0.45% NaCl may be used to provide free water to compensate for GIT losses and manage hypernatremia. This therapy should be used with caution in patients with chronic or unknown duration of hypernatremia, as rapid decreases in serum sodium concentration may result.

- Serum sodium levels should be monitored every 2–4 hours to ensure safe, gradual decreases in serum sodium concentration.
- For patients with chronic hypernatremia who have a rapid decrease in serum sodium and develop signs of depressed mentation, decreased PLR, decreased responsiveness, or seizures, cerebral edema should be suspected and treated appropriately.
- For patients with **acute** (<18 hour) duration of hypernatremia, serum sodium concentration can be decreased more rapidly, as idiogenic osmoles will not yet have formed and there is little risk of cerebral edema developing secondary to changes in serum sodium concentration.

■ For patients that develop seizures secondary to fluid shifts from paintball toxicosis, as well as iatrogenically from fluid therapy and rapid serum sodium concentration decrease, seizures should be controlled with diazepam (0.5–1 mg/kg IV) or midazolam (0.2–0.5 mg/kg IV).

■ Seizures must be aggressively controlled to prevent cerebral edema, noncardiogenic pulmonary edema, and aspiration of GIT contents. Any patient for whom the ability to protect their airway is questionable should be intubated.

■ In neurologically impaired patients, serum potassium and blood glucose should be monitored and appropriately supplemented as needed. Hyperglycemia should be avoided.

■ Antiemetic therapy:
- Ondansetron 0.1–0.2 mg/kg IV q 8–12 hours
- Dolasetron 0.5–0.6 mg/kg IV q 24 hours
- Metoclopramide CRI 1–2 mg/kg/day
- Maropitant 1.0 mg/kg SQ q 24 hours

Drug(s) and Antidotes of Choice

■ There are no specific antidotes for paintball toxicosis.

■ If there is any concern that a patient's neurologic signs could be secondary to ethylene glycol ingestion, then treatment for this fatal toxicosis must take priority. See chapter 6 for specific information on the treatment and management of patients with ethylene glycol toxicosis.

Precautions/Interactions

■ Treatment with activated charcoal with a cathartic, such as sorbitol, is contraindicated, as the cathartic will exacerbate fluid flux into the GIT and could further contribute to hypernatremia.

■ Since none of the components of paintballs are themselves toxic, administration of activated charcoal is of little value, especially in patients with altered mentation or neurologic status, which have an increased risk of aspiration.

■ Warm water enemas are contraindicated in patients with chronic hypernatremia.

Nursing Care

- Intensive nursing care and neurologic monitoring should be carried out every 2–4 hours.
- Care for recumbent patients, including frequent turning, passive range of motion, bladder and colon care, and eye and oral care, should be provided.
- For patients with seizures and concerns for cerebral edema, a board under the head and neck, positioned at a 15–30-degree angle, should be used to help decrease intracranial pressure. Compression of the jugular veins (especially for venipuncture) and hyperthermia should be avoided in such patients. Mannitol (0.5–2 g/kg, IV, to effect) can also be considered but may contribute to hyperosmolality and should be used judiciously.

Follow-up

- It is likely that follow-up care and monitoring will not be necessary after discharge, provided the sodium levels have normalized.

Diet

- For patients with neurologic compromise, vomiting, regurgitation, or those that are sedated, oral food and water should be withheld until the patient is neurologically appropriate and GIT signs have resolved.
- Due to gastric irritation from vomiting, a bland diet should be implemented for 3–5 days.

Activity

- Activity restriction is not necessary, as the patient's neurologic status will likely determine its activity level.

Prevention

- Proper storage of paintballs in an area inaccessible to pets will help prevent exposure. Those involved with paintball sports should be advised of the risks to pets, and pets should not be allowed access to areas where paintball games are played. Any paintball remnants in the environment should be disposed of properly.

 COMMENTS

Client Education

- Clients should be educated on the mechanism of action of paintball toxicosis, as well as given recommendations for safe storage and use options.

- Information about the gradual reintroduction of a bland diet, monitoring for ongoing GIT and neurologic signs, and general observation instructions should be provided.

Patient Monitoring

- See Appropriate Health Care

Possible Complications

- In most patients, a full recovery is made after appropriate monitoring and supportive care.

Expected Course and Prognosis

- Since a toxic dose of ingested paintballs is not known, every exposure should be managed very aggressively.
- Between 2002 and 2009, Pet Poison Helpline and the ASPCA Animal Poison Control Center received over 400 calls for paintball ingestion by dogs, cats, and ferrets. Euthanasia or death was uncommon. For the vast majority of pets exposed, complete recovery was often within 24 hours. The overall prognosis for paintball toxicosis is good to excellent with appropriate treatment.

Synonyms

paintball ingestion, paintball toxicity, paintball toxicosis

Abbreviations

ADH = antidiuretic hormone
CNS = central nervous system
CRI   = continuous rate infusion
D5W = dextrose in water
GIT   = gastrointestinal tract
IM   = intramuscular
IV   = intravenous
PCV = packed cell volume
PEG = polyethylene glycol
PLR = pupillary light reflex
q   = every
SQ   = subcutaneous
TS   = total solids
UOP = urine output

See Also

Diuretics
Ethylene Glycol

Suggested Reading

DiBartola, SP. Disorders of sodium and water: hypernatremia and hyponatremia. In: DiBartola SP, ed. Fluid, Electrolyte, and Acid-Base Disorders in Small Animal Practice, 3rd ed. St. Louis: Elsevier, 1996.

Donaldson CW. Paintball toxicosis in dogs. Vet Med 2003; 98(12):995–998.

Howard J. Paintball toxicosis. Vet Tech 2007; 28(5):336–337, 340.

King JB, Grant DC. Paintball intoxication in a pug. J Vet Emerg Crit Care 2007; 17(3): 290–293.

Authors: Dana L. Clarke, VMD; Justine A. Lee, DVM, DACVECC
Consulting Editor: Ahna G. Brutlag, DVM

chapter 78

Phenols/Pine Oils

DEFINITION/OVERVIEW

- Phenol, phenolic compounds, and pine oil are used in household cleaning products, disinfectants, medicated shampoos, scents, and rarely, insecticides.
- **Phenol** is an aromatic alcohol originally derived from coal tar.
  - Phenols are highly corrosive in all species and can cause neurologic, renal, and liver disease.
- **Phenolic derivatives** include creosote, creosol, hexachlorophene (Phisohex), phenylphenol, chlorophenol, dinitrophenol, alkyl phenols, phenolic resins and epoxy (bisphenol A), and others (see Synonyms).
  - Phenolic disinfectants may contain chlorophenols (3%–8%), phenyl phenol (2%–10%) or pure phenol (20%–50%).
  - Phenolic derivatives are generally less corrosive than phenol.
- **Pine oil** is an essential oil derived from pine trees. Pine oil contains alpha-terpineol, terpene ethers, and phenolic compounds.
  - Pine Sol, a popular home cleaning product, contains up to 20% pine oil.
  - Pine oil is a gastric irritant for most species, but when ingested in large amounts, in high concentrations, or by cats, it can cause GI signs followed by changes in mentation, respiratory depression, ataxia, anemia, and nephritis.
- Cats are very sensitive to these chemicals due to their limited glucuronide transferase activity and develop toxicosis at lower doses than dogs.
- Toxicosis can follow all routes of exposure (dermal, inhalation, ingestion, etc.).

ETIOLOGY/PATHOPHYSIOLOGY

Mechanism of Action

- **Pine oils** are a direct irritant to the mucous membranes. The mode of action is poorly understood.
- **Phenols** are corrosive to the skin and mucous membranes. The true mode of action is unknown, but theories include a cardiac sodium channel blockade, a direct toxic effect on the CNS and the myocardium, or CNS stimulation from an increased acetylcholine release.
- **Phenolic derivatives** have a similar MOA as phenols but are less corrosive.

Pharmacokinetics/Absorption, Distribution, Metabolism, and Excretion

- Pine oil
  - Dermal and GIT absorption occurs (extent varies).
  - Well distributed with highest concentrations in the brain, lungs, and kidneys
  - Metabolized via epoxide pathway, then oxidized in the liver by cytochrome P-450 and conjugated with glucuronic acid
  - Excreted in the urine
- Phenol and phenolic derivatives
  - Rapidly absorbed following oral, dermal, or inhalation exposures. Absorption begins within 5 minutes and is complete within a few hours.
  - Distributed to all tissues with peak concentration within 1 hour of oral ingestion and 6–10 hours of dermal exposure. The highest concentrations are found in the liver.
  - Metabolized by glucuronyl and sulfotransferases. The metabolites are excreted via the kidneys in 24–72 hours.

Toxicity

- Toxicity is dependent upon the concentration, the volume ingested/applied, and the amount of exposed body surface area.
- Cats are more sensitive than dogs (limited glucuronide transferase activity).
- Pine oil
  - $LD_{50} = 1$–$2.5\,mL/kg$
  - Severe toxicosis develops at much lower doses.
  - One cat ingesting $100\,mL$ of undiluted Pine Sol died within 12 hours.
  - $0.5\,oz$ of pure oil fatal in a child; $8\,oz$ fatal in an adult human being (ingestion)
- Phenol
  - Cat LD_{50} (unknown route) = $80\,mg/kg$
  - Dog LD_{50} (oral) = $500\,mg/kg$
  - Mouse and rat LD_{50} (oral) = 270–$317\,mg/kg$
  - Rat LD_{50} (dermal) = $669\,mg/kg$
  - Concentrations 1%–5%: Expect tissue irritation. May result in dermal burns.
  - Concentrations 5%–10%: Dermal burns possible. May result in oral/GI burns.
  - Concentrations >10%: Expect corrosive damage to all tissues.
- Hexachlorophene
  - Concentrations above 3% can cause severe dermal damage.
  - Rat and mouse LD_{50} (oral) = 56–$67\,mg/kg$
  - Mice LD_{50} (dermal) = $270\,mg/kg$
  - Rate LD_{50} (dermal) = $1840\,mg/kg$

Systems Affected

- Gastrointestinal—irritation at low concentration and ulcerations at high concentrations. Salivation, emesis, diarrhea, laryngeal edema, and esophageal strictures may result.
- Skin/exocrine—deep caustic burns to the dermis with prolonged exposure. Burns may not be painful initially due to local anesthetic properties of some phenols.
- Nervous—ataxia, tremors, CNS stimulation or depression, seizures, or coma
- Hepatobiliary—hepatic failure as early as 12 hours postexposure
- Renal—renal failure as early as 12 hours postexposure
- Respiratory—respiratory depression and panting (in dogs) followed by pulmonary edema and cardiac muscle damage. Aspiration pneumonia.
- Cardiovascular—prolonged CRT with very pale to muddy mucous membranes
- Hemic—methemoglobinemia, hemoglobinemia, and Heinz body anemia (especially cats).
- Ophthalmic—ulcers with direct exposure to the cornea

 # SIGNALMENT/HISTORY

Risk Factors

- Compared to dogs, cats develop toxicosis at lower doses due to their limited glucuronide transferase activity.

Historical Findings

- Witnessed ingestion of pine oil/phenol–based products (most common)
- Drooling, gagging, or emesis are typically reported by the owner.
- Chewed mop heads after phenol-based cleaners were used. (Water evaporates faster than phenols resulting in a potentially corrosive concentration of phenols.)
- History of chewing on pine needles/cones
- Pine oil/phenol products applied directly to pets (often by children)
- Animals enclosed in a garage/utility room without other water sources.

Location and Circumstances of Poisoning

- Exposure usually occurs within the home and is rarely intentional.

 # CLINICAL FEATURES

- All chemicals may create deep, penetrating ulcers.
  - Phenols have anesthetic properties that may render the injury initially painless.

- Common clinical signs following oral exposure include drooling, gagging, or vomiting.
- Inhalation may cause tissue irritation/damage leading to dyspnea, panting, and increased respiratory effort.
- CNS abnormalities may develop within 5 minutes of ingestion and 1 hour of dermal exposure.
  - Ataxia, mydriasis, muscle tremors, CNS stimulation or depression, seizures, or coma.
  - Convulsions, coma, or death are most common in the following:
    - □ Significant dermal exposures (>25% body surface area)
    - □ Exposures to highly concentrated products (see Toxicology)
- Hepatic or renal failure may develop within 12–24 hours.
- Animals that remain asymptomatic for 6 hours or more following exposure are not expected to develop clinical signs.

DIFFERENTIAL DIAGNOSIS

- Corrosive injury from acid or alkaline products
- Dermal or GI exposures to other essential oils/liquid potpourri
- Ethylene glycol toxicosis
- Primary renal failure

DIAGNOSTICS

- Diagnosis is usually made based on the history, an odor of the animal's breath or coat, or postmortem evaluation of the liver, kidneys, or GIT.
- A CBC, UA, chemistry panel, and acid/base analysis should be performed upon presentation and again 12–24 hours after the exposure (in symptomatic animals).
  - CBC: hemolysis, Heinz body formation, hemolytic anemia, methemoglobinemia, thrombocytopenia, and Döhle bodies in neutrophils
  - UA: The urine may have a dark green to black discoloration from the passage of phenolic intermediates or due to methemoglobinemia, hematuria, albuminuria, and casts.
  - Chemistry panel: used to establish a baseline (liver, kidneys). Elevation of liver enzymes, BUN, and creatinine may develop 12–24 hours after exposure. The chemistry may show multiple changes such as elevations in CPK, Mg, or K.
  - Acid-base status: metabolic acidosis or a respiratory alkalosis
- Cautious endoscopic examination of the esophagus and stomach to evaluate for ulceration or stricture

- If ocular or respiratory exposure occurred, further diagnostics may include corneal stain/slit lamp examination, thoracic radiographs, arterial blood gas, or bronchoscopy.

Pathological Findings

- Necropsy may reveal an enlarged, congested, and friable liver with hepatocellular necrosis; severe renal proximal tubular and cortical necrosis; pulmonary edema and congestion; a hyperemic gastrointestinal tract; or edema of the cerebral cortices.

 # THERAPEUTICS

- The primary goals of therapy include decontamination, stabilization, correction of laboratory abnormalities, liver and kidney support, and the treatment of corrosive injury.

Detoxification

- Protect human caregivers: Gloves and other protective equipment should be worn to prevent dermal contact.
- Dermal:
  - Blot visible material.
  - Use polyethylene glycol (PEG) 300 or 400 to initially dilute and remove the product. (*Water may increase dermal absorption and is not recommended.*) Follow this by washing the animal with a mild liquid dishwashing detergent and then rinse with water.
  - If PEG is not available, isopropyl alcohol can be used on small areas. Alternatively, use liquid dishwashing detergents and copious amounts of water.
    - □ Lavage the skin until the smell of the product has gone away.
    - □ Multiple reapplications of soap and water will be needed.
    - □ Monitor body temperature.
- GI:
  - Do not induce emesis (risk of corrosive injury and aspiration).
  - Activated charcoal: not proven to bind pine oil but may have some benefit against phenols. It is not often recommended because of the risk of vomiting.
  - Pine oil: If the pet is presented within 1 hour of a large ingestion, gastric lavage with an inflated endotracheal tube is recommended, provided no tissue damage is present.
  - Phenol: Because phenols are highly corrosive, gastric lavage could increase the risk of ulceration and stricture. The decision to lavage should be made

based on the amount ingested and the concentration of that product. If gastric lavage is not indicated, dilute the product with water or saline and prevent emesis.
- Some sources recommend oral mineral oil (10 mL/kg lavage) to dilute (vs. water).
- Ocular: Flush the eye for 20 minutes with tepid water or saline.

Appropriate Health Care

- Stabilize:
  - If hydration or tissue perfusion is inadequate, provide a balanced electrolyte solution IV.
  - Evaluate neurological activity. For seizures, give diazepam 0.25–1 mg/kg IV or phenobarbital 2–5 mg/kg IV (increase if needed).
  - Evaluate body temperature. Slowly return to normal using standard methods.
- Address blood work abnormalities:
  - Correct acid/base imbalances. Metabolic acidosis should be alleviated with sodium bicarbonate administration if pH is less than 7.2.
  - Methemoglobinemia
    - Methylene blue 1–4 mg/kg slowly IV in dogs or 1.5 mg/kg slowly IV in cats one time. Use cautiously.
    - Ascorbic acid 20–50 mg/kg PO in dogs or 20 mg/kg PO in cats
- Support the liver and kidney:
  - Intravenous fluids—since metabolic acidosis is common, consider a non-acidic fluid such as saline or Normasol-R.
  - Supportive medications for the liver have been tried with varying success.
    - SAMe: loading dose of 40 mg/kg PO q 24 hours 2–4 days, then 20 mg/kg PO q 24 hours. Give on an empty stomach.
    - N-acetylcysteine: loading dose of 140 mg/kg PO or IV as a 5% solution, then 70 mg/kg q 4–6 hours
- Treat ulcerations:
  - Topical therapy (triple antibiotic ointment or silversulfadiazine cream) and bandaging (bandages to prevent soiling or wet to dry bandages pending severity)
  - Antibiotics for gastrointestinal or dermal lesions
    - Metronidazole 15 mg/kg PO or IV q 12 hours
    - Cephalexin 22 mg/kg PO q 8 hours or cefazolin 22 mg/kg IV q 8 hours
  - GI ulcerations
    - H_2 blockers (e.g., famotidine 0.5 mg/kg IV, IM, or SQ q 12 hours)
    - Sucralfate 0.25–1 g PO on an empty stomach q 8 hours

- Consider anti-inflammatory therapy, but use cautiously and weigh against risk of worsening GI ulcerations.
    - Carprofen 2.2 mg/kg PO or SQ q 12 hours
    - Prednisone 0.5 mg/kg PO or dexamethasone 0.5 mg/kg SQ or IV. Use is controversial.
- Analgesia. Although these chemicals often have an initial anesthetic effect, it is short-lived, and discomfort from oral, gastric, or dermal ulceration should be controlled with opiate therapy.
    - Buprenorphine 0.005 mg/kg IV, IM, or SQ q 8–12 hours
    - Tramadol 1–4 mg/kg PO q 8 hours

Drug(s) and Antidotes of Choice

- No antidote exists.
- See Appropriate Health Care

Precautions/Interactions

- Methylene blue—May affect accuracy of urinalysis due to green/blue discoloration of urine. May also increase Heinz body formation. Use is controversial.

Nursing Care

- The patient must be kept clean to prevent infection of dermal ulcerations.
- Body temperature should be monitored closely, especially after bathing.

Follow-up

- Patient will require regular evaluation of skin ulcerations until healed. Recheck initial ulcerations 2–5 days after flushing, then as needed pending progression.
- Continue to recheck liver and kidney values q 24–48 hours while hospitalized or until they return to normal and the patient is stable.
- Esophageal ulcers may take weeks to heal. Also, it takes weeks to months before clinical evidence of a stricture may be noted. Repeated esophageal endoscopy is recommended to follow progress.

Diet

- NPO for up to 72 hours after ingestion if oropharyngeal damage is severe and patient can tolerate fasting. Obese cats should not be fasted for greater than 24 hours. Consider feeding a liquid diet while ulcerations heal. Consider stomach tube placement if eating is painful. Diet modification may be needed if renal or liver failure develops.

Activity

- No changes needed

Surgical Considerations

- Endoscopy may be needed to determine the full extent of gastrointestinal damage or to remove pinecones or pine needles lodged in the stomach. Careful consideration of anesthetic protocol, coupled with recent renal and liver chemistry evaluation, is needed.
- Endoscopy should be done carefully as tissues may be fragile and risk of perforation is high.
- Surgical correction of gastrointestinal perforation may be needed.

Prevention

- Do not prescribe pine oil–based insecticides to cats, and caution owners not to use canine products on cats.
- See Client Education

Public Health

- Humans can absorb these chemicals from the skin, eyes, and gastrointestinal tract. Protect caregivers from accidental exposure to contaminated vomit or skin. If an exposure does occur, clean the area immediately, flush with PEG solution or water, and contact a human poison control center for further recommendations.
- Death has occurred in children following accidental ingestion of pine oil, phenol, and phenolic derivatives.

 COMMENTS

- Animals that remain asymptomatic for 6 hours or more following exposure are not expected to develop clinical signs. Their prognosis is excellent.

Client Education

- Do not allow pets to have access to products that contain phenol or pine oil.
- Secure used mops or mop water out of the reach of children and pets. Rinse mops well before drying.
- Even if pet makes a full recovery, subclinical damage may have been done to the liver or kidneys.

Patient Monitoring

- If liver or renal disease, methemoglobinemia, or metabolic acidosis occurs, hospitalization until resolution is recommended.
- Chemistry panel and CBC should be checked every 24–48 hours pending the severity and clinical course.

▪ Blood pH will need to be reevaluated frequently during treatment with sodium bicarbonate, then rechecked 12–24 hours later to ensure stability.

Possible Complications

▪ Liver failure/necrosis, renal failure/necrosis, methemoglobinemia, metabolic acidosis, esophageal strictures, GI perforation with septic peritonitis, and aspiration pneumonia
▪ Pine needle or pinecone foreign body.

Expected Course and Prognosis

▪ Prognosis for cats exposed to phenol/phenolic derivatives is poor; that for pine oil is guarded. Small ingestions can quickly result in rapidly progressive signs and require aggressive medical intervention. Even with excellent medical management, death from liver or renal necrosis can occur.
▪ Most dogs recover uneventfully.

Synonyms

Pine oil: alpha terpineol, arizole, oleum abietis, terpentinoel, unipine, yarmor

Phenol: benzenol, carbolic acid, carbolic oil, fenosmolin, fenosmoline, hydroxybenzene, monohydroxybenzene, monophenol, oxybenzene, phenic acid, phenol alcohol, phenyl alcohol, phenyl hydrate, phenyl hydroxide, phenylic acid , phenylic alcohol

Phenolic derivatives: cade oil, chlorinated phenols, creosote, creosol, coal tar, cresolic acid, hexachlorophene, hydroquinone, juniper tar (*Juniperus oxycedrus*), paraphenol, phenylphenol, phlorglucinol, pyrocatechol, pyrogallol, resorcin, resorcinol, sulfurated phenols, xylenol

Abbreviations

BUN = blood urea nitrogen
CBC = complete blood count
CNS = central nervous system
CPK = creatinine phosphokinase
CRT = capillary refill time
GI   = gastrointestinal
GIT   = gastrointestinal tract
IV   = intravenous
K   = potassium
LD_{50} = median lethal dose
Mg   = magnesium
MOA = mechanism of action

NPO = *nil per os* (nothing by mouth)
PEG = polyethylene glycol
PO   = *per os* (by mouth)
q   = every
SAMe = S-adenosyl-L-methionine
UA   = urinalysis

See Also

Acids
Alkalis
Essential Oils/Liquid Potpourri
Tea Tree Oil/Melaleuca Oil

Suggested Reading

Chan TY, Sung JJ, Crichley JA. Chemical gastro-oesophagitis, upper gastrointestinal haemorrhage and gastroscopic findings following Dettol poisoning. Hum Exp Toxicol 1995; 14:18–19.

Coppock RW, Mostrom MS, Lillie MS, Lillie LE. The toxicology of detergents, bleaches, antiseptics, and disinfectants in small animals. Vet Hum Topical 1988; 30:463–473.

Debone R, Lasting G. Phenolic household disinfectant: further precautions required. Burns 1997; 23:182–185.

Oehme FW, Kore AM. Miscellaneous indoor toxicants. In: Peterson ME, Talcott PA, eds. Small Animal Toxicology, 2nd ed. St. Louis: Elsevier, 2006; p 223.

Pine Oil. In: POISINDEX® System [Internet database]. Thompson Healthcare. Updated periodically. Available at http://www.thomsonhc.com/hcs/librarian/ND_T/HCS/ND_CPR/ToxicSubstanceLists/ND_PR/Toxicology/CS/DB47B1/DUPLICATIONSHIELDSYNC/11DFB5/ND_PG/PRIH/ND_B/HCS/ND_P/Toxicology/PFActionId/hcs.common.RetrieveDocumentCommon/DocId/345/ContentSetId/51#TopOfPage. Accessed Jan 31, 2010.

Phenol and Related Agents. In: POISINDEX® System [Internet database]. Thompson Healthcare. Updated periodically. Available at http://www.thomsonhc.com/hcs/librarian/ND_T/HCS/ND_CPR/ToxicSubstanceLists/ND_PR/Toxicology/CS/4E4D7C/DUPLICATIONSHIELDSYNC/5DB9FF/ND_PG/PRIH/ND_B/HCS/ND_P/Toxicology/PFActionId/hcs.common.RetrieveDocumentCommon/DocId/40/ContentSetId/51#TopOfPage. Accessed Jan 31, 2010.

Rousseax CG, Smith RA. Acute pinesol toxicity in a domestic cat. Vet Hum Toxicol 1986; 28:316–317.

Welker JA, Zaloga GP. Pine oil ingestion: a common cause of poisoning. Chest 1999; 116:1822–1826.

Author: Catherine Angle, DVM, MPH; Ahna G. Brutlag, DVM
Consulting Editor: Ahna G. Brutlag, DVM

Soaps, Detergents, Fabric Softeners, Enzymatic Cleaners, and Deodorizers

chapter 79

DEFINITION/OVERVIEW

- Soaps, detergents, fabric softeners, and enzymatic cleaners are composed mainly of anionic, cationic, nonionic, or amphoteric surfactants. Some also contain builders such as complex phosphates, sodium carbonate, and sodium silicate; or enzymes such as proteases, amylases, or lipases. Deodorizers and soaps contain perfume oils, and select products contain alcohol(s) (e.g., alcohol ethoxylate, ethanol, isopropanol).
- Most of these products can cause a variety of clinical symptoms but generally produce a low level of toxicity in veterinary species. The exceptions are the cationic detergents and automatic dishwashing detergents (ADWD).
- Clinical signs of toxicity from these products include nausea, vomiting, diarrhea, drooling, or more serious but uncommon complications such as CNS depression, renal insufficiency, oral or esophageal burns, GI bleeds, convulsions, and coma.

ETIOLOGY/PATHOPHYSIOLOGY

Mechanism of Action

- With polar and nonpolar ends, surfactants reduce water surface tension, thus allowing surfaces to be wet more efficiently.
- Builders reduce water hardness, emulsify grease and oil, and maintain alkalinity. High concentrations of certain builders (e.g., trisodium phosphate) bind up calcium and can cause hypocalcemia.
- With catalytic action, enzymes in enzymatic cleaners break down organic stains to enhance cleaning efficacy. Enzymes cause release of bradykinin and histamine, resulting in dermal irritation and possible respiratory sensitization/bronchospasm if inhaled.
- ADWD cause toxicity through a direct effect on tissue and may lead to necrosis. Muscle weakness and paralysis can result from the ganglion-blocking and curare-like activity of quaternary ammonium compounds.

Pharmacokinetics/Absorption, Distribution, Metabolism, Excretion

- These products produce their effects on GI mucosa and are generally well absorbed, with peak levels 1 hour postingestion. Dermal irritant effects can occur almost immediately.
- Topical absorption is limited with ≤1% absorption in some cases.
- Surfactants are metabolized in the liver, and resulting metabolites are excreted mainly in the urine and minimally in feces.

Toxicity

- Cationic surfactants are the most toxic, followed by anionic surfactants, and then nonionic and amphoteric surfactants. See table 79.1 for a list of common surfactants.
  - Animals licking or grooming skin surfaces exposed to cationic detergents may develop toxicity.
  - Products containing >7.5% cationic surfactants may be corrosive and cause serious complications. Fatalities have been reported from >20% dermal exposure to cationic products.

TABLE 79.1. Common surfactants.

Anionic

- Alkyl sodium sulfate
- Alkyl sodium sulfonate
- Dioctyl sodium sulfosuccinate
- Linear alkyl benzene sulfonate
- Sodium lauryl sulfate
- Tetrapropylene benzene sulfonate

Nonionic

- Alkyl ethoxylate
- Alkyl phenoxy polyethoxy ethanols
- Polyethylene glycol stearate

Cationic

- Quaternary ammonium compounds
  - Benzalkonium chloride
  - Benzethonium chloride
- Pyridinium compounds
  - Cetylpyridinium chloride
- Quinolinium compounds
  - Dequalinium chloride

Amphoteric

- Imidazolines
- Betaines

- There is risk of corrosive damage at pH <2 or pH >12, but pH should not be the only determining factor, especially with the cationic detergents where the pH may be neutral or only slightly alkaline.
- LD_{50} mouse (oral): 1400–4600 mg/kg (anionic and nonionic detergents)
- LD_{50} rat (oral): 420 mg/kg (cationic detergents)

■ Personal care soap, hand dishwashing soaps, laundry detergents, deodorizers, and enzymatic cleaners may be irritants causing nausea, vomiting, and diarrhea.

■ Median emetic dose in dogs (oral): 6–25 mg/kg (laundry products)

■ Builders are irritants at low concentrations but corrosive at high concentrations.

■ Perfume oils and alcohols cause irritant effects and drying/defatting of skin.

■ Fatal automatic dishwashing detergent dose in dogs is 500–2500 mg/kg.

Systems Affected

■ Gastrointestinal—nausea, vomiting, diarrhea, and gastritis are common. There is potential for corrosive injury leading to drooling, dysphagia, epigastric pain, and bleeding from cationic surfactants and highly concentrated products.

■ Skin—dryness, dermatitis, and irritation. Hair loss, chemical burns, and necrosis are uncommon except with high concentration cationic surfactants and ADWD.

■ Respiratory—coughing, stridor, dyspnea, and respiratory muscle paralysis (with severe exposures to cationic surfactants)

■ Ophthalmic—conjunctive erythema, irritation, pain, stinging, tearing, and potentially corneal damage

■ Cardiovascular—hypotension and shock (only in severe exposures with cationic surfactants)

■ Nervous—lethargy, CNS depression, coma (severe poisoning), and seizures (cationic surfactants)

■ Endocrine/metabolic—metabolic acidosis (severe poisoning)

■ Hemic/immune—hypersensitivity reactions and intravascular hemolysis (rare)

 # SIGNALMENT/HISTORY

■ Any age or breed of animal can be affected.

Risk Factors

■ Preexisting liver disease may slow metabolism of surfactants.

■ Preexisting chronic skin conditions (e.g., allergic dermatitis) may be exacerbated.

■ Preexisting respiratory illnesses (e.g., asthma) may be exacerbated.

Historical Findings

- Exposures to these products is frequently but not always witnessed. Discovery of spilled detergent, soap, or enzymatic cleaners, or chewed-up bars of soap or fabric softeners, is common.

 # CLINICAL FEATURES

- **Ingestion:** Initial clinical signs of nausea, vomiting, or diarrhea and drooling are immediate and common. As toxicity with cationic or other corrosive products progresses, lethargy, vocalization, stridor, or dysphagia may occur. Oral or esophageal burns, with bleeding, are possible. Serious but uncommon systemic symptoms include restlessness, CNS depression, renal insufficiency, convulsions, and coma.
- **Inhalation/aspiration of powdered products or mist deodorizers:** Initially, coughing, shortness of breath, drooling, stridor, and retractions. As toxicity progresses, respiratory depression or airway compromise may occur but are unlikely with acute exposure.
- **Ocular exposure:** Initially, irritation, redness, and tearing. With delays in treatment and highly concentrated products, there is an increased risk of corneal damage from cationic surfactants and more corrosive products.
- **Dermal exposure:** initial signs of irritation, pruritis, and erythema, but more serious dermal necrosis with some highly concentrated cationic detergents
- Fatalities are usually associated with respiratory failure, aspiration, asphyxia, and corrosive gastrointestinal injuries resulting from ingestion.

 # DIFFERENTIAL DIAGNOSIS

- Toxicities
  - Pesticides
  - Bleaches (notably, highly concentrated or "ultra" bleaches)
  - Corrosives
- Primary hypersensitivity to topical products
- Primary respiratory disease

 # DIAGNOSTICS

- Diagnosis should be made based on patient history, physical examination, symptoms, and clinical suspicion. No specific laboratory testing is useful in confirming the diagnosis.
- Endoscopy should be performed within 12–24 hours of cationic surfactant ingestion if signs of tissue injury are present (drooling, stridor, anorexia, etc.).

- Animals with respiratory symptoms should be evaluated with a thoracic radiograph.

Pathological Findings

- Gross examination at necropsy may reveal mucosal ulceration in fatal cases of corrosive product ingestion.
- There are no specific histopathologic findings associated with soap, detergent, fabric softener, enzymatic cleaner, or deodorizer toxicity.

 # THERAPEUTICS

- Treatment and care following exposures to most soaps, hand dishwashing soaps, detergents, laundry detergents, and deodorizers can be handled at home.
- Goals of treatment include removal from exposure site, prevention of further absorption, and providing necessary supportive and symptomatic care.
- Emesis is not generally indicated or necessary (see Detoxification).
- Exposure to cationic surfactants and ADWD should be carefully evaluated and assessed for potential corrosive and systemic toxicity.
  - Minimal ingestions of low concentrations of cationic detergents (<7.5%) can be handled similarly to hand dishwashing soaps and laundry detergents.
  - Sizable ingestions of cationic detergents, especially with concentrations >7.5%, should be handled as corrosive exposures.

Detoxification

- Emesis is not generally indicated or necessary.
- Evacuation of stomach contents should be considered only when product ingredients, history, and assessment indicate a high potential for serious systemic toxicity.
- Emesis may be induced if the animal has not spontaneously vomited within 30 minutes after ingestion of >20 g/kg of a noncorrosive product.
- Ocular: Flush the eyes with normal saline (preferred) or room temp water for ≥20 minutes or until the pH of conjunctival sac is 8 or less (for alkaline exposures). If ocular irritation progresses for >2 hours, if the product's pH >12, if cationic concentration is >2% or if an ADWD is involved, the animal should be referred to an ophthalmic specialist.
- Dermal: Irrigate the exposed topical area(s) for ≥10 minutes with room temp water (initially use soap in cases of deodorizer or cationic product exposure).

Appropriate Health Care

- Maintain vital functions: Secure and protect airway, supply oxygen, and provide respiratory supportive care as needed.

- Aggressively monitor and replace fluids and electrolytes when necessary.
- Ingestion:
  - Oral dilution with water or milk
  - Monitor for GI bleeding.
  - If excessive vomiting and/or diarrhea occur, consider an antiemetic or antidiarrheal as needed.
  - In cases with a significant potential for gastritis, corrosive injury, or GI bleeding, NSAIDs should be avoided.
- Inhalation of powder or deodorizer mist:
  - No treatment usually necessary other than monitoring for symptom development
  - Oral or IV corticosteroids (e.g., prednisone 1–2 mg/kg PO q 12–24 hours or dexamethasone 0.5–1 mg/kg IV or IM, dogs) and inhaled beta$_2$ agonists (e.g., albuterol 0.05 mg/kg PO q 8 hours, dogs) may help control bronchospasm.
  - Analgesic administration as needed following exposure (e.g., buprenorphine 0.005–0.02 mg/kg IV, IM, SQ q 6–12 hours)

Drug(s) of Choice

- There are no known effective antidotes.

Precautions/Interactions

- Do NOT try to neutralize the exposure with additional chemicals.
- Do not orally dilute with large volumes of water postingestion as this may increase the risk of vomiting, "sudsing," and aspiration.
- Avoid topical oil-based creams, lotions, or ointments if exposed to potentially corrosive products.
- Do not induce emesis or administer activated charcoal if you suspect ingestion of a corrosive product (cationic concentration >7.5% or ADWD) or if vomiting has already occurred.
- Be alert to interactions with strong oxidizers, strong reducing agents, strong acids, and metals.
- In cases with a significant potential for gastritis, corrosive injury, or GI bleeding, NSAIDs should be avoided.

Alternative Drugs

- Ingestion of sizable quantities of phosphate-containing products may require treatment with sevelamer or another oral phosphate–binding medication. Monitor blood levels of calcium, magnesium, and phosphorous until symptoms have abated.

- Calcium gluconate 10% solution (0.5–1.5 mL/kg IV, slowly over 15–30 min) or calcium chloride 10% (0.15–0.50 mL/kg IV, slowly) is indicated as needed for hypocalcemia following ingestion of builder-containing detergents.
- Animal studies have shown corticosteroid (prednisone 0.25–0.5 mg/kg PO q 24 hours x 3–5 days, then q 48 hours x 2 weeks) and prophylactic antibiotic treatment within 48 hours of exposure or ingestion to be helpful in cases of severe burns or esophageal injury.
- Topical hydrocortisone cream, aloe vera gel, lotion, and cold packs are additional options for dermal relief.
- Seizures should be controlled with anticonvulsants (e.g., diazepam 0.5–1mg/kg IV to effect).

Diet

- If the animal is vomiting or unconscious, keep NPO until signs resolve.

Activity

- Base on signs and severity of exposure.

Surgical Considerations

- Surgical resection of damaged tissue in cases of severe corrosive damage.
- Severely injured patients may need PEG tube placement for nutritional support.

 COMMENTS

Client Education

- Readmit patient if pain or signs return/worsen despite appropriate treatment or if the animal is not eating and drinking.

Patient Monitoring

- Monitor electrolytes, fluids, and acid-base status postingestion.
- Monitor 6–8 hours postvomiting for signs of aspiration, coughing, gagging, or stridor.
- Monitor for intravascular hemolysis. If this occurs, monitor renal function and PCV/TS.
- Monitor serum calcium levels following ingestion of detergents containing builders.
- Monitor respiratory signs for up to 12 hours postinhalation.

Prevention/Avoidance

- Prevent access to products in the home, particularly while cleaning or doing laundry.

Possible Complications

- Aspiration postvomiting
- Irreversible ocular damage, changes in vision
- Development of esophageal or intestinal strictures
- Intravascular hemolysis, though uncommon, may occur, especially in animals with liver disease.

Expected Course and Prognosis

- Prognosis depends mainly on the specific ingredients, product pH, concentration, and quantity of exposure (see Toxicology).
- For animals with exposure to personal care soap, hand dishwashing detergent, laundry detergent, deodorizers, enzymatic cleaners, and other noncorrosive products, the prognosis is generally excellent and the course uneventful.
- For animals with clinical signs such as hypotension, CNS depression, coma, seizures, necrosis, GI bleeds, metabolic acidosis, or dysphagia, the prognosis is guarded. The animal should be monitored for stricture development.

Synonyms

air fresheners, surfactants, builders

Abbreviations

ADWD = automatic dishwashing detergents
CNS   = central nervous system
GI   = gastrointestinal
IM   = intramuscular
IV   = intravenous
LD_{50} = median lethal dose
NPO   = *nil per os* (nothing by mouth)
NSAID = nonsteroidal anti-inflammatory drugs
PCV   = packed cell volume
PEG   = percutaneous endoscopic gastrostomy
PO   = *per os* (by mouth)
q   = every
SQ   = subcutaneous
TS   = total solids

See Also

Acids
Alkalis
Essential Oils/Liquid Potpourri

Suggested Reading

DiCarlo MA. Scientific reviews. Household products: a review. Vet Human Toxicol 2003; 45(2):256–261.

Gfeller RW, Messonnier SP. Handbook of Small Animal Toxicology and Poisonings, 2nd ed. St. Louis: Mosby/Elsevier, 2004; pp. 125–126, 151–156, 299–300.

Oehme FW, Kore AM. Miscellaneous indoor toxicants. In: Peterson ME, Talcott PA, eds. Small Animal Toxicology, 2nd ed. St. Louis: Elsevier, 2006; 223.

Sioris LJ, Schuller HK. Soaps, detergents, and bleaches. In: Shannon MW, Borron SW, Burns MJ, eds. Haddad and Winchester's Clinical Management of Poisoning and Drug Overdose, 4th ed. Philadelphia: Saunders/Elsevier, 2007; p. 1443.

Authors: Leo J. Sioris, PharmD; Lauren E. Haak, PharmD
Consulting Editor: Ahna G. Brutlag, DVM

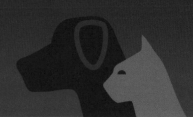

Insecticides and Molluscacides

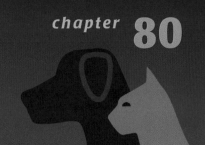

chapter 80

Amitraz

DEFINITION/OVERVIEW

- Amitraz is a formamidine derivative insecticide which is used as an acaracide and immiticide in veterinary medicine.
- Product is available in various forms and concentrations, including powders, collars, sprays, dips, and topicals for both companion animals and industrial and agricultural use.
- The most common trade names include Amitraz, Francodex, Mitaban, Mitac, Mitacur, Ovasyn, Preventic, Taktic, Triatox, and Zema.
- Exposures are often due to animals' ingesting collars or from product misuse.
- Clinical signs depend on the route of toxicosis. Topical overdose usually results in transient sedation lasting from 48 to 72 hours. The signs associated with oral exposure are more severe and include depression, head pressing, ataxia, seizures, coma, ileus, diarrhea, vomiting, hypersalivation, polyuria, hypothermia, bradycardia, hyper- or hypotension, and mydriasis.

ETIOLOGY/PATHOPHYSIOLOGY

Mechanism of Action

- Amitraz is a diamide topical parasiticide with a poorly understood mechanism of action.
- It primarily acts as a CNS alpha$_2$-adrenergic agonist and as a weak monoamine oxidase inhibitor (MAOI).
- Other suspected actions include a mild serotonin and antiplatelet effect.

Pharmacokinetics/Absorption, Distribution, Metabolism, and Excretion

- The pharmacologic action of amitraz is not well understood in veterinary patients but is well documented in human patients. Animals do appear to follow human models closely.
- Rapidly absorbed orally, taking as little as 30 minutes to 2 hours to produce signs
- Dermal absorption is minimal, although some healthy animals dipped in amitraz have developed toxicosis.

- Tissues found to contain the highest concentrations of amitraz are bile, the liver, the eye, and the intestines.
- Metabolized in the liver to active and inactive metabolites
- Metabolites are excreted primarily in urine; some fecal excretion occurs.

Toxicity

- LD_{50} PO in dogs: 100 mg/kg
- 4 mg/kg/day PO for 90 days in beagles resulted in CNS depression, ataxia, hypothermia, hyperglycemia, and increased pulse rates. No dogs died during the study.
- Toxicosis associated with ingestion of amitraz-containing collars is significant in all species studied.

Systems Affected

- CNS—depression, ataxia, coma, seizures
- Gastrointestinal—bloat or ileus secondary to anticholinergic-like effects, hypersalivation, vomiting, diarrhea
- Cardiovascular—hypertension or hypotension, bradycardia secondary to alpha$_2$-adrenergic receptor activity
- Endocrine/metabolic—hyperglycemia, presumably by inhibiting insulin release; hypothermia (or hyperthermia)
- Respiratory—respiratory depression due to depression of the respiratory center of the brain
- Ophthalmic—mydriasis due to alpha$_2$-adrenergic receptor activity
- Renal/urologic—polyuria may result at higher overdoses due to suppression of ADH.
- Hemic/lymphatic/immune—DIC secondary to severe hyperthermia from prolonged seizures/tremors

 # SIGNALMENT/HISTORY

- All breeds of dogs are affected. Toy breeds are reported to be more susceptible to the CNS effects.
- Cats are very sensitive to toxicosis and develop signs at much lower doses.

Risk Factors

- Amitraz is contraindicated for canine patients ≤4 months of age.
- Geriatric and debilitated animals are at greater risk of toxicosis even at normal doses.
- Amitraz is not suitable for patients with seizure disorders as it may potentially lower the seizure threshold.

Historical Findings

- History of exposure, which may be witnessed. Pet owners may find chewed amitraz collars in the household, along with symptomatic pets if enough time has elapsed.
- Owners may be directly responsible for toxicosis in their feline or rabbit pets when canine products are inadvertently or inappropriately applied.

Location and Circumstances of Poisoning

- Exposures generally occur in the home due to unsecured products or via direct application.
- The potential does exist for exposures in the farm environment due to its use in agriculture.

Interactions with Drugs, Nutrients or Environment

- Corticosteroids and other immune-suppressing drugs (e.g., azathioprine, cyclophosphamide)
- MAOI (e.g., selegiline) and those with MAOI-type activity
- Tricyclic antidepressants (e.g., amitriptyline and clomipramine)
- SSRIs (e.g., fluoxetine and fluvoxamine)
- Atypical antipsychotic agents
- Anesthetic drugs with known adrenergic activity (e.g., xylazine or medetomidine)
- Cats ingesting amitraz should not have emesis induced with xylaxine due to risks of severe CNS depression with secondary aspiration pneumonia.

 # CLINICAL FEATURES

- Onset of signs generally occurs within 30 minutes to 2 hours after ingestion although they may be delayed for up to 10–12 hours.
- Animals generally present with CNS depression, tremors, ataxia, and GI signs (including hypersalivation and bloat). Hypothermia or hyperthermia may also be present.
- Some pets may present seizuring or with an owner history of having seized. They are often mydriatic.
- The duration of clinical signs is generally quite long (3–7 days) if reversal agents have not been used.

 # DIFFERENTIAL DIAGNOSIS

- Toxicities
  - 5-HTP
  - Atypical antipsychotic agents

- Benzodiazepines
- Imidazoline
- Methionine
- Tremorgenic mycotoxins
- Nicotine
- SSRIs
- TCAs
- Primary or secondary neurologic disease
- Primary metabolic disease (e.g., renal, hepatic, hypoglycemia)

 # DIAGNOSTICS

- ECG and blood pressure monitoring for bradycardia and hypotension
- Baseline chemistry, including renal values and CBC, should be performed.
- Monitor blood glucose levels frequently, especially for those patients that are known diabetics.

Pathological Findings

- None specific

 # THERAPEUTICS

Detoxification

- Induction of emesis is not recommended in animals with clinical signs.
- If the patient is asymptomatic in the early stages of ingestion or does not pose an aspiration hazard at the time of veterinary evaluation, a one-time dose of activated charcoal (with a cathartic) may be administered.
- If the patient is stable and if exposure was topical, decontaminate with warm water and dish detergent to remove the product.
- Ingested collars or collar pieces will need to be removed (e.g., surgery, endoscopy).

Appropriate Health Care

- Frequent monitoring of TPR is imperative.

Drug(s) and Antidotes of Choice

- No specific antidotes are available; however, alpha$_2$-adrenergic antagonists may be helpful in these cases. They enjoy a broad range of safety but may have to be administered multiple times during the course of treatment as their half-life may not be as long as the amitraz agent that the clinician is seeking to reverse.
  - Atipamezole (Antisedan) 50 µg/kg IM may be used to reverse severe sedation and bradycardia.

- Yohimbine 0.1 mg/kg IV may be used to reverse severe sedation and bradycardia.
- Crystalloid IV fluids should be administered to help maintain hydration and treat hypotension. Important to note that diuresis does not speed elimination, and fluids are strictly to aid in support of the cardiovascular system.
- If the patient remains hypotensive, additional therapy may be necessary, including colloid therapy (Hetastarch) and/or vasopressor therapy.
- Tremors/seizures may be treated with diazepam or barbiturates, but the lowest effective dose should be used due to severe sedation.
  - Diazepam 0.1–0.25 mg/kg, IV to effect PRN
  - Phenobarbital 2–4 mg/kg, IV to effect PRN
- If vomiting is protracted, consider antiemetic therapy:
  - Ondansetron 0.1–0.2 mg/kg SQ, IV q 8–12 hours
  - Maropitant 1 mg/kg SQ q 24 hours
  - Metoclopramide 0.2–0.5 mg/kg SQ, IM q 8–12 hours

Precautions/Interactions

- Clinicians should not use xylazine or medetomidine as emetic agents in patients exposed to amitraz.
- Atropine should not be used for treatment of bradycardia, as it may exacerbate hypertension and GI stasis.

Follow-up

- Generally minimal in uncomplicated cases once signs have resolved

Diet

- Animal may return to normal diet at discharge or may be given several days of bland diet if GI irritation is persistent.

Activity

- Patient should be kept quiet and secure while symptomatic but may return to normal activity with successful resolution of the case.

Surgical Considerations

- Endoscopic or surgical removal of amitraz-containing collars is necessary.

 COMMENTS

Client Education

- Secure all medications where they cannot be accessed by pets or children.

Patient Monitoring

- Observation may be required for as long as 24–72 hours. More severe cases may persist for 5–7 days.

Possible Complications

- Animals allowed to tremor or seizure for prolonged periods of time can potentially develop myoglobinuric renal failure and DIC if symptoms are not controlled.
- Equids that develop ileus secondary to amitraz toxicosis are prone to a poorer prognosis.

Expected Course of Prognosis

- Generally good if treated early. Animals exhibiting CNS symptoms generally have a poorer prognosis.

Synonyms

N,N-(methyliminodimethylidyne) bis-2,4-xylidine; N'-(2,4-Dimethylphenyl)-N-[(2,4-dimethylphenyl)iminomethyl]-N-methylmethanimidamide; N,N' ((Methylimino)dimethylidyne) di-2,4-xylidine, 2-methyl-1,3-di(2,4-xylylimino)-2-azapropane; ENT 27967; BTS 27419; U-36059; CAS 33089-61-1; BAAM, BTS 27419; methylmethanimidamide; 1,5 di(2,4-dimethylphenyl)-3-methyl-1,3,5-, trizapenta-1,4-diene

Abbreviations

5-HTP = 5-hydroxytryptophan
ADH = antidiuretic hormone
CBC = complete blood count
CNS = central nervous system
DIC = disseminated intravascular coagulation
ECG = electrocardiogram
GI = gastrointestinal
IM = intramuscular
IV = intravenous
MAOI = monoamine oxidase inhibitor
q = every
PO = *per os* (by mouth)
PRN = *pro re nata* (as needed)
SQ = subcutaneous
SSRI = selective serotonin reuptake inhibitor
TCA = tri-cyclic antidepressant
TPR = temperature, pulse, respiration

See Also

Atyical Antipyschotics
Benzodiazepines
Methionine
Selective Serotonin Reuptake Inhibitors (SSRIs)

Suggested Reading

Andrade SF, Sakate M. The comparative efficacy of yohimbine and atipamezole to treat amitraz intoxication in dogs. Vet Hum Toxicol 2003; 45(3):124–127.
Demirel YA, Yilmaz S, Gursoy K, et al. Acute amitraz intoxication: retrospective analysis of 45 cases. Hum Experiml Tox 2006; 25: 613–617.
Gupta RC. Veterinary Toxicology Basic and Clinical Principles. New York: Academic, 2007.
Hellmann KK, Adler L, Parker K, et al. Evaluation of the efficacy and safety of a novel formulation of metaflumizone plus amitraz in dogs naturally infested with fleas and ticks in Europe. Vet Parasit 2007; 150:239–245.
Oglesby PA, Joubert KE, Meiring R. Canine renal cortical necrosis and haemorrhage following ingestion of an amitraz formulated insecticide dip. J S Afr Vet Assoc 2006; 77(3):160–163.

Author: Nancy M. Gruber, DVM
Consulting Editors: Justine A. Lee, DVM, DACVECC; Lynn R. Hovda, DVM, MS, DACVIM; Gary D. Osweiler, DVM, PhD, DABVT

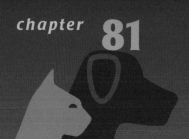

chapter 81

Metaldehyde Snail and Slug Bait

DEFINITION/OVERVIEW

- Metaldehyde is a polycyclic polymer of acetaldehyde.
- Primarily affects the CNS
- Ingredient of slug and snail baits; also used as solid fuel for some camp stoves and is marketed as a color flame tablet for party goods
- Snail and slug baits
  - Purchased as liquids, granules, wettable powders, or pelleted baits
  - May also contain other toxicants such as arsenate or insecticides

ETIOLOGY/PATHOPHYSIOLOGY

Mechanism of Action

- The exact mechanism is unknown.
  - It has been proposed that metaldehyde is converted to acetaldehyde after ingestion and that acetaldehyde is the primary toxic agent.
  - However, acetaldehyde was not found in the serum of rats during a dosing study and the authors recommended that this theory be reevaluated.
- Recent evidence suggests that metaldehyde may increase excitatory neurotransmitters or decrease inhibitory neurotransmitters; seizure threshold may be decreased.
  - Decreased levels of GABA, NE, and 5-HT are found in experimental mice.
  - MAO concentrations increased in treated mice.
- Metabolic acidosis and hyperthermia may be additional factors in clinical effects.

Pharmacokinetics/Absorption, Distribution, Metabolism, and Excretion

- Low water solubility
- Hydrolyzed, in part, in acid environment of the stomach
- Likely metabolized and detoxified by cytochrome P450
- Acetaldehyde is metabolized to carbon dioxide and eliminated by the lungs.
- Urinary excretion as metaldehyde is less than 1% of dose.

Toxicity

- LD_{50} values
  - Canine LD_{50}: 210–600 mg/kg BW
  - Feline LD_{50}: 207 mg/kg BW
  - Rabbit LD_{50}: 290–1250 mg/kg BW
  - Guinea pig LD_{50}: 175–700 mg/kg BW
- Bait concentration ranges from 2.75% to 3.25%.
- At 210 mg/kg (lowest canine LD_{50}) and 3.25% bait, dosage for LD_{50} is 6.5 grams bait/kg BW.

Systems Affected

- Neuromuscular—seizures and muscle tremors
- Hepatobiliary—delayed hepatotoxicosis has been reported but is not common.
- Multiple organ failure is possible secondary to convulsions and hyperthermia.

 SIGNALMENT/HISTORY

Risk Factors

- Increased poisoning during predominant gardening and growing season
- Increased risk when baits are overused or placed without protection from pets, or containers are left available or open
- Dogs are much more likely to be poisoned than cats.
- Breed, age, or sex predilections are not known.

Historical Findings

- Recent history of pets with access to treated garden areas
- Recent purchase of slug baits
- Baits not protected from access by pets
- Occasionally, access to camp stove fuels or other metaldehyde sources

Location and Circumstances of Poisoning

- Prevalence is highest where slugs are a pest problem.
- Most common usage of baits is in coastal and low-lying areas with high prevalence of snails.
- Most consistent problems are also in warmer temperate to subtropical areas of United States.

Interactions with Drugs, Nutrients, or Environment

- None reported
- Conditions that inhibit cytochrome P450 might enhance toxicity.

CLINICAL FEATURES

General Comments

- May occur immediately after ingestion or may be delayed for up to 3 hours.

Historical Findings

- Anxiety and panting are early signs.
- Hypersalivation and/or vomiting may occur.
- Ataxia
- Muscle tremors
- Convulsions

Physical Examination Findings

- Seizures—may be intermittent early but progress to continuous; not necessarily evoked by external stimuli
- Hyperthermia—temperature up to 108°F (42.2°C) common; probably caused by excessive muscle activity from convulsions; may lead to DIC or multiple organ failure if uncontrolled
- Tachycardia and hyperpnea between convulsions—may note muscle tremors and anxiety; may be hyperesthetic to sounds, light, and/or touch
- Nystagmus or mydriasis possible
- Hypersalivation, vomiting, or diarrhea possible
- Ataxia prior to or between seizures

 ## DIFFERENTIAL DIAGNOSIS

- Strychnine toxicosis—causes intermittent seizures that can be evoked by external stimuli
- Penitrem A—mycotoxin usually found in moldy English walnuts or cream cheese; has been reported in other foodstuffs; causes a tremorgenic syndrome
- Roquefortine—mycotoxin found in moldy bleu cheese and other foodstuffs; causes a tremorgenic syndrome
- Lead toxicosis—may cause seizures, behavior changes, blindness, vomiting, diarrhea
- Zinc phosphide rodenticide—may cause seizures and hyperesthesia
- Bromethalin rodenticide—may cause seizures
- Organochlorine insecticides—cause seizures in most mammals
- Anticholinesterase insecticides—organophosphates and carbamates; may cause seizures; often accompanied by excessive salivation, miosis, lacrimation, dyspnea, urination, and defecation

- Seizures—may be the result of a host of nontoxic conditions (e.g., neoplasia, trauma, infection, metabolic disorder, and congenital disorder)

 # DIAGNOSTICS

- No specific or diagnostic features on CBC, chemistry, or UA
- Increased serum muscle enzyme activities
- Metabolic acidosis is typical.
- Changes in renal or hepatic values are possible but most likely secondary to uncontrolled hyperthermia.
- Radiographs may be indicated to evaluate for the presence of gastric material or severity of ingestion. Some metaldehyde bait pellets are radiopaque and may show up on radiographs.

Pathological Findings

- Lesions are not consistent or pathognomonic.
- Odor of acetaldehyde or formaldehyde in stomach contents
- Hepatic, renal, or pulmonary congestion
- Pulmonary edema and/or hemorrhage
- Nonspecific agonal hemorrhages on heart and mucosal surfaces
- Traumatic bruising or hemorrhage secondary to seizures

Toxicological Testing

- Metaldehyde testing can be performed on vomitus, stomach contents, serum, urine, or liver.
- Keep samples frozen after collection.
- Urine may yield low or negative values (see Pharmacokinetics).
- Testing capabilities vary widely among laboratories, so check first to see what samples are recommended.

 # THERAPEUTICS

Detoxification

- Recommend emesis at home if ingestion is reported less than 2 hours previous and animal is asymptomatic.
- Use hydrogen peroxide PO at 1–3 mL/kg BW; if no response, send patient to veterinary hospital.
- In hospital, use apomorphine 0.03 mg/kg IV (preferred) or 0.04 mg/kg IM in dog or cat.
  - Note: some authorities recommend not using apomorphine in cats.

- Do *not* administer emetic to patients in seizures or that are comatose or hyperesthetic.
- Alternative to emetic is gastric lavage with water at 3–5 mL/kg, repeated until lavage fluid is clear.
- Follow gastric clearing with activated charcoal (1–3 g/kg BW) and sorbitol cathartic (4 g/kg BW PO).
- Symptomatic patients should have their symptoms controlled (e.g., muscle relaxant, anticonvulsant, thermoregulation, cooling measures, etc.), and once stabilized, they should be gastric lavaged under sedation or general anesthesia. The airway should be protected with an inflated ETT, and the stomach gastric lavaged to remove any remaining product.
- Tepid-water enemas may be necessary to aid in promotion of removal from the GIT.

Appropriate Health Care

- Emergency inpatient intensive care management until convulsions cease and hyperthermia is controlled
- Acute care for metabolic acidosis may be essential to successful treatment.
- Treat according to laboratory blood gas results.
- If venous blood gas analysis reveals a severe metabolic acidosis (pH <7.0, BE <−15, HCO_3 <11), sodium bicarbonate should be considered (0.5–1 mEq/kg slowly over 1–3 hours, IV).

Drug(s) and Antidotes of Choice

- No antidote available
- Decrease absorption in asymptomatic or stabilized patient with emetics, gastric lavage, and/or activated charcoal as appropriate.
- Convulsions are controlled with diazepam, barbiturates, general anesthesia, methocarbamol, or guaifenesin as a single agent or in combination if necessary. Seizures are frequently resistant to anticonvulsants and require general inhalant anesthesia for control.
    - Diazepam: 0.5–1 mg/kg IV bolus; repeat 5 minutes later if seizure has not subsided. Supplement with other control methods if seizures continue.
    - Barbiturates: phenobarbital 4–16 mg/kg IV; if control not adequate, consider pentobarbital 3–15 mg/kg IV to effect.
    - Methocarbamol: 50–150 mg/kg IV; do not exceed 330 mg/kg/day
    - Guaifenesin 5%: 100 mg/kg IV; *do not use in cats*

Precautions/Interactions

- Never induce vomiting in a convulsing patient.

Nursing Care

- Control hyperthermia with cool water baths, ice packs, IV fluids, etc., until temperature reaches 103.5°F; cooling measures should be discontinued at this temperature and regulated frequently.
- Monitor to prevent aspiration of vomitus. Consider the use of antiemetics or prokinetics if necessary.
- Aggressive IV fluid therapy is often necessary to aid in cooling measures, to treat the underlying metabolic acidosis, to correct dehydration, to correct electrolyte imbalances, and to aid in perfusion.

Follow-up

- Monitor for possible liver or renal damage during convalescence.

Diet

- Do not feed patients that are vomiting, convulsing, or heavily sedated.

Activity

- Restrict activity so that patient is not injured during convulsions.

Prevention

- Instruct owners/guardians on risks of metaldehyde.
- Advise clients on proper use, placement, and protection of metaldehyde from access by pets.

Public Health

- Humans are susceptible.
- Advise, especially, prevention of access to baits by young children.

    COMMENTS

Client Education

- Provide client education information about pesticide threats, including metaldehyde.
- Periodically remind clients of dangers from pesticides, especially during seasons of high usage.

Patient Monitoring

- Periodically allow anticonvulsants to wear off to reevaluate seizure condition.

Prevention/Avoidance

- Do not apply metaldehyde in areas accessible to pets.
- Some manufacturers dye the product green or blue to assist with identification, which can result in confusion with other products (e.g., rodenticides).
- Some states require manufacturers to adjust the formulation to decrease palatability to pets.

Possible Complications

- Liver or renal dysfunction are possible several days after recovery from the initial signs and are probably sequelae to the convulsions and hyperthermia.
- Aspiration pneumonia is a concern with any convulsing patient.
- Hyperthermia may lead to DIC or multiple organ failure.
- Temporary blindness or memory loss may occur.
- Concurrent toxicoses from additional ingredients (arsenate or insecticides) if they are present in the molluscacide

Expected Course and Prognosis

- Prognosis principally depends on the amount ingested, time to treatment, and quality of care.
- Delayed or nonaggressive treatment may result in death within hours of exposure.

Synonyms

- Molluscacide
- Slug bait
- Snail bait

Abbreviations

5HT = 5 hydroxy tryptamine
BW = body weight
CBC = complete blood count
DIC = disseminated intravascular coagulation
ETT = endotracheal tube
GABA = gamma amino butyric acid
GIT = gastrointestinal tract
IM = intramuscular
IV = intravenous
LD_{50} = median lethal dose
MAO = monamine oxidase
NE = norepinephrine
PO = *per os* (by mouth)
q = every
UA = urinalysis

Suggested Reading

Booze TF, Oehme FW. An investigation of metaldehyde and acetaldehyde toxicities in dogs. Fundam Appl Toxicol 1986; 6(3):440–446.

Kitchell RL, Schubert TA, Mull RL, et al. Palatability studies of snail and slug poison baits, using dogs. J Am Vet Med Assoc 1978; 173(1):85–90.

Studdert VP. Epidemiological features of snail and slug bait poisoning in dogs and cats. Aust Vet J 1985; 62(8):269–271.

Von Burg R, Stout T. Metaldehyde. J Appl Toxicol 1991; 11:377–378.

Yas-Natan E, Segev G, Aroch I. Clinical, neurological and clinicopathological signs, treatment and outcome of metaldehyde intoxication in 18 dogs. J Small Anim Pract 2007; 48(8): 438–443.

Author: Konnie H. Plumlee, DVM, MS, DABVT, DACVIM
Editor: Gary D. Osweiler, DVM, PhD, DABVT

chapter 82

Organophosphate and Carbamate Insecticides

 DEFINITION/OVERVIEW

- Organophosphate (OP) and carbamate insecticides are still common causes of toxicosis in dogs and cats, although the incidence has been steadily decreasing. This is likely due to the removal of several products from the home market and the introduction of several other less toxic pesticides.
  - Chlorpyrifos, once found in flea collars and other animal products, was withdrawn in 2000, and diazinon followed in 2004. Older products are still found and used in homes, garages, and attics and remain a source of poisoning.
- Products currently licensed for use on animals, in the house, on the lawn and garden, or for farm or agricultural use are all potential sources of poisoning.
- Carbamate *fungicides* are in a different category and not discussed in this chapter.

 ETIOLOGY/PATHOPHYSIOLOGY

- In addition to systemic exposure, dogs and cats can be poisoned through the ophthalmic, respiratory, and dermal route. Clinical signs and toxicity vary depending on the particular OP or carbamate as well as the route of exposure.

Mechanism of Action

- Competitive inhibitors of cholinesterase enzymes. Enzyme inhibition allows acetylcholine, a neurotransmitter, to accumulate at nerve junctions in parasympathetic/sympathetic nervous systems, peripheral nervous systems, and the CNS. This results in stimulation of muscarinic, nicotinic, and CNS cholinergic synapses.
- Two main enzymes with cholinesterase activity:
  - Acetylcholinesterase ("true" cholinesterase)—present in the RBC membrane
  - Pseudocholinesterase (plasma cholinesterase)—found in the plasma, liver, pancreas, and CNS

Pharmacokinetics/Absorption, Distribution, Metabolism, and Excretion

- Precise pharmacokinetics vary with each compound.
  - Well absorbed across skin, lungs, cornea, and GIT
  - Widely distributed and many accumulate in fat
  - Metabolized in liver
  - Excreted in urine as metabolites
- Organophosphates
  - Liver microsomal enzymes convert OPs to an "oxon" compound. Oxons irreversibly bind to cholinesterase enzymes, increasing the toxicity and duration of action.
  - Different OPs bind with different affinity. Some "age" or become more strongly bound with the passage of time.
- Carbamates
  - Inhibition of cholinesterase enzymes is due to carbamylation of the enzyme esters. Binding is labile, reversible, and not as long lasting as OPs.

Toxicity

- Varies widely depending on the compound
- Oral LD_{50} of chlorpyrifos in cats is very low (10–40 mg/kg).
- Organophosphate compounds
  - Very highly toxic compounds include disulfoton, fensulfothion, parathion, terbufos, TEPP (tetraethyl pyrophosphate), and others.
  - Compounds with intermediate toxicity include coumaphos, famphur, trichlorfon, and others.
  - Intermediate- to low-order-toxicity compounds include chlorpyrifos, diazinon, dichlorvos, fenthion, malathion, and others.
- Carbamate compounds
  - Extremely toxic compounds include aldicarb, carbofuran, methomyl, carbofuran, and others.
  - Aminocarb, bendiocarb, and propuxur are among the highly toxic compounds.
  - Moderately toxic compounds include carbaryl and others.

Systems Affected

- Virtually all systems in the body are affected to some extent by OP or carbamate poisoning, with effects dependent on specific neuro effector junction.
  - Accumulation of acetylcholine at autonomic junctions results in excessive stimulation of end organs, with secretion and smooth muscle contractions the expected outcome.
  - Variable effects are observed at skeletal muscle junctions where both stimulatory and inhibitory effects occur.

- Gastrointestinal—Stimulation of muscarinic synapses results in the acute onset of salivation, lacrimation, urination, defecation, and gastroenteritis.
- Nervous—Stimulation results in variable and diverse signs.
- Neuromuscular—Tremors and muscle weakness as part of nicotinic stimulation; paresis or frank paralysis following the acute cholinergic crisis (intermediate syndrome)
- Cardiovascular—Inhibitory effect on SA node results in bradycardia.
- Ophthalmic—Mydriasis or miosis from either muscarinic or nicotinic stimulation
- Respiratory—Vapors produce irritation to mucous membranes and bronchospasm.

 # SIGNALMENT/HISTORY

- Cats are more susceptible to intoxication than dogs, especially to chlorpyrifos.
- Younger animals may be at greater risk.
- Thin animals or those with a naturally occurring lean body mass may be more susceptible to intoxication from lipophilic OPs.

Historical Findings

- Chewed up containers or disturbed earth around recently treated rose bushes and shrubs
- Rapid onset of SLUDGE syndrome

 # CLINICAL FEATURES

- Local effects from direct contact with the product. Signs may be seen in just a few moments or delayed for days with dermal exposure.
  - Ophthalmic—irritation, lacrimation, photophobia, and miosis or mydriasis. Pupil size generally returns to normal in 12–36 hours.
  - Respiratory—respiratory irritation with bronchospasm; absorption across mucous membranes
  - Dermal—irritation; absorption can occur across intact skin with systemic toxicity if concentration and duration of exposure is high enough.
- Systemic effects may occur as early as 30–60 minutes, usually occur by 6 hours, and rarely after 12 hours.
  - CNS—agitation or depression, aggression, seizures, respiratory depression and failure (centrally mediated), death
  - Muscarinic signs—most commonly observed and generally associated with the SLUDGE syndrome. Other signs include bradycardia, dyspnea, and miosis.

- Nicotinic signs—facial twitching (especially in cats), weakness, ataxia, muscle tremors, tachycardia, paralysis, and mydriasis
- Intermediate syndrome: Signs generally occur 24–72 hours after the onset of acute signs and may last from 7 to 14 days up to several months.
  - Occurs most commonly with lipophilic OPs
  - Acute or chronic; prolonged dermal exposure
  - Neuromuscular weakness predominantly affects the thoracic limb, neck, and respiratory muscles. Cervical ventroflexion is common.
  - Other signs include cranial nerve deficits, anorexia, diarrhea, muscle tremors, abnormal postures or behaviors, miosis or mydriasis, depression, and seizures.
  - Death from hypoventilation and respiratory depression

 DIFFERENTIAL DIAGNOSIS

- Amphetamine, methylphenidate, and other human CNS stimulant pharmaceuticals
- Concentrated pyrethrin/permethrin topical products
- Metaldehyde
- Mushrooms
- Severe gastroenteritis or pancreatitis from infectious, environmental, or other causes
- Street drugs (methamphetamine, cocaine, etc.)
- Tremorgenic mycotoxins may produce vomiting, salivation, and neuromuscular signs.
- Zinc phosphide–containing rodenticides

 DIAGNOSTICS

- Positive analysis of stomach contents or vomitus
- Positive response to a test dose of atropine (0.02 mg/kg IV)
- Brain cholinesterase level at necropsy. Levels less than 50% of normal are considered suspicious and less than 25% of normal are diagnostic.
- Cholinesterase testing: cautious interpretation of levels, considering onset of signs and when sample was taken. Levels less than 50% of normal are considered suspicious and less than 25% of normal are diagnostic.
  - Plasma cholinesterase—may be more appropriate for cats and avian species; can be used for other species
  - Whole blood cholinesterase—measures cholinesterase in plasma and RBC membranes; can be used for all species, including cats
- Modern analytical methods can detect OP poisoning residues in body organs such as liver or kidney.

Pathological Findings

- Nonspecific lesions; endocardial and epicardial petechial hemorrhages; pulmonary edema; pancreatitis in dogs

 # THERAPEUTICS

Detoxification

- Oral exposure
  - Early induction of emesis depending on the carrier. Many liquid products have petroleum-based carriers, and emesis is NOT indicated for these.
  - Gastric lavage followed by one dose of activated charcoal with or without a cathartic (depends on diarrhea)
  - Flea collars that are ingested will need to be removed either by emesis, whole bowel irrigation, endoscopy, or surgery.
- Dermal exposure
  - Clip hair if possible.
  - Bathe thoroughly in warm water and soap. Rinse and repeat several times.
  - Personal protection important when bathing.
- Ophthalmic exposure
  - Lavage with tepid water for 10–15 minutes.
  - Ophthalmic ointment for irritation
- Respiratory exposure
  - Move to fresh air
  - Humidified oxygen as needed for severe dyspnea

Appropriate Health Care

- Close monitoring of heart rate. Bradycardia is most common; tachycardia can occur.
- Blood pressure support as needed
- Oxygen as needed for dyspnea or hypoxemia
- Severe respiratory depression or secondary aspiration pneumonia can occur; be prepared to provide ventilator support as needed.
- Venous blood gas monitoring to detect metabolic acidosis; bicarbonate only if severe.
- Monitor closely for pancreatitis (dogs) and HGE (dogs and cats).

Drug(s) and Antidotes of Choice

- Atropine—effective ONLY for SLUDGE symptoms. Primarily used to control bronchial secretions and bradycardia. Dosage range for this is very wide.
  - Mild to moderate OP toxicity:
    - Dosage range of 0.1 to 0.5 mg/kg BW

- □ Give ¼ of dose IV and remainder IM or SQ.
      - □ Repeat every 1 to 2 hours as needed until the animal is stable and secretions are controlled.
    - Serious and life-threatening OP toxicity:
      - □ Use the high end of the dosage range (1–2 mg/kg BW).
      - □ Give ¼ of the dose IV, wait 15 minutes and give the remainder SQ or IM.
      - □ Repeat every 1–2 hours until animal is stable and secretions are controlled.
    - Secretions and then heart rate should be the guide to redosing.
    - Pay particular attention to secretions as animals can drown in their own secretions if not enough atropine is administered. It is important to use enough atropine to counteract the effects of acetylcholine.
- Pralidoxime chloride (2PAM)—used for OP toxicity to reverse the initial binding with acetylcholinesterase
    - 20 mg/kg BW IV or SQ q 12 hours slowly over 15–30 minutes
    - Rapid IV administration of 2PAM is associated with tachycardia, laryngospasm, neuromuscular blockade, muscle rigidity, and death.
    - Must be given within the first 24 hours to be effective for acute syndrome.
    - Generally see effects after 1 or 2 doses; if no response after 3–4 doses, then discontinue use.
    - Has been suggested to be beneficial in treatment of intermediate syndrome, even when signs occur later than 24 hours postexposure. It appears to work well on the most commonly affected muscles, that is, diaphragm and cervical muscles.
- Fluid therapy: IV fluids to maintain hydration. Use the PCV/TPP to monitor, but generally run fluids at 2–3 x maintenance or greater as significant amounts of fluid are lost with secretions.
- Seizures
    - Diazepam 0.25–0.5 mg/kg IV
    - Phenobarbital 3–5 mg/kg IV
- Antiemetics if vomiting is severe or persists
    - Maropitant 1 mg/kg SQ q 24 hours, not labeled for cats
    - Ondansetron 0.1–0.2 mg/kg IV q 8–12 hours
- GI protectants as needed
    - H₂ blockers
      - □ Famotidine 0.5–1 mg/kg PO, SQ, IM, IV q 12 hours
      - □ Ranitidine 1–2 mg/kg PO, SQ, IM, IV q 8–12 hours
      - □ Cimetidine 5–10 mg/kg PO, SQ, IM, IV q 6 hours
    - Omeprazole 0.5–1 mg/kg daily
    - Sucralfate 0.25–1 g PO TID x 5–7 days if evidence of active ulcer disease

Precautions/Interactions

- Do NOT use 2 PAM in combination with phenothiazines, morphine, or succinylcholine.
- Judicious use of atropine. Use enough to keep the animal from drowning in secretions. Initial tachycardia should not preclude the use of atropine.

Surgical Considerations

- Endoscopic or surgical removal may be necessary if the animal has swallowed a flea collar or older cattle ear tag.

Environmental Issues

- ▢ Properly dispose of these pesticides to avoid groundwater contamination.

 # COMMENTS

Patient Monitoring

- Pay close attentions to secretions. Use an appropriate amount of atropine so the animal does not drown in secretions. Replace IV fluids to correct fluid losses from secretions.
- Monitor heart rate—bradycardia occurs most commonly, tachycardia less so.

Prevention/Avoidance

- Keep pesticides away from pets, follow label directions, and properly dispose of old or unused product.
- Fence or otherwise keep pets out of rose gardens and shrubs when pesticides are applied.

Expected Course and Prognosis

- Good with early and aggressive care. Animals developing the intermediate syndrome may need care for several weeks. Pancreatitis and HGE complicate the recovery.

Abbreviations

2PAM	= pralidoxime chloride
BW	= body weight
CNS	= central nervous system
HGE	= hemorrhagic gastroenteritis
GI	= gastrointestinal
IM	= intramuscular

IV   = intravenous
OP   = organophosphate
PCV   = packed cell volume
PO   = *per os* (by mouth)
q   = every
RBC   = red blood cell
SA   = sinoatrial
SLUDGE = salivation, lacrimation, urination, diarrhea, gastroenteritis
SQ   = subcutaneous
TEPP   = tetraethyl pyrophosphate
TID   = three times a day

Suggested Reading

Bahri L. Pralidoxime. Compend Contin Educ Vet 2002; 24(11):884–886.

Fikes J. Organophosphorus and carbamate insecticides. Toxicology of selected pesticides, drugs and chemicals. Vet Clin North Am Small Anim Pract 1990; 20(2):353–367.

Frick TW, Dalo S, O'Leary JF, et al. Effects of the insecticide diazinon on pancreas of dog, cat, and guinea pig. J Environ Pathol Toxicol 1987; 7(4):1–11.

Hopper K, Aldrich J, Haskins C. The recognition and treatment of the intermediate syndrome of organophosphate poisoning in a dog. J Vet Emerg Crit Care 2002; 12(2): 99–102.

Tecles F, Panizo C, Subiela SM, et al; Effects of different variables on whole blood cholinesterase analysis in dogs. J Vet Diagn Invest 2002; 14:132–139.

Author Name: John Gualtieri, PharmD, MT (ASCP)
Consulting Editors: Gary D. Osweiler, DVM, PhD, DABVT; Lynn R. Hovda, RPH, DVM, MS, DACVIM

83

Pyrethrins and Pyrethroids

DEFINITION/OVERVIEW

- Pyrethrins are a class of drug derived from flowers in the genus *Chrysanthemum*, while pyrethroids are synthetic derivatives. They are commonly used as topical and environmental insecticides and come in a variety of formulations.
- Synthetic pyrethroids were created to further fortify the product due to the rapid breakdown that natural pyrethrins experience when exposed to light, heat, and air.
- Depending on formulation and route of exposure, symptoms associated with toxicosis may include hypersalivation, hyper- or hypothermia, dyspnea, paraesthesia, vomiting, hyperexcitability, tremors, ataxia, weakness, seizures, and death.
- Formulations vary in concentration and synergists depending on intended use but occur in three general classifications: pyrethrin, Type I pyrethroid, and Type II pyrethroid.
  - Pyrethrins: Pyrethrin I & II, cinerin I & II, and jasmolin I & II
  - Type I pyrethroids: allethrin, bifenthrin, permethrin, phenothrin, remethrin, sumithrin, tefluthrin, tetramethrin
  - Type II pyrethroids: cyfluthrin, cyhalothrin, cypermethrin, deltamethrin, fenvalerate, flumethrin, fluvalinate, and tralomethrin

ETIOLOGY/PATHOPHYSIOLOGY

Mechanism of Action

- Pyrethrins and pyrethroids cause hyperexcitability of cells by slowing the opening and closing of sodium channels. The duration of action is much longer in Type II versus Type I pyrethroids. Type II pyrethroids may also exhibit activity on GABA-gated chloride channels. Calcium channels may also be affected. These channels are found in large numbers in peripheral muscle, salivary glands, and the CNS, which explains the manifestation of symptoms seen with overdoses.
- Pyrethrins and pyrethroids are highly lipophilic and readily distribute to those tissues that contain high lipid concentrations such as the CNS, adipose tissue,

liver, and kidneys. No concrete studies were found that demonstrate whether or not pyrethrins and pyrethroids are excreted into milk, but the high lipid concentration in milk poses a concern for potential residues.
- The paraesthesia effect associated with topical applications is caused in large part by the hyperactivity of the cutaneous sensory nerves.

Pharmacokinetics/Absorption, Distribution, Metabolic, Excretion

- Pyrethrins and pyrethroids are poorly absorbed dermally but largely absorbed orally; this explains the significant difference in the severity of symptoms when topical products are ingested compared with when they are topically applied. One study conducted in humans showed 2% dermal absorption compared with 40%–60% oral absorption.
- Pyrethrins and pyrethroids have a wide distribution in the body due to their lipophilic nature.
- Pyrethrins and pyrethroids are rapidly metabolized in mammalian patients by specific plasma esterases and oxidation via conjugation of glucuronides; as cats lack the ability to efficiently conjugate glucuronides, they are particularly sensitive.
- Inactive metabolites are excreted primarily and completely in the urine.

Toxicity

- Toxicity varies depending on the species involved and the product, concentration, synergists, or propellants included. For this reason, it is imperative that products containing pyrethrins and pyrethroids are used only in the manner in which they are intended.
- Onset may be as rapid as 30 minutes but may take several hours to occur.
- Oral toxicosis—may result in GI signs (e.g., hypersalivation, vomiting, etc.)
- Ocular toxicosis—ocular irritation with potential for secondary self-trauma
- Dermal toxicosis—paresthesia (dogs), localized dermal hypersensitivity reactions (dogs); tremors, seizures (cats)

Systems Affected

- Endocrine/metabolic—stimulation of the adrenal gland resulting in potential hyperglycemia
- Gastrointestinal—hypersalivation (particularly with Type II pyrethroids), vomiting, diarrhea, gastritis
- Nervous—paresthesia, hyperexcitability, tremors, seizures. Type I pyrethroids result in the "T" or "tremor" syndrome, which is characterized by tremors, seizures, collapse, ataxia, and even death. Type II pyrethroids result in the "CS" or "choreoathetosis/salivation" syndrome, which is characterized by hypersalivation, hyperexcitability, tremors, and ataxia.

- Ophthalmic—significant ocular irritation due often in part to the carrier agents included in the product's formulation
- Renal/urologic—myoglobinuria secondary to uncontrolled/prolonged tremors or seizures, resulting in potential ARF
- Respiratory—respiratory distress secondary to unmanaged neurological symptoms. True anaphylactic or allergic responses generally only occur with natural pyrethrins.
- Skin/exocrine—paresthesia, localized dermal hypersensitivity reactions

 SIGNALMENT/HISTORY

Risk Factors

- Fish are exquisitely sensitive to pyrethrins and pyrethroids and may die from even the most minimal exposures. Dogs that had a pyrethrin product applied should not be allowed to swim with fish until the product is completely dried (e.g., koi pond in yard).
- Feline patients are especially sensitive to pyrethrins and pyrethroids due to their inability to conjugate glucuronides (see Pharmacokinetics).
- Mammals (other than cats) are fairly resistant to toxicosis and generally rapidly recover from exposures.

Historical Findings

- Patient may present with a history of product application/misuse within the previous 12–24 hours. In the case of cats, some may present after a canine strength product was applied to another pet in the house with which they have had physical contact. Some dogs may present after having ingested the contents of one or more tubes.

Location and Circumstances of Poisoning

- Intentional or accidental exposures generally occur in the home but may occur in farming environments where topical drenches are used on livestock.

Interactions with Drugs, Nutrients, or Environment

- Pyrethrins should never be mixed with other drugs that have anticholinesterase activity.
- Methoprene and piperonyl butoxide potentiate the effects of pyrethrins; these agents are often paired together to slow the process of pyrethrin degradation.
- Pyrethrins should not be combined with other pyrethrins due to a potential additive effect, resulting in toxicosis. Owners commonly bathe pets with shampoos containing pyrethrins and pyrethroids, only to use additional topical products, resulting in a cummulative overdose.

CLINICAL FEATURES

- Onset of clinical signs varies based on formulation of product and route of exposure.
- Symptoms common at presentation are hypersalivation, hyper- or hypothermia, parasthesia, "paw flicking," vomiting, hyperexcitability, tremors, ataxia, weakness, dyspnea, seizures, and death. Some dogs will develop "acute paralysis" after they have scratched at the area of application with their paws. This is generally not a true neurological event but rather a dog reluctant to walk due to a paresthesia response occurring from secondary contact to the topical product.

 # DIFFERENTIAL DIAGNOSIS

- Toxicities—organophosphates, carbamates, 5-fluorouracil, metaldehyde, cocaine, amphetamines, mycotoxins, aflatoxins, phenylpropanolamine, pseudoephedrine, bromethalin, TCAs, SSRIs, antipsychotics, DEET concentrates, hexachlorophene, methylxanthines, strychnine, etc.
- Primary neurologic disease—inflammatory, infectious, neoplastic, structural
- Primary metabolic disease—renal, hepatic, hypoglycemic

 # DIAGNOSTICS

- Baseline PCV/TS and blood glucose
- CBC, chemistry, UA, particularly in geriatric patients or those with metabolic disease
- With severe cases (e.g., tremoring, seizuring), a CK and coagulation panel may be helpful in determining other underlying etiologies or secondary complications (e.g., DIC).
- Hair sample analysis may help to identify active ingredients in un-witnessed exposures but are rarely practical.
- Cholinesterase tests are of no use.
- In dead animals, gas chromatographic assay for pyrethroids (not pyrethrins) may verify exposure, but tissue concentrations do not correlate well with severity of clinical signs.
- Brain, hair, and insecticide samples are preferred specimens.
- Chemical analysis for pyrethrins is not generally available.

Pathological Findings

- None specific

THERAPEUTICS

Detoxification

- No antidote available
- Emesis induction should not occur in symptomatic animals due to the risk of aspiration pneumonia.
- Oral toxicosis:
  - Thoroughly irrigate oral cavity if the ingestion has been recent.
  - Activated charcoal may be administered in those pets that ingested a large amount and are asymptomatic.
- Ocular toxicosis:
  - Eyes should be irrigated copiously with saline or lukewarm water for 10–15 minutes.
  - Fluorescein stain should be performed to rule out corneal damage.
- Dermal:
  - Affected pets should be bathed with a liquid degreasing dish detergent several times to remove the product.

Appropriate Health Care

- Treatment should be specific to the route of exposure:
  - Fluid therapy (e.g., IV, SQ) may be administered to cool hyperthermic patients and maintain hydration in those pets with secondary losses to vomiting, diarrhea, and hypersalivation.
  - Hyperthermic patients should be cooled with cooling measures (e.g., fans, cold water baths) if temperatures exceed 105.5°F. Cooling measures should be discontinued at 103.5°F.
  - Vitamin E oil may be applied to areas of dermal irritation as needed.
  - With dermal exposure, cool compresses may also provide some soothing comfort to the affected area.
  - Discontinuation of the use of pyrethroids or pyrethrins in those pets exhibiting any adverse reactions

Drugs and Antidotes of Choice

- Patients with tremors or seizures should be administered methocarbamol, diphenhydramine, or barbiturates.
  - Methocarbamol 55–220 mg/kg, IV slowly to effect PRN, not to exceed 330 mg/kg/day. PO administration can also be used but is not as effective nor as rapid in onset in symptomatic patients.
  - Diphenhydramine 1–2 mg/kg, IM q 8 hours or 2–4 mg/kg PO q 8–12 hours
  - Phenobarbital 4–16 mg/kg, IV slow to effect for seizures PRN
  - Pentobarbital 3–15 mg/kg, IV to effect PRN

Precautions/Interactions

- Mechanism of action is entirely separate from those of organophosphates or carbamates; therefore, atropine is *not* helpful. The salivation exhibited by these patients is not indicative of SLUDGE symptoms.
- Tremors and seizures often do not respond well to diazepam; they should generally only be used if no other anticonvulsants are readily available.

Follow-up

- Typically unnecessary unless rare, secondary complications (e.g., rhabdomyolysis, DIC, or renal damage) occur.

Diet

- Animal may return to normal diet at discharge or may be given several days of bland diet if GI irritation is present.

Activity

- Patient should be kept quiet and secure while symptomatic but may return to normal activity with successful resolution of the case.

Surgical Considerations

- No surgical considerations necessarily unless foreign body obstruction risk (from ingesting large amounts of plastic containers, etc.)

Prevention

- Secure all topical medications where they cannot be accessed by pets or children.
- Pet owners should be informed to read and follow product directions to avoid accidental poisonings (e.g., application of dog product onto a cat).

 COMMENTS

Client Education

- Educate clients about securing all medications, including topical flea and tick products.
- Due to the potential for drug interactions, pet owners should be informed not to combine topical flea and tick products (e.g., powders, sprays, and squeeze-on products concurrently). Pre-packed products are not intended to be drawn up in aliquots or divided (e.g., large dog product divided for three smaller dogs). Even when only a portion of a larger pet product is administered, it may result in serious medical complications.

- Apply products only on the species and in the manner for which it is intended.
- Apply only the appropriately sized product on the appropriately sized pet.
- Veterinary products are never intended for human use.

Patient Monitoring

- Patients should be monitored for seizures or tremors. TPR should be carefully monitored.
- Patients exhibiting neurological symptoms such as tremors and seizures should be monitored for a minimum of 48–72 hours. Animals often improve for a period of time only to have symptoms return, particularly if appropriate dermal decontamination has not occurred.

Possible Complications

- Myglobinuric renal failure and DIC following prolonged seizures/tremors

Expected Course and Prognosis

- Generally good if treated early
- Animals developing DIC or myoglobinuria have a poor prognosis.

Abbreviations

ARF	= acute renal failure
CBC	= complete blood count
CK	= creatine kinase
CNS	= central nervous system
DEET	= N,N-diethyl-m-toluamide
DIC	= disseminated intravascular coagulation
GI	= gastrointestinal
IM	= intramuscular
IV	= intravenous
PCV	= packed cell volume
PO	= *per os* (by mouth)
PRN	= *pro re nata* (as needed)
q	= every
SLUDGE	= salivation, lacrimation, urination, defecation, gastroenteritis
SQ	= subcutaneous
SSRI	= selective serotonin reuptake inhibitor
TCA	= tricyclic antidepressant
TPR	= temperature, pulse rate, respiratory rate
TS	= total solids
UA	= urinalysis

Suggested Reading

Gupta RC. Veterinary Toxicology Basic and Clinical Principles. New York: Academic, 2007.
Peterson ME, Talcott PA. Small Animal Toxicology with Veterinary Consult Access. Philadelphia: Saunders, 2007.
Plumb DC. Plumb's Veterinary Drug Handbook. Ames, Iowa: Blackwell, 2008.

Author: Nancy M. Gruber, DVM
Consulting Editors: Gary D. Osweiler, DVM, PhD, DABVT; Justine A. Lee, DVM, DACVECC

Metals and Metalloids

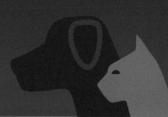

chapter 84

Iron

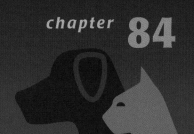

DEFINITION/OVERVIEW

- Iron is an essential element for living organisms in that it is essential for the transport and binding of oxygen, as well as its requirement for many oxidation-reduction reactions.
- In companion animals, oral toxicosis is predominant, but iron can be toxic by injectable routes as well.
- Iron may be lethal when ingested in large quantities due to oxidation-reduction properties.
- Sources of large concentrations of readily ionizable iron include multivitamins, dietary mineral supplements, human gestational supplements, fertilizers, and some types of hand warmers.
- Large doses of ionizable iron can result in loss of the normal mucosal limitations of iron absorption, likely due to the corrosive effect to the GI mucosa.
- Circulating iron in excess of the total iron-binding capacity (TIBC), also referred to as free iron, is very reactive. It can cause oxidative damage to any cell type, as well as subcellular organelles.
- Damage to mitochondria results in loss of oxidative metabolism.
- Primary systems affected are GI, hepatic, cardiovascular, and CNS.

ETIOLOGY/PATHOPHYSIOLOGY

- Iron toxicosis is generally associated with ingestion of iron-fortified pills (e.g., vitamin/minerals or gestational supplements), but other sources include iron-fortified fertilizers and some types of hand warmers.
- In order for iron to be absorbed and be toxic, it must be in a readily ionizable form.
- Metallic iron, iron-containing alloys, and iron oxide (rust) are not readily ionizable. Thus, they are not associated with iron toxicoses.
- Take care when calculating iron ingestion; iron salts in supplements and medications vary in elemental iron content (between 12% and 63%; see table 84.1)

Table 84.1. Percentage of elemental iron in common soluble iron salts.	
Salt	Percentage of Elemental Iron
Iron (as ferric salt)	100
Iron (as ferrous salt)	100
Ferric ammonium citrate	15
Ferric chloride	34
Ferric hydroxide	63
Ferric phosphate	37
Ferric pyrophosphate	30
Ferrocholinate	12
Ferroglycine sulfate	16
Ferrous fumarate	33
Ferrous carbonate	48
Ferrous gluconate	12
Ferrous lactate	24
Ferrous sulfate (anhydrous)	37
Ferrous sulfate (hydrate)	20
Peptonized iron	16

Mechanism of Action

- Large oral doses of ionizable iron can result in loss of the normal mucosal limitations of iron absorption, likely due to the corrosive effect to the GI mucosa.
- Circulating iron in excess of the TIBC (i.e., free iron) is very reactive. It can cause oxidative damage to any cell type, as well as subcellular organelles.
- Reduction-oxidation cycling of iron from ferric to ferrous states and back can result in free radicals that are highly reactive.
- Free circulating iron causes oxidative damage to membranes, resulting in highly reactive hydroxyl ions and hydroxyl radicals. These reactive byproducts cause further membrane damage.
- Predominant damage is focused on tissues of highest exposure to the free iron: GI, cardiovascular, and hepatic.
- Vasodilatation and vascular damage result in systemic shock, resulting in a metabolic acidosis.
- Vascular damage can result in hemorrhage.
- Damage to mitochondria results in loss of oxidative metabolism and further contributes to systemic metabolic acidosis.

Pharmacokinetics/Absorption, Distribution, Metabolism, and Excretion

- Iron absorption is typically limited at the site of the GI mucosa.
- Iron must be ionized in order to be absorbed.
- Ferrous iron is more bioavailable than ferric, but ferric can be absorbed to a lesser degree if it is ionized.
- Once absorbed, iron is distributed to tissues bound to iron-binding proteins.
- Saturation of these iron-binding proteins results in "free iron" being circulated in the serum to tissues.
- Unused iron is sequestered in tissues as ferritin molecules.
- Unlike most metals, animal systems have an inability to excrete excess iron. Even in overdose situations, excess iron is incorporated into ferritin in cells as a means of sequestering it.
- Minimal amounts of iron are lost from the body, primarily via exfoliation of GIT cells or via blood loss.

Toxicity

- Oral toxic dose (dogs)
    - <20 mg/kg of ionizable iron is nontoxic.
    - 20–60 mg/kg of ionizable iron can result in clinical signs.
    - >60 mg/kg of ionizable iron can result in serious clinical disease.
- Injectable iron is more toxic due to much greater bioavailability.

Systems Affected

- Cardiovascular
    - Free circulating iron reacts with the lipids in cell membranes with which it comes in contact.
    - Oxidative damage occurs to the vascular endothelial cells.
    - Cellular damage results in vasodilatation, vascular leakage, and hemorrhage.
- Metabolic
    - Hypovolemia and hypotension result in a lactic acidosis, contributing to acid-base imbalances (e.g., metabolic acidosis).
    - Mitochondrial damage by free iron inhibits oxidative metabolism.
- Gastrointestinal
    - Direct oxidative damage to the mucosal cells results in GI erosions, ulcerations, and hemorrhage.
    - Pills may adhere to mucosal surfaces, resulting in significant localized erosions even when systemic toxic doses have not been ingested.
    - Corrosive damage allows iron to move more freely into systemic circulation.
    - Potential long-term effects are stricture formation in the esophagus or GIT.

- Hepatobiliary
  - Free iron absorbed from the GIT has a great exposure to hepatocytes via portal blood flow.
  - Hepatocytes and Kupffer cells extract free iron from circulation.
  - Free iron damages hepatocellular membranes and subcellular organelles.
  - Cellular damage can result in coagulation deficits.
- Nervous
  - CNS effects typically secondary to effects on other systems
  - Vascular damage can result in CNS edema.
  - Hepatic damage can result in hepatic encephalopathy.

 # SIGNALMENT/HISTORY

- All species are potentially susceptible, with no age-associated difference in susceptibility.
- Dogs are likely to ingest large amounts of the described iron-containing materials, owing to relatively indiscriminate eating behavior.

Historical Findings

- Owners frequently report ingestion of large numbers of vitamin/mineral pills.

Location and Circumstances of Poisoning

- Most frequent ingestion occurs inside households when dogs gain access to bottles of vitamin/mineral pills.
- Much rarer exposures that result in toxic effects include ingestions of iron-fortified fertilizers or some types of iron-containing hand warmers.

 # CLINICAL FEATURES

- Toxicosis is unlikely to develop in animals that remain asymptomatic for 6 to 8 hours.
- Iron toxicosis occurs in four phases outlined below.
- Severity and timing of the phases is dependent on the dose and differing amounts of damage among tissues.
- Clinical stages initially present in the GIT, due to first presentation for oral exposures.

Stage I (0–6 hours)
- Vomiting
- Diarrhea
- Lethargy

- GI hemorrhage
- Abdominal pain

Stage II (6–24 hours)
- Apparent recovery

Stage III (12–96 hours)
- Vomiting
- Diarrhea
- Lethargy
- GI hemorrhage
- Shock
- Tremors
- Abdominal pain
- Metabolic acidosis

Stage IV (2–6 weeks)
- GI obstruction from stricture formation is a secondary effect of the massive mucosal damage that occurs early in the syndrome.

DIFFERENTIAL DIAGNOSIS

- Primary gastrointestinal disease—mesenteric torsion, GDV, foreign body obstruction, pancreatitis, septic peritonitis, hemorrhagic gastroenteritis, viral enteritis, bacterial enteritis, gastroenteritis, infectious, parasitic
- Secondary gastrointestinal disease—hypoadrenocorticism, endotoxin ingestion from garbage, caustic/corrosive ingestion, heat stroke, "shock gut"
- Primary metabolic disease—renal, hepatic, etc.

DIAGNOSTICS

- CBC, chemistry, UA, venous blood gas analysis—evidence of leukocytosis, hyperglycemia, metabolic acidosis, normal to high AST, ALT, ALP, and serum bilirubin
- Serum analysis for total iron and TIBC
    - Often available through local human hospitals
    - Normal serum iron binding capacity is 3–4 times the serum iron concentration.
    - Serum iron in excess of TIBC indicates poisoning such that treatment is required.
    - If chewable tablets or a liquid solution are involved, serum iron levels should be checked 2–3 hours postingestion.
        - Normal level in dogs: 94–122 µg/dL
        - Level at which chelation is necessary: >350–500 µg/dL

- Monitor at 2–3 hours and at 5–6 hours postingestion in asymptomatic patients (absorption rates vary with tablet dissolution and serum iron concentrations may change rapidly).
  - Monitor every 6 to 8 hours in patients on chelation therapy.
- Radiography may be beneficial, as intact iron-containing pills can be radio dense. One may be able to visualize pill bezoars or pills adhered to the esophageal/gastric mucosa.

Pathological Findings

- Primary gross lesions are of damage to the GIT, liver, and vascular systems.
- Damage to the GIT can range from erythema to complete denudation of epithelial cells.
- Hemorrhage in the GIT and liver are often observed, but hemorrhage can be seen in any organ system. Hepatomegaly may also be evident.
- Pathologic lesions of edema and hemorrhage in any organ system can occur due to damage to vasculature.
- Cellular damage to vascular endothelium, hepatocytes, and myocardial cells may be seen histologically.

 # THERAPEUTICS

- General therapy is aimed at minimizing further iron absorption, correcting hypovolemic shock, correcting metabolic acidosis, treating GI signs, and eliminating free iron.

Detoxification

- Activated charcoal does not bind to iron and should not be used.
- Prevent further GI and systemic damage by removal of unabsorbed iron from the stomach. This will lessen the duration and severity of clinical signs.
- Induce emesis in asymptomatic patient, early postingestion. Caution is advised if evidence of gastric damage is already present.
- Gastric lavage to decrease absorption. This should be performed when emesis is contraindicated or when pill bezoars are identified (e.g., radiographically).
- Emergency gastrotomy may be indicated if lavage fails to remove adherent pills or bezoars, and a toxic amount of iron is ingested.

Appropriate Health Care

- Treat shock and metabolic acidosis appropriately. (See chap. 2, "Emergency Management of the Poisoned Patient," for more information.)

- IV fluids as needed for dehydration and hypovolemia for 24–72 hours or as needed until clinical signs abate; this will also enhance urinary elimination of chelated iron.
- Treat GI damage with gastric antiulcer medication, demulcents, or sucralfate. Maintain gastric demulcents/protectants to decrease GI damage and decrease the potential for stricture formation. This care should continue beyond the use of chelation to remove free iron.
- Chelation therapy as appropriate
  - Chelate the systemic free iron to prevent further oxidative damage to tissues.
  - Deferoxamine mesylate is an effective iron chelator.
  - Duration of chelation therapy is until TIBC is greater than serum iron.
  - Monitor serum iron and TIBC every 6–8 hours while on chelation therapy.

Drug(s) and Antidotes of Choice

- Deferoxamine mesylate 15 mg/kg/h, slow IV infusion or 40 mg/kg IM q 4–6 hours or 40 mg/kg, slow IV q 4–6 hours
  - For chelation when indicated by serum iron exceeding TIBC, or when serum iron levels are >350–500 µg/dL
- Antiemetics
  - Maropitant 1 mg/kg, SQ q 24 hours (not labeled for cats)
  - Ondansetron 0.1–0.2 mg/kg, SQ, IV q 8–12 hours
  - Metoclopramide 0.2–0.5 mg/kg, PO, IM, SQ q 8 hours or 1–2 mg/kg/day, CRI IV
- H$_2$ antagonists
  - Famotidine 0.5–1.0 mg/kg, PO, SQ, IM, or IV q 12–24 hours
- Proton pump inhibitors
  - Omeprazole 0.5–1.0 mg/kg, PO q 24 hours in dogs; 0.7 mg/kg, PO q 24 hours in cats
  - Pantoprazole 1 mg/kg, IV q 24 hours in dogs
- Sucralfate 0.5–1 g, PO q 8 hours
- Oral milk of magnesia or aluminum hydroxide will precipitate iron in the GIT as insoluble iron hydroxide. See *Plumb's Veterinary Drug Handbook* for further drug dosing.

Precautions/Interactions

- Gastric lavage is contraindicated when hematemesis is present, owing to increased risk of perforation.
- Intravenous deferoxamine must be given slowly or may precipitate cardiac arrhythmias.
- Deferoxamine is teratogenic. Use in pregnant patients only if the benefits outweigh the risks.

- Deferoxamine-iron chelates are eliminated in the urine. Caution is advised for patients with poor renal function.

Alternative Drugs

- New iron chelation agents are in development for human therapies, but they currently have not been investigated for acute iron overload in companion animals.

Follow-up

- After chelation therapy is discontinued, appropriate supportive care should be provided for an additional 24 hours in order to monitor the serum iron and TIBC at least one time 24 hours postchelation therapy.
- In severely affected animals, owners should be informed to monitor their pet for normal dietary intake and fecal production for up to 6–8 weeks in order to evaluate for the development of strictures.

Diet

- Oral intake should be limited during the first 24 hours in severely affected animals. After thorough evaluation of GI damage, one can determine whether the patient can return to a normal diet or should be placed on a bland, easily digestible, soft food diet for a period of time to allow mucosal repair.

Activity

- Once clinical signs have abated, activity does not need to be limited.

Surgical Considerations

- In cases where a toxic dose has been ingested and (1) pill bezoars are adherent to mucosa, (2) pills are visualized by radiography, or (3) lavage fails to remove materials, emergency gastrotomy is indicated.

Prevention

- Prevention is only achieved by limiting the potential animal exposure.

 COMMENTS

- Care must be taken with induction of emesis or gastric lavage, as cellular damage can predispose to perforating injuries during these procedures.
- It is critical that remaining iron material or pills be removed to prevent further absorption or GI damage.

Client Education

- Clients should be educated as to changes in dietary intake, recurrent vomiting, or poor stool production as indicators of potential stricture formation secondary to the mucosal damage.

Patient Monitoring

- Primary monitoring involves evaluation of serum iron and TIBC as previously outlined.
- Monitor hydration status, serum hepatic enzymes, acid-base status, and GIT effects.

Prevention/Avoidance

- Prevention of reexposure

Possible Complications

- As previously outlined, stricture formation is a possible sequel to GI mucosal damage.

Expected Course and Prognosis

- In patients that do not develop clinical signs by 8 hours, the prognosis is very good. These animals are unlikely to develop clinical signs.
- In patients that are adequately decontaminated prior to development of clinical signs, the prognosis is fair to guarded until there is a lack of signs for 8 hours or until the serum iron is less than the TIBC at 6–8 hours postingestion.
- In symptomatic patients, the prognosis is guarded until chelation therapy results in serum iron levels less than the TIBC. The prognosis is based on the severity of clinical signs and the amount of damage already done.

Abbreviations

ALT = alanine transaminase
ALP = alkaline phosphatase
AST = aspartate transaminase
CBC = complete blood count
CNS = central nervous system
CRI = continuous rate infusion
GDV = gastric dilatation volvulus
GI   = gastrointestinal
GIT = gastrointestinal tract
IM   = intramuscular
IV   = intravenous

PO = *per os* (by mouth)
q = every
SQ = subcutaneous
TIBC = total iron-binding capacity
UA = urinalysis

Suggested Reading

Albretsen JC. Iron. In: Plumlee H ed. Clinical Veterinary Toxicology. St. Louis: Mosby, 2004; pp. 202–204.

Greentree WF, Hall JO. Iron toxicosis. In: Bonagura JD, ed. Current Veterinary Therapy VII. Philadelphia: WB Saunders, 1995; pp. 240–242.

Hall JO. Iron. In: Peterson ME, Talcott PA, eds. Small Animal Toxicology, 2nd ed. Philadelphia: Saunders, 2006; pp. 777–784.

Hooser. Iron. In: Veterinary Toxicology Basic and Clinical Principles. New York: Elsevier, 2007; pp. 433–437.

Author: Jeffery O. Hall, DVM, PhD, DABVT
Editors: Gary D. Osweiler, DVM, PhD, DABVT; Justine A. Lee, DVM, DACVECC

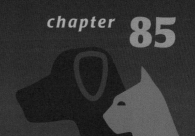

chapter 85

Lead

DEFINITION/OVERVIEW

- Multisystemic intoxication (blood lead >0.4 ppm) following acute or chronic exposure to some form of lead
- Both acute and chronic intoxications are possible depending on exposure amounts and duration.
- Primarily GI and neurologic signs. Gastrointestinal signs often precede CNS signs and are more likely with chronic, low-level lead exposure. CNS signs are more common with acute exposures and in younger animals.
- Sources for lead exposure include lead paint and paint residues or dust from sanding; car batteries; linoleum; solder; plumbing materials and supplies; lubricating compounds; putty; tar paper; lead foil; golf balls; lead object (e.g., shot, fishing sinkers, drapery weights); leaded glass; use of improperly glazed ceramic food or water bowls, etc.
- The most common sources of exposure for dogs and cats are lead paint or lead-contaminated dust or soil.

ETIOLOGY/PATHOPHYSIOLOGY

Mechanism of Action

- Cell damage is due to the ability of lead to substitute for other polyvalent cations (especially divalent cations such as calcium and zinc) important for cell homeostasis.
- Diverse biological processes are affected, including metal transport, energy metabolism, apoptosis, ion conduction, cell adhesion, inter- and intracellular signaling, enzymatic processes, protein maturation, and genetic regulation.

Pharmacokinetics/Absorption, Distribution, Metabolism, Excretion

- Bioavailability of lead is dependent on its form (inorganic or organic; if inorganic, salt or pure metal).
- Lead has higher bioavailability in young animals due to absorption via calcium-binding proteins.
- More than 90% of absorbed lead is bound to RBCs.

657

- Unbound lead is widely distributed in tissues.
- Bone serves as a long-term storage site for lead.
- A significant percentage of ingested lead is eliminated via the feces without being absorbed; absorbed lead is eliminated via the urine and bile.
- The half-life of lead is multiphasic; in dogs, lead elimination is tri-phasic with half-lives of 12 days (blood), 184 days (soft tissues), and >4500 days (bone).

Toxicity

- Not well defined in cats; toxicity noted in cats at 1000 ppm in diet or 3 mg/kg
- An acutely toxic dose for dogs is approximately 190 to 1000 mg/kg (dependent on lead form), whereas a chronic cumulative toxic dose is 1.8 to 2.6 mg/kg/day.

Systems Affected

- Gastrointestinal—unknown mechanism, likely damage to peripheral nerves
- Nervous—capillary damage; alteration of membrane ionic channels and signaling molecules
- Renal/urologic—damage to proximal tubule cells due to enzyme disruption and oxidative damage
- Hemic/lymph/immune—interference with hemoglobin synthesis, increased fragility and decreased survival of RBCs, release of reticulocytes and nucleated RBCs from bone marrow, inhibition of 5'-pyrimidine nucleotidase causing retention of RNA degradation products and aggregation of ribosomes resulting in basophilic stippling

 SIGNALMENT/HISTORY

Risk Factors

- Housing in older, nonrenovated buildings where lead-based paint was used
- Housing in older buildings undergoing renovation where environmental lead contamination is more likely to occur
- Low socioeconomic status of pet owner
- Younger animals (<1 year) have higher risk due to greater lead bioavailability.
- Dogs more commonly affected than cats
- No breed or sex predilections

Historical Findings

- History of renovation of older house or building or ingestion of lead objects.

Location and Circumstances of Poisoning

- Dogs more likely to ingest lead-containing paint or objects; cats are exposed to lead-containing dusts as a result of grooming.

Interaction with Drugs, Nutrients or Environment

- Lead bioavailablity is enhanced in animals that are fasting or are deficient in calcium, zinc, iron, or vitamin D.
- High dietary zinc and calcium decrease lead bioavailability.

 # CLINICAL FEATURES

- Primarily GI and CNS signs
- Signs are often insidious in onset and vague, and include vomiting, diarrhea, anorexia, weight loss, abdominal pain, colic, regurgitation (secondary to megaesophagus), lethargy, hysteria, seizures, blindness, anemia, and PU/PD.
- Cats—central vestibular abnormalities such as vertical nystagmus and ataxia have been reported.

 # DIFFERENTIAL DIAGNOSIS

Dogs
- Canine distemper
- Infectious encephalitides
- Epilepsy
- Bromethalin, methylxanthine, or tremorgenic mycotoxin toxicosis
- NSAID toxicosis
- Heat stroke
- Intestinal parasitism
- Intussusception
- Foreign body
- Pancreatitis
- Infectious canine hepatitis

Cats
- Degenerative or storage diseases
- Hepatic encephalopathy
- Infectious encephalitides
- Organophosphate, bromethalin, or methylxanthine toxicosis

 # DIAGNOSTICS

CBC/Biochemistry/Urinalysis
- Between 5 and 40 nucleated RBCs/100 WBCs without anemia; absence of nucleated RBCs does not rule out the diagnosis.
- Anisocytosis, polychromasia, poikilocytosis, target cells, hypochromasia
- Basophilic stippling of RBCs; often difficult to detect

- Neutrophilic leukocytosis
- Cats—elevated AST and ALP reported
- Urinalysis—mild nonspecific renal damage; glucosuria; hemoglobinuria

Imaging

- Presence of radio-opaque material in the GIT (not diagnostic)
- Lead lines (precipitation of lead salts) within the epiphyseal plate of long bones are uncommon.

Lead Detection

- Toxic—antemortem whole blood: >0.4 ppm (40 μg/dL); postmortem liver and/or kidney: >5 ppm (wet weight)
- Lower values—must be interpreted in conjunction with history and clinical signs
- No normal "background" blood lead concentrations; typically <0.05 ppm
- Blood concentrations—do not correlate with occurrence or severity of clinical signs
- $CaNa_2EDTA$ mobilization test—collect one 24-hour urine sample; administer $CaNa_2EDTA$ (75 mg/kg IM); collect a second 24-hour urine sample; with toxicosis, urine lead increases 10–60-fold post-EDTA (succimer could conceivably be substituted for $CaNa_2EDTA$).

Pathological Findings

- Grossly—might note paint chips or lead objects in GIT
- Intranuclear inclusion bodies—may occur infrequently in hepatocytes or renal tubular epithelial cells; intracellular storage form of lead; considered pathognomonic
- Cerebrocortical lesions—spongiosis, vascular hypertrophy, gliosis, neuronal necrosis, demyelination

 # THERAPEUTICS

Detoxification

- Evacuation of GIT—saline cathartics; sodium or magnesium sulfate (dogs, 2–25 g; cats 2–5 g PO as 20% solution or less)
- Sulfate-containing cathartics potentially precipitate lead in the GIT to the less-bioavailable lead sulfate form.
- Endoscopic or surgical removal of lead objects in the GIT might be warranted in some cases.

Appropriate Health Care

- Inpatient—first course of chelation, depending on severity of clinical signs
- Outpatient—orally administered chelators

Drug(s) and Antidotes of Choice

- Control of seizures—diazepam (given to effect; dogs and cats, 0.5 mg/kg IV) or phenobarbital sodium (administer in increments of 10 to 20 mg/kg IV to effect)
- Alleviation of cerebral edema—mannitol (0.25–2 g/kg of 15% to 25% IV, slow infusion over 30–60 minutes)
- Some evidence that antioxidants or thiol-containing drugs might be useful—vitamins C and E, α-lipoic acid, N-acetylcysteine; optimal doses not determined
- B vitamins, especially thiamine, may also be useful; optimal doses not determined
- Reduction of lead body burden-chelation therapy
  - $CaNa_2EDTA$ (dogs and cats, 25 mg/kg SQ, IM, IV q 6 hours for 2–5 days): dilute to a 1% solution with D_5W before administration; may need multiple treatment courses if blood lead concentration is high; allow 5-day rest period between treatment courses.
  - Succimer: alternative to $CaNa_2$ EDTA; orally administered chelating agent; 10 mg/kg PO q 8 hours for 5 days followed by 10 mg/kg PO q 12 hours for 2 weeks; allow 2-week rest period between treatments; may administer per rectum if clinical signs such as emesis preclude oral administration; cats successfully treated with 10 mg/kg PO q 8 hours for 17 days. Advantages over other chelators: can be given PO allowing for outpatient treatment, does not increase lead absorption from the GIT, not reported to be nephrotoxic, and chelation of essential elements such as zinc and copper is not clinically significant.

Precautions/Interactions

- $CaNa_2EDTA$—do not administer to patients with renal impairment or anuria; establish urine flow before administration; do not administer orally.
- $CaNa_2EDTA$—safety in pregnancy not established; teratogenic at therapeutic doses, although in human medicine is recommended over succimer for use in pregnant patients.
- Succimer—safety in pregnancy not established; fetotoxic at doses much higher (100–1000 mg/kg) than recommended therapeutic dose
- $CaNa_2EDTA$—depletion of zinc, iron, and manganese with long-term therapy; although succimer also chelates zinc and copper, the degree of chelation is not clinically significant.

Nursing Care

- Balanced electrolyte fluids; replacement of hydration deficit

Follow-up

- Assess blood lead values before additional courses of chelation therapy or 10–14 days after cessation of chelation therapy.
- Identify sources for lead exposure and eliminate or restrict access.

Diet

- Provide good quality, nutritionally complete diet.

Surgical Considerations

- Removal of lead objects from the GIT might be warranted in some cases.

Prevention

- Client awareness of potential sources for exposure and avoidance of contact with those sources
- Test paint, dust, soil prior to animal access if likelihood of lead contamination

Public Health

- Environmental lead contamination and exposure is a significant public health problem.
- Families of affected pets should consult their physicians and have lead determinations made.

Environmental Issues

- Depending on the circumstances of exposure, environmental clean-up might be warranted.

 COMMENTS

Prevention/Avoidance

- Test paint, dust, soil prior to animal access if likelihood of lead contamination
- Determine source of lead and remove it from the patient's environment.

Possible Complications

- Uncontrolled seizures can result in permanent neurologic deficits.
- Blindness

Expected Course and Prognosis

- Signs should dramatically improve within 24–48 hours after initiating chelation therapy.
- Prognosis–favorable with treatment
- Uncontrolled seizures—guarded prognosis

Synonyms

Plumbism

Abbreviations

CaNa$_2$EDTA = calcium disodium ethylene diamine tetraacetate
CNS   = central nervous system
GI   = gastrointestinal
GIT   = gastrointestinal tract
IM   = intramuscular
IV   = intravenous
PO   = *per os* (by mouth)
PU/PD   = polyuria/polydypsia
ppm   = parts per million
q   = every
RBC   = red blood cell
SQ   = subcutaneous
WBC   = white blood cell

Suggested Reading

Knight TE, Kent M, Junk JE. Succimer for treatment of lead toxicosis in two cats. J Am Vet Med Assoc 2001; 218:1946–1948.

Knight TE, Kumar MSA. Lead toxicosis in cats: a review. J Feline Med Surg 2003; 249–255.

Morgan, RV. Lead poisoning in small companion animals: an update (1987–1992). Vet Hum Toxicol 1994; 36:18–22.

Ramsey DT, Casteel SW, Fagella AM, et al. Use of orally administered succimer (meso-2,3-dimercaptosuccinic acid) for treatment of lead poisoning in dogs. J Am Vet Med Assoc 1996; 208:371–375.

VanAlstine WG, Wickliffe LW, Everson RJ, et al. Acute lead toxicosis in a household of cats. J Vet Diagn Invest 1993; 5:496–498.

Author: Robert H. Poppenga, DVM, PhD, DABVT
Consulting Editor: Gary D. Osweiler, DVM, PhD, DABVT

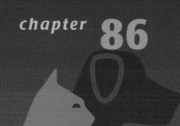

chapter **86**

Zinc

DEFINITION/OVERVIEW

- Zinc (Zn) toxicity results from the ingestion of zinc-containing objects and products such as pennies (see below), metallic nuts, bolts, staples, galvanized metal (e.g., nails), pieces from board games, zippers, toys, and jewelry.
- The most common cause of Zn toxicity is penny ingestion.
  - U.S. pennies minted after 1982 contain 97.5% Zn.
  - Canadian pennies minted from 1997 through 2001 contain 96% Zn.
- Zinc oxide, a common ingredient in skin protectants (e.g., diaper rash cream), is not expected to cause Zn toxicity in acute ingestions.
- Toxicity initially presents as gastrointestinal upset with vomiting and anorexia but progresses to hemolytic anemia. Secondary multiorgan failure (e.g., renal, hepatic, pancreatic, and cardiac), DIC, and cardiopulmonary arrest can occur in severe toxicities.

ETIOLOGY/PATHOPHYSIOLOGY

Mechanism of Action

- Unknown; mechanisms have been proposed but none confirmed.
- Intravascular hemolysis is the most common effect from zinc toxicosis.
- High concentrations of zinc may be found in the serum, RBCs, liver, kidney, and pancreas following toxicosis.

Pharmacokinetic/Absorption, Distribution, Metabolism, and Excretion

- Zinc is absorbed primarily through the small intestine after oral exposure. The acidic environment within the stomach promotes leaching of zinc from the ingested substance, allowing for zinc to be absorbed.
- It is metabolized by the liver where metallothionein plays a significant role in metabolism.
- Excretion occurs primarily in the feces with a small amount excreted in the urine; urinary excretion can increase with chelation therapy.

Toxicity

- The LD_{50} in dogs has been reported at 100 mg/kg for acute Zn salt ingestion.
- One ingested penny (2.5 g) can cause toxicity, even in larger dogs (see Definition/Overview).
- Toxicity depends on the bioavailability of the Zn compound ingested and can come in the following forms:
  - Zinc carbonate and gluconate (dietary supplements); acetate (throat lozenges)
  - Zinc chloride (deodorants); pyrithione (shampoo), oxide (sunblock, Desitin, calamine lotion)
  - Zinc sulfide (paints)
  - Metallic zinc (coins, nuts and bolts); brass (alloy of copper and zinc)
- Zinc-containing topical preparations generally cause only gastrointestinal upset, but chronic exposure has been documented to cause zinc toxicity.

Systems Affected

- Hemic—intravascular hemolysis, Heinz body anemia, prolonged PT/PTT, DIC, leukocytosis with neutrophilia, left shift, monocytosis, lymphopenia
- Gastrointestinal—vomiting, anorexia, diarrhea
- Renal—hemoglobinuria, azotemia, oliguria/anuria, bilirubinuria
- Nervous—depression, ataxia, seizures
- Hepatic—elevated liver enzymes, hyperbilirubinemia

 SIGNALMENT/HISTORY

- While toxicity may occur in any species, it is most frequently reported in young, small dogs (<25 pounds) because they are often unable to pass the metallic object out of the stomach.

Risk Factors

- Young animals have a tendency to eat indiscriminately and may ingest more foreign objects.

Historical Findings

- Owners frequently do not witness the ingestion of the object but will report vomiting, lethargy, anorexia, jaundice, and abnormal or red-colored urine.
- Dogs that ingest topical creams and lotions will typically vomit shortly after ingestion.

Location and Circumstance of Poisoning

■ Most exposures occur in the home with coin or zinc oxide (cream/ointment) ingestion. Kennels or garages/workplaces may pose added risks if there are metallic objects present.

Interactions with Drugs, Nutrients, or Environment

■ Zinc toxicity may interfere with copper or iron absorption.
■ Absorption will be decreased with high levels of dietary phytates, calcium, and phosphorus and increased with certain amino acids and EDTA.

 # CLINICAL FEATURES

■ GI signs may begin minutes after ingestion; however, the onset of hemolysis is dependent upon the rate at which the zinc-containing object breaks down in the GIT and may take hours to days.
■ The most common signs are anorexia, vomiting, diarrhea, lethargy, depression, pale or icteric mucous membranes, and icteric sclera and skin. Orange-tinged feces and hemoglobinuria may be noted.
■ Animals with anemia will often be tachycardic with hypodynamic pulses. A heart murmur may be noted on auscultation.
■ Severe depression and seizures can develop at later stages.
■ Death is often due to cardiovascular collapse and multiorgan failure.

 # DIFFERENTIAL DIAGNOSIS

■ Hemolysis can occur secondary to IMHA, *Babesiosis*, onions, garlic, chives, naphthalene mothballs, acetaminophen, snake and spider envenomation, propylene glycol, and caval syndrome.
■ Gastrointestinal signs can be due to numerous infectious and inflammatory causes as well as foreign body ingestion, dietary indiscretion, and secondary to metabolic disease.

 # DIAGNOSTICS

■ CBC—Hemolytic anemia with possible Heinz body formation with evidence of regeneration. Other RBC morphologies include target cells and spherocytosis.
  • Thrombocytopenia can be noted in animals with DIC.
  • Leukocytosis with neutrophilia, monocytosis, lymphopenia

- Serum chemistry—Hyperbilirubinemia with elevated AST, ALP; less common elevations in GGT, ALT
  - Azotemia
  - Elevated amylase and lipase
- Urinalysis—Bilirubinuria, hemoglobinurina, isosthenuria, proteinuria, tubular casts
- Serum zinc levels often exceed 5 ppm (normal range: 0.70–2 ppm for dogs and cats). Contact reference lab as blood must be collected in tubes specific for zinc testing.
- Coagulation panel may indicate DIC with prolonged PT /PTT, hypofibrinogenemia, thrombocytopenia, and high FDPs.
- Abdominal radiographs may reveal metallic object(s) in the GIT. Repeat radiographs after object removal should be done to ensure all objects are removed.

Pathological Findings

- Gross lesions include icterus, splenomegaly, hepatomegaly, and dark stained urine.
- Histologic lesions include evidence of pigmentary nephropathy, hepatic necrosis, and pancreatic necrosis. Macrophages in these organs may contain hemosiderin.
- Tissue zinc levels may be measured from the liver, kidney, and pancreas.

 THERAPEUTICS

- The goal of treatment is rapid removal of the zinc object(s) along with symptomatic and supportive care.

Detoxification

- Induce emesis in asymptomatic animals.
- Activated charcoal does not bind to Zn and should not be given.
- Rapid removal of the object via endoscopy or laparotomy/gastrotomy is imperative, though stabilization prior to anesthesia should be attempted. Zinc levels will decrease rapidly once the source is removed.

Appropriate Health Care

- IV fluid therapy to maintain hydration and tissue perfusion (as ARF is a potential complication)
- Colloid therapy (e.g., Hetastarch) and vasopressors (e.g., dopamine 2–10 µg/kg/min IV CRI) may be necessary for persistent hypotension.

- Animals with severe anemia and clinical signs associated with anemia may require red blood cell transfusion(s) and oxygen-carrying substances such as Oxyglobin.

Alternative Drugs

- If famotidine is unavailable, other acceptable gastroprotectants include:
  - Omeprazole, a proton pump inhibitor, 0.5–1.0 mg/kg, PO q 24 hours
  - Pantoprazole, a proton pump inhibitor, 0.7–1 mg/kg IV q 24 hours
  - Calcium carbonate, an oral antacid calcium salt, 25–50 mg/kg, PO q 2–4 hours until object removal in nonvomiting animals

Drug(s) and Antidotes of Choice

- Chelation is controversial and should not be necessary once the object or source has been removed. Zinc levels will rapidly decrease once the source is removed.
  - Ca EDTA 100 mg/kg diluted in D5W, divided into 4 SQ doses per day.
  - Penicillamine 110 mg/kg/day PO divided 6–8 hours for 5–14 days
- H_2-receptor antagonists, such as famotidine 0.5–1 mg/kg IV, SQ, IM, PO q 12–24 hours, can be given to help reduce stomach acidity, thereby decreasing the rate of Zn release from ingested metallic object(s).
- Antiemetics, such as maropitant 1 mg/kg SQ q 24 hours, can be given for protracted vomiting.

Precautions/Interactions

- Avoid nephrotoxic drugs such as NSAIDs and aminoglycosides because of the risk of ARF.
- Transfusion reactions may occur because a cross-match cannot be performed prior to administration due to severity of hemolysis. The use of blood products from a universal donor (DEA 1.1 negative) is recommended.

Nursing Care

- Minimize patient stress. Recumbent animals will need soft bedding and positional rotation q 4 hours to prevent atelectasis.
- Urinary catheters may need to be placed to monitor urine output.

Follow-up

- Animals will need to be hospitalized and monitored until clinical signs resolve, which is often 48–72 hours following object removal.
  Follow-up blood work can be done to assess the patient's improvement and response to therapy 1–2 weeks after discharge.
- Blood and urine zinc levels typically decrease rapidly within days following the removal of zinc objects. If a significant decrease is not noted, the presence of additional zinc in GIT should be considered.

COMMENTS

Client Education

- Make sure clients are aware of the dangers of both metallic zinc objects and zinc-containing ointments. Have owners check the environment for zinc objects in garages, kennels, and work areas.
- Inform client about the hazards of ingesting zinc-containing objects (especially pennies).
- Advise owners to not use topical preparations on animals without veterinarian approval.

Patient Monitoring

- Coagulation profile, CBC, serum chemistry will need to be monitored for the first 72 hours after zinc removal with special attention to the PCV and kidney values.
- ECG and BP should be monitored frequently as cardiopulmonary arrest can occur in severely affected animals.
- Serum zinc levels can be monitored, but clinical signs and lack of hemolysis may be better indicators of recovery.

Possible Complications

- Multiple organ failure (especially liver and renal), DIC, pancreatic disease, cardiopulmonary arrest, and seizures can occur even with aggressive therapy.

Expected Course and Prognosis

- Animals may show improvement within 48–72 hours after object removal.
- Prognosis can be good to grave depending on the duration of clinical signs and the animal's condition on presentation. Complete recovery is possible.
- If multiple organ failure (especially liver and renal), DIC, pancreatic disease, cardiopulmonary arrest, and seizures are present, prognosis is poor.

Abbreviations

ALT = alanine aminotransferase
ALP = alkaline phosphatase
ARF = acute renal failure
AST = aspartate aminotransferase
BP   = blood pressure
CBC = complete blood count
CRI = continuous rate infusion
DIC = disseminated intravascular coagulation

ECG   = electrocardiogram
EDTA = ethylenediaminetetraacetic acid
FDP   = fibrin degradation product
GGT   = gamma-glutamyl transpeptidase
IM   = intramuscular
IMHA = immune-mediated hemolytic anemia
IV   = intravenous
LD   = lethal dose
NSAID = nonsteroidal anti-inflammatory drug
PCV   = packed cell volume
PO   = *per os* (by mouth)
ppm   = parts per million
PT   = prothrombin time
PTT   = partial thromboplastin time
q   = every
RBC   = red blood cell
SQ   = subcutaneous
Zn   = zinc

See Also

Batteries
Foreign Bodies
Lead
Matches and Fireworks
Metallic Toxicants (appendix)

Suggested Reading

Dziwenka MM, Coppock R. Zinc. In: Plumlee KH, ed. Clinical Veterinary Toxicology. St. Louis: Elsevier Mosby, 2004; pp. 221–230.
Gurnee CM, Drobatz KJ. Zinc intoxication in dogs: 19 cases (1991–2003). JAVMA 2007; 230(8):1174–1179.
Talcott PA. Zinc poisoning. In: Peterson ME, Talcott PA, eds. Small Animal Toxicology. St. Louis: Elsevier Saunders, 2006; pp. 1094–1100.

Acknowledgment: The authors and editors acknowledge the prior contributions of Dr. Kathryn M. Meurs, who authored this topic in previous editions.
Authors: Katherine L. Peterson, DVM; Patricia A. Talcott, DVM, PhD, DAVBT
Consulting Editors: Gary D. Osweiler, DVM, PhD, DABVT; Ahna G. Brutlag, DVM

Nondrug Consumer Products

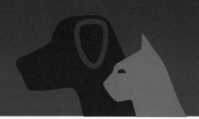

chapter 87

Glow Jewelry (Dibutyl Phthalate)

DEFINITION/OVERVIEW

- Most glow jewelry or glow-in-the-dark jewelry contains an oily, chemilumines-cent substance known as dibutyl phthalate.
- Types of glow jewelry include plastic wands, sticks, necklaces, earrings, and other pieces that are commonly worn at Halloween, Fourth of July, and other holidays (fig. 87.1).
- Other kinds of glow jewelry that contain small batteries or other luminescent substances are not covered in this chapter.

ETIOLOGY/PATHOPHYSIOLOGY

Mechanism of Action

- Dibutyl phthalate is widely used in the manufacture of a number of products including plastics, glues, dyes, printing ink, solvents for perfume, safety glass, and as insect repellants for use in clothing.
- Dibutyl phthalate is an irritant to the eyes, skin, and mucous membranes.
- Dibutyl phthalate has an unpleasant, bitter taste that tends to limit oral exposure.

Toxicity

- Dibutyl phthalate has a low order of acute toxicity with a wide margin of safety.
- Oral LD_{50} (rats) >8 g/kg.
- Rats receiving an oral dose of 1 mg/kg twice a week for 6 weeks developed no abnormalities; a similar study evaluated this same oral dose for 1.5 years and found no abnormalities either.
- Rats and other laboratory animals tolerated 2 g/kg orally once daily for 10 days in a reproductive study.
- Minimum lethal exposure for other species, including human beings, is unknown.
- Glow jewelry contains small amounts of dibutyl phthalate, with most pieces containing less than 5 mL of liquid. The exterior packaging often states the exact amount (fig. 87.2).
  - Earrings and bracelets contain approximately 0.3–0.5 mL.
  - Necklaces contain approximately 1–2 mL.
  - Large wands contain approximately 3–5 mL.

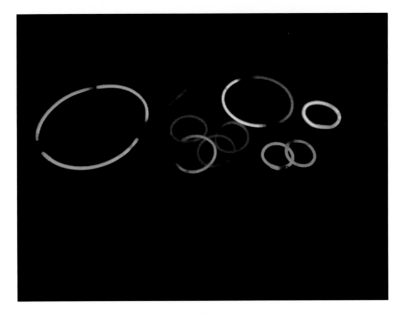

■ **Fig. 87.1.** Glow jewelry. (Photo courtesy of Tyne K. Hovda)

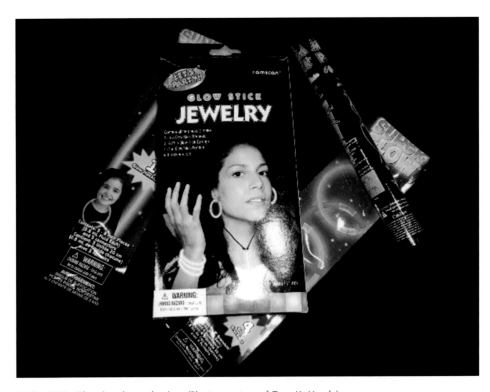

■ **Fig. 87.2.** Glow jewelry packaging. (Photo courtesy of Tyne K. Hovda)

Systems Affected

- Gastrointestinal—oral irritation and discomfort, profuse hypersalivation, agitation secondary to oropharyngeal discomfort, GI upset, vomiting
- Skin/exocrine—stinging sensation, irritation, burning, redness, contact dermatitis reported in humans
- Ophthalmic—stinging and burning sensation, profuse lacrimation, photophobia, conjunctival edema, conjunctivitis
- Respiratory—typically not seen with glow jewelry products purchased for personal use; however, with very large experimental doses, labored breathing and respiratory paralysis has been noted in fatally poisoned animals.

 # SIGNALMENT/HISTORY

- History of biting or chewing product
- Any age or breed of dog or cat may be affected.
- Self-grooming increases potential for oral and ocular exposure, especially in cats, due to fastidious grooming habits.

Location and Circumstances of Poisoning

- The presence of children in the household may increase exposure, as children use glow jewelry as part of costumes or toys.
- The presence of glowing liquid may be present in the area of ingestion—turning off the light may reveal spilled dibutyl phthalate, which should be promptly cleaned to prevent additional reexposure.
- Pets ingesting glowing liquid should also be evaluated in a dark room to make sure dibutyl phthalate present on their fur is cleaned off appropriately.

 # CLINICAL FEATURES

- Cats generally seem to be more exposed to dibutyl phthalate due to their curious, chewing nature, exposing them to toxicosis from direct ingestion, direct skin exposure, or ocular exposure.
- Generally just a small amount is ingested due to the bitter taste of dibutyl phthalate; most of the liquid remains in the stick or jewelry, but it may also spill on the floor or onto the pet's fur.
- Clinical symptoms are typically due to the unpleasant chemical taste of the product, resulting in acute onset of profuse hypersalivation or vomition.
- Other clinical signs include agitation, aggressiveness, and other neurological abnormalities may be seen.
- Direct skin exposure may also occur due to accidental splash contact or by cat's rubbing or rolling in the contaminated environment. Rare intentional or accidental application by children or unknowledgeable adults have been reported.

- A pet's hair coat provides some protection, but contact with thin or hairless areas results in a rapid onset of a burning and stinging sensation.
- Cats may develop severe pruritis secondary to skin irritation and can further excoriate themselves to the point of developing open wounds.
- Finally, ocular exposure may occur secondary to self-grooming. Evidence of conjunctivitis, ocular pruritis (rubbing the face on the carpet or grooming excessively), or any corneal lesions should be thoroughly evaluated. The presence of corneal ulceration should be ruled out with fluorescein staining.
- In general, dogs are rarely exposed, but clinical signs tend to be similar; however, symptoms are typically more transient in nature and resolve sooner. Treatment is similar for both species.

 # DIFFERENTIAL DIAGNOSIS

- Other irritant products such as perfumes and alcohols
- Oxalate-containing plants
- Oral ingestion of pyrethrin and permethrin products

 # DIAGNOSTICS

- In general, diagnostics are not necessary due to the rapid response to therapy. However, pediatric, geriatric, or patients with underlying metabolic or endocrine disorders may need baseline blood work performed to evaluate for the presence of hypoglycemia, severity of dehydration, etc.

 # THERAPEUTICS

- Goals of treatment include decontamination, oropharyngeal lavage to remove the presence of dibutyl phthalate, whole body bathing (or bathing of the affected "glowing" area), and potential subcutaneous fluids to maintain hydration.

Detoxification

- Emesis should not be induced, as it is unnecessary. Due to the bitter taste, cats rarely ingest more than just a small amount. Gastric lavage and the use of activated charcoal are also unnecessary.
- Treatment includes removal of the product by rinsing or lavaging the mouth out several times with cool water. If this is not possible by the pet owner, the use of dilution with a small amount of a palatable liquid can be used (e.g., chicken broth, milk, canned tuna water, or canned cat food).
- The signs are generally self-limiting and related to the taste of dibutyl phthalate; once that is gone, the signs resolve quickly.

- Detoxification of the hair coat is also necessary. The patient should ideally be bathed with a mild, noninsecticidal pet shampoo and rinsed well with tepid water.
- The pet should be further examined in a darkened room to ensure that all of the "glow" product has been completely removed.

Appropriate Health Care

- A thorough ocular exam may be necessary if ophthalmic signs are present. This generally requires veterinary care, as it is difficult for owners to adequately rinse or evaluate a cat's eyes without adequate restraint.
- If there is ocular exposure to dibutyl phthalate, the eyes should be lavaged thoroughly with ophthalmic saline for 10–15 minutes.
- Slit-lamp or fluorescein testing may be necessary to evaluate for the presence of corneal ulceration. Ulceration should be treated with ophthalmic medication as deemed medically appropriate.

Drug(s) and Antidotes of Choice

- No antidote exists.

 COMMENTS

Client Education

- Pet owners should be informed on this toxicity, particularly during seasonal holidays or events.
- Most reactions are self-limiting and can be treated at home without veterinary intervention.
- Many of the signs are behavioral changes associated with the bitter taste of the product.
- Pets with ocular exposures often have to be seen and treated by a veterinarian.

Expected Course and Prognosis

- Most exposures, especially those by cats, involve a very small amount of dibutyl phthalate and little treatment is required.
- The clinical signs associated with oral exposure resolve quickly once the bitter taste is gone.
- No laboratory tests are recommended for these exposures, and the prognosis for complete recovery is excellent.
- Animals exposed to large doses should be monitored closely and treated with appropriate decontamination followed by supportive care.

Abbreviations

GI   = gastrointestinal
LD_{50} = median lethal dose

Suggested Reading

Kamrin MA. Phthalate risks, phthalate regulation, and public health: a review. J Toxicol Environ
    Health B Crit Rev 2009; 12(2):157–174.
Keys N, Erickson T, Lipscomb J. Glow compound exposure. J Toxicol Clin Toxicol 1995; 33:488.
Merola V, Dunayer E. Toxicology brief: the 10 most common toxicoses in cats. Vet Med 2006;
    101(6):339–342.
Rosendale ME. Glow jewelry (dibutyl phthalate) ingestion in cats. Vet Med 1999; 94(8):703.

Authors: Tyne K. Hovda; Justine A. Lee, DVM, DACVECC
Consulting Editor: Justine A. Lee, DVM, DACVECC

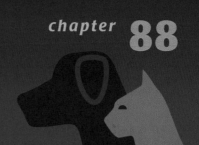
Fluoride

DEFINITION/OVERVIEW

- Fluoride toxicosis develops after the ingestion of products that contain fluoride compounds. Many fluoride-containing products are used for prophylactic dental care, as multivitamins, for treatment of osteoporosis, and as insecticides.
- When ingested acutely in large enough quantities, fluoride salts can be caustic to the GIT and lead to metabolic disturbances that result in arrhythmias and respiratory muscle paralysis. Long-term chronic overdoses without calcium supplementation can cause skeletal fluorosis, which is a weakening of the bone, leading to fractures and malformations.

ETIOLOGY/PATHOPHYSIOLOGY

Mechanism of Action

- When fluoride salts are ingested, they react in the acid environment of the stomach to create hydrofluoric acid, which is highly corrosive. Once absorbed, fluoride interferes with electrolyte concentrations and can result in hypocalcemia and hypokalemia.
- With large or high concentration ingestions, hypokalemia can be severe enough to cause ECG changes (prolonged QT intervals), and secondary cardiac symptoms may result. Respiratory muscle paralysis from hypocalcemia or cardiac arrest from hypokalemia are the most common causes of death.

Pharmacokinetics/Absorption, Distribution, Metabolism, and Excretion

- Sodium fluoride and other soluble fluorides are rapidly absorbed from the GIT and reach peak plasma levels 30 minutes after ingestion.
- Fluoride is not protein bound but instead circulates as a free ion until it is bound to the bone gradually over the next few hours.
- Fluoride is excreted very slowly, with half the ingested amount eliminated by the kidneys daily. The remainder is excreted in feces, sweat, and milk or retained by the bone.
- Elimination half-life is 2–9 hours in people with normal kidney function and up to 2 years in people with kidney failure.

Toxicity

- Fluoride salts react with the acids in the stomach to produce highly caustic hydrofluoric acid.
- Once absorbed, hydrofluoric acid interferes with calcium metabolism and induces efflux of potassium from red blood cells, resulting in profound clinical symptoms from electrolyte abnormalities.
- Most pets will have mild symptoms when the amount of elemental fluoride ingested is less than 5 mg/kg. This dose is extrapolated from the human pediatric dose, as little veterinary literature exists regarding fluoride toxicosis in animals.
- Fluoride toothpaste typically contains a maximum of 1.1 mg of fluoride per gram of toothpaste. Mouthwashes or rinses typically contain 0.2% sodium fluoride and have approximately 9.1 mg of fluoride/mL of rinse.

Systems Affected

- Gastrointestinal—oral corrosive injury, GI irritation, nausea, vomiting, anorexia, pain, pancreatitis, HGE
- Cardiovascular—potentially fatal cardiac arrhythmias secondary to profound hypokalemia and hypocalcemia
- Respiratory—coughing, choking, respiratory irritation, respiratory muscle paralysis
- Hemic/lymphatic/immune—hypocalcemia, interference with normal calcium metabolism, secondary coagulopathy due to hypocalcemia, hypokalemia
- Hepatobiliary—increased liver enzymes
- Nervous—hyperactive reflexes
- Musculoskeletal—painful muscle spasms, weakness and titanic contractures (secondary to hypocalcemia), skeletal fluorosis (weak, brittle bones and calcified ligaments)
- Gastrointestinal—pitted tooth enamel, discolored teeth (chronic toxicity), primarily when exposure precedes dental eruption
- Skin/exocrine—dermal irritation after prolonged topical exposure

 SIGNALMENT/HISTORY

Risk Factors

- Any age, sex, and breed of pet
- Young animals that are more curious may be more likely to chew on household items.
- Animals drinking water from a well or water source with high fluoride content
- Chronic exposure of young animals impairs dentin and enamel formation resulting in enamel pitting and excessive tooth wear.

Historical Findings

- Witnessed ingestion
- Discovery of chewed up packaging; owner may notice clinical symptoms of drooling, vomiting, and anorexia.
- Frequent fractures and boney injury with minimal trauma may be indicative of chronic fluoride toxicosis.
- Chronic lameness and exostosis may be early signs of chronic fluorosis.

Location and Circumstances of Poisoning

- This poisoning typically occurs within the owner's home, specifically in the bathroom, where the pet has access to toothpaste or mouthwash containing fluoride.

Interactions with Drugs, Nutrients, or Environment

- Fluoride is present in many products, and pets that already receive high levels of fluoride from their water source are at higher risk.

 # CLINICAL FEATURES

- Initial clinical signs of hypersalivation, nausea, depression, abdominal pain, frequent swallowing, gagging, or lip licking will be present.
- Ulcers or erythma may be present in the mouth, but this may not be initially evident within the first 1–2 hours.
- Cardiac arrhythmia may be detectable on auscultation.

 # DIFFERENTIAL DIAGNOSIS

- Toxicities—corrosive:
  - Oven and toilet cleaners
  - Ultra-concentrated bleach
- Permethrin ingestion or application
- Toxicities—plant:
  - Azalea or rhododendron, calcium oxalate–containing plants, etc.

 # DIAGNOSTICS

- Electrolytes—Potassium, calcium, and magnesium need to be monitored frequently and supplemented appropriately.
- ECG—Arrhythmias secondary to potassium and calcium abnormalities are a frequent cause of cardiac arrest with large ingestions.

Pathological Findings

- Primarily limited to damage in the GIT. Chronic fluorosis causes exostosis of long bones (e.g., legs, ribs) as well as mottled, pitted, or excessively worn teeth.

 THERAPEUTICS

- Treatment for fluoride toxicosis includes aggressive decontamination, neutralization of the fluoride with calcium, fluid therapy, correction of electrolyte abnormalities, gastroprotectants, antiemetics, analgesics, and overall supportive care.

Detoxification

- Before decontamination is initiated, determine which type of fluoride was ingested (e.g., corrosive vs. noncorrosive), if possible.
    - Noncorrosive:
        - Emesis should be induced only if the fluoride product ingested is not corrosive.
        - If ingestion was within 2 hours for a tablet-based product or 1 hour for a gel or powder, prompt decontamination should be attempted.
        - If emesis return is low yield, consider gastric lavage with a large-bore stomach tube and an inflated endotracheal tube to protect the airway.
    - Corrosive:
        - If the type of fluoride is corrosive, emesis is not recommended.
        - Careful gastric lavage with a calcium gluconate solution to bind the fluoride ion should be performed, followed by an additional product that will neutralize the fluoride.
            - Aluminum- or magnesium-based antacid: aluminum hydroxide 30–90 mg/kg PO q 24 hours x 5–7 days

Appropriate Health Care

- Maintain hydration and perfusion with IV fluid therapy until clinical symptoms resolve.
- Correct electrolyte abnormalities.
    - Calcium supplementation: calcium gluconate 10% 50–150 mg/kg over 20–30 minutes, IV to effect
    - Potassium supplementation: potassium chloride diluted in IV fluids. Do not exceed 0.5 mEq/kg/hr.
- Monitor cardiac function with a continuous ECG to evaluate for the presence of arrhythmias.

- Treat GI signs with antiemetic therapy, H_2 blockers, and gastroprotectants, particularly if the product was corrosive. The additional use of dairy products (e.g., milk, yogurt, etc.) and/or aluminum hydroxide agents to neutralize the fluoride may be beneficial, provided the patient is not vomiting.

Drug(s) and Antidotes of Choice

- No particular antidote

Precautions/Interactions

- Electrolyte supplementation needs to be performed slowly, with cardiac monitoring and regular rechecks of serum levels to determine if further supplementation is necessary.
- Patients with renal failure should be supplemented with potassium cautiously.
- Aluminum hydroxide supplementation can alter the absorption of other drugs and should be administered 1 hour apart from other oral medications.

Diet

- Calcium supplementation may be needed initially, but no long-term diet changes are recommended.

Prevention

- Pet owners should be informed about the risks of fluoride toxicosis.
- Appropriate pet-proofing of household consumer products, bathroom products, etc. will aid in preventing pet exposure to these products.

 COMMENTS

Patient Monitoring

- Serum electrolytes should be monitored every 2–4 hours during initial management. Frequent monitoring is needed to ensure that the amount of supplementation is appropriate, to ensure the pet is not being oversupplemented, and to detect trends and response to treatment.

Prevention/Avoidance

- Store fluoride-containing products away from pets.

Possible Complications

- Ulcerations of the GIT could potentially cause perforation, necessitating surgical intervention.

- If electrolyte abnormalities cannot be corrected quickly, death from cardiac arrest or respiratory muscle paralysis is possible. Mechanical ventilation may be necessary until respiratory muscle paralysis resolves.

Expected Course and Prognosis

- Prognosis is good with small ingestions or with early intervention and appropriate management. Large ingestions with late intervention have a guarded prognosis.

Synonyms

skeletal fluorosis, sodium fluoride toxicosis, fluoride silicate toxicosis, fluoridosis

Abbreviations

CBC = complete blood count
ECG = electrocardiogram
GI   = gastrointestinal
GIT = gastrointestinal tract
HGE = hemorrhagic gastroenteritis
IV   = intravenous
PO   = *per os* (by mouth)
q   = every

See Also

Hydrofluoric Acid

Suggested Reading

Augenstein WL, Spoerke DG, Kulig KW. Fluoride ingestion in children: a review of 87 cases. Pediatrics 1991; 88:907–912.
Boink AB, Wemer J, Meulenbelt J, et al. The mechanism of fluoride-induced hypocalcaemia. Hum Exp Toxicol 1994; 13:149–155.

Author: Catherine Angle, DVM, MPH
Consulting Editor: Justine A. Lee, DVM, DACVECC

Plants and Biotoxins

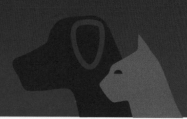

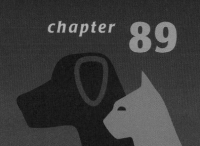

chapter **89**

Blue-green Algae (Cyanobacteria)

DEFINITION/OVERVIEW

- Blue-green algal (cyanobacterial) proliferations occur in freshwater and brackish ecosystems under certain environmental conditions, potentially resulting in toxin production and leading to harmful algal blooms (fig. 89.1).
- Most blue-green algal blooms do not produce toxins. However, determining toxin production and severity is not possible with the naked eye. All blooms are potentially toxic.
- Blue-green algae exposure can lead to an acute intoxication affecting either the liver or the CNS. Hepatotoxic blue-green algae poisonings are more frequently reported than neurotoxic algal intoxication.
- Toxigenic blue-green algae include *Microcystis*, *Anabena*, *Aphanizomenon*, *Oscillatoria*, *Lyngbya*, and *Planktothrix*.
- Microcystins are hepatotoxic blue-green algae toxins that have been found worldwide and are produced by *Microcystis*, *Anabaena*, *Planktothrix*, and other genera.
- Anatoxins, which include anatoxin-a and anatoxin-a$_s$, are neurotoxic blue-green algae toxins produced by *Anabaena*, *Planktothrix*, *Oscillatoria*, *Microcystis*, and other genera.
- Cyanotoxin poisoning has occurred in animals and humans.
- The overall prognosis is poor, with death occurring minutes to hours (neurotoxin) or hours to days (hepatotoxin) after exposure.

ETIOLOGY/PATHOPHYSIOLOGY

Mechanism of Action

- Microcystins are specifically toxic to the liver by inhibiting protein phosphatases 1 and 2A. The resulting disruption of cytoskeletal components and associated rearrangement of filamentous actin within hepatocytes account for the severe liver damage. Free radical formation and mitochondrial alterations may also contribute to the pathological changes, most notably acute centrilobular necrosis.
- Anatoxin-a is a potent cholinergic agonist at nicotinic acetylcholine receptors that results in continuous electrical stimulation at the neuromuscular junctions.

687

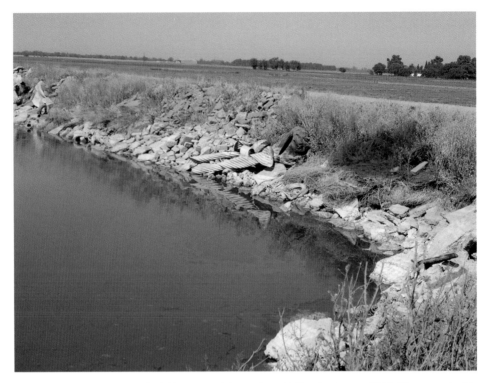

■ **Fig. 89.1.** *Microcystis* sp. algal bloom; pond in Northern California, August 2008. Bloom resulted in illness and death of cattle. Outbreak occurred during a period of high ambient temperature (above 100°F for days) after strong winds had concentrated the algal material at one side of the pond, which was the only water access these cattle had. (Photo courtesy of Birgit Puschner)

- Anatoxin-a$_s$ is a naturally occurring irreversible acetylcholinesterase inhibitor that leads to increased acetylcholine concentrations in the synapse. The mechanism of action is similar to acetylcholinesterase inhibition caused by organophosphorus and carbamate insecticides. A major difference, however, is that anatoxin-a$_s$ is incapable of crossing the blood brain barrier; therefore, effects and clinical signs are peripheral.

Pharmacokinetics/Absorption, Distribution, Metabolism, and Excretion

- There is very limited data on the kinetics of microcystins. Some data suggest conjugation with glutathione and cystine as major detoxification pathways.
- Data on the toxicokinetics of anatoxin-a and anatoxin-a$_s$ do not exist.

Toxicity

- The LD$_{50}$ for microcystins varies between 50 and 11,000 µg/kg, depending on the exact microcystin structure, the species affected, and the route of administra-

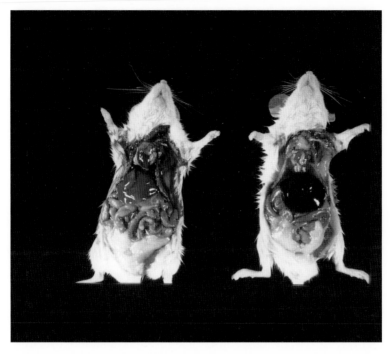

■ **Fig. 89.2.** Mouse bioassay: massive hepatic enlargement with dark discoloration subsequent to intraperitoneal injection with 0.5 mL of algal extract (R mouse). Control mouse (L) was given 0.5 mL of deionized water IP. Algal boom had resulted in illness and death of cattle in Northern California and was identified morphologically as a *Microcystis* sp. (Photo courtesy of Birgit Puschner)

tion. In mice, the oral LD_{50} value for microcystin-LR is 10.9 mg/kg, while the IP LD_{50} is 50 μg/kg. Most algal blooms contain a number of structural variants of microcystins, and thus it is difficult to estimate the potential toxicity of a bloom.

■ The reported IP LD_{50} of anatoxin-a in mice is 200 μg/kg while the IV LD_{50} is estimated at less than 100 μg/kg. The oral toxicity of anatoxin-a is much higher, with an oral LD_{50} in mice reported as greater than 5,000 μg/kg (see fig. 89.2).

■ Anatoxin-a_s is much more toxic than anatoxin-a. The reported IP LD_{50} in mice is 20 μg/kg.

Systems Affected

■ Microcystins
   • Hepatobiliary—diarrhea, weakness, pale mucous membranes, icterus, shock
■ Anatoxin-a and anatoxin-a_s
   • Nervous—muscle tremors, muscle rigidity, paralysis, cyanosis, salivation with anatoxin-a_s

SIGNALMENT/HISTORY

- Dogs are the most common species to be affected by microcystins and anatoxin-a, although many species may develop toxicosis if a sufficient dose is ingested.
- Backyard ponds that are poorly maintained and allow for cyanobacterial proliferation may pose a risk to dogs.

Risk Factors

- Dogs that enjoy swimming are more likely to consume toxic amounts of an algal bloom than dogs that refrain from water.
- Algal bloom prevalence is higher during increased water temperature and elevated nutrient concentrations in the water.

Historical Findings

- Witnessed exposure to water with or without visible algal bloom. Toxins may persist in the water post-bloom.
- Algal material on coat or present in vomit
- Owners frequently report rapid onset of clinical presentation, usually within 30 minutes of access to water.
- Other animals (especially livestock) may be found dead near the water source.

Location and Circumstances of Poisoning

- Lakes, streams, ponds, removed algal material (bucket)
- Most microcystin-producing algal blooms are found in freshwater, but they have also occurred in saline environments.
- Algal bloom prevalence is highest during increased water temperature and elevated nutrient concentrations in the water.
- Steady winds that propel toxic blooms to shore allow for ingestion by thirsty animals.
- Different algal species reside in the benthic zone (i.e., on the sediment) or in the pelagic zone (water column). Blooms of pelagic species are usually easily detected at the water surface of ponds, rivers, or lakes. Blooms of benthic species are difficult to detect as the algae are on the surface of sediment and stones in rivers or lakes.

CLINICAL FEATURES

- Microcystins—acute hepatotoxicosis with clinical signs of diarrhea, weakness, pale mucous membranes, and shock. Progression of disease is rapid and death generally occurs within several hours of exposure.

- Anatoxin-a—Clinical signs include rapid onset of rigidity and muscle tremors, followed by paralysis, cyanosis, and death as a result of potent cholinergic stimulation. Progression is very rapid and death usually occurs within minutes to a few hours of exposure.
- Anatoxin-a$_s$—rapid onset of excessive salivation (the "s" stands for salivation), lacrimation, diarrhea, and urination associated with muscarinic overstimulation. Clinical signs of nicotinic overstimulation include tremors, incoordination, and convulsions. Respiratory arrest and recumbency may be seen prior to death. Progression is very rapid and animals may die within 30 minutes of exposure.

 # DIFFERENTIAL DIAGNOSIS

- Microcystin toxicosis—other causes of acute liver failure such as amanitins, aflatoxins, cocklebur, xylitol, cycad palms, acetaminophen
- Anatoxin-a—strychnine, metaldehyde, avitrol, penitrem A/roquefortine mycotoxins, methylxanthines, pyrethrin/pyrethroid insecticides, organochlorine insecticides, poisonous plants (cyanide, oleander, poison hemlock), illicit substances (amphetamine derivatives), ephedra-containing compounds
- Anatoxin-a$_s$—organophosphorus and carbamate insecticides, slaframine

DIAGNOSTICS

- Save gastric contents and water source samples for diagnostic testing
- Clinical pathology
  - Microcystins—increase in serum ALP, AST, ALT and in bilirubin, hyperkalemia, hypoglycemia
  - Anatoxin-a and anatoxin-a$_s$—no significant findings
- Toxicology testing
  - Toxicity is strain specific and identification of a potential toxin-producing strain should be followed up by toxicant detection to predict toxicity level.
  - Anatoxin-a$_s$—depressed blood cholinesterase activity
  - Identification of the algae in the suspect water source or stomach contents; however, positive identification does not confirm intoxication because the toxicity of the cyanobacteria is strain specific, and morphological observations alone cannot predict the hazard level.
  - Detection of microcystins in gastric contents and suspect source material
  - Detection of anatoxin-a in gastric contents, urine, bile, and suspect source material
  - Mouse bioassay (IP injection of algal bloom extract) was used in the past to determine the toxicity of crude algal biomass in suspicious blue-green algae poisonings (fig. 89.2).

Pathological Findings

- Microcystins—detection of algal bloom material in GI tract and/or on legs. Grossly evident liver enlargement; histologic lesions include progressive centrilobular hepatocyte rounding, dissociation, and necrosis; breakdown of the sinusoidal endothelium; and intrahepatic hemorrhage.
- Anatoxin-a and anatoxin-a$_s$—detection of algal bloom material in GI tract and/or on legs. No lesions are usually present.

 # THERAPEUTICS

- The treatment goals are to prevent further exposure and absorption, control CNS signs, and provide supportive care.
- Treatment is often unsuccessful due to the rapid onset of clinical signs and death.
- Microcystin toxicosis—Provide supportive therapy to treat hypovolemia and electrolyte imbalances.
- Anatoxin-a toxicosis—General supportive care and specific measures to control seizures should be performed.
- Anatoxin-a$_s$ toxicosis—Atropine should be given at a test dose to determine its efficacy in animals with life-threatening clinical signs. After the test dose, atropine can be given repeatedly until cessation of salivation.

Detoxification

- Emesis may be induced in asymptomatic animals with recent exposures.
- Activated charcoal can be attempted, but efficacy is questionable.
- Bathe all animals with dermal exposure very thoroughly. Protective clothing must be worn by staff members during bathing (risk of dermatitis).

Appropriate Health Care

- All intoxicated animals will need aggressive and intensive care.
- Ventilation should be closely monitored in patients with severe neurologic impairment using venous or arterial (preferred) pCO$_2$ or end-tidal capnography. Mechanical ventilation is indicated for patients with hypoventilation.

Drug(s) and Antidotes of Choice

- No antidote available
- Manage acute signs of hepatic hemorrhagic shock with IV crystalloids, colloids, and blood products as needed. Initial shock boluses of 20 mL/kg of crystalloids can be given over 10–20 minutes during initial stabilization.

- The use of blood products (pRBC, WB, FFP, or FP) may be necessary to increase oxygen carrying capacity and to replace coagulation factors. Patients should be blood typed prior to transfusion.
  - Blood products (whole blood, pRBC, etc.) 10–20 mL/kg IV to effect
  - FFP or FP 10–20 mL/kg IV over 1–4 hours
- Seizures
  - Diazepam 2–5 mg/kg IV. These doses are much higher than normally used for seizure control. In general, if a 2-mg/kg IV dose does not control seizures, switch to phenobarbital.
  - Phenobarbital 2–20 mg/kg IV q 6–12 hours
- Tremors
  - Methocarbamol 55–220 mg/kg IV
- Atropine 0.02–0.04 mg/kg IV to effect in anatoxin-a$_s$ intoxication
- Vitamin K$_1$ (phytonadione) 1–5 mg/kg q 24 hours PO, SQ to address clotting issues
- Hepatoprotectants
  - SAMe 18–20 mg/kg PO q 24 hours
  - Silymarin 20–50 mg/kg PO q 24 hours

Precautions/Interactions

- Wear protective clothing while handling/bathing affected animals. Significant contact dermatitis may occur.

Nursing Care

- Intensive care and monitoring may be needed.
- Anatoxin-a and anatoxin-a$_s$—thermoregulation and minimize sensory stimulation

Prevention

- Dogs should be denied access to water with visible algal blooms.
- Reduce fertilizer runoff and applications in fields surrounding ponds used for drinking water.
- Remove algal blooms from ponds immediately and discard material safely.

Public Health

- Toxin-producing algal blooms also pose a significant human health risk. Cases of human contact dermatitis, upper respiratory irritation, and death have occurred.
- Suspect blooms should be reported to local environmental regulatory authorities.

COMMENTS

Client Education

- Though most algae blooms do not produce toxins, determining toxicity is not possible with the naked eye. Therefore, warn clients to avoid all visible algal blooms.
- Toxin-producing algal blooms also pose a risk to humans. Do not allow children to play in or near suspect blooms.

Patient Monitoring

- Microcystin toxicosis—monitor liver function, coagulation status
- Anatoxin-a and anatoxin-a$_s$—monitor biochemical profile, blood gases, and respiratory function

Prevention/Avoidance

- Dogs should be denied access to water with visible algal blooms.
- Reduce fertilizer runoff and applications in fields surrounding ponds used for drinking water.
- Remove algal blooms from ponds immediately and discard material safely.

Possible Complications

- DIC, rhabdomyolysis, and myoglobinuria with subsequent renal failure are possible if prolonged, untreated tremors/seizures or hyperthermia present.

Expected Course and Prognosis

- Animals poisoned with blue-green algae toxins are often found dead.
- Blue-green algae intoxications progress so rapidly that treatment is often too late.
- Prognosis is poor.

Abbreviations

ALP = alkaline phosphatase
ALT = alanine transaminase
AST = aspartate transaminase
CNS = central nervous system
CO_2 = carbon dioxide
DIC = disseminated intravascular coagulation
FFP = fresh frozen plasma
FP = frozen plasma

GI   = gastrointestinal
IM   = intramuscular
IP   = intraperitoneal
IV   = intravenous
LD_{50} = median lethal dose
PO   = *per os* (by mouth)
q   = every
pRBC = packed red blood cells
SAMe = s-adenosyl-methionine
SQ   = subcutaneous
WB   = whole blood

Suggested Reading

Puschner B. Cyanobacterial (blue-green algae) toxins. In: Gupta RC, ed. Veterinary Toxicology: Basic and Clinical Principles. New York: Elsevier, 2007; pp. 714–724.

Puschner B, Brent H, Tor ER. Diagnosis of anatoxin-a poisoning in dogs from North America. J Vet Diagn Invest 2008; 20:89–92.

Authors: Amber Roegner, BS; Birgit Puschner, DVM, PhD, DABVT
Consulting Editor: Lynn R. Hovda, RPH, DVM, MS, DACVIM

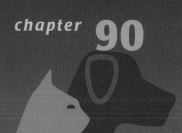

chapter 90

Cardiac Glycosides

DEFINITION/OVERVIEW

- Several plants and animals contain naturally occurring cardiotoxic cardenolides or bufadienolides that cause GI disturbances as well as severe cardiac arrhythmias. Approximately 400 cardiac cardenolides have been reported. Digoxin and digitoxin, the most widely known of these toxins, were originally used to treat congestive heart failure in human beings.
- Common plants containing cardiac glycoside toxins include:
  - Desert rose (*Adenium obesum*)
  - Dogbane (*Apocynum* spp.)
  - Purple or common foxglove (*Digitalis purpurea*; fig. 90.1)
  - Giant milkweed (*Calatropis* spp.)
  - Kalanchoe (*Kalanchoe* spp.; fig. 90.2)
  - Lily of the valley (*Convallaria majalis*; fig. 90.3)
  - Milkweed (*Asclepias* spp.)
  - Oleander (*Nerium oleander*; figs. 90.4 and 90.5)
  - Star of Bethlehem (*Ornithogalum umbellatum*)
  - Wooly foxglove (*Digitalis lantana*)
  - Yellow oleander (*Thevetia peruviana*)
- Common names are often used for several different plants, making the scientific names essential for accurate identification.
- Different plants may have varying levels of toxicity, and concentrations of these glycosides will differ in separate parts of the plant (i.e., stem, leaves, seeds, or fruit).
- Plants can be cultivated for indoor and outdoor uses (landscape plants) and are also found in nature.

ETIOLOGY/PATHOPHYSIOLOGY

Mechanism of Action

- Consuming cardiac glycoside–containing plants causes interference with the sodium-potassium pump mediated by ATPase, resulting in an increase in intracellular sodium and decrease in intracellular potassium.
- The decrease in intracellular potassium interferes with electrical conduction, resulting in progressive electrical changes. The normal resting membrane

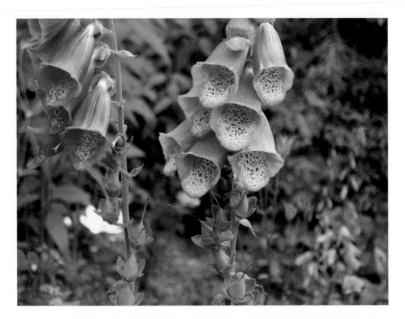

■ **Fig. 90.1.** Common foxglove (*Digitalis purpurea*). (photo courtesy of Tyne K. Hovda)

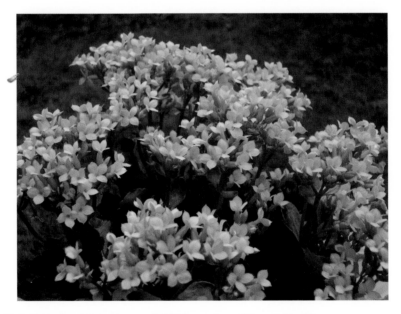

■ **Fig. 90.2.** Kalanchoe (*Kalanchoe* spp.). (photo courtesy of Tyne K. Hovda)

potential is decreased and eventually a complete loss of normal myocardial electrical function occurs.
■ Hyperkalemia may be marked with a loss of cardiac excitability and response.

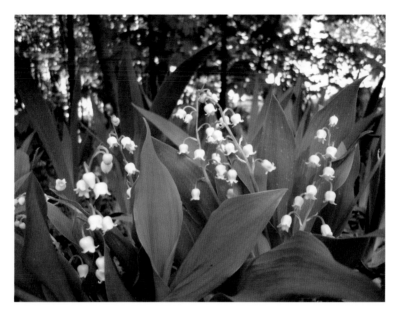

■ Fig. 90.3. Lily of the valley (*Convallaria majalis*). (photo courtesy of Tyne K. Hovda)

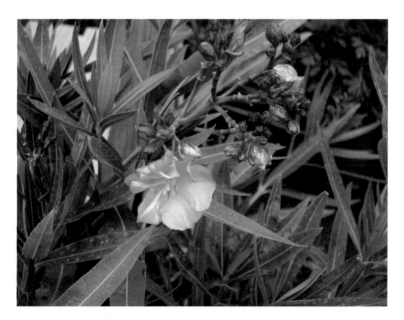

■ Fig. 90.4. Oleander flower (*Nerium oleander*). (photo courtesy of Tyne K. Hovda)

Pharmacokinetics/Absorption, Distribution, Metabolism, and Excretion

■ Absorption is rapid, with signs occurring from 30–45 minutes to a few hours after ingestion.

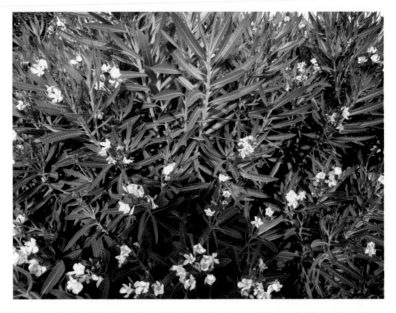

■ **Fig. 90.5.** Oleander plant (*Nerium oleander*). This plant was photographed growing along a sidewalk in downtown Las Vegas, Nevada. (photo courtesy of Tyne K. Hovda)

Toxicity

- Toxins are structurally similar to digitalis (steroidal glycosides) and present the same toxic profile.
- Several hundred different toxins have been identified, most specific to a particular plant.
  - The degree of toxicity varies depending on the particular plant, plant part, and amount consumed.
  - Most of the cardiac glycoside plants cause toxicosis in either fresh or dried form when consumed.
  - All plant parts are considered toxic—even water in vases containing bouquets. Ingestion of just a few seeds or one to two leaves may be enough to cause serious clinical signs.

Systems Affected

- Gastrointestinal—Signs occur more frequently and include hypersalivation and vomiting and diarrhea with or without blood.
- Cardiovascular—Abnormalities include bradycardia, all degrees of AV block, and a variety of arrhythmias. Rarely, tachycardia occurs. Death is from asytole.
- Neuromuscular—Signs are vague and may be related to decreased cardiac output and hypotension.
- Ophthalmic—Mydriasis

SIGNALMENT/HISTORY

- No breed or species predilection; cats may be more sensitive than dogs.
- Dogs with ABCB1 (formerly referred to MDR-1) gene mutation (e.g., Collies, Australian Shepherds, etc.) are more sensitive to the CNS effects of glycoside toxicity.
- Common clinical signs include vomiting and diarrhea, weakness and depression, and cardiac abnormalities.

Risk Factors

- Animals with a prior history of renal disease or cardiac disease, especially those currently receiving digoxin or other cardiac drugs

Historical Findings

- Owner often reports that the animal chewed or dug up plants or knocked over a vase and drank the water

Location and Circumstances of Poisoning

- Can be anywhere as some species of the plants are found throughout the United States
- Oleander tends to occur with greater frequency in the warmer portions of the country.
- Most of the plants are unpalatable but may be ingested by bored or confined animals.

CLINICAL FEATURES

- Vomiting with or without blood, diarrhea with or without blood, and hypersalivation are the most commonly reported signs, often occurring with 30–45 minutes of ingestion. Weakness and depression often precede the onset of cardiac abnormalities. Varying degrees of bradycardia or tachycardia, weak and irregular pulses, hypotension, AV block, and arrhythmias can occur. Other signs include mydriasis, tremors, and coma.
- Males may exhibit clinical signs more often than females.
- Some animals may be found dead.

DIFFERENTIAL DIAGNOSIS

- Cardiac disease of any origin
- Digoxin or digitoxin ingestion
- Calcium channel blocker or beta-blocker ingestion

- Ingestion of *Taxus* spp. or plants in *Ericaceae* family (azaleas, rhododendrons)
- Ingestion of animal or human pharmaceuticals with known cardiac effects
- Severe GI disease associated with viral, bacterial, or other diseases

 # DIAGNOSTICS

- Presence of plant in stomach or GIT
- Serum chemistry with early and marked hyperkalemia. May change to hypokalemia as time passes.
- Serum digoxin levels available from human hospitals; be sure the laboratory is running an assay that includes the toxin associated with the specific plant in question.
- Detection of cardiac glycoside in tissue or urine is rarely performed but available by use of chromatography if specific glycoside is known.

Pathological Findings

- Gross findings depend on the time of death, but often plant pieces are found in the stomach and small intestine. The epicardium may have a mottled appearance with clotted blood in the ventricles.
- Histopathological findings include venous and capillary congestion throughout the body with severe, diffuse hepatic congestion and marked caudal vena cava distention.

Detoxification

- Induction of emesis if early and the animal is not already vomiting
- Activated charcoal with a cathartic × 1 dose followed by activated charcoal every 4–6 hours for 2–3 doses

Appropriate Health Care

- Hospitalize animals with known ingestions for at least 12 hours. Clinical signs are often evident at 30–45 minutes but may be delayed for several hours depending on particular plant ingested.
- ECG monitoring for minimum of 24 hours in animals with clinical signs. Treat arrhythmias as they develop.
- Baseline serum chemistry with special attention to potassium and renal indices. Hyperkalemia may be severe. Correct electrolyte abnormalities as needed.
- Judicious use of IV fluids to support but not overload the cardiovascular system

Drugs and Antidotes of Choice

- Digoxin-specific Fab fragments (Digibind) have been used in dogs to reverse the cardiac effects of oleander and may be effective for other cardiac glycoside toxins as well. The cost often precludes their use.

- Early, yet cautious, use of IV fluids to maintain blood pressure and cardiovascular system but not overload the cardiovascular system
- Bradycardia
  - Atropine 0.02–0.04 mg/kg IV, IM, or SQ
  - Glycopyrrolate 0.01–0.02 mg/kg SQ, IM, or IV
  - In severe cases of bradycardia unresponsive to medical management, the use of a temporary pacemaker may be indicated.
- The use of antiarrhythmics (lidocaine, procainamide) may be necessary if the patient is persistently tachycardic and nonresponsive to IV fluids, has severe ventricular dysrhythmias, or has evidence of poor perfusion (hypotension, pulse deficits, tachycardia, pale mucous membranes, prolonged CRT).
  - Lidocaine
    - Dogs: 2–8 mg/kg IV to effect while monitoring ECG
    - Cats: 0.25–0.5 mg/kg slow IV while monitoring ECG. Use judiciously in cats!
  - Procainamide
    - Dogs: 2 mg/kg IV over 3–5 minutes (up to 20 mg/kg IV bolus), followed by 25–50 µg/kg/min CRI
    - Cats: 1–2 mg/kg IV once, followed by 10–20 µg/kg IV CRI
- Antiemetics if vomiting is severe or persists
  - Maropitant 1 mg/kg SQ q 24 hours, not labeled for cats
  - Ondansetron 0.1–0.2 mg/kg IV q 8–12 hours
- GI protectants as needed
  - H$_2$ blockers
    - Famotidine 0.5–1 mg/kg PO, SQ, IM, IV q 12 hours
    - Ranitidine 1–2 mg/kg PO, SQ, IM, IV q 8–12 hours
    - Cimetidine 5–10 mg/kg PO, SQ, IM, IV q 6 hours
  - Omeprazole 0.5–1 mg/kg daily
  - Sucralfate 0.25–1 g PO q 8 hours for 5–7 days if evidence of active ulcer disease

Alternative Drugs

- Fructose-1, 6-diphosphate has been used experimentally to prevent the severity of cardiac effects in dogs. The mechanism of action is not understood.

Precautions/Interactions

- Hawthorne, an herbal supplement, should not be used as it exacerbates the toxicity of cardiac glycosides.
- Calcium channel blockers and beta-blockers can have additive effects on AV conduction and may result in complete heart block.

Nursing Care

- Palpation of extremities for coldness; may indicate decreased perfusion and onset of hypotension
- Often required for 5–6 days

 # COMMENTS

Client Education

- Avoid the use of use of herbal or alternative supplements such as hawthorne until the animal has recovered completely.

Patient Monitoring

- Frequent ECG strips for first 24 hours and then as needed to monitor effect of cardiac drugs
- Blood pressure monitoring, especially early in toxicity. Hypotension may become severe.
- Baseline and repeat serum electrolytes. Hyperkalemia may be early and marked; hypokalemia has been reported but often occurs later.

Prevention/Avoidance

- Learn to recognize the common plants in your house and geographical location.
- Oleander commonly grows wild in the Southwest, especially Arizona, California, and Texas. Off-leash dogs should be watched carefully for any signs of exposure.

Expected Course and Prognosis

- Prognosis is good with appropriate care and timely intervention
- The occurrence of cardiac arrhythmias complicates recovery but is not insurmountable if treated early.

Abbreviations

AV	= atrioventricular
CNS	= central nervous system
CRI	= constant rate infusion
CRT	= capillary refill time
ECG	= electrocardiogram
Fab	= fragment antigen binding
GI	= gastrointestinal tract

IM   = intramuscular
IV   = intravenous
MDR-1 = Multidrug Resistance 1 gene
PO   = *per os* (by mouth)
q   = every
SQ   = subcutaneous

See Also

Beta Blockers
Calcium Channel Blockers
Rhododendrons/Azaleas
Yew

Suggested Reading

Burrows GE, Tyrl RJ. Toxic Plants of North America. Ames: Iowa State Press; 2001; pp. 68–70, 1093–1095.

Clark RF, Selden BS, Curry SC. Digoxin-specific Fab fragments in the treatment of oleander toxicity in a canine model. Ann Emerg Med 1991; 20(10):1073–1077.

Hamlin RL. Digitalis toxicosis. Clinical toxicology of cardiovascular drugs. Vet Clin North Am Small Anim Pract 1990; 20(2):474–476.

Milweski LM, Safda AK. An overview of potentially life-threatening poisonous plants in dogs and cats. J Vet Emerg Criti Care 2006; 16(1):25–33.

Smith G. Kalanchoe species poisoning in pets. Vet Med 2004; 99(11):913–936.

Authors: Erica Cargill, CVT; Krishona L. Martinson, PhD
Consulting Editor: Lynn R. Hovda, RPH, DVM, MS, DACVIM

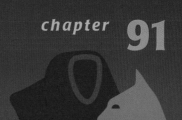
Lilies

DEFINITION/OVERVIEW

- Toxicity is associated with ingestion of many plants in the genera *Lilium* and *Hemerocallis*.
- The target organ is the kidney. Ingestion of plant parts can result in vomiting, anorexia, lethargy, oliguria or anuria, acute renal failure, and rarely, pancreatitis in cats.
- Lilies are frequently cultivated as garden and house plants, found growing in nature, and used in many floral bouquets and baskets.

ETIOLOGY/PATHOPHYSIOLOGY

- Ingestion of plant material (leaves, stems, and flowers)
- Ingestion of pollen and water contaminated with pollen or plant material
- Floral extract contains the highest amounts of toxic compound.
- Includes Easter lily (*Lilium longiflorum*; fig. 91.1), tiger lily (*L. tigrinum*), rubrum lily (*L. speciosum*), stargazer lily (*L. auratum*), Japanese show lily (*L. lancifolimu*), Asiatic hybrid lilies (*Lilium* spp.; fig. 91.2), red lily (*L. umbellantum*), Western lily (*L. umbellantum*), wood lily (L. umbellantum), and daylily (*Hemerocallis* spp.; fig. 91.3)

SIGNALMENT/HISTORY

- Most cases are reported in cats.
- Dogs are thought to be affected, but attempts to reproduce the disease in dogs (and rabbits) have been unsuccessful.
- Most exposure occurs during holidays or other festive occasions where lilies are used as house plants or found in floral arrangements.

Mechanism of Action

- Renal tubular necrosis with intact basement membrane

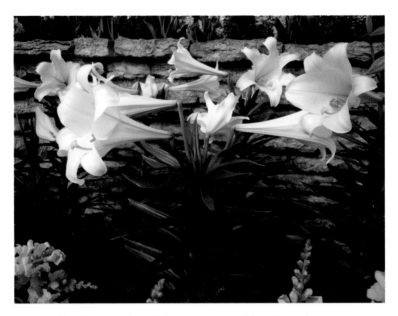

■ **Fig. 91.1.** Easter lily (*Lilium longiflorum*). (photo courtesy of Tyne K. Hovda)

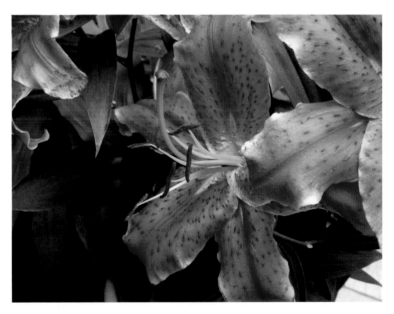

■ **Fig. 91.2.** Asiatic hybrid liliy (*Lilium* spp.). (photo courtesy of Tyne K. Hovda)

Toxicity

- The toxin has not been identified but is known to be water soluble.
- A dose of 568 mg/kg of aqueous leaf extract and 291 mg/kg of aqueous flower extract of Easter lily has elicited toxicosis in cats.
- Deaths have occurred after ingestion of only 1 or 2 plant pieces.

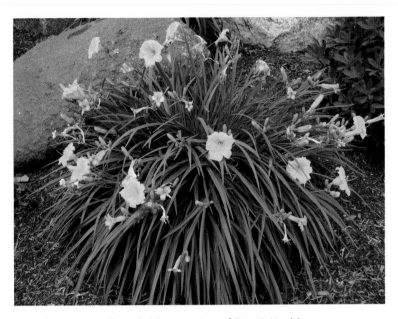

■ Fig. 91.3. Daylily (*Hemerocallis* spp.). (photo courtesy of Tyne K. Hovda)

Systems Affected

- Renal—acute renal failure
- Gastrointestinal—vomiting, diarrhea
- Neurological—ataxia, tremors, seizures

 # CLINICAL FEATURES

- All parts of the lily are considered toxic; however, the leaves are most commonly ingested.
- Signs usually develop within 6–12 hours of exposure.
- Early signs include vomiting, anorexia, and lethargy followed by acute renal failure.
- Clinical signs of renal failure include polyuria, oliguria, or anuria, dehydration, vomiting, diarrhea, and depression.
- Some cats also presented with CNS signs such as ataxia, head pressing, disorientation, tremors, and seizures.

 # DIFFERENTIAL DIAGNOSIS

- Toxins
  - Ethylene glycol
  - Grapes or raisins

- - Nonsteroidal anti-inflammatory drugs and nephrotoxic drugs
  - Soluble oxalate plants
- Infectious diseases
- Physical abnormalities (ureteral obstruction, nephrolith)

 # DIAGNOSTICS

- Serum chemistry findings include increases in blood urea nitrogen (BUN), creatinine, phosphorus, and potassium. BUN and creatinine generally increase within 18–24 hours of exposure. Creatine kinase may be disproportionately elevated.
- Urinalysis typically shows glucosuria, proteinuria, and isosthenuria. Epithelial casts usually can be seen in urine 12 hours after exposure.
- Renal ultrasound reveals changes consistent with acute tubular necrosis.

Pathological Findings

- Gross examination shows swollen, edematous kidneys and systemic congestion. Pancreatic necrosis may be present.
- Histopathologic examination of the kidneys shows acute proximal convoluted renal tubular necrosis with or without mineralization. The collecting ducts may contain granular or hyaline casts, and the basement membrane, while intact, may contain mitotic figures.

 # THERAPEUTICS

- Treatment of lily toxicosis consists primarily of early and aggressive supportive care including early decontamination, prevention of renal failure, and maintenance of fluid, electrolyte, and acid-base balance.
- Baseline BUN, creatinine, and electrolytes should be obtained on admission and repeated daily until they have returned normal.

Detoxification

- Bathe cats contaminated with pollen.
- Emesis within 1–2 hours of ingestion. Hydrogen peroxide is not recommended in cats. Xylazine (0.44–1.1 mg/kg IM or SQ) is effective and can be reversed with yohimbine or atipamezole after emesis.
- Activated charcoal with a cathartic × 1 dose only

Appropriate Healthcare

- Early and aggressive use of IV fluids to prevent renal damage
- Baseline serum chemistries to include BUN and creatinine. Monitor daily.
- Monitor urine output and add diuretics as needed.

Drugs of Choice and Antidote

- No antidote available
- IV fluid therapy at 2–3 times maintenance for 48 hours, then decrease depending on BUN and creatinine levels. Choice of fluid therapy depends on electrolyte and glucose levels. Generally 0.9% NaCl is an effective first line choice. IV fluids should be started within 18 hours of exposure; SQ fluids are not effective.
- Diuresis in oliguric cats once they are well hydrated
  - Furosemide CRI at 1–2 mg/kg/hour
  - Mannitol bolus at 1–2 g/kg
- GI protectants as needed
  - H₂ blockers
    - Famotidine 0.5–1 mg/kg PO, SQ, IM, IV q 12 hours
    - Ranitidine 1–2 mg/kg PO, SQ, IM, IV q 8–12 hours
    - Cimetidine 5–10 mg/kg PO, SQ, IM, IV q 6 hours
  - Omeprazole 0.5–1 mg/kg daily
  - Sucralfate 0.25–1 g PO q 8 hours × 5–7 days if evidence of active ulcer disease
- Peritoneal or renal dialysis may be useful in anuric cats.

 COMMENTS

Client Education

- Any exposure to lilies, regardless of the amount, should be considered harmful, and immediate veterinary intervention sought.

Prevention

- Keep Easter lilies and floral arrangements with lilies out of households with cats.
- Do not plant or maintain lilies in a garden if an outside cat can gain access to them.

Expected Course and Prognosis

- A delay in treatment of 18 hours or longer after exposure usually results in renal failure.
- The prognosis for cats aggressively treated prior to 18 hours is good. Once oliguria or anuria develops, the prognosis becomes fair to grave. Chronic renal impairment may occur in these cats even after treatment.
- Mortality rate from Easter lily toxicosis is reported to be as high as 100% if treatment is delayed and renal failure occurs.

Abbreviations

BUN = blood urea nitrogen
CNS = central nervous system
CRI = continuous rate infusion
GI = gastrointestinal
IM = intramuscular
IV = intravenous
NaCl = sodium chloride
PO = *per os* (by mouth)
q = every
SQ = subcutaneous

See Also

Ethylene Glycol
Grapes and Raisins

Suggested Reading

Berg RI, Francey T, Segev G. Resolution of acute kidney injury in a cat after lily (Lilium lancifolium) intoxication. J Vet Intern Med 2007; 21(4):857–859.

Hadley RM, Richardson JA, Gwaltney-Brand SM. A retrospective study of daylily toxicosis in cats. Vet Hum Toxicol 2003; 45(1):38–39.

Langston CE. Acute renal failure caused by lily ingestion in six cats. J Am Vet Med Assoc 2002; 220(1):49–52.

Milweski LM, Safdar AK. An overview of potentially life-threatening poisonous plants in dogs and cats. J Vet Emerg Crit Care 2006; 16(1):25–33.

Rumbeiha WK, Jayaraj AF, Fitzgerald SD, et al. A comprehensive study of Easter lily poisoning in cats. J Vet Diagn Invest 2004; 16(6):527–541.

Authors: Krishona L. Martinson, PhD; Lynn R. Hovda, DVM, MS, ACVIM
Consulting Editor: Lynn R. Hovda, RPH, DVM, MS, ACVIM

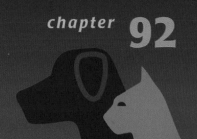

chapter 92

Mushrooms

DEFINITION/OVERVIEW

- Several thousand species of mushrooms are found in North America, but fewer than 100 are toxic.
- There is no simple test that distinguishes poisonous from nonpoisonous mushrooms.
- The most toxic mushrooms contain amanitin toxins.
- The number of reported mushroom poisonings in animals is low, although this is likely to be a result of the lack of diagnostic work-up and methods to confirm exposure.
- Amanitins:
    - The majority of confirmed mushroom poisonings in animals are caused by hepatotoxic mushrooms that contain amanitins.
    - Poisoned animals develop gastrointestinal signs between 6 and 24 hours after ingestion. After a period of "false recovery," fulminant liver failure develops generally 36 to 48 hours after exposure. During the final stage, renal failure can also develop.
    - While a number of mushroom genera (*Amanita*, *Galerina*, and *Lepiota*) contain the hepatotoxic cyclopeptides, *Amanita phalloides* (fig. 92.1), also known as death cap or death angel, and *A. ocreata* (fig. 92.2), also known as the destroying angel, are the species most frequently reported in poisonings.
    - Aggressive therapeutic measures are required to improve prognosis and include decontamination, supportive care, and administration of drugs that may reduce the toxin uptake into hepatocytes.
- Other toxic mushrooms (not further discussed in detail in this chapter):
    - Mushrooms that contain muscarine (e.g., *Inocybe* spp., *Clitocybe* spp.) are relatively common but do not appear to be a major risk for poisoning in animals. Poisoned animals show signs of salivation, lacrimation, vomiting, diarrhea, bradycardia, and miosis. Atropine and decontamination procedures are important treatment strategies.
    - Mushrooms that contain muscimol and ibotenic acid (e.g., *Amanita muscaria*, *Amanita pantherina*) are common in the Pacific Northwest. Ingestion

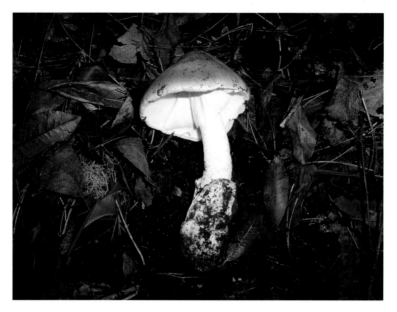

■ **Fig. 92.1.** *Amanita phalloides.* (Photo courtesy of R. Michael Davis)

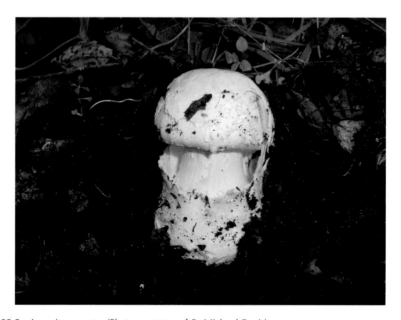

■ **Fig. 92.2.** *Amanita ocreata.* (Photo courtesy of R. Michael Davis)

can result in ataxia, sedation, muscle spasms, and seizures, but with aggressive supportive care, full recovery is expected within 1 to 2 days.

• False morel (*Gyromitra* spp.) ingestion can lead to vomiting, abdominal pain, and diarrhea followed by convulsions. With supportive care, poisoned animals are likely to recover within several days of exposure.

- Hallucinogenic mushrooms (*Psilocybe*, *Panaeolus*, *Conocybe*, and *Gymnopilus* spp.) contain psilocybin. Poisoned animals can develop ataxia, vocalization, overt aggression, nystagmus, and increased body temperature. The management of hallucinogenic mushroom poisoning is essentially supportive, and in most cases, treatment is not necessary.
- Many mushrooms are capable of causing gastrointestinal irritation (*Agaricus*, *Boletus*, *Chlorophyllum*, *Entoloma*, *Lactarius*, *Omphalotus*, *Rhodophyllus*, *Scleroderma*, and *Tricholoma* spp.). In most exposures, vomiting and diarrhea develop between 1 and 6 hours after ingestion, with complete recovery within 24 to 48 hours.

 ## ETIOLOGY/PATHOPHYSIOLOGY

- *A. phalloides* (commonly known as death cap; fig. 92.1) is found throughout North America and grows most commonly under oak, birch, pine, and other hardwoods. It can also be found in open pastures.
- *A. ocreata* (commonly known as Western North American destroying angel; fig. 92.2) grows from Baja California, Mexico, along the Pacific Coast to Washington. *A. ocreata* is most commonly found in sandy soils under oak or pine.
- Amanitins (α-, β-, γ-, and ε-amanitins) are bicyclic octapeptides that are found in approximately 35 mushroom species from three different genera: *Amanita*, *Galerina*, and *Lepiota*. The toxins are not degraded by cooking, freezing, or the acidic environment of the stomach.

Mechanism of Action

- Amanitins inhibit nuclear RNA polymerase II, resulting in decreased protein synthesis and cell death. Hepatocytes, crypt cells, and proximal convoluted tubules are especially susceptible to the effect because of their high metabolic rate.
- Other toxic mechanisms are likely to play an important role in the toxicity of amanitins.

Pharmacokinetics/Absorption, Distribution, Metabolism, and Excretion

- After exposure, amanitins exert toxic effects to intestinal cells. Amanitins are rapidly absorbed from the gastrointestinal tract and distributed (not plasma protein bound) to liver and kidney. The plasma half-life of amanitins in dogs is short ranging, from 25 to 50 minutes. Amanitins are largely excreted unchanged in urine and can be detected in urine well before clinical signs occur. Only a small amount of amanitins is excreted in the bile.
- Species-specific data on the bioavailability of amanitins are largely unavailable, but it appears that the absorption rate in dogs is much greater than in mice and rabbits and much less than in people. Rodents appear resistant to the effects of amanitins.

Toxicity

- Amanitins are extremely toxic. The IV LD_{50} of α-amanitin in dogs is 0.1 mg/kg BW. An oral LD_{50} for methyl-γ-amanitin was estimated to be 0.5 mg/kg BW. In humans, the estimated oral LD_{50} of α-amanitin is 0.1 mg/kg BW.
- Toxin concentrations in *Amanita* spp. vary depending on growing conditions, moisture, and time of year. Hence, it is very difficult to estimate the minimum amount of mushroom material needed to cause poisoning. Considering the average concentration of amanitins per mushroom of 4 mg/g, the ingestion of two *A. phalloides* has the potential to be lethal to an adult dog, while a smaller amount may kill a puppy.

Systems Affected

- Gastrointestinal—Vomiting, diarrhea, and severe abdominal pain begin approximately 8 to 12 hours after exposure.
- Hepatobiliary—Fulminant liver failure develops approximately 36 to 48 hours after exposure.
- Renal/urologic—If the animal survives liver failure, renal- and multiorgan failure can develop.
- Hemic—Coagulopathy can develop as a result of liver failure.
- Nervous—Encephalopathy can develop as a result of liver failure.

 # SIGNALMENT/HISTORY

- All breeds and genders are equally susceptible.
- Puppies are at greater risk to be poisoned than adults.
- There are no known genetic predispositions.
- Severe gastrointestinal signs such as vomiting, diarrhea, and abdominal pain occurring hours after an observed mushroom ingestion.
- Severe gastrointestinal signs such as vomiting, diarrhea, and abdominal pain present hours after unobserved roaming in the woods, especially during mushroom season.
- Liver failure occurring after a period of recovery, although gastrointestinal signs were present prior to the recovery phase.

Location and Circumstances of Poisoning:

- Amanitin-containing mushrooms are very common in the San Francisco Bay area, the Santa Cruz Mountains, the Pacific Northwest, and the Northeast.
- Toxic mushrooms are most abundant in warm, wet years and are often found under certain trees (oak, cork, spruce, birch, pine).
- In California, toxic mushrooms are typically found from mid-autumn through late winter.

- In the Northeast, toxic mushrooms are most commonly found from late September through late October.

 CLINICAL FEATURES

- The chief complaints of amanitin poisoning are vomiting and diarrhea within 24 hours of mushroom exposure and icterus, lethargy, ataxia, seizures, and coma approximately 36 to 48 hours after exposure.
- The clinical course of amanitin toxicosis can be separated into four phases with characteristic clinical features for each phase. However, not every case presents with the classic four stages.
  - The first phase is a latency period of approximately 8 to 12 hours after ingestion of amanitin-containing mushrooms without any clinical signs.
  - The second phase begins approximately 6 to 24 hours after mushroom exposure and is characterized by vomiting, diarrhea, and abdominal pain.
  - The third phase is a period of false recovery during which the animal appears to have recovered. This phase can last from several hours to a few days. During this third phase, close monitoring of liver and kidney function is essential in order to prevent misdiagnosis. In this phase, the breakdown of liver glycogen can lead to severe hypoglycemia.
  - The last phase is characterized by fulminant liver failure and begins between 36 and 84 hours after exposure to amanitins. In this stage, renal and multiorgan failure can also occur and affected animals are icteric, lethargic, and ataxic and have polyuria, polydipsia, anorexia, clotting abnormalities, seizures, or coma. Seizures and coma can also be a direct result of severe hypoglycemia. If large amounts of amanitin-containing mushrooms are ingested, or if a puppy ingested a toxic mushroom, it is possible that the animal may die acutely within 24 hours or just be found dead.

 DIFFERENTIAL DIAGNOSIS

- Caustics
- Viral, bacterial, rickettsial, and parasitic diseases
- Mushrooms that cause gastrointestinal signs (without liver involvement)—collect mushrooms in area of exposure and have identified
- Dietary indiscretion such as ingestion of garbage or spoiled food
- Other causes of acute liver failure
- Severe acute pancreatitis
- Toxicants
  - Acetaminophen overdose
  - Aflatoxins

- Cocklebur (*Xanthium* spp.)
- Cycad palms (*Cycas* spp.)
- Heavy metals (e.g., lead, zinc)
- Microcystins (hepatotoxic blue-green algae toxins)
- Organophosphate and carbamate insecticides
- Ricin and abrin

 DIAGNOSTICS

- Identification of mushrooms found in the environment or gastric contents. Accurate mushroom identification will require consultation with an experienced mycologist. DNA sequencing of mushroom material is also possible.
- Serum chemistry: beginning with the 2nd or 3rd phase see increases in AST, ALT, ALP, and bilirubin; hypoglycemia develops
- Coagulation panel: beginning with the 3rd phase see prolonged PT and PTT
- Detection of α-amanitin in serum, urine, gastric contents, liver, or kidney. This testing is provided by select veterinary toxicology laboratories.
  - In live animals, urine is considered of superior diagnostic use compared to serum. Amanitins can be detected in urine well before any clinical sign has developed, whereas routine laboratory tests such as serum chemistry profiles are unremarkable until liver or kidney damage has occurred. Amanitins are excreted in urine for several days (up to 72 hours) postexposure. Because of the short half-life of amanitins in plasma, amanitins are usually only detected for approximately 36 hours postexposure. Plasma and urine amanitin concentrations do not seem to correlate with clinical severity or outcome.
  - Postmortem, kidney contains higher amanitin concentrations than liver and is considered the sample of choice, especially if the animal survived for a longer period of time.

Pathological Findings

- The liver may be swollen and distended. No other significant gross abnormalities may be noticed. Histopathologically, the liver has massive hepatocellular necrosis with collapse of hepatic cords. Acute tubular necrosis is seen in dogs that develop renal failure.

 THERAPEUTICS

- No specific therapy has proven to be effective. Even with supportive measures, the mortality rate from amanita poisoning in dogs is high. Amanitin poisoning requires immediate and aggressive treatment to improve prognosis.

The key components of therapy are close monitoring, fluid replacement, and supportive care.

Detoxification

- Emesis in animals where exposure occurred less than 2 hours prior to presentation
- Activated charcoal: multidose activated charcoal at 1–4 g/kg PO q 2–6 hours until 2–3 days postingestion

Drug(s) and Antidotes of Choice

- No specific antidote is available.
- Intravenous fluids—Maintain hydration, induce diuresis, correct hypoglycemia.
- 50% dextrose 1 mL/kg IV slow bolus (1–3 min)
- Furosemide 2–4 mg/kg IV q 8–12 hours
- Vitamin K_1 0.5–1.5 mg/kg SQ or IM q 12 hours; 1–5 mg/kg PO q 24 hours
- Blood products—dependent on haemostatic test results
- Silibinin—may be beneficial, but controlled studies are lacking. Experimentally, silibinin was shown to be effective when given twice to dogs at a dose of 50 mg/kg IV, 5 and 24 hours after exposure to *A. phalloides*. An oral form is available that can be given at 2–5 mg/kg PO q 24 hours (silibinin complexed with phosphatidylcholine).
- Penicillin G—reduces the uptake of amanitins into hepatocytes; 1000 mg/kg IV as soon as possible after exposure.

Alternative Drugs

- N-acetylcysteine (NAC)—antioxidant; no data on efficacy in amanitin toxicosis available. This glutathione precursor can be included in the treatment regimen for acute fulminant hepatic failure at 140 mg/kg IV load, followed by 70 mg/kg IV q 6 hours for 7 treatments.
- S-adenosylmethionine (SAMe)—antioxidant and hepatoprotectant; no data on efficacy in amanitin toxicosis available. 20 mg/kg PO q 24 hours
- Ascorbic acid and cimetidine—hepatocyte protectors; no data on efficacy in amanitin toxicosis available. Can be given for supportive therapy

Precautions/Interactions

- A variety of decontamination procedures are used in humans, including hemodialysis, hemoperfusion, plasmapherisis, forced diuresis, and nasoduodenal suctioning. Controversy remains about the efficacy of these procedures, as specific data do not exist.
- The use of steroids and thioctic acid is no longer recommended in the treatment of amanitin poisoning.

Prevention

- Advise owner to closely scrutinize the environment for mushrooms. Suggest that owner have mushrooms identified by mycology expert and get additional information on the seasonality of amanita mushrooms in their geographic region.

Public Health

- Amanitins are very toxic to humans. Even with supportive measures, the reported mortality rate from amanita poisoning in humans is 20% to 40%.

 COMMENTS

Client Education

- Warn client that temporary improvement can be followed by severe hepatic and renal failure.
- Monitoring in the clinical setting for the first 2 to 3 days in a suspect amanitin exposure

Patient Monitoring

- Monitor blood glucose, electrolytes, CBC, serum biochemistry, and coagulation parameters at least daily.
- Prevent hypothermia.
- Monitor urine output.

Possible Complications

- DIC
- Hepatic encephalopathy
- Progressive hepatic failure
- Renal failure

Expected Course and Prognosis

- It takes 3 to 5 days to estimate prognosis.
- Progressive worsening of liver and kidney function and unresponsiveness to supportive treatments are negative indicators.

Synonyms

amanita toxicosis, death cap intoxication, amatoxin poisoning, hepatotoxic mushroom poisoning, amanitin poisoning

Abbreviations

ALP = alkaline phosphatase
ALT = alanine transaminase
AST = aspartate aminotransferase
BW = body weight
CBC = complete blood count
DIC = disseminated intravascular coagulation
IM   = intramuscular
IV   = intravenous
LD_{50} = median lethal dose
PO = *per os* (by mouth)
PT   = prothrombin time
PTT = partial thromboplastin time
q   = every
SQ = subcutaneous

See Also

Acetaminophen
Organophosphate and Carbamate Insecticides
Sago Palm

Suggested Reading

Enjalbert F, Rapior S, Nouguier-Soule J, et al. Treatment of amatoxin poisoning: 20-year retrospective analysis. J Toxicol Clin Toxicol 2002; 40:715–757.
Magdalan J, Ostrowska A, Piotrowska A, et al. Failure of benzylpenicillin, N-acetylcysteine and silibinin to reduce alpha-amanitin hepatotoxicity. In Vivo 2009; 23:393–399.
Puschner B. Mushroom toxins. In: Gupta RC, ed. Veterinary Toxicology: Basic and Clinical Principles, 1st ed. San Diego: Elsevier, 2007; pp. 915–925.
Puschner B, Rose HH, Filigenzi MS. Diagnosis of amanita toxicosis in a dog with acute hepatic necrosis. J Vet Diagn Invest 2007; 19:312–317.

Author: Birgit Puschner, DVM, PhD, DABVT
Consulting Editor: Lynn R. Hovda, RPH, DVM, MS, DACVIM

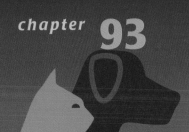

chapter **93**

Oxalates–Insoluble

DEFINITION/OVERVIEW

- Insoluble oxalate crystals are found naturally in plants of the *Araceae* family.
- There are roughly 200 species that contain insoluble oxalate crystals.
- *Dieffenbachia* spp. are most commonly associated with problems in animals.
  - Oxalate crystals occur in more layers in leaves and stems.
  - The plants are present in many homes and offices.
- Most commonly reported plants associated with toxicity include the following:
  - Anthurium, flamingo flower (*Anthurium* spp.; fig. 93.1)
  - Arrowhead vine (*Syngonium* spp.; fig. 93.2)
  - Calla lily (*Zantedeschia* spp.; fig. 93.3)
  - Chinese evergreen (*Aglaonema commutatum*; fig. 93.4)
  - Dumbcane (*Dieffenbachia* spp.; fig. 93.5)
  - Peace lily (*Spathiphyllum* spp.; fig. 93.6)
  - Philodendron, sweetheart vine (*Philodendron* spp.; fig. 93.7)
  - Pothos, hunter's robe, devil's ivy (*Epipremnum* spp.; fig. 93.8)
  - Umbrella plant (*Schefflera actinophylla*; fig. 93.9)
  - Upright elephant's ear (*Xanthosoma* spp.; fig. 93.10)
- Common names vary tremendously from plant to plant and accurate plant identification must include the scientific name.

ETIOLOGY/PATHOPHYSIOLOGY

Mechanism of Action

- Insoluble crystals are needle sharp and generally arranged in bundles called raphides. In many plants, bundles of raphides are organized into specialized cells called idioblasts.
- Chewing or biting into plant material releases the crystals in rapid succession until the idioblast is emptied.
  - The double-edged crystals, acting much like miniature spears, are believed to function primarily as a mechanical irritant to the mucous membranes.
  - They also act as chemical irritants, penetrating cells and allowing the entrance of other substances such as prostaglandins, histamine, proteolytic enzymes, or oxalic acid.

720

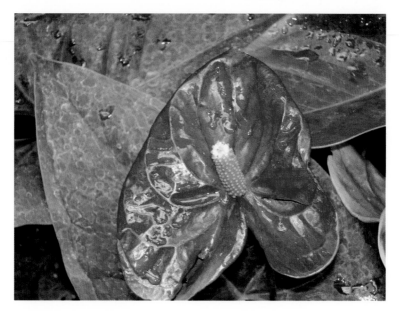

■ **Fig. 93.1.** Anthurium (*Anthurium* spp.) (photo courtesy of Tyne K. Hovda)

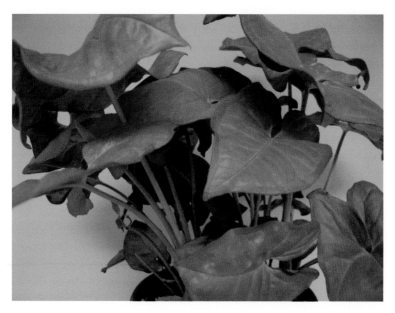

■ **Fig. 93.2.** Arrowhead (*Syngonium* spp.). (photo courtesy of Tyne K. Hovda)

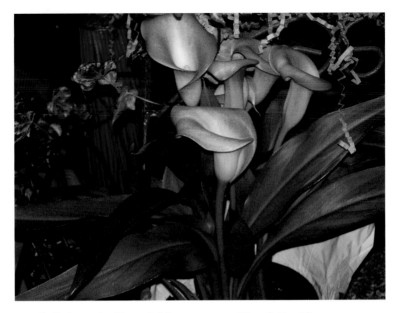

■ **Fig. 93.3.** Calla lily (*Zantedeschia* spp.). (photo courtesy of Tyne K. Hovda)

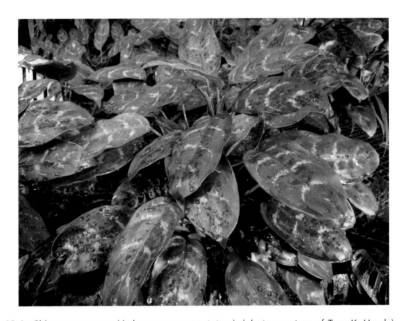

■ **Fig. 93.4.** Chinese evergreen (*Aglaonema commutatum*). (photo courtesy of Tyne K. Hovda)

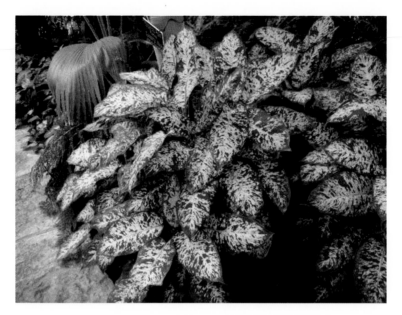

■ **Fig. 93.5.** Dumbcane (*Dieffenbachia* spp.). (photo courtesy of Tyne K. Hovda)

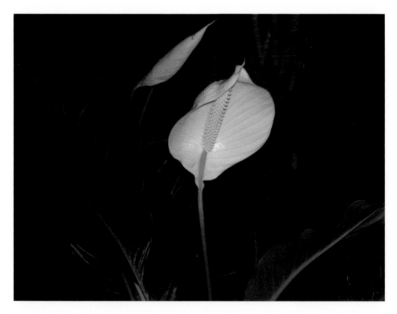

■ **Fig. 93.6.** Peace lily (*Spathiphyllum* spp.). (photo courtesy of Tyne K. Hovda)

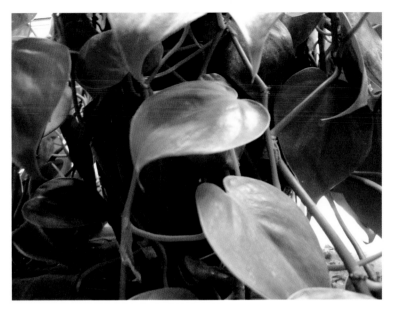

■ **Fig. 93.7.** Philodendron vine (*Philodendron* spp.). (photo courtesy of Tyne K. Hovda)

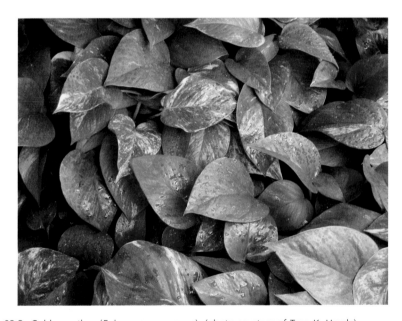

■ **Fig. 93.8.** Golden pothos (*Epipremnum aureum*). (photo courtesy of Tyne K. Hovda)

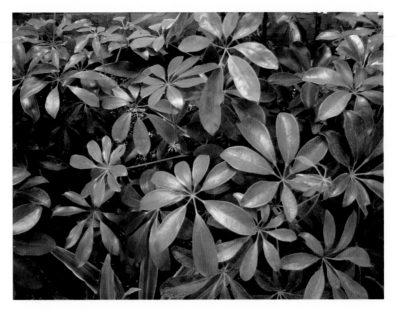

■ **Fig. 93.9.** Umbrella plant (*Schefflera actinophylla*). (photo courtesy of Tyne K. Hovda)

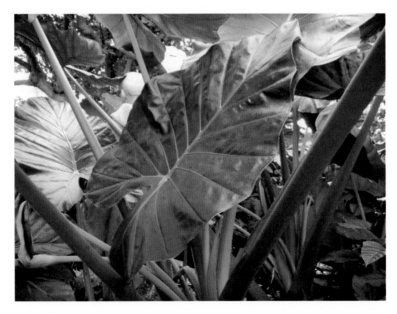

■ **Fig. 93.10.** Upright elephant ear (*Xanthosoma* spp.). (photo courtesy of Tyne K. Hovda)

Pharmacokinetics/Absorption, Distribution, Metabolism, and Excretion

- Onset of action is very rapid, occurring within minutes of chewing on the plant.

Toxicity

- Generally regarded as mild to moderate toxicants
- Severe cases have occurred, and rarely, death has been reported.
- *Dieffenbachia* spp. has been associated with more serious outcomes, including death, in dogs and cats.
- Cats ingesting philodendrons often exhibit a wider array of clinical signs.

Systems Affected

- Gastrointestinal—immediate onset of oral pain with vocalization, pawing at the muzzle, and hypersalivation; anorexia and vomiting; and edema of lips, tongue, and/or pharynx
- Respiratory—rarely dyspnea from inflammation and laryngeal swelling
- Ophthalmic—Plant juices in the eye are associated with severe pain, photophobia, and conjunctival swelling; crystals may be present on the corneal epithelium.

 # SIGNALMENT/HISTORY

- Indoor dogs and cats are at a higher risk, as most of these are houseplants.
  - Dogs tend to chew and destroy the entire plant, often ingesting leaves and stems.
  - Cats, more fastidious, tend to nibble on the leaves.
- All ages can be affected, although ingestions by younger pets, curious or bored by confinement, tend to occur more often.
- The most common immediate signs are related to the severe pain in the oropharynx and include hypersalivation, headshaking, and pawing at the muzzle area. Signs occurring shortly after exposure include edema of the lips and tongue, vomiting, and anorexia. Airway obstruction and dyspnea are more rare occurrences. Ophthalmic exposure results in severe pain, photophobia, lacrimation, blepharospasm, and swelling of the lids.

Risk Factors

- Presence of plants in animal's environment
- Boredom, confinement

 # CLINICAL FEATURES

- Gastrointestinal—evidence of immediate oral pain (hypersalivation, head shaking, pawing at muzzle) within minutes of exposure; redness or irritation to

mucous membranes in oropharynx occurring a short time later; vomiting minutes to hours after exposure
- Respiratory—dyspnea and airway obstruction if inflammation is severe (rare)
- Ophthalmic—issues only if plant juices have been squirted or rubbed into the eye

 DIFFERENTIAL DIAGNOSIS

- Exposure to other agents causing oral irritation (capsaicin, topically applied permethrins, detergents)
- Ingestion of caustic agents (alkalis, acids in household, and drain cleaners)
- Systemic diseases associated with oral lesions and GI signs
- Ingestion of plants containing bitter volatile oils
- Stinging nettle ingestion

 DIAGNOSTICS

- Rarely performed as crystals are insoluble and not absorbed; signs are primarily local in nature and self-limiting.
- Serum electrolytes and chemistry if vomiting persists

Pathological Findings

- Death rarely occurs, and in the few reported cases, severe and extensive erosive and ulcerative glossitis was present.

 THERAPEUTICS

- Therapy is generally limited and includes appropriate detoxification and supportive care. Many animals respond in 2–4 hours, while some may take 12–24 hours for a complete response.

Detoxification

- Wash the mouth and oral cavity with copious amounts of cool fluids.
- Provide small amounts of milk, yogurt, or other calcium-containing products to bind the oxalate crystals. Give enough to coat the oropharynx but not cause GI upset and diarrhea.
- If ophthalmic exposure is evident, lavage the eye for 15 minutes.

Appropriate Health Care

- Observe closely for evidence of dyspnea, especially those animals that chewed up or ingested large amounts of plants
- Thorough ophthalmic examination after lavage; fluoroscein dye or slit lamp examination

Drugs and Antidotes of Choice

- No specific antidote is available.
- Antiemetic agents as needed
  - Maropitant 1 mg/kg SQ q 24 hours, not labeled for cats
  - Ondansetron 0.1–0.2 mg/kg IV q 8–12 hours
- GI protectants as needed
  - H₂ blockers
    - ☐ Famotidine 0.5 mg/kg PO, SQ, IM, IV q 12–24 hours
    - ☐ Ranitidine 1–2 mg/kg PO, SQ, IM, IV q 8–12 hours
    - ☐ Cimetidine 5–10 mg/kg PO, SQ, IM, IV q 6 hours
  - Omeprazole 0.5–1 mg/kg daily
  - Sucralfate 0.25–1 g PO q 8 hours × 5–7 days if evidence of active ulcer disease
- IV fluids if dehydration occurs secondary to hypersalivation and vomiting
- Nonsteroidal anti-inflammatory agents if needed for pain and inflammation
  - Carprofen
    - ☐ Dogs: 2.2 mg/kg PO q 12–24 hours
    - ☐ Cats: 1–2 mg/kg SQ q 24 hours. Limit dosing to 2 days.
  - Deracoxib 1–2 mg/kg PO q 24 hours (dogs)
- Corticosteroid use is controversial, but dexamethasone phosphate 0.125–0.5 mg/kg IV, IM, or SQ may be useful in cases with severe inflammation.

Public Health

- Human beings, especially young children and vulnerable adults, are equally at risk if they chew or ingest plant pieces.

 COMMENTS

Expected Course and Prognosis

- Prognosis is excellent as most signs are mild to moderate, have a short duration of action, and require no therapy.

Prevention/Avoidance

- Identify plants presently in the household and place them far out of the animal's reach.
- Learn the scientific names of poisonous plants and keep them out of the household.

Abbreviations

GI = gastrointestinal
IM = intramuscular

IV = intravenous
PO = *per os* (by mouth)
q   = every
SQ = subcutaneous

Suggested Reading

Ellis W, Barfort T, Mastman GJ. Keratoconjunctivitis with corneal crystals caused by Dieffenbachia plant. Am J Ophthalmol 1973; 76:143–146.

Hornfeldt CS. Plant toxicity in small animals: oxalate-containing plants. Vet Prac Staff 1993; 5(5):2–5.

Knight AP. A Guide to Poisonous House and Garden Plants. Jackson Hole, WY: Teton NewMedia, 2006; pp. 203–204.

Peterson K, Beymer J, Rudloff E, et al. Airway obstruction in a dog after Dieffenbachia ingestion. J Vet Emerg Crit Care 2009; 19(6):635–639.

Spoerke DG, Smolinske SC. Toxicity of Houseplants. Boca Raton, FL: CRC Press, 1990; 29–32, 192–193.

Authors: Lynn R. Hovda, RPH, DVM, MS, ACVIM; Erica Cargill, CVT
Consulting Editor: Ahna G. Brutlag, DVM; Lynn R. Hovda, RPH, DVM, MS, DACVIM

chapter 94

Oxalates–Soluble

DEFINITION/OVERVIEW

- Oxalate toxicity includes both oxalic acid and oxalate salts.
  - Oxalic acid is a dicarboxylic acid found naturally in plants of the Araceae, Oxalidaceae, Liliaceae, Polygonaceae, Chenopodiaceae, and Amaranthus families.
  - Soluble salts (ammonium, calcium, potassium, sodium) of oxalic acid are found as well in a number of plants in these families.
- Most of these plants are weeds growing in pastures and are only associated with problems in livestock grazing on them. A few have been cultivated as houseplants and if ingested in large enough quantities are a potential source of poisoning to dogs and cats.
- Common household plants with soluble oxalates include the following:
  - Common or garden rhubarb (*Rheum rhabarbarum*; fig. 94.1)
  - Shamrock plant (*Oxalis* spp.; fig. 94.2)
  - Star fruit (*Averrhoa carambola*; figs. 94.3, 94.4)
  - Hybrid plants, *Oxalis* spp.

ETIOLOGY/PATHOPHYSIOLOGY

Mechanism of Action

- Soluble oxalates and free oxalic acid are present to varying degrees in all parts of the plant. Total oxalate material in many of the pasture plants is about 16%, with 7% to 10% of this in the form of an oxalate salt.
- Rhubarb stems are edible, the leaves are not.
- Star fruit presents an interesting dilemma, with soluble oxalates found in much greater concentrations in the sour fruit versus sweet fruit. The sour fruit is generally recognized as inedible, the sweet fruit and juices as edible.
- Ingestion of plants results in both free oxalic acid and soluble salts.
- Soluble oxalate salts are absorbed through the GI tract and bind with systemic calcium, resulting in a sudden drop in serum calcium. The accumulation of calcium oxalate crystals causes nephrosis and renal failure.
- Free oxalic acid may be responsible for GI irritation.

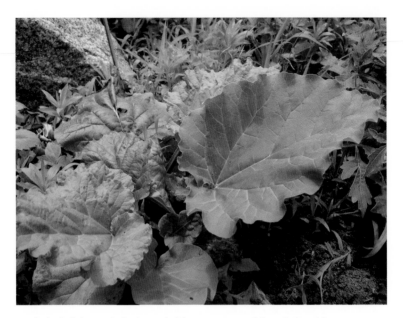

■ **Fig. 94.1.** Rhubarb (*Rheum rhabarbarum*). (Photo courtesy of Tyne K. Hovda)

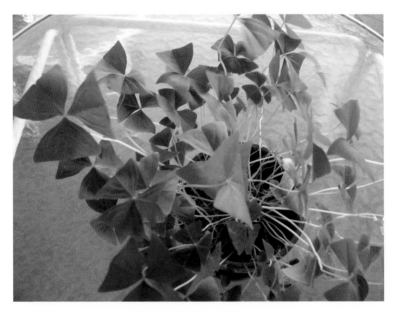

■ **Fig. 94.2.** Shamrock (*Oxalis* spp.). (Photo courtesy of Tyne K. Hovda)

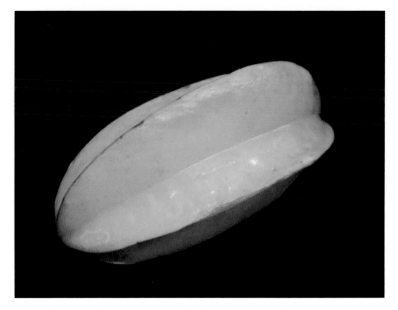

■ **Fig. 94.3.** Star fruit intact (*Averrhoa carambola*). (Photo courtesy of Tyne K. Hovda)

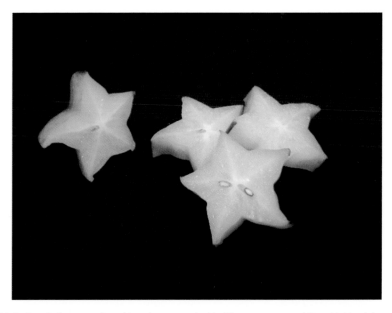

■ **Fig. 94.4.** Star fruit cut sections (*Averrhoa carambola*). (Photo courtesy of Tyne K. Hovda)

Pharmacokinetics/Absorption, Distribution, Metabolism, and Excretion

- Little is known about the true pharmacokinetics in animals.

Toxicity

- Unlikely to be an issue unless large amounts are ingested. The sap is very bitter tasting and this may limit absorption in most animals.
- Stems or stalks of rhubarb are edible; leaves are not.
- Star fruit and star fruit juices are usually only a problem when ingested in large quantities or in the presence of dehydration or underlying renal disease.

Systems Affected

- Gastrointestinal—GI irritation with vomiting (with or without blood) and diarrhea (with or without blood)
- Renal/urological—renal failure from formation of calcium oxalate crystals
- Neuromuscular—signs associated with hypocalcemia
- Musculoskeletal—tetany secondary to hypocalcemia

 SIGNALMENT/HISTORY

- All small animals, indoors and out, are susceptible to toxicity.

Risk Factors

- Preexisting GI or chronic renal disease
- Boredom in confined animal

Historical Findings

- Confirmation of chewed up plant in animal's environment
- Leaves from rhubarb plants that have not been adequately disposed of and are ingested
- Ingestion of many star fruits or large volumes of juices

 CLINICAL FEATURES

- Hypersalivation and anorexia are the earliest signs, followed by vomiting with or without blood and diarrhea with or without blood.
- Depression, weakness, tremors, tetany, and coma follow if the ingestion is large enough to result in systemic hypocalcemia.
- Acute renal failure secondary to calcium oxalate crystal formation results in polydypsia, polyuria, or oliguria with oxaluria, hematuria, and albuminuria. Signs develop at 24–36 hours postingestion.

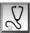 **DIFFERENTIAL DIAGNOSIS**

- Diabetes mellitus (ketoacidosis or hypoglycemic shock)
- Toxicants
  - Calcipotriene (Dovonex)
  - Cholecalciferol rodenticides
  - Ethylene glycol
  - Other plant ingestions, including lilies in cats
- Underlying diseases such as acute renal failure, pancreatitis, or diabetes mellitus
- Viral or bacterial gastroenteritis (garbage can toxicosis)

 DIAGNOSTICS

- Serum chemistry with early attention to calcium, magnesium, BUN, and creatinine
- Urinalysis initially may be normal but later will show crystaluria (oxaluria), hematuria, and albuminuria.

Pathological Findings

- Gross pathology yields only renal lesions (swollen and edematous kidneys) and systemic congestion. Histopathologic lesions include moderate to severe, diffuse acute renal tubular necrosis.

 THERAPEUTICS

Detoxification

- Emesis early after ingestion
- Activated charcoal with cathartic × 1 dose

Appropriate Health Care

- In severe cases with systemic hypocalcemia and oxaluria, aggressive IV fluid therapy for a minimum of 48 hours is needed to preserve renal function.
- Monitor serum calcium and electrolytes, BUN, and creatinine daily until they have returned to normal limits.

Drug(s) and Antidote of Choice

- No true specific antidote, although some may consider the administration of IV calcium an antidote

- Hypocalcemia
  - 10% calcium gluconate IV at 50–150 mg/kg (0.5–1.5 mL/kg) over 20–30 minutes
  - Stop if bradycardia or arrhythmias develop; once CV system is stable, reinstitute slower rate.
- Vigorous IV fluid therapy at 2–3x maintenance and adjust as needed for dehydration, electrolyte changes, and urine output. SQ fluids will not be effective in preventing renal damage if oxaluria is present.
- Monitor urine output for development of oliguria (0.5 mL/kg/hr of urine) or anuria (<0.5 mL/kg/hr of urine). If decreased urinary output, consider individually or in combination.
  - Furosemide 2–4 mg/kg IV intermittent boluses in both dogs and cats
  - Dopamine 2–5 µg/kg/min IV
  - Mannitol 1–2 g/kg IV
- Antiemetics if vomiting is severe or persists
  - Maropitant 1 mg/kg SQ q 24 hours, not labeled for cats
  - Ondansetron 0.1–0.2 mg/kg IV q 8–12 hours
- GI protectants as needed
  - H_2 blockers
    - Famotidine 0.5–1 mg/kg PO, SQ, IM, IV q 12 hours
    - Ranitidine 1–2 mg/kg PO, SQ, IM, IV q 8–12 hours
    - Cimetidine 5–10 mg/kg PO, SQ, IM, IV q 6 hours
  - Omeprazole 0.5–1 mg/kg daily PO
  - Sucralfate 0.25–1 g PO q 8 hours × 5–7 days if evidence of active ulcer disease
- Non steroidal anti-inflammatory agents or other analgesics for pain
  - Carprofen
    - Dogs: 2.2 mg/kg PO q 12–24 hours
    - Cats: 1–2 mg/kg SQ q 24 hours. Limit dosing to 2 days.
  - Deracoxib 1–2 mg/kg PO q 24 hours (dogs)

COMMENTS

Prevention/Avoidance

- Keep these and other toxic plants out of the reach of animals.
- Properly dispose of rhubarb leaves after picking the stems.

Possible Complications

- Chronic renal disease

Expected Course and Prognosis

- In general, few problems other than GI irritation occur with ingestion of these plants by healthy animals, and the prognosis for recovery is excellent.

■ Rarely, systemic hypocalcemia with secondary renal disease develops. If treated early, the prognosis is very good for a full recovery. The prognosis decreases considerably for those animals treated after acute renal disease has occurred.

Abbreviations

BUN = blood urine nitrogen
CV   = cardiovascular
GI   = gastrointestinal
IM   = intramuscular
IV   = intravenous
PO   = *per os* (by mouth)
q   = every
SQ   = subcutaneous

See Also

Ethylene Glycol

Suggested Reading

Chen CL, Fang HC, Chou KJ. Acute oxalate nephropathy after ingestion of a star fruit. Am J Kidney Disease 2001; 37:418–422.

Knight AP. A Guide to Poisonous House and Garden Plants. Jackson Hole, WY: Teton NewMedia, 2006; pp. 203–204.

Spoerke DG, Smolinske SC. Toxicity of Houseplants. Boca Raton, FL: CRC Press, 1990; pp. 29–32.

Authors: Lynn R. Hovda, RPH, DVM, MS, ACVIM; Erica Cargill, CVT
Consulting Editors: Justine A. Lee, DVM, ACVECC; Lynn R. Hovda, RPH, DVM, MS, ACVIM

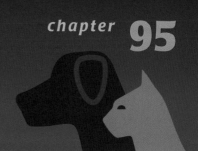

chapter **95**

Rhododendrons/ Azaleas

DEFINITION/OVERVIEW

- There are over 1,000 species of rhododendrons/azaleas in the Ericaceae family. The small, deciduous plants are generally referred to as azaleas (fig. 95.1) and the large, woody shrubs as rhododendrons (fig. 95.2). Both produce showy flowers.
- Rhododendrons/azaleas are found in nature throughout the Northern hemisphere, cultivated as shrubs and small trees, and used as ornamental plants.
- Toxic diterpenoids, now referred to as grayanotoxins, are found to some extent in every plant species in the Ericaceae family.
- All parts of the plant are toxic.
- Clinical signs may occur within an hour after ingestion but can be delayed up to 12 hours.

ETIOLOGY/PATHOPHYSIOLOGY

Mechanism of Action

- Grayanotoxins bind to sodium channels and increase their permeability, resulting in prolonged depolarization of cardiac muscle.

Pharmacokinetics/Absorption, Distribution, Metabolism, and Excretion

- Absorption is rapid and clinical signs generally occur within a few hours.

Toxicity

- Grayanotoxins I and II (formerly called acetylandromedol, andromedotoxin, and rhodotoxin) are water-soluble diterpenoids responsible for the majority of clinical signs.
- Other grayanotoxins (III through XVIII) and compounds may be present in some species and play a role as well.
- ALL parts of the plant, including nectar and flowers, are toxic.
- Ingestion of 0.2% of animal's body weight can result in signs.

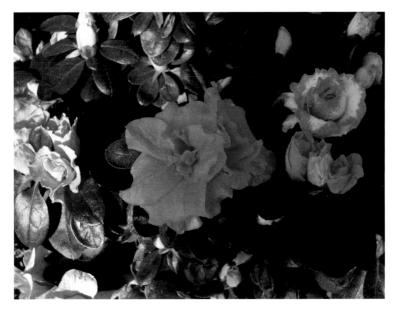

■ **Fig. 95.1.** Azalea (Ericaceae family). (Photo courtesy of Tyne K. Hovda)

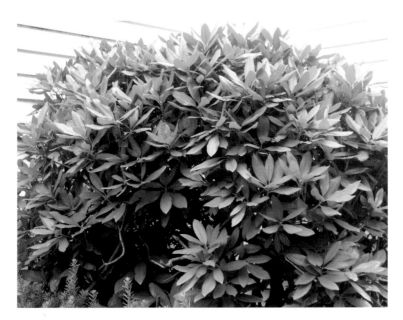

■ **Fig. 95.2.** Rhododendron (Ericaceae family). (Photo courtesy of Tyne K. Hovda)

Systems Affected

- Gastrointestinal—early onset of hypersalivation and gastroenteritis
- Cardiovascular—changes in heart rate and rhythm; hypotension
- Nervous—ranges from depression to coma. Signs can persist for days.

SIGNALMENT/HISTORY

- No breed or species predilection
- Animals with underlying cardiac disease are at increased risk for toxicity.

CLINICAL FEATURES

- The onset of signs is generally rapid, occurring within the first 1–2 hours after exposure. In some instances, signs may be delayed for up to 12 hours. Gastrointestinal signs tend to predominate, with severe cardiovascular signs occurring less frequently.
- Gastrointestinal abnormalities include hypersalivation, vomiting, diarrhea, abdominal pain, anorexia, and possible hemorrhagic enteritis.
- Cardiovascular changes include bradycardia or tachycardia, arrhythmias, hypotension, weakness, and cardiopulmonary arrest.
- Neurological signs include depression, tremors, seizures, paralysis, and coma.
- Other signs include blurred vision, transient blindness, dyspnea, and vocalization.

DIFFERENTIAL DIAGNOSIS

- Infectious or metabolic diseases (viral, bacterial, HGE)
- Toxicants
  - *Taxus* spp. and cardiac glycoside–containing plants (foxglove, oleander, others)
  - Human and veterinary prescription medications used for cardiac disease (especially digitalis)
  - Human and veterinary prescription medications not specifically used for cardiac disease but with known cardiac effects
  - Organophosphate- and carbamate containing pesticides
- Underlying cardiac disease

DIAGNOSTICS

- Clinical laboratory tests (serum chemistry and CBC) do not show any specific abnormalities.
- Diagnosis is most often made by plant identification.
- Liquid chromatography–mass spectrometry is available to determine presence of grayanotoxins (stomach contents, serum, urine).

Pathological Findings

- Gross and microscopic abnormalities are nonspecific.

THERAPEUTICS

Detoxification

- Bathe the animal if it is contaminated with nectar.
- Early emesis if CNS signs have not yet developed
- Gastric lavage should be used to remove large amounts of plant material. Keep returned lavage material for toxin identification.
- Activated charcoal with a cathartic x 1 dose

Appropriate Health Care

- Frequent blood pressure monitoring and ECG for first 12–18 hours
- Close attention to hydration status as vomiting may be severe
- Keep in darkened area without excess stimulation as seizures may occur at any time and neurological signs persist for several days

Drug(s) and Antidotes of Choice

- No specific antidote is available.
- Early, yet cautious, use of IV fluids to maintain blood pressure and cardiovascular system but not overload the cardiovascular system
- For bradycardia:
  - Atropine 0.02–0.04 mg/kg IV, IM, or SQ
  - Glycopyrrolate 0.01–0.02 mg/kg SC, IM, or IV
  - In severe cases of bradycardia unresponsive to medical management, the use of a temporary pacemaker may be indicated.
- The use of antiarrhythmics (lidocaine, procainamide) may be necessary if the patient is persistently tachycardic and nonresponsive to IV fluids, has severe ventricular dysrhythmias, or has evidence of poor perfusion (hypotension, pulse deficits, tachycardia, pale mucous membranes, prolonged CRT)
  - Lidocaine
    - Dogs: 2–8 mg/kg IV to effect while monitoring ECG
    - Cats: 0.25–0.5 mg/kg slow IV while monitoring ECG. Use judiciously in cats!
  - Procainamide
    - Dogs: 2 mg/kg IV over 3–5 minutes (up to 20 mg/kg IV bolus), followed by 25–50 µg/kg/min CRI
    - Cats: 1–2 mg/kg IV once, followed by 10–20 µg/kg IV CRI
- Diazepam or other anticonvulsant medications for seizures
  - Diazepam 0.25–0.5 mg/kg IV PRN
  - Phenobarbital 3–5 mg/kg IV PRN
- Antiemetics if vomiting is severe or persists
  - Maropitant 1 mg/kg SQ q 24 hours, not labeled for cats
  - Ondansetron 0.1–0.2 mg/kg IV q 8–12 hours

- GI protectants as needed
  - H₂ blockers
    - ☐ Famotidine 0.5–1 mg/kg PO, SQ, IM, IV q 12–24 hours
    - ☐ Ranitidine 1–2 mg/kg PO, SQ, IM, IV q 8–12 hours
    - ☐ Cimetidine 5–10 mg/kg PO, SQ, IM, IV q 6 hours
  - Omeprazole 0.5–1 mg/kg daily
  - Sucralfate 0.25–1 g PO q 8 hours x 5–7 days if evidence of active ulcer disease

 COMMENTS

Prevention/Avoidance

- Azaleas and rhododendrons should be kept out of a pet's environment and clippings should not be left in areas where dogs can play with them.
- Flowering plants are often a temptation to house pets, particularly cats, and should be placed well out of their reach.

Expected Course and Prognosis

- The prognosis is good with early and appropriate therapy.
- The development of cardiac arrhythmias complicates therapy and lowers the prognosis.
- Neurological signs may persist for days.

Abbreviations

CBC = complete blood count
CNS = central nervous system
CRI = continuous rate infusion
ECG = electrocardiogram
HGE = hemorrhagic gastroenteritis
IM   = intramuscular
IV   = intravenous
PO   = *per os* (by mouth)
PRN = *pro re nata* (as needed)
q   = every
SQ   = subcutaneous

See Also

Beta-Blockers
Calcium Channel Blockers
Cardiac Glycosides
Organophosphate and Carbamate Insecticides
Yew

Suggested Reading

Burrows GE, Tyrl RJ. Toxic Plants of North America. Ames, IA: ISU Press, 2006; pp. 80–82.

Knight AP. A Guide to Poisonous House and Garden Plants. Jackson, WY: Teton NewMedia, 2006; pp. 235–237.

Milewski LM, Khan SA. An overview of potentially life threatening poisonous plants in dogs and cats. J Vet Emerg Crit Care 2006; 16(1):25–33.

Puschner B. Grayanotoxins. In: Plumlee KH, ed. Clinical Veterinary Toxicology. St. Louis: Mosby, 2004; pp. 412–414.

Authors: Erica Cargill, CVT; Lynn R. Hovda, RPH, DVM, MS, DACVIM

Consulting Editors: Lynn R. Hovda, RPH, DVM, MS, DACVIM; Justine A. Lee, DVM, DACVECC

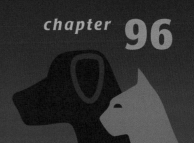

chapter 96

Sago Palm

DEFINITION/OVERVIEW

- Toxicosis caused by ingestion of any part of the sago/cycad palm plant (fig. 96.1)
  - Order Cycadaceae; genera *Cycads*, *Zamias*, and *Macrozamia*
  - The sago palm is not really a palm. It belongs to a group of plants that date back to the dinosaur era and are often referred to as "living fossils."
  - All parts of the plant are toxic; the seeds (nuts) are the most toxic part of the plant as they contain the highest amounts of cycasin, the principle toxin.
- The degree of illness is dependent upon what part of the plant and how much has been ingested.
- The liver is the target organ. The most common response to exposure is an early onset of vomiting followed by severe, acute liver failure.

ETIOLOGY/PATHOPHYSIOLOGY

- The incidence of sago palm toxicosis is most common in the southern United States and Hawaii due to the geographic location of the plant.
- Toxicosis also occurs in those situations where sago palms are grown as household "container" plants.

Mechanism of Action

- Toxin is ingested orally and absorbed through the gastrointestinal tract.

Pharmacokinetics/Absorption, Distribution, Metabolism, and Excretion

- Cycasin contains a glucose molecule that is hydrolyzed by an enzyme in the gut, yielding compounds that cause gastrointestinal and hepatotoxic effects.

Toxicity

- Due to azoglycoside toxins cycasin and methylazomethanol

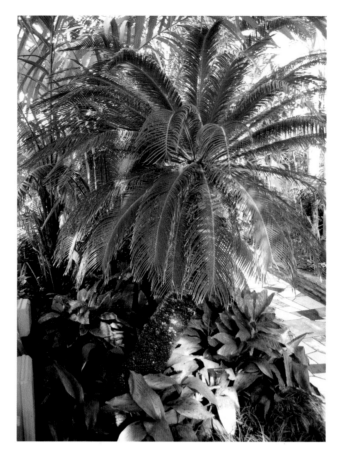

■ **Fig. 96.1.** Sago palm (*Cycas* spp.). (Photo courtesy of Tyne K. Hovda)

Systems Affected

- Hepatobiliary—Acute, severe hepatic necrosis develops at 2–3 days.
- Gastrointestinal—Irritation with vomiting and diarrhea occurs early (15 minutes to several hours).
- Neurological—Weakness and ataxia to seizures or coma may occur early or with the onset of hepatic disease.

 # SIGNALMENT/HISTORY

- Dogs are the species known to be affected by this toxicity.
- No breed or sex predilection
- Ages reported to be affected range from 8 weeks to 11 years, although any age can be affected if the plant is ingested.

- Signs associated with this condition include the following:
  - Vomiting (with or without blood)
  - Diarrhea (with or without blood)
  - Icterus secondary to massive elevations in liver enzymes
  - Lethargy
  - Anorexia
  - Abdominal pain
  - Ascites
  - Neurologic signs; vary from weakness and ataxia to coma and seizure

Risk Factors

- Environmental exposure to sago palm trees or plants

Historical Findings

- History of ingesting sago palm plant or seeds followed by vomiting

Location and Circumstances of Poisoning

- Most cases occur in the southern United States and Hawaii due to the sandy soil and natural geographic location of the plant.
- Toxicosis is becoming more common in other areas as the plant can now be found as a dwarf or bonsai ornamental houseplant.

 # CLINICAL FEATURES

- Onset of clinical signs ranges from 15 minutes to 3 days, and duration ranges from 24 hours to 9 days. Gastrointestinal signs occur first, followed by hepatic enzyme changes (2–3 days).
- Systems most commonly affected include the following:
  - Gastrointestinal tract—vomiting and/or diarrhea (with or without blood), abdominal tenderness, anorexia
  - Hepatobiliary system—icterus and abdominal pain
  - Nervous system—ranges from weakness and ataxia to coma and seizures

 # DIFFERENTIAL DIAGNOSIS

- Any toxin or disease process that would cause vomiting and acute hepatic necrosis
  - Common toxicants
    - Acetaminophen
    - Amanita mushrooms

       ☐ Nonsteroidal anti-inflammatory drugs
       ☐ Xylitol
- Disease processes
       ☐ Chronic hepatic necrosis/fibrosis
       ☐ Foreign body obstruction
       ☐ Hepatic shunts
       ☐ Severe pancreatitis

DIAGNOSTICS

- Abdominal/hepatic ultrasound is usually normal shortly after ingestion but by 24–72 hours may show ascites and evidence of severe liver damage.
- Serum chemistry abnormalities primarily indicate liver damage.
  - Liver enzyme elevations can be very large.
    - ☐ Increased ALT; may be well into thousands
    - ☐ Increased AST
    - ☐ Increased ALP
    - ☐ Increased conjugated bilirubin
    - ☐ Increased bile acids
  - Azotemia—increases in BUN and creatinine
  - Electrolyte abnormalities
  - Hypoalbuminemia
  - Hypoglycemia
- Complete blood count
  - Leukocytosis (generally neutrophilia)
  - Neutropenia rarely occurs
  - Increased hematocrit and decreased total protein
- Coagulation abnormalities
  - Thrombocytopenia
  - Increased PTT
  - Increased PT
  - Increased ACT
- Urinalysis
  - Bilirubinuria
  - Hematuria
  - Glucosuria

Pathological Findings

- Gross findings include icterus; petechial and ecchymotic hemorrhage; dark, tarry ingesta in the stomach; and evidence of liver damage.
- Histopathological findings include cirrhosis with focal centrolobular and mid-zonal necrosis and evidence of generalized hemorrhagic disease.

THERAPEUTICS

■ The primary objectives of treatment are to prevent further toxin absorption, provide supportive care, and correct clotting abnormalities.

Detoxification

■ Induce emesis if within several hours of ingestion.
■ Administer activated charcoal with a cathartic x 1 dose; repeat activated charcoal every 4–6 hours x 2 additional doses.

Appropriate Health Care

■ Monitor closely for signs of liver or renal failure and abnormal bleeding.
■ Repeat serum chemistries daily until stabilized.
■ Liver protectants may need to be administered for a minimum of 4–6 weeks; some dogs may require them for the remainder of their lives.

Drug(s) and Antidotes of Choice

■ No antidote is available.
■ Aggressive IV fluid therapy with frequent monitoring of plasma proteins
  • Crystalloids—supply dextrose and B vitamins in addition to maintaining hydration
  • Colloids or plasma as needed
■ Seizure control
  • Diazepam 0.25–0.5 mg/kg IV PRN
  • Phenobarbital 3–5 mg/kg IV PRN
■ Antiemetics (maropitant, metoclopramide, ondansetron) if vomiting is severe or persists
  • Maropitant 1 mg/kg SQ every 24 hours, not labeled for cats
  • Ondansetron 0.1–0.2 mg/kg IV q 8–12 hours
■ GI protectants as needed
  • H$_2$ blockers
    □ Famotidine 0.5 mg/kg PO, SQ, IM, IV q 12–24 hours
    □ Ranitidine 1–2 mg/kg PO, SQ, IM, IV q 8–12 hours
    □ Cimetidine 5–10 mg/kg PO, SQ, IM, IV q 6 hours
  • Omeprazole 0.5–1 mg/kg daily
  • Sucralfate 0.25–1 g PO TID x 5–7 days if evidence of active ulcer disease
■ Vitamin K$_1$ 2–5 mg/kg PO q 24 hours or divided q 12 hours as needed for clotting disorders
■ Blood transfusion for cases of severe hemorrhage
■ Hepatic protectants
  • SAMe 20 mg/kg/day PO

- Silymarin (milk thistle) 20–50 mg/kg/day orally PO
- Vitamin E 100–400 IU q 12 hours orally PO
- Broad spectrum antibiotics if liver necrosis occurs

Alternative Drugs

- Acetylcysteine (anecdotal use): Loading dose of 140 mg/kg IV or PO followed by 70 mg/kg q 6 hours IV or PO for 7 doses

Follow-up

- Once stable, monitor liver enzymes every 1–2 weeks until they normalize.

Diet

- Oral intake should be avoided until vomiting is controlled, after which a low-protein diet should be fed.

COMMENTS

Client Education

- Educate the client on the serious consequences associated with ingestion of sago palm plant pieces and seeds.

Patient Monitoring

- Liver enzymes should be monitored at 24, 48, and 72 hours postexposure. If no elevations have occurred by 48–72 hours the animal is unlikely to develop further problems.
- Symptomatic animals should have liver enzymes monitored until clinical signs have resolved, and then every 1–2 weeks until they normalize.

Prevention/Avoidance

- Remove sago palm plants from the environment or restrict the dog's access to them.

Possible Complications

- Severe chronic active hepatitis
- Permanent hepatic dysfunction

Expected Course and Prognosis

- Varies depending on the use of early and aggressive therapy and the quantity and part of the plant material ingested. The seeds are more toxic than the rest of the plant.
- If vomiting and diarrhea can be controlled and liver function is not dramatically affected, animals usually recover.

- Prognosis for recovery is good if liver enzymes are not elevated by 48–72 hours.
- The reported recovery rate after treatment is approximately 42%.
- Long term survival may be poor. Methylazomethanol, one of the toxins associated with sago palm toxicosis, damages neuronal DNA and death may occur in recovered animals 8–12 weeks after initial toxic exposure.

Synonyms

- Cycad palm toxicity

Abbreviations

ACT = activated clotting time
ALP = alkaline phosphatase
ALT = alanine aminotransferase
AST = aspartate aminotransferase
BUN = blood urea nitrogen
IM   = intramuscular
IV   = intravenous
PO   = *per os* (by mouth)
PRN = *pro re nata* (as needed)
PT   = prothrombin time
PTT = partial prothromboplastin time
q   = every
SAMe = S-adenosylmethionine
SQ   = subcutaneous

See Also

Acetaminophen
Mushrooms
Xylitol

Suggested Reading

Albretsen JC, Khan SA, Richardson JA. Cycad palm toxicosis in dogs: 60 cases (1987–1997). J Am Vet Med Assoc 1998; 213(1):99–101.
Ferguson D, Crowe M, Acierno M, et al. Cycad intoxication in dogs: survival and prognostic indicators. Proceedings of American College of Veterinary Internal Medicine Forum, Anaheim, CA, 2010.
Milewski LM, Khan SA. An overview of potentially life-threatening poisonous plants in dogs and cats. J Vet Emerg Crit Care 2006; 16(1):25–33.
Senior DF, et al. Cycad intoxication in the dog. J Am Animal Hosp Assoc 1985; 21:103–109.
Youssef H. Cycad toxicity in dogs. Vet Med 2008; 103(5):242–244.

Author: Christy A. Klatt, DVM
Consulting Editor: Lynn R. Hovda, RPH, DVM, MS, DACVIM

chapter 97

Yew

DEFINITION/OVERVIEW

- Japanese yew (*Taxus cuspidata*), English yew (*Taxus baccata*), and Chinese yew (*Taxus chinensis*) are the most toxic members of the yew family found in the United States.
- Yew is referred to as "the tree of death," and prevention of exposure is critical.
- Yew is commonly introduced as a landscape evergreen, likely because of its winter-hardiness.
- Yews are dioceous plants, with the male tree considered more toxic than the female.
- The leaves, bark, and seed inside the red fruit are toxic; the fleshy part of the red fruit is not (see fig. 97.1).
- Toxicosis in small animals is rare.

ETIOLOGY/PATHOPHYSIOLOGY

- Ingestion of plant material (fresh or dried) from yew species (*Taxus* spp.)
- Leaves are easily identified. They are simple, alternate, spirally arrange, needle-like, and 2–3 cm in length (see fig. 97.1).
- Yew is generally an upright plant growing adjacent to buildings and foundations (see fig. 97.2).

Mechanism of Action

- Taxine A and B are the toxic agents.
- Both taxine A and B are cardiotoxic, but taxine B is more potent and associated with atrioventricular conduction delays, resulting in widening of the QRS complex and depressed p waves on an ECG.
- In addition, taxine B reduces cardiac contractility and the rate of cardiac depolarization.
- Both taxine A and B are direct calcium and sodium channel blockers at the cardiac cellular level.

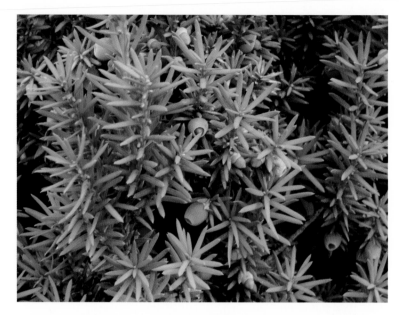

■ **Fig. 97.1.** Japanese yew berry (*Taxus cuspidata*). (Photo courtesy of Tyne K. Hovda)

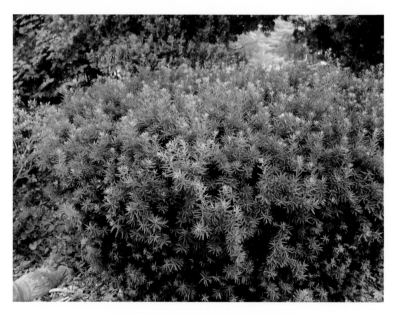

■ **Fig. 97.2.** Yew shrub (*Taxus* spp.). (Photo courtesy of Krishona Martinson)

Pharmacokinetic/Absorption, Distribution, Metabolism, and Excretion

- Once ingested, the toxins are rapidly absorbed and distributed.
- Generally referred to as alkaloids, taxines are technically pseudoalkaloids, metabolized by the liver and excreted as benzoic acid.

Toxicity

- Taxine alkaloids are the toxic compounds.
- Cardiotoxic taxine A and taxine B are considered the primary toxicants.
- LD_{min} in dogs is 2.3 g leaves/kg BW (11.5 mg/kg BW taxine alkaloids).
- An average-size dog could obtain a lethal dose by chewing on yew branches or eating about an ounce of leaves.

Systems Affected

- Cardiovascular—cardiovascular collapse
- Gastrointestinal—gastroenteritis
- Nervous—behavior changes, ataxia, seizures

 # SIGNALMENT/HISTORY

- Yew is toxic to all species. Toxicosis occurs far more frequently in horses and ruminants than small animals and human beings.
- The bitter, irritant oil in the bark and leaves limits ingestion in small animals.

Location and Circumstances of Poisoning

- The incidence and degree of intoxication depends on the particular *Taxus* species. The Pacific yew (*Taxus brevifolia*) has very low levels of taxine alkaloids and thus a much lower potential for toxicity.

 # CLINICAL FEATURES

- The overall effect of taxine alkaloids in poisoned animals is peracute cardiovascular collapse and death due to disruption of cardiovascular function with arterial vasodilatation and hypotension.
- Subacute poisoning has been observed and clinical signs include bradycardia, ventricular fibrillation, nonspecific cardiac dysrhythmias, dyspnea, hyperthermia, ataxia, muscle tremors, aggressive behavior, mydriasis, recumbency, seizure, collapse, and death.
- Surviving animals develop gastroenteritis secondary to the volatile oil irritants found in the bark and leaves.

 # DIFFERENTIAL DIAGNOSIS

- Cardiac disease
- Toxicants
  - Arsenic, cyanide, and nitrate either in plant material or as direct toxins

- Cardiac glycoside–containing plants such as foxglove, rhododendron, oleander, and others
- Human and veterinary pharmaceutical agents specific to the cardiovascular system, including digoxin, calcium channel blockers, and beta-blockers
- Other pharmaceutical agents not specific to the cardiovascular system but with known cardiac side effects

DIAGNOSTICS

- The presence of *Taxus* spp. should be confirmed in the animal's environment and the stomach contents examined for the presence of the plant. Recovered lavage material should examined for yew and submitted for taxine alkaloid determination.
- CBC and serum chemistry abnormalities in surviving dogs may include an increased hematocrit, decreased total protein, hyponatremia, hypochloremia, hypoalbuminemia, and elevated alkaline phosphatase.

Pathological Findings

- Gross and histopathological lesions are generally absent due to the sudden onset of toxicity and death.
- Yew leaves and bark may be found in the stomach, and the mucous membranes of the gastrointestinal tract may be red and inflamed from the volatile irritant oils.
- Other nonspecific findings include pulmonary congestion or edema and hemorrhage secondary to cardiovascular collapse.

THERAPEUTICS

- Death often occurs immediately, leaving little opportunity for therapeutic intervention.
- Additional supportive treatment for surviving animals may be required for several weeks.

Detoxification

- Emesis only if within minutes of witnessed ingestion
- Gastric lavage followed by activated charcoal with a cathartic x 1 dose

Appropriate Health Care

- ECG monitoring for several days with appropriate use of cardiac specific drugs as needed

- Monitor and treat hyperthermia if it develops
- Close attention to CNS signs as seizures occur without warning

Drug(s) and Antidotes of Choice

- No specific antidote available
- Early yet cautious use of IV fluids to maintain blood pressure and cardiovascular system but not overload the cardiovascular system. Severe bradycardia may result in forward-pump failure, so IV fluids must be used judiciously.
- For bradycardia:
  - Atropine 0.02–0.04 mg/kg IV, IM, or SQ
  - Glycopyrrolate 0.01–0.02 mg/kg SQ, IM, or IV
  - In severe cases of bradycardia unresponsive to medical management, the use of a temporary pacemaker may be indicated.
- The use of antiarrhythmics (lidocaine, procainamide) may be necessary if the patient is persistently tachycardic and nonresponsive to IV fluids, has severe ventricular dysrhythmias, or evidence of poor perfusion (hypotension, pulse deficits, tachycardia, pale mucous membranes, prolonged CRT).
  - Lidocaine
    - Dogs: 2–8 mg/kg IV to effect while monitoring ECG
    - Cats: 0.25–0.5 mg/kg slow IV while monitoring ECG. Use judiciously in cats!
  - Procainamide
    - Dogs: 2 mg/kg IV over 3–5 minutes (up to 20 mg/kg IV bolus), followed by 25–50 µg/kg/min CRI
    - Cats: 1–2 mg/kg IV once followed by 10–20 µg/kg IV CRI
- Seizure control as needed
  - Diazepam 0.25–0.5 mg/kg IV PRN
  - Phenobarbital 2–5 mg/kg IV PRN
- Antiemetics if vomiting is severe or persists
  - Maropitant 1 mg/kg SQ q 24 hours, not labeled for cats
  - Ondansetron 0.1–0.2 mg/kg IV q 8–12 hours
- GI protectants as needed
  - H$_2$ blockers
    - Famotidine 0.5 mg/kg PO, SQ, IM, IV q 12–24 hours
    - Ranitidine 1–2 mg/kg PO, SQ, IM, IV every 8–12 hours
    - Cimetidine 5–10 mg/kg PO, SQ, IM, IV q 6 hours
  - Omeprazole 0.5–1 mg/kg daily
  - Sucralfate 0.25–1 g PO q 8 hours x 5–7 days if evidence of active ulcer disease

Nursing Care

- Additional stresses, excitement, and exercise should be avoided for several days.

COMMENTS

Client Education

▪ Prevention of exposure to yew is critical. Yew should not be planted where pets have access. Yew branches should not be used as playthings or chew sticks for pets.

Patient Monitoring

▪ ECG monitoring should occur for several days after the initial insult.

Expected Course and Prognosis

▪ Peracute death usually occurs, although a few dogs and cats have survived.

Abbreviations

BW = body weight
CBC = complete blood count
CRI = continuous rate infusion
CRT = capillary refill time
ECG = electrocardiogram
IM   = intramuscular
IV   = intravenous
LD = lethal dose
PO = *per os* (by mouth)
PRN = *pro re nata* (as needed)
q   = every
SQ = subcutaneous

See Also

Beta-Blockers
Calcium Channel Blockers
Cardiac Glycosides

Suggested Reading

Cope RB. The dangers of yew ingestion. Vet Med 2005; 100(9):646–650.
Evans KL, Cook JR. Japanese yew poisoning in a dog. J Am Animal Hosp Assoc 1991; 27:300–302.
Ogden L. Taxus (yews): a highly toxic plant. Vet Hum Toxicol 1988; 30(6):563–564.
Pierog J, Kane B, Kane K, et al. Management of isolated yew berry toxicity with sodium bicarbonate: a case report in treatment efficacy. J Med Toxicol 2009; 5(2):84–89.
Wilson CR, Sauer JM, Hooser, SB. 2001. Taxines: a review of the mechanism and toxicity of yew (Taxus sp) alkaloids. Toxicon 2001; 39:175–185.

Authors: Krishona L. Martinson, PhD; Lynn R. Hovda, RPH, DVM, MS, DACVIM
Consulting Editor: Lynn R. Hovda, RPH, DVM, MS, DACVIM

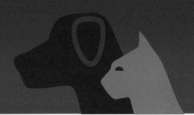

Rodenticides

chapter 98

Anticoagulants

DEFINITION/OVERVIEW

- Anticoagulant rodenticides result in a coagulopathy caused by reduced vitamin K_1–dependent clotting factors in the circulation after exposure.
- Second-generation anticoagulants were more recently developed; they are generally more toxic and some persist longer in the liver, resulting in greater risk (and requirement for a longer duration of treatment) than older (first-generation) anticoagulants.
- Commonly marketed as pellets or blocks under a variety of trade names (fig. 98.1)

ETIOLOGY/PATHOPHYSIOLOGY

Mechanism of Action

- Reduced Vitamin K_1 is required for carboxylation to activated vitamin K–dependent clotting factors: II, VI, IX, and X.
- Carboxylation of clotting factors oxidizes vitamin K_1 to the inactive epoxide form.
- Anticoagulants inhibit vitamin K_1 epoxide reductase, DT diaphorase, and possibly other enzymes involved in the reduction of vitamin K_1–epoxide to vitamin K_1.
- Uncarboxylated clotting factors do not bind calcium sufficiently to participate in clot formation.
- Carboxylated clotting factors decline with time after anticoagulant rodenticide exposure to a point after which coagulation function is inadequate.

Pharmacokinetics/Absorption, Distribution, Metabolism, and Excretion

- Readily absorbed (90%) from GIT
- Peak plasma concentrations occur 1–12 hours post-ingestion.
- Bind to plasma proteins providing an inactive reservoir until released and transported to liver
- Concentrated in liver; may involve enterohepatic recycling

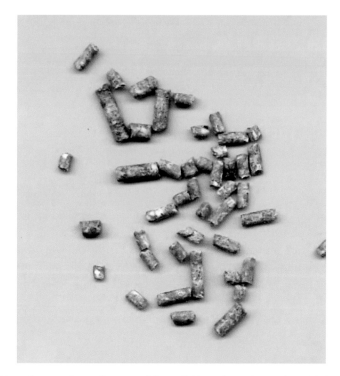

■ **Fig. 98.1.** Common form of commercially available anticoagulant rodenticide bait pellets.

- Some are metabolized in the liver to hydroxyl metabolites that are excreted in urine.
- Plasma half-life ranges from hours (for first-generation products like warfarin) to days (for brodifacoum, chlorphacinone, diphacinone, or other long-lasting compounds).
- Humans pass warfarin into milk; evidence of secretion of anticoagulant rodenticides in milk of animals is well documented. It is best to assume that nursing puppies or kittens could be at risk.

Toxicity

- General
  - Exposure to anticoagulant rodenticide products
  - First-generation coumarin anticoagulants (i.e., warfarin, pindone) have been largely replaced by more potent second-generation anticoagulants.
  - Second-generation anticoagulants (i.e., brodifacoum, bromadiolone, diphacinone, and chlorophacinone) are generally more toxic and persist longer before excretion than first-generation agents.
  - Consumption of bait often precedes clinical hemorrhage by 2–3 days.

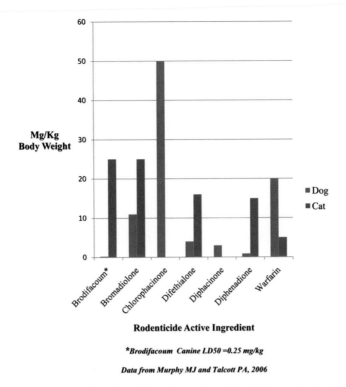

Brodifacoum Canine LD50 =0.25 mg/kg

Data from Murphy MJ and Talcott PA, 2006

■ **Fig. 98.2.** Comparative LD$_{50}$ values for anticoagulant rodenticides in dogs and cats. Cats are generally more resistant to second-generation (long-acting) anticoagulants than are dogs.

- Dogs
  - Difethialone (D-Cease)—highly toxic to rats and mice (0.52 mg/kg and 0.47 mg/kg, respectively); toxic to dogs (LD$_{50}$ = 4 mg/kg)
  - Brodifacoum: LD$_{50}$ = 0.25–2.5 mg/kg
  - Bromadiolone: LD$_{50}$ = 11–20 mg/kg
  - Chlorophacinone: LD$_{50}$ = 50–100 mg/kg
  - Warfarin: LD$_{50}$ = 20–50 mg/kg
  - Diphacinone: LD$_{50}$ = 3–7.5 mg/kg
  - See figure 98. 2 for a graphic comparison of toxicity from common rodenticides.
- Cats
  - Difethialone (D-Cease): LD$_{50}$ >16 mg/kg
    - Concentration in baits lower (0.0025% or 25 ppm) than that of other second-generation rodenticide baits (0.005% or 50 ppm)
    - Dogs and cats may tolerate higher intake of bait material.

Systems Affected

- Hemic/lymphatic/immune—depletion of activated clotting factors resulting in hemorrhage

- Gastrointestinal—oral, gastric, intestinal or colonic bleeding
- Respiratory—Massive pulmonary hemorrhage and hemothorax often cause sudden death.
- Neuromuscular—Hemorrhage within the CNS compresses neural tissue in the cranium or spinal canal, causing ataxia, tetraparesis, and seizures in rare cases; muscle hemorrhage occurs in response to trauma.
- Musculoskeletal—lameness secondary to hemarthrosis
- Renal hemorrhage—leads to hematuria
- Reproductive—Placental hemorrhage can lead to abortion; vaginal bleeding may also occur.

 # SIGNALMENT/HISTORY

Risk Factors

- Common—many types of bait are sold OTC and widely used in homes.
- Major market share of rodenticides in North America is second-generation anticoagulants.
- Rodenticide products are more commonly used in the spring and fall, so exposure increases during these times.
- Dogs and cats primarily affected, with higher prevalence in dogs
- No breed or gender predilections
- Younger animals may ingest bait more readily than older animals, due to their curious nature.

Historical Findings

- Baits are often sold as pellets or blocks of various sizes.
- Most baits are colored to distinguish them as a pesticide. However, specific identification of one type of product is difficult based on color alone. Colors: green, blue-green, red, or brown/tan.
- Coughing, dyspnea, tachypnea, or exercise intolerance are often the first clinical signs.
- Less commonly, SQ swellings, joint swelling, or bleeding from body orifices are observed.
- Rarely, death is the first evidence of poisoning.

Location and Circumstances of Poisoning

- Often in or around buildings where rodent baits are placed
- Prevalence increased by careless placement without protective bait stations
- Exposure may be acute with single large dose or multiple small doses.

Interactions with Drugs, Nutrients, or Environment

- Sulfonamides and phenylbutazone may displace anticoagulant rodenticides from plasma binding sites, leading to more free toxicant and toxicosis.
- Concurrent use of NSAIDs or other drugs that inhibit platelet function is discouraged due to the risks of exacerbated coagulopathy or bleeding.

 # CLINICAL FEATURES

Physical Examination

- Evidence of hemorrhagic shock (i.e., tachycardia, hypovolemic, hypotensive, poor pulse quality, pallor)
- Coughing, dyspnea, tachypnea, pale mucous membranes
- Hemarthrosis, lameness, presence of SQ hematomas
- Exercise intolerance, lethargy, depression
- Hematomas—often ventral and at venipuncture sites
- Bleeding from body orifices, periorbital bleeding
- Epistaxis, vaginal or rectal bleeding
- Muffled heart or lung sounds

Systemic Signs

- Hemic/lymphatic/immune—clotting factor depletion results in generalized ecchymotic hemorrhages and occasional frank bleeding from many body sites.
- Gastrointestinal—oral, gastric, intestinal, or colonic bleeding characterized by epistaxis, hemoptysis, hematemesis, melena, or hemorrhagic diarrhea; severe hemorrhage can result in anemia.
- Respiratory
  - Coughing, dyspnea, abnormal auscultation (i.e., moist rales, increased bronchovesicular sounds, dull ventral lung sounds, etc.), muffled heart sounds, massive pulmonary hemorrhage, hemothorax, exercise intolerance
  - Acute anemia, hypoxemia, respiratory arrest, and sudden death may follow acute pulmonary bleeding.
- Cardiovascular
  - Evidence of hemorrhagic shock secondary to blood loss, hypovolemia, or poor cardiac filling may be seen.
  - Pericardial effusion (seen as muffled heart sounds, presence of VPCs, pulse deficits, vomiting, collapse, etc.) may be seen with toxicity, resulting in poor cardiac filling and signs of hypovolemic shock.
- Neuromuscular
  - Hemarthrosis results in general or asymmetrical lameness.
  - Rarely, hemorrhage compresses neural tissue in cranium or spinal canal,

resulting in CNS signs including ataxia, lethargy, blindness, and occasionally seizures. Spinal bleeding can cause paraplegia or quadriplegia.
- Muscle hemorrhage occurs in response to trauma or IM injection.
■ Renal—Hemorrhage results in hematuria.
■ Reproductive—placental Hemorrhage can lead to abortion; vaginal bleeding possible.

DIFFERENTIAL DIAGNOSIS

■ IMT—platelet count <10,000–15,000 × 10^3/μL
■ Coagulation factor deficiency from prolonged liver disease: Assay for related factor deficiencies, for example, factor VII, liver function, bile acids.
■ DIC—association with neoplasia, sepsis, pancreatitis, concurrent disease; laboratory evidence of elevated PT, PTT, FDP, d-dimers with thrombocytopenia
■ Hemophilia—congenital clotting factor deficiencies: Assay for related factor deficiencies, for example, factor VIII.
■ Fat malabsorption
■ Hemorrhagic shock from trauma, neoplasia, bone marrow suppression, IMHA

DIAGNOSTICS

Clinical Laboratory Findings

■ Anemia—with marked hemorrhage, often acute and nonregenerative
■ Thrombocytopenia from consumptive bleeding (typically 50,000–150,000 × 10^3/μL)
■ Prolonged PT and PTT—support exposure to rodenticide; PT/PTT prolongation seen at 36–48 hours after ingestion but will normalize with vitamin K$_1$ therapy. Typically, PT is prolonged more extensively and earlier (6–18 hours earlier) than PTT.
■ ACT >150 seconds—supports coagulopathy
■ PIVKA assay, although this is rarely used
■ Anticoagulant analysis of blood or liver—confirms exposure to a specific product
■ Anticoagulant assay of stomach or intestinal contents is not reliable because of delay between consumption of bait and appearance of clinical signs.

Imaging

■ Thoracic radiography may detect pleural effusion (i.e., hemothorax), multilobular, alveolar infiltration (i.e., pulmonary hemorrhage), or an enlarged cardiac silhouette (i.e., pericardial effusion).

Diagnostic Procedures

- Thoracentesis in dyspneic patients; may confirm hemothorax
- Preliminary ultrasound of both the pleural and peritoneal cavities may reveal effusion consistent with hemorrhage.

Pathological Findings

- Free blood in the thoracic cavity, lungs, and abdominal cavity—common finding
- Hemorrhage into the cranial vault, GIT, and urinary tract—less common; may also see hemorrhage in the subcutaneous space or within muscle bellies

 THERAPEUTICS

Detoxification

- If recent ingestion has occurred, immediate emesis induction followed by activated charcoal with a cathartic can be performed.
- If clinical signs have already developed, or if the patient is already coagulopathic (based on diagnostic testing), oral detoxification is ineffective and too late.

Appropriate Health Care

- Inpatient—acute crisis
- Outpatient—consider once the coagulopathy is stabilized
- Correct acute signs of hemorrhagic shock with IV crystalloids, colloids, and blood products as needed. Initial shock boluses of 20 mL/kg of crystalloids can be given over 15–20 minutes during initial stabilization. Repeat 2–3x as needed to effect to increase blood pressure.
- The use of pRBC, WB, FFP, or FP may be necessary to increase oxygen carrying capacity (increasing RBC count) and to replace coagulation factors. Patients should be blood typed prior to transfusion.
- Correct life-threatening cardiac tamponade or hemothorax. If volume resuscitation (listed above) does not improve clinical signs of hemorrhagic shock, or if dyspnea is severe, pericardiocentesis or thoracocentesis may be indicated. If the patient is stable and responding to therapy, these procedures should be avoided due to the coagulopathic state of the patient. With time, the blood will be reabsorbed and clinical signs should improve. If, however, there is no response to therapy, an autotransfusion of the patient's blood from the pericardial sac or thoracic cavity can be performed via aseptic technique.
- Administration of vitamin K_1—avoid IM injections, and give orally (if there are no contraindications such as vomiting) or SQ (with a small needle, in multiple locations if needed). Bioavailability of oral absorption is enhanced by the concurrent feeding of a small amount of a fatty meal, such as canned dog food.

Drug(s) and Antidotes of Choice

- Vitamin K$_1$—2.5–5.0 mg/kg PO q 24 h 5 days to 6 weeks (depending on the specific product) or divided PO q 12 h for first-generation anticoagulant toxicosis
- Vitamin K$_1$ administration—continued for 3–4 weeks with suspected second-generation anticoagulant toxicosis

Precautions/Interactions

- Vitamin K$_3$—not efficacious in the treatment of anticoagulant rodenticide toxicosis; contraindicated
- Intravenous vitamin K$_1$—reported anaphylactic reactions; avoid this route of administration.
- Avoid unnecessary surgical procedures and unnecessary parenteral injections until coagulation parameters are within normal limits (e.g., PT, PTT).
- Minimize stress, trauma, and jugular venipuncture or cystocentesis. Catastrophic bleeding may occur as a result.
- Use the smallest possible needle when giving an injection or collecting samples. Phlebotomy sites should be held off adequately to ensure appropriate clot formation.
- Sulfonamides and phenylbutazone may displace anticoagulant rodenticides from plasma binding sites, leading to more free toxicant and toxicosis.

Follow-up

- Recheck PT 36 to 48 hours after vitamin K$_1$ therapy is discontinued.
- There is no need to check a PT, ACT, or PTT while patients are on vitamin K$_1$ therapy, as these coagulation panels should be normal while on therapy. Follow-up blood work should be monitored upon discontinuing vitamin K$_1$ therapy.

Activity

- Confine patient during the early stages; activity enhances blood loss.

Surgical Considerations

- Thoracentesis may be important for removing free thoracic blood, which causes dyspnea and respiratory failure, but should only be performed when life-threatening, severe dyspnea, or hypoxemia is evident.
- Coagulopathies must be corrected prior to surgery.

Public Health

- Children who accidentally consume anticoagulant baits could be at risk.
- Anticoagulants may be excreted in human milk; the extent of milk as a source from exposed animals (milking goats, cows) is not well known.

Environmental Issues

- Anticoagulant rodenticides appear to be relatively weak environmental toxicants.
- Baits transported and hoarded by rodents could be consumed by desirable non-target species.

 COMMENTS

Client Education

- Feed a nutritious high-quality protein diet to support coagulation factor synthesis.
- Do not discontinue vitamin K_1 medication, even if the patient appears completely healthy without treating for the adequate duration of time.

Patient Monitoring

- ACT and PT—assess efficacy of therapy; monitor for 48–72 hours after discontinuation of treatment; if PT is still prolonged, an additional 1–2 weeks of vitamin K_1 therapy should be given.

Prevention/Avoidance

- Do not allow animals access to anticoagulant rodenticides.
- Recommend covered bait stations or placement out of reach of pets.

Possible Complications

- Warn client that reexposure could be a serious problem—remove all the bait from the environment!
- Stress importance of continuing vitamin K_1 for the full time of prescribed period—if not, serious recurrence of hemorrhage can occur.
- Pregnant animal can abort after acute crisis due to placental hemorrhage and detachment.
- A nursing mother that ingested a toxic amount should be treated; the puppies or kittens will also need to be treated for the full duration of time with vitamin K_1 therapy.

Expected Course and Prognosis

- If the patient survives the first 48 hours of acute coagulopathy, the prognosis improves.
- Prolonged vitamin K_1 therapy is important to continued improvement.

Abbreviations

ACT   = activated clotting time
CBC   = complete blood count
CNS   = central nervous system
DIC   = disseminated intravascular coagulation
GIT   = gastrointestinal tract
FDP   = fibrin degradation product
FFP   = fresh frozen plasma
FP   = frozen plasma
IM   = intramuscularly
IMHA   = immune-mediated hemolytic anemia
IMT   = immune-mediated thrombocytopenia
IV   = intravenous
NSAIDs = nonsteroidal anti-inflammatory drugs
OTC   = over-the-counter
PIVKA   = proteins induced by vitamin K antagonism
PO   = *per os* (by mouth)
pRBC   = packed red blood cells
PT   = prothrombin time
PTT   = activated partial thromboplastin time
q   = every
SQ   = subcutaneous
VPC   = ventricular premature contraction
WB   = whole blood

Suggested Reading

Haines B. Anticoagulant rodenticide ingestion and toxicity: a retrospective study of 252 canine cases. Aust Vet Practit 2008; 38:38–50.

Luiz JA, Heseltine J. Five common toxins ingested by dogs and cats. Comp Cont Ed Pract Vet 2008; 30:578–587.

Murphy MJ. Rodenticides. Vet Clin North Am Small Animal Pract 2002; 32(2):469–484.

Murphy MJ, Gerken D. The anticoagulant rodenticides. In: Kirk RW and Bonagura J, eds. Current Veterinary Therapy X. Philadelphia: Saunders, 1989; pp 143–146.

Murphy MJ, Talcott PA. Anticoagulant rodenticides. In Peterson ME and Talcott PA, eds. Small Animal Toxicology, 2nd ed. St. Louis: Elsevier Saunders, 2006; pp 563–577.

Author: Michael Murphy, DVM, PhD, DABVT, DABT, JD
Editor: Gary D. Osweiler, DVM, PhD, DABVT

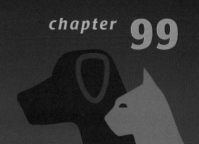

chapter 99

Bromethalin

DEFINITION/OVERVIEW

- Bromethalin (N-methyl-2,4-dinitro-N-[2,4,6-tribromophenyl]-6-[trifluoromethyl] benzeneamine) is a neurotoxic rodenticide marketed under a number of trade names, including Assault, Clout, Fastrac, No Pest Rat and Mice Killer, Real Kill, Talpirid, Tomcat Mole Killer, Vengeance, and others.
- It is usually sold as green, greenish-blue, or tan pellets, blocks, or worms (mole baits) with an active ingredient of 0.01% or 0.025% bromethalin.
  - 0.01% baits contain 2.84 mg bromethalin/ounce bait (0.1 mg/g).
- It is *not* an anticoagulant rodenticide and vitamin K_1 is *not* an antidote.

ETIOLOGY/PATHOPHYSIOLOGY

Mechanism of Action

- Bromethalin uncouples oxidative phosphorylation primarily in the CNS.
- ATP production is decreased, sodium and potassium pumps are inhibited, electrolyte imbalances occur, and lipid peroxidation develops.
- The net result is sodium accumulation inside the cell with edema formation in the brain and spinal cord.

Pharmacokinetics/Absorption, Distribution, Metabolism, and Excretion

- Very little scientific small animal data; information is largely based on rats.
- Bromethalin is rapidly absorbed from the GIT.
- Peak plasma concentrations occur within 4–6 hours of ingestion.
- Widely distributed to brain, fat, liver, and kidney; lipophilic and crosses the BBB
- Metabolism occurs in the liver to a toxic N-demethylated metabolite.
- Enterohepatic recirculation occurs.
- Excretion occurs primarily through the biliary system (feces).
- T½ in rats is 5–6 days.

Toxicity

- Dogs
  - LD_{50} in dogs is 2.38–3.65 mg bromethalin/kg.

769

- Minimum lethal dose is 2.5 mg bromethalin/kg.
- Clinical signs, including death, have occurred at dosages from 0.95 to 1.05 mg bromethalin/kg.
  - Cats
    - LD_{50} in cats is 0.54 mg bromethalin/kg.
    - Minimum lethal dose is 0.45 mg bromethalin/kg.
    - Clinical signs have occurred with dosages as low as 0.24 mg bromethalin/kg.

Systems Affected

- Nervous—CNS depression or stimulation, cerebral edema, seizures, coma
- Neuromuscular—paralytic syndrome with weakness, tremors, ataxia, paresis
- Ophthalmic—abnormal PLR, anisocoria, nystagmus
- Gastrointestinal—anorexia, vomiting (not a consistent finding)
- Endocrine/metabolic—hyperthermia
- Respiratory—respiratory depression (may be cause of death)

 # SIGNALMENT/HISTORY

- Diagnosis is based on history of exposure and clinical signs.
- No breed or age specificity is seen.

Risk Factors

- Cats are much more sensitive to toxicosis than dogs.
- Cats may be at risk of relay toxicity from ingestion of poisoned rodents.
- Smaller ingestions on a chronic basis may produce clinical signs of toxicosis.

Historical Findings

- Owners may report tan, green, or greenish blue material in the feces. Rarely, chunks of the blocks, pellets, or worms are passed.

Location and Circumstances of Poisoning

- Witnessed ingestion
- Bait boxes chewed or bait scattered around

 # CLINICAL FEATURES

- Clinical signs are dose dependent, and onset varies depending on amount ingested.
  - Acute ingestions of large doses will show clinical signs within 2–24 hours.
  - Subacute or chronic ingestions may not show clinical signs for several days.

- Acute ingestions show signs primarily related to the CNS—stimulation or depression, abnormal behavior, hyperesthesia, seizures, coma. Neuromuscular signs include paresis, hind limb paralysis, tremors, ataxia, anisocoria, nystagmus, and changes in PLR. Other acute signs are variable but include vomiting and hyperthermia.
- Clinical signs with a much slower onset (1–2 weeks after ingestion) include hind limb ataxia, paresis or paralysis, loss of deep pain response, and bladder paralysis.

 # DIFFERENTIAL DIAGNOSIS

- Primary neurologic disease—trauma, infection, inflammatory, neoplastic, congenital, structural, vascular events
- Drug-related toxicity
  - Amphetamines/methamphetamine
  - Atypical antipsychotics
  - Baclofen
  - Lead
  - Metaldehyde
  - SSRIs

 # DIAGNOSTICS

- Based on history of ingestion. Accurate product identification is essential as bromethalin is easily confused with other rodenticides that are similar in color.
- Identification of product returned in emesis is difficult.
- Early clinicopatholgical changes are unremarkable.
- Serum chemistry and electrolyte abnormalities may occur secondary to dehydration.
- Bromethalin assay in tissue of animals may be useful for final diagnosis. Best specimens are liver and brain.

Pathological Findings

- Lesions are usually confined to the CNS. Cerebral edema may or may not be grossly visible. Spongy degeneration of CNS white matter tracts (diffuse white matter vacuolization) is evident on histopathology.

 # THERAPEUTICS

- The goal of therapy is to provide early decontamination and prevention of cerebral edema.

Detoxification

- Emesis up to several hours after ingestion in the absence of clinical signs
- Activated charcoal with a cathartic for one dose followed by activated charcoal without a cathartic q 6–8 hours for 24 hours to reduce enterohepatic cycling.

Appropriate Health Care

- Baseline laboratory work (CBC, chemistry panel, UA) to rule out complications from dehydration, anorexia
- IV fluids are needed to maintain cerebral perfusion and to correct any dehydration prior to use of mannitol.
- If cerebral edema, keep head elevated to 15–30 degrees
- Oxygen therapy PRN
- Monitor vitals, mentation, blood pressure, hydration, urine output

Drug(s) and Antidotes of Choice

- No specific antidote is available.
- IV fluids for dehydration. Their use will not promote excretion.
- Mannitol 0.5–2 g/kg IV q 4–6 hours, slowly over 20–30 minutes, PRN to treat cerebral edema. Discontinue IV fluids during administration. Use only when patient is stabilized and adequately hydrated.
- Anticonvulsant therapy:
  - Diazepam 0.25–0.5 mg/kg IV, to effect PRN
  - Phenobarbital 3–5 mg/kg IV, to effect PRN
- Tremors:
  - Methocarbamol 55–220 mg/kg IV, to effect PRN. Do not exceed 330 mg/kg in 24 hours. Monitor for excessive sedation and respiratory depression with high-dose therapy.

Precautions/Interactions

- Steroid use is controversial and has been shown to be of little benefit in reversing signs in experimental animals. The use of steroids in humans with cerebral ischemia has been associated with a poor outcome and is currently not recommended in the use of treatment for cerebral edema.

Alternate Drugs

- *Ginkgo biloba* extract 100 mg/kg PO has been used in rats, but the benefit in animals has not been evaluated.

Nursing Care

- Monitor temperature frequently and treat appropriately. Elevate head at 15–30 degrees if patient is laterally recumbent and showing signs of cerebral edema; turn every 6 hours to prevent atelectasis. Lubricate eyes every 6 hours PRN.

Follow-up

▪ Monitor until clinical signs resolve, which may be up to several weeks in severely affected animals.

Diet

▪ Animals with CNS impairment, depression, or vomiting should have food and water withheld to prevent aspiration pneumonia.
▪ Enteral or parenteral feeding if prolonged neurologic complications preclude oral nutrition

COMMENTS

Client Education

▪ Owners should be instructed to keep all rodenticides out of reach of animals, and if an ingestion occurs to bring the packaging along with the animal.

Patient Monitoring

▪ Monitor hydration, heart rate, blood pressure, and body temperature. Frequency of monitoring will vary with severity of clinical signs.

Possible Complications

▪ DIC, rhabdomyolysis, and myoglobinuria with subsequent renal failure are possible if seizures occur and are left untreated.
▪ Neurological deficits may persist for an extended period of time.

Expected Course and Prognosis

▪ Pet Poison Helpline recorded 1,845 cases of bromethalin toxicity reported from 2006 to 2009. Overall, the prognosis for bromethalin toxicity was fair with prompt aggressive medical treatment but guarded if persistent seizures or paralytic syndrome had developed.
▪ Prognosis varies depending on the amount ingested and whether appropriate decontamination occurred in a timely manner.
▪ Prognosis deteriorates if seizures or coma develop.

Abbreviations

ATP = adenosine triphosphate
BBB = blood brain barrier
CBC = complete blood count
CNS = central nervous system
DIC = disseminated intravascular coagulation

GIT = gastrointestinal tract
IM   = intramuscular
IV   = intravenous
LD_{50} = median lethal dose
PLR = pupillary light reflex
PO   = *per os* (by mouth)
PRN = *pro re nata* (as needed)
q   = every
SQ   = subcutaneous
SSRI = selective serotonin reuptake inhibitor
UA   = urinalysis

Suggested Reading

Dorman D. Bromethalin. In: Talcott PA, Peterson ME, eds. Small animal toxicology, 2nd ed. St. Louis: Elsevier, 2006; pp 609–618.

Dunayer R. Bromethalin: the other rodenticide. Vet Med 2003; 98(9):732–739.

Pasquale-Styles MA, Sochaski MA, Dorman DC. Fatal bromethalin poisoning. J Forensic Sci 2006; 51(5):1154–1157.

Van Lier RB, Cherry LD. The toxicity and mechanism of action of bromethalin: a new single feeding rodenticide. Fundam Appl Toxicol 1988; 11(4):664–672.

Authors: Catherine M. Adams, DVM; Lynn R. Hovda, RPH, DVM, MS, DACVIM
Consulting Editors: Justine A. Lee, DVM, DACVECC; Lynn R. Hovda, RPH, DVM, MS, DACVIM

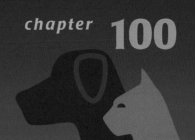

Cholecalciferol

chapter **100**

DEFINITION/OVERVIEW

- Cholecalciferol, the chemical name for vitamin D_3, is a necessary part of dietary requirements. Sources are through ingested food, vitamin supplements, and dermal exposure to the sun.
- Rodenticides are another source of cholecalciferol and are the primary cause of vitamin D_3 toxicosis in dogs and cats.
- Vitamin D_3 is expressed either as mg/kg or as IU; $1\,\mu g$ vitamin D_3 is equivalent to 40 IU.

ETIOLOGY/PATHOPHYSIOLOGY

Mechanism of Action

- 1,25-dihydroxycholecalciferol (calcitriol) is the most active metabolite of cholecalciferol.
- Cholecalciferol is converted in the liver by 25-hydroxylase to 25-hydroxycholecalciferol (calcifediol). This is then converted to 1,25-dihydroxycholecalciferol (calcitriol) in the kidneys by 1-alpha-hydroxylase.
- In toxic exposures, calcitriol exerts negative feedback and suppresses renal hydroxylase. There is almost no feedback by calcium, calcitriol, or calcifediol to liver hydroxylase, so calcifediol continues to be produced.
- Calcitriol increases calcium absorption from the GIT, stimulates bone resorption, and increases calcium absorption in the renal distal tubules. This results in increased serum calcium and increased serum phosphorus, causing mineralization of soft tissues.

Pharmacokinetics/Absorption, Distribution, Metabolism, and Excretion

- Cholecalciferol undergoes enterohepatic recirculation.
- Cholecalciferol half-life is 19–25 hours. The terminal half-life is weeks to months because it is highly fat soluble.
- Calcifediol plasma half-life is ≥10 days.
- Calcitriol plasma half-life is 3–5 days.

775

Toxicity

- The LD_{50} in dogs is 85 mg/kg. These calculations are based on a cholecalciferol rodenticide concentration of 0.075%.
- Clinically, normal dogs and cats have developed hypercalcemia at dosages of 0.5 mg/kg (20,000 IU/kg).
- Signs of toxicosis (i.e., vomiting, anorexia, weakness) have occurred in clinically normal dogs and cats at 0.1 mg/kg (4000 IU/kg).

Systems Affected

- Renal—renal tubular necrosis, impaired calcium and phosphorus homeostasis, metastatic calcification
- Cardiovascular—bradycardia, ventricular arrhythmias, ECG changes (e.g., shortened QT interval and prolonged PR interval), metastatic calcification
- Gastrointestinal—metastatic calcification of muscularis in stomach and GIT
- Respiratory—pulmonary metastatic calcification, decreased lung compliance
- CNS—variable from depression and lethargy to seizures
- Musculoskeletal—excessive calcium mobilization from bones, metastatic calcification, periarticular calcification

 SIGNALMENT/HISTORY

- All breeds and ages of cats and dogs are susceptible to this toxicity.
- Cats and dogs under 6 months of age may be more susceptible.

 CLINICAL FEATURES

- The overt clinical signs are vomiting, weakness, lethargy, melena, hemorrhagic diarrhea, depression, PU/PD, and death.
- With examination and diagnostics, hypercalcemia, hyperphosphatemia, renal failure, metabolic acidosis, and bradycardia are found.
- Clinical signs usually begin to occur within 12–36 hours of ingestion.
- Renal failure will occur at 12–36 hours with toxic ingestion.
- Surviving animal may have renal impairment and may develop cardiac and GI complications because of calcium deposition and bradycardia.
- Clinical signs may last for weeks because of the slow release of the product from fat stores.

 DIFFERENTIAL DIAGNOSIS

- Chronic renal failure
- Ethylene glycol toxicosis

- Grape/raisin toxicosis
- Idiopathic hypercalcemia of cats
- Hypercalcemia of malignancy
- Primary hyperparathyroidism
- Ingestion of prescription skin products containing calcipotriene or tacalcitol
- Ingestion of high-dose oral vitamin D supplements
- Hypoadrenocorticism
- Juvenile hypercalcemia

 # DIAGNOSTICS

- Toxicosis is potentially life threatening when the serum calcium is greater than 12.5 mg/dL, serum phosphorus levels are over 7 mg/dL, and hyposthenuria is documented.
- Phosphorus levels show an increase about 12 hours prior to the calcium level increase and act as a good indicator for treatment with pamidronate or salmon calcitonin.
- Radiographs or ultrasound may show calcification of renal, GI, or vascular tissues.
- Specific tests for levels of calcipotriene, tacalcitol, and calcitriol are not available.
- Calcifediol levels are available but are not routinely used in veterinary medicine.

Pathological Findings

- At necropsy, renal tubular degeneration and necrosis; mineralization of the renal tubules, coronary arteries, GIT, and other soft tissues; hemorrhage of gastric mucosa may be evident.
- Concentration of calcifediol levels can be found in renal tissue.

 # THERAPEUTICS

Detoxification

- Early emesis or gastric lavage
- Activated charcoal with a cathartic initially, followed by activated charcoal *without* a cathartic q 8 hours for 1–2 days to decrease enterohepatic circulation.

Appropriate Health Care

- Baseline laboratory work (CBC, chemistry panel, venous blood gas, UA, and USG)

- Repeat calcium and phosphorus daily
- The goal of treatment is to keep the calcium level at less than 12.5 mg/dL and the phosphorus level at less than 7 mg/dL.

Drug(s) and Antidotes of Choice

- No specific antidote is available for calcipotriene toxicity.
- Aggressive 0.9% NaCl diuresis at 2–3 times maintenance until calcium levels decrease.
- If urine output decreases in face of adequate hydration, add the following:
  - Furosemide CRI at 1–2 mg/kg/hour IV
  - Mannitol bolus at 1–2 g/kg
- To increase calcium excretion:
  - Furosemide 0.5 mg/kg/hr IV or 2.5–4.5 mg/kg PO TID
  - Dexamethasone 0.2 mg/kg IV q 12 hours *or* prednisone 2–3 mg/kg PO BID
- Phosphate binders to keep the calcium x phosphorus product at less than 60 or 70.
  - Aluminum hydroxide 2–10 mL PO q 6 hours if phosphorus levels are high
- Bisphosphonates to inhibit bone reabsorption and minimize hypercalcemia
  - Currently, pamidronate is the most widely used, although others have been tried.
  - Pamidronate disodium (Aredia).
    - 1.3–2 mg/kg IV diluted in saline and infused over 2 hours for one dose only.
    - Expect serum calcium and phosphorus levels to decrease in 24–48 hours.
    - If levels decrease and then rebound, a second dose may be needed in 5–7 days. Anecdotally, extremely large ingestions have needed redosing in just 3–4 days.
- Antiemetics as needed for persistent vomiting
  - Maropitant 1 mg/kg SQ q 24 hours, not labeled for cats
  - Ondansetron 0.1–0.2 mg/kg IV q 8–12 hours
- GI protectants
  - H$_2$ blockers
    - Famotidine 0.5–1 mg/kg PO, SQ, IM, IV q 12 hours
    - Ranitidine 1–2 mg/kg PO, SQ, IM, IV q 8–12 hours
    - Cimetidine 5–10 mg/kg PO, SQ, IM, IV q 6 hours
  - Omeprazole 0.5–1 mg/kg daily
  - Sucralfate 0.25–1 g PO TID x 5–7 days if evidence of active ulcer disease

Precautions/Interactions

- Thiazide diuretics are contraindicated as they decrease clearance of calcium.

- Bisphosphonates should rarely be used in combination with calcitonin and then only in the most refractory cases. There is some evidence that the combined use may increase soft tissue mineralization.
- Excessive doses of pamidronate can cause hypocalcemia, and treatment with calcium carbonate may be needed. In severe cases IV calcium gluconate may be used.

Alternative Drugs

- Salmon calcitonin (Trade Names: Calcimar, Micalcin) at 4–7 IU/kg SQ q 8–12 hours
- Currently used less often than pamidronate due to inconsistencies in treatment and development of resistance after several days of treatment
- Used instead of pamidronate. All other treatment recommendations remain the same.
- Occasionally both pamidronate and salmon calcitonin must be used to get non-responsive animals to respond to treatment, but there is some concern for possible soft tissue calcification as a result. Pamidronate is used as the first treatment. If recalcitrant, the pet may then receive salmon calcitonin.

Diet

- Low-calcium diet

 COMMENTS

Expected Course and Prognosis

- Pet Poison Helpline documented 884 cases of cholecalciferol toxicity reported from 2006 to 2009.
- Outcome depends on the length of and severity of hypercalcemia.
- If calcification has already occurred in the cardiac tissue or GIT, prognosis is guarded.
- The full course of treatment may take from 1 week to several weeks.

Abbreviations

BID   = twice a day
CBC   = complete blood count
CNS   = central nervous system
CRI   = continuous rate infusion
GI   = gastrointestinal
GIT   = gastrointestinal tract
IM   = intramuscular
IU   = international units

IV   = intravenous
PO   = *per os* (by mouth)
PU/PD = polyuria/polydipsia
q   = every
SQ   = subcutaneous
TID   = three times a day
UA   = urinalysis
USG   = urine specific gravity

Suggested Reading

Hare WR et al. Calcipotriene poisoning in dogs. Vet Med 2000; 10:770–778.

Hostutler RA et al. Uses and effectiveness of pamidronate disodium for treatment of dogs and cats with hypercalcemia. J Vet Int Med 2005; 19:29–33.

Martin TM, De Lorimer LP, Fan TM, et al. Pharmacokinetics and pharmacodynamics of a single dose of zoledronate in healthy dogs. J Vet Pharmacol Therap 2007; 30:492–495.

Pesillo SA et al. Calcipotriene toxicosis in a dog successfully treated with pamidronate disodium. J Vet Emerg Crit Care 2002; 12(3):177–181.

Rumbeiha WK et al. Use of pamidronate disodium to reduce cholicalciferol-induced toxicosis in dogs. Am J Vet Res 2000; 61(1):9–13.

Author: Catherine M. Adams, DVM
Consulting Editor: Gary D. Osweiler, DVM, PhD, DABVT

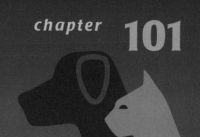

chapter **101**

Phosphides

DEFINITION/OVERVIEW

- Zinc phosphide has been used as a rodenticide since the 1930s and is used to control rats, mice, voles, ground squirrels, prairie dogs, nutria, muskrats, feral rabbits, and gophers.
- Aluminum phosphide is also used as a fumigant in grain storage silos and grain transport vehicles.
- OTC products containing 2% zinc phosphide are available in many states; often they are labeled only for below-ground use to control gophers and moles.
- Zinc phosphide is a grey crystalline powder commonly available in 2%–10% concentrations as grain or sugar-based baits in a powder, pellet, paste, or tablet formulation.
- Formulations of phosphides commonly have a distinctive odor described as similar to acetylene, rotten fish, or garlic.
- Trade names of commercially available products include the following: Arrex, Commando, Denkarin Grains, Gopha-Rid, Phosvin, Pollux, Ridall, Ratol, Rodenticide AG, Zinc-Tox and ZP.
- Toxicity is secondary to the production of phosphine gas production following ingestion, which leads to GI, respiratory, or CNS effects.

ETIOLOGY/PATHOPHYSIOLOGY

- Zinc (or aluminum and magnesium) phosphide exerts toxic effects due to ingestion, inhalation, or by absorption through broken skin. The most common type of exposure is ingestion with subsequent phosphine gas production.
- Phosphine gas is produced by hydrolysis in a moist or acid environment. The phosphine gas is considered a corrosive and is a direct irritant to the GIT, which leads to anorexia, vomiting, possible hematemesis, or melena. The production of phosphine gas within the stomach may lead to gastric or abdominal distension ("bloat") and often pain.
- Profound cardiovascular and respiratory effects can lead to circulatory collapse, possible arrhythmia development, pulmonary edema, or pleural effusion.
- The smell of rotten fish or acetylene may be noted on the patient's breath or from the vomitus.

Mechanism of Action

- Zinc phosphine gas is produced by hydrolysis in a moist or acid environment.
- Significant hydrolysis of zinc phosphide occurs at a pH of less than 4, whereas aluminum or magnesium phosphide will undergo hydrolysis at a neutral pH.
- Phosphine gas is considered to have direct corrosive effects on the GIT (esophagus, stomach, and duodenum).
- Phosphine is rapidly absorbed from the GI mucosa and systemically distributed.
- Phosphine may lead to the production of free radicals and oxidative stress, which also directly causes cellular damage and inhibits aerobic respiration (see fig. 101.1).

Pharmacokinetics/Absorption, Distribution, Metabolism, and Excretion

- Toxicokinetics of zinc (or aluminum and magnesium) phosphides are not well described.
- Given the rapid onset of clinical signs and the broad range of effects typically seen, there is presumed rapid GI absorption and broad distribution of the phosphine gas.
- Oral doses of phosphides result in significant elimination in expired air; available information suggests this may occur within 12 hours after ingestion.

Toxicity

- The approximate toxic dosage of zinc phosphide is believed to be 20–40 mg/kg.
- Several factors affect toxicity, including the amount of food in the stomach, the gastric acid level, and the different formulations of zinc phosphides; therefore, the toxic dose can vary depending on when the animal last ate.

BAIT	STOMACH	SYSTEMIC
$ZN_3P_2 \rightarrow$	$ZN_3P_2 + H_2O + H^+ \rightarrow 3\,Zn^{2+} + 2\,PH_3 \rightarrow$	$\rightarrow$ROS + Cellular damage $PH_3 \rightarrow$ Cyt C Oxidase $\rightarrow //$

■ Fig. 101.1. Zinc phosphide or other metal phosphides rapidly hydrolyze in stomach acids or a moist environment to form toxic phosphine gas. Phosphine generates reactive oxygen species (ROS) and blocks aerobic respiration, leading to metabolic acidosis and multiple organ damage. It should be considered a toxicological emergency. This is one of the few poisons where a full stomach increases toxicity.

- Animals that have ingested up to 300 mg/kg on an empty stomach have survived, while consumption of much lower dosages are toxic when consumed with food, which releases the acids that promote hydrolysis.
- Zinc phosphide ingestion can lead to emesis; therefore, the toxicity may be self-limiting in some cases.
- The dose that may produce clinical signs is estimated to be 1/10 the lethal dose.
- Clinical signs often occur within 15 minutes to 4 hours; death has been reported to occur within 3–48 hours.

Systems Affected

- Gastrointestinal—anorexia, vomiting, hematemesis, melena
- Cardiovascular—direct myocardial damage, arrhythmias, decreased contractility, hypotension
- Respiratory—pulmonary edema, pleural effusion
- Hemic/lymphatic/immune—methemoglobinemia, Heinz body production
- Nervous—ataxia, weakness, tremors, hyperesthesia, seizures
- Renal/urologic—azotemia, acute renal failure
- Hepatobiliary—increased ALT, AST, and total bilirubin
- Endocrine/metabolic—metabolic acidosis; electrolyte imbalances (e.g., potassium and magnesium)
- Musculoskeletal—weakness, ataxia

 SIGNALMENT/HISTORY

- There is no known breed or sex predilection.
- Common presenting complaints may include the following:
  - Acute GI signs of vomiting, hematemesis, anorexia, bloating, abdominal pain, and melena
  - Respiratory distress
  - Neurological signs of ataxia, tremors, seizures, coma, or sudden death

Risk Factors

- Ingestion of food will decrease the gastric pH and lead to rapid phosphine gas release.
- Pet owners should be told not to feed their affected pet immediately after toxin exposure (e.g., piece of bread).

Historical Findings

- Determine if there has been potential exposure to rodenticide, and if so, determine the active ingredient of the product used.

- Owners may report acute abdominal distension, pain, vomition, and a malodor noted on the animal's breath.
- In severe cases, respiratory distress, ataxia, seizures, and sudden death have occurred.

Location and Circumstances of Poisoning

- These may be used as household, environmental, or commercially placed baits.

Interactions with Drugs, Nutrients, or Environment

- The toxicity of this product varies depending on the exposure parameters.
- Zinc phosphide will remain stable when placed in a dry environment for 2 weeks, but excessive heat will lead to decreased efficacy of the baits (>122°F).
- Exposure to moisture will cause deterioration of the product.
- Exposure to acid will lead to rapid hydrolysis and phosphine production.
- Some products are formulated to preserve stability in outdoor environments, so occasionally toxicity can persist for more extended periods.

 ## CLINICAL FEATURES

- The most common initial clinical signs are vomiting, nausea, and hematemesis.
- The animal may have considerable abdominal distension or pain on palpation.
- A rotten fish odor from the animal's breath or the vomitus is characteristic.
- As phosphine gas is absorbed, there is progression to respiratory distress with labored or raspy breathing and tachypnea.
- Signs may progress to include neurological signs such as ataxia, agitation, aimless wandering or pacing, wild running and barking, tremors, and seizures.
- Occasionally phosphide poisoned dogs become excited and exhibit loud barking and wild and aimless running.
- On PE, the gums may appear cyanotic (due to severe hypoxemia) or brown (due to methemoglobinemia).
- On thoracic auscultation there may be crackles noted.
- Heart rate may be rapid or slow, and arrhythmias may be evident.
- Shock, as demonstrated by rapid heart rate, decreased pulse quality, and cool extremities, can occur.
- Neurological assessment will vary depending on the degree of CNS effects.

 ## DIFFERENTIAL DIAGNOSIS

- Organophosphate toxicosis
- Metaldehyde toxicosis

- Serotonin syndrome
- NSAID toxicosis
- Tremogenic mycotoxins
- Primary gastrointestinal disease (e.g., HGE, acute gastroenteritis, parvovirus, etc.)
- Primary cardiac disease (e.g., congestive heart failure)
- Secondary cardiopulmonary disease (e.g., noncardiogenic pulmonary edema from near drowning, seizures, electrocution, ARDS)
- Metabolic disease (renal, hepatic, pancreas)

 # DIAGNOSTICS

- There is no in-house confirmatory test for phosphide rodenticide exposure.
- A suspected exposure, along with consistent clinical signs and an acetylene or rotten fish smell, may support the diagnosis.
- Confirmation using gas chromatography or a Dräger detector tube test can be performed through a diagnostic laboratory. The Dräger detection tube test has been validated using canine stomach contents and vomitus. Other postmortem samples for detection of zinc phosphide include the liver and kidney.
- Blood work findings may include the following:
  - Methemoglobinemia or Heinz body formation with evidence of secondary hemolysis on a CBC
  - Clinical chemistry panel may reveal azotemia, increased liver enzymes (ALT, AST, and total bilirubin)
  - Electrolyte abnormalities, such as hypokalemia and hypomagnesemia
  - Other changes may include decreased cholinesterase activity, increased myocardial troponin, metabolic acidosis, and hypoxemia.

Pathological Findings

- Postmortem findings are nonspecific and include venous congestion, capillary breakdown, pulmonary congestion, interlobar lung edema, pleural effusion, hepatic and renal congestion, renal tubular necrosis (in some cases), myocardial necrosis with mononuclear infiltration and fragmentation of fibers, valvular (mitral and aortic) inflammation, and desquamated respiratory epithelium.

 # THERAPEUTICS

- There is no antidote.
- Treatment goals are to perform a safe and effective decontamination followed by symptomatic and supportive care.

- Given the risk of phosphine gas exposure to veterinary staff (and owners), clinical judgment and treatment in a well-ventilated area is an important consideration. Depending on the patient's clinical presentation, detoxification may include induction of emesis or gastric lavage.
- Administration of a liquid antacid to try to limit the amount of phosphine gas production may help decrease risk to the patient and veterinary staff.
- Activated charcoal may decrease toxic effects in zinc phosphide cases.
- Treatment should include gastroprotectants; monitoring for any respiratory, CNS, electrolyte, liver, or kidney effects; and subsequent supportive care.

Detoxification

- Increasing the gastric pH with the administration of a liquid antacid may decrease or stop the production of phosphine gas.
- Activated charcoal may help decrease the toxicity of zinc phosphide.

Appropriate Health Care

- Care should be symptomatic and supportive.
- Monitoring for the development of signs in the asymptomatic patient for 12 hours is warranted.
- Hospitalization and care should be continued until life-threatening signs and symptoms resolve.

Drug(s) and Antidotes of Choice

- There is no antidote available.
- Oral adsorption detoxification with one dose of charcoal at 2–4 g/kg PO.
- Liquid antacids (such as aluminum hydroxide, magnesium hydroxide, or calcium carbonate) or 5% sodium bicarbonate administered at a dose of 0.5 mL/kg to 1 mL/kg orally may help increase the gastric pH, which may slow or stop the production of phosphine gas. These given prior to emesis induction or at the time of gastric lavage may also protect the veterinary staff from exposure to phosphine gas.
- Respiratory—If there is evidence of hypoxemia, then oxygen supplementation or mechanical ventilation may be indicated.
- In the presence of shock and for renal protection, IV fluid therapy with either crystalloids or colloids is warranted.
- Gastroprotectants should be used due to the corrosive effects of phosphine gas on the GI mucosa.
    - Famotidine 0.5–1 mg/kg IV q 24 hours
    - Omeprazole 0.5–1 mg/kg PO q 24 hours
    - Misoprostol (synthetic prostaglandin analog) may be helpful, 2–5 μg/kg PO q 8 hours
    - Sucralfate 0.25–1 g PO q 8–12 hours

- Anticonvulsants that may be indicated to control seizures:
  - Diazepam 0.5 mg/kg IV to effect or at 0.5–1 mg/kg/hr IV, CRI
  - Phenobarbital 4–16 mg/kg IV to effect
  - Propofol 1–8 mg/kg IV to effect followed by 0.1–0.6 mg/kg/hr IV, CRI
- Methocarbamol 50–220 mg/kg IV, to effect; up to 330 mg/kg/day may be effective for tremors.
- Hepatic support should include the use of the following:
  - S-adenosyl-methionine 18 mg/kg PO q 24 hours
  - Silymarin/milk thistle 50–250 mg/day PO q 24 hours
  - Vitamin K_1 2–3 mg/kg PO q 12–24 hours
  - Low-protein diet
- Antioxidants:
  - Free radical scavengers and antioxidants may protect tissues from damage.
  - N-acetylcysteine (NAC) may help replace depleted glutathione stores, be directly cytoprotective to the myocardium, and may prevent damage by reactive oxygen species formed due to phosphine gas toxicity.
- Methemoglobinemia can be treated with NAC to help resolve this abnormality.
  - NAC should be loaded (140 mg/kg, IV or PO) followed by intermittent dosing (50–70 mg/kg IV or PO q 4–6 hours for up to 72 hours).
- Analgesics may be indicated if the patient is still exhibiting pain after initial stabilization.

Precautions/Interactions

- Examination and emesis should be performed in a well-ventilated area to avoid human exposure to the phosphine gas.
- Do not feed these animals prior to induction of emesis as it may lead to increased phosphine gas production due the lowering of the gastric pH.

Alternative Drugs

- Magnesium supplementation—There are some reports of hypomagnesemia as a result of zinc phosphine toxicity, and controversy regarding supplementation exists.
  - Magnesium plays a key role in the synthesis and activity of glutathione and other antioxidants, which may help counteract some of the damage caused by zinc phosphine gas exposure.
- Pralidoxime (2-PAM):
  - Rat studies have shown phosphine causes some acetylcholinesterase inhibition.
  - Improved survival is reported with administration of pralidoxime (and atropine) in rats poisoned with aluminum phosphide.

- Melatonin has been shown to decrease tissue damage caused in several organs (brain, heart, liver, kidney, and lungs) by phosphine gas production.
- Lipids:
  - There are a few clinical reports of the use of coconut oil to decrease phosphine gas production.
  - Studies on the administration of oil (vegetable or paraffin) have been shown *in vitro* to decrease phosphine gas release.

Nursing Care

- Monitor acid base status, electrolytes, liver and kidney function, and signs of hypoxemia; intervention should be based on clinical presentation and progression.

Follow-up

- Will be case dependent

Diet

- Due to the GI effects and irritation, a bland diet is indicated for 5–7 days.

Activity

- Case-dependent, but should be able to return to normal activity level

Surgical Considerations

- None

Prevention

- Client education to allow safe use or placements of baits in the animal's environment.

Public Health

- Risk of exposure to phosphine gas by owners (or veterinary staff) if emesis is induced at home, in the car, or in the clinic and not in a well-ventilated area.

 COMMENTS

- This can be a very serious or lethal toxicosis.
- Decontamination should take priority, followed by symptomatic and supportive care.
- Close monitoring of the patient will help guide treatment.

Client Education

- At-home monitoring for any evidence of GI ulceration or possible perforation.
  - Signs such as weakness, lethargy, anorexia, vomiting, retching, malaise, labored breathing, painful abdomen, etc., should prompt an immediate recheck.
- Delayed hepatic insults have been reported.
  - Owners should watch for PU/PD, anorexia, vomiting, weight loss, icterus, etc.
- Acute tubular necrosis is also possible.
  - Animals should be monitored for evidence of renal failure, PU/PD, vomiting, anorexia, and decreased urine production.

Patient Monitoring

- Evaluation of respiratory status and hypoxemia should be done frequently on initial presentation.
- Pulse oximetry monitoring and arterial blood gas analysis may help direct therapy.
- Presence of hypoxemia and brown-appearing blood should alert the clinician to possible methemoglobinemia.
- Monitoring of the acid-base status and electrolytes (i.e., ionized calcium, ionized magnesium, sodium, potassium, and chloride) may be indicated.
- Evaluation of liver and kidney function should be repeated to assess for delayed injury.

Prevention/Avoidance

- Discontinue use, remove all baits, or discontinue access to bait.

Possible Complications

- Acute renal failure and hepatic damage may follow sublethal exposures.
- A follow-up clinical chemistry should be evaluated following discharge.

Expected Course and Prognosis

- Asymptomatic patients should be monitored for up to 12 hours.
- Symptomatic patients should be monitored for 48–72 hours or until life-threatening signs resolve and the dog is stable enough for at-home care.

Synonyms

- Trizinc diphosphide
- Zn_3P_2
- Metallophosphide

Abbreviations

ALT   = alanine aminotransferase
ARDS = acute respiratory distress syndrome
AST   = aspartate aminotransferase
CBC   = complete blood count
CNS   = central nervous system
GI   = gastrointestinal
GIT   = gastrointestinal tract
HGE   = hemorrhagic gastroenteritis
IV   = intravenous
NAC   = N-acetylcysteine
NSAID = nonsteroidal anti-inflammatory
OTC   = over-the-counter
PE   = physical exam
PO   = *per os* (by mouth)
PU/PD = polyuria/polydyspia
q   = every
ROS   = reactive oxygen species (fig. 101.1)

Suggested Reading

Casteel SW, Bailey EM. A review of zinc phosphide poisoning. Vet Hum Toxicol 1986; 28:151–153.

Fessesswork GG, Stair EL, Johnson BW, et al. Laboratory diagnosis of zinc phosphide poisoning. Vet Hum Toxicol 1994; 36:517–518.

Knight MW. Zinc phosphide. In: Peterson ME, Talcott PA, eds. Small Animal Toxicology, 2nd ed. St. Louis: Elsevier Saunders, 2006.

Proudfoot AT. Aluminum and zinc phosphide poisoning. Clin Toxicol 2009; 47:89–100.

Rodenberg HD, Chang CC, Watson WA. Zinc phosphide ingestion: a case report and review. Vet Hum Toxicol 1989; 31:559–562.

Author: Sarah Gray, DVM
Consulting Editor: Gary D. Osweiler, DVM, PhD, DABVT

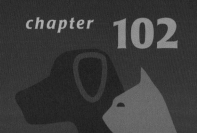

chapter 102

Strychnine

DEFINITION/OVERVIEW

- Strychnine is a very potent alkaloid toxin, derived from the seeds of *Strychnos nux-vomica* and *S. ignatii*. It is used to kill/control ground squirrels, mice, chipmunks, prairie dogs, rats, moles, gophers, birds, and occasionally used on larger predators (e.g., coyotes, wolves, dogs).
- Strychnine is very rapidly absorbed, with onset of clinical signs within 10 minutes to 2 hours.
- Strychnine reversibly blocks the binding of the inhibitory neurotransmitter glycine, resulting in an unchecked reflex stimulation.
- Clinical signs progress from hyperextension of all limbs, extensive muscle rigidity (i.e., with the extensor muscles being more severely affected due to more dominance), seizures, and finally respiratory arrest from paralysis of muscles or respiration.
- Strychnine is eliminated as hepatic metabolites; the parent compound is eliminated in the urine.
- Cause of death is due to apnea, hypoxemia, and respiratory arrest.
- Baits are available in multiple forms and concentrations, and typically range from <0.5 to >0.5%. Lower concentrations are available to the general public in some states, but concentrations >0.5% are limited to use by certified applicators.

ETIOLOGY/PATHOPHYSIOLOGY

- Malicious poisoning is a relatively common means of exposure.
- Direct exposure to baits is more common in dogs than other domestic species, due to their indiscriminant feeding behavior.
- Relay toxicosis can occur via the ingestion of poisoned rodents and birds.
- Due to more rigid state control and regulation, strychnine toxicosis is less commonly seen.

Mechanism of Action

- Strychnine reversibly blocks the binding of glycine, an inhibitory neurotransmitter in the dorsal horn of the spinal cord and in the CNS.

- The loss of the inhibitory effect in the nervous system results in unchecked spinal reflexes and nerve excitability to the skeletal muscles.
- Muscle tremors, extensor rigidity, seizures, and respiratory failure develop secondary to toxicosis.

Pharmacokinetics/Absorption, Distribution, Metabolism, and Excretion

- Strychnine absorption is very rapid and occurs primarily from the small intestine. A significant amount may also be absorbed from the stomach as well.
- It is widely distributed in the tissues.
- Strychnine is actively metabolized by the liver.
- Parent compound is excreted in the urine.
- Complete elimination should occur by 48 to 72 hours postingestion.

Toxicity

- Oral lethal dosage:
  - Dogs: 0.2 mg/kg
  - Cats: 0.5 mg/kg
  - Rodents: 1–20 mg/kg

Systems Affected

- Neuromuscular
  - Uninhibited nerve stimulation leads to continuous muscle stimulation and eventually to tetanic contracture.
- Nervous
  - Uninhibited nerve stimulation leads to seizures.
- Metabolic
  - Continual muscle stimulation leads to metabolic acidosis.
- Musculoskeletal
  - Trauma from the seizure activity can lead to musculoskeletal damage.
- Respiratory
  - Terminal rigidity of respiratory musculature results in apnea and death.

 SIGNALMENT/HISTORY

- Occasional history of "rodenticide exposure," but more commonly owners do not know of the exposure.
- Dogs and cats are quite susceptible, as well as all other species.
- All ages of animals are equally susceptible. Unsupervised, outdoor dogs that roam pastures, fields, etc., are at higher risk.
- The most common clinical sign is seizure activity.
- Often, owners do not see the initial signs of muscle tremors.

- Hyperthermia and metabolic acidosis are commonly observed, secondary to the extreme muscle exertion.

Historical Findings

- In the author's experience, the most common history is of malicious poisoning suspicions.
- Occasionally, histories of carcass ingestion are reported.

Location and Circumstances of Poisoning

- Most strychnine poisonings occur in rural areas and agricultural communities. However, it could occur in any area.

 CLINICAL FEATURES

- Clinical signs can develop within 10 to 120 minutes of ingestion.
- Violent tetanic seizures may be initiated by physical, visible, or auditory stimuli.
- Extensor rigidity
- Muscle stiffness
- Opisthotonus
- Tachycardia
- Hyperthermia
- Metabolic acidosis
- Apnea
- Vomiting—very rare
- Death
- Recovery should be less than 48–72 hours.

 DIFFERENTIAL DIAGNOSIS

- Other toxicants:
  - 1080 (fluoroacetate)
  - 4-aminopyridine
  - Amphetamines
  - Antidepressants
  - Caffeine
  - Chocolate
  - Cocaine
  - Lead
  - LSD
  - Metaldehyde
  - Nicotine

- Organochlorine insecticides
- Pyrethrins or pyrethroids
- Tremorgenic mycotoxins
- Zinc phosphide

■ Systemic diseases: uremia, electrolyte abnormalities (e.g., hypocalcemia) and hepatic encephalopathy, CNS neoplasia, hypoglycemia, encephalitides, heat stroke, trauma, ischemia, tetanus, epilepsy

 # DIAGNOSTICS

■ Serum chemistries will identify high CK and lactate dehydrogenase, as well as a systemic metabolic acidosis on venous blood gas analysis.
■ Evidence of myoglobinuria may be present on UA.
■ Analysis of stomach contents, liver, kidney, blood, or urine for the presence of strychnine
  - If death is too rapid, kidney and urine may be negative.
■ Death from strychnine intoxication is often rapid, with significant bait material still present in the stomach on autopsy.
  - Often, the color-coded grains or pellets (red or green) are obvious in the stomach contents.
  - The sample of choice for testing is generally stomach contents.

Pathological Findings

■ Gross and histologic pathology is associated with trauma from the seizure activity.
■ Red or green pellets or bait stations are often found in the stomach contents.

 # THERAPEUTICS

■ Inpatient therapy may require treatment for as long as 48–72 hours.
■ Primary goals are preventing dehydration, controlling seizures, maintaining cerebral perfusion, reducing ICP, preventing hypoxemia, and treating muscle rigidity. This often requires care in a 24-7 facility, mechanical ventilation with aggressive sedation, the use of mannitol (to decrease ICP), oxygen therapy, IV fluid therapy, thermoregulation, and nursing care.

Detoxification

■ Early decontamination is imperative to minimize duration and severity of clinical signs.
■ In asymptomatic patients, immediate emesis induction should be performed, followed by activated charcoal with a cathartic. Because strychnine undergoes

enterohepatic recirculation, an additional dose of activated charcoal, this time without a cathartic, should be given orally q 6–8 hours for 24 hours.

■ In symptomatic patients, sedation, control of the airway (with an inflated ETT), and gastric lavage are imperative for recent ingestion. Activated charcoal should be administered with a gastric tube once the stomach has been thoroughly lavaged.

Appropriate Health Care

■ Patients should be sedated in a quiet, dimly lit room, with cotton earplugs in place to prevent auditory stimulation.

■ Patients should be treated with IV fluid therapy q 8 hours for 24 hours to maintain hydration, perfusion, and aid in strychnine elimination and urinary excretion.

■ Control tremors and seizures. The use of anticonvulsants is imperative with strychnine toxicosis.

■ Supportive care and nursing care:
  • Minimize animal stimulation to avoid inducing a seizure.
  • Control hyperthermia. Monitor temperature q 2–4 hours; implement cooling measures when temperatures exceed 105.5°F. Cooling measures should be stopped when temperatures reach 103.5°F.
  • Change body position and lubricate eyes q 4–6 hours.
  • Avoid nutritional feeding (orally) until clinical signs resolve in order to prevent aspiration pneumonia.

Drug(s) and Antidotes of Choice

■ Decontamination—activated charcoal (2 g/kg PO); cathartic (sorbitol at 2.1 g/kg PO; magnesium sulfate at 0.5 g/kg PO)

■ Seizure control
  • Phenobarbital 4–16 mg/kg IV q 2–6 hours PRN
  • Potassium bromide 100 mg/kg PO or rectally q 6 hours x 4 doses
  • Diazepam 0.5–1 mg/kg IV to effect

■ Tremor control
  • Methocarbamol 55–100 mg/kg IV q 2–6 hours PRN
  • Glycerol guaiacolate 110 mg/kg IV, repeated as needed

■ Urinary acidification—Ammonium chloride (150 mg/kg) is reported to enhance elimination, based on the principle of ion trapping, but this has not been shown to be a practical clinical application and is not commonly done.

Precautions/Interactions

■ Do not induce emesis in symptomatic patients due to risks of aspiration pneumonia and seizure stimulation.

■ Do not acidify with ammonium chloride if the patient is acidotic, based on venous blood gas analysis.

Follow-up

- Monitor for secondary renal damage from myoglobinuria and possible tubular cast development. Aggressive treatment with IV fluids should be used to prevent this.
- Prognosis—guarded until seizures are controlled; good after seizures are controlled

Activity

- Normal activity should resume upon recovery, unless traumatic injuries limit activity.

Prevention

- Prevention is limited to keeping animals away from baits or poisoned carcasses, and dogs supervised at all times (instead of free-roaming).

Public Health

- Due to potential exposure to and poisoning of children, the source of the exposure should be investigated and eliminated.

Environmental Issues

- Strychnine is degraded by soil organisms.

COMMENTS

- Although anesthetic intervention does not directly treat the cause of the seizures, it provides the time necessary for the animals to eliminate the offending compound.
- CAUTION: Do not induce a seizure with a stimulus as a means of diagnosing strychnine. This is *not* diagnostic and may be lethal.

Client Education

- Strychnine poisoning is NOT treatable at home. If exposure has occurred, have the owner bring the animal to the clinic immediately. If clients wait until clinical signs occur, the animal may be dead before it reaches the clinic.

Patient Monitoring

- With sedation/anesthesia to control the seizures, the animal can be gradually withdrawn periodically to evaluate the reoccurrence of seizure activity as a means of determining how long the treatment must be continued.
- Early significant decontamination will significantly shorten the duration of required treatment.

Prevention/Avoidance

- Prevent reexposure by removing the source of the toxin.

Possible Complications

- Dependent on the initiation of therapy, hypoxemia that occurred prior to therapy can have permanent neurologic effects.
- Renal damage secondary to myoglobinuria will gradually repair.

Expected Course and Prognosis

- Prognosis is poor until seizures are controlled.
- Prognosis is good after seizures are controlled, but prior hypoxemia and secondary renal effects should be discussed with the owner.
- Animals that have normal neurologic function at 48 to 72 hours should have no permanent effect.

See Also

Decontamination and Detoxification of the Poisoned Patient
Emergency Management of the Poisoned Patient

Abbreviations

CK = creatine kinase
CNS = central nervous system
ETT = endotracheal tube
ICP = intracranial pressure
IV   = intravenous
PO = *per os* (by mouth)
PRN = *pro re nata* (as needed)
q   = every
UA = urinalysis

Suggested Reading

Gupta RC. Non-anticoagulant rodenticides. In: Veterinary Toxicology Basic and Clinical Principles. New York: Elsevier, 2007; pp. 548–560.
Osweiler GD. Strychnine poisoning. In: Kirk RW, ed. Current Veterinary Therapy VIII. Philadelphia: Saunders, 1983; pp. 98–100.
Talcott PA. Strychnine. In: Peterson ME, Talcott PA, eds. Small Animal Toxicology. Philadelphia: Saunders, 2006; 1076–1082.

Author: Jeffery O. Hall, DVM, PhD, DABVT
Consulting Editor: Gary D. Osweiler, DVM, PhD, DABVT

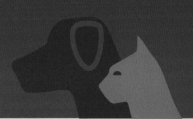

Toxic Gases

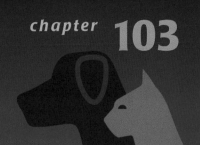

Carbon Monoxide

DEFINITION/OVERVIEW

- Carbon monoxide (CO) is a noxious gas that, when inhaled in high enough concentrations, leads to fatal hypoxia.
- CO is a product of incomplete fuel combustion and is a gas that is odorless, colorless, and nonirritating.
- CO is produced in fires, from generators, from car exhaust systems, and endogenously, as a neurotransmitter.
- Reports in veterinary medicine include toxicosis secondary to fires as well as one report of 4 dogs and 2 cats that experienced CO toxicosis from a generator system.
- Inhalation of 0.1% CO can result in carboxyhemoglobin (COHb) levels of greater than 50%.

ETIOLOGY/PATHOPHYSIOLOGY

- CO has an affinity for Hb that is 260 times greater than oxygen (O_2) and is readily absorbed across the alveolar membrane. CO displaces O_2 and forms COHb. With the presence of enough COHb, not enough O_2 reaches the tissues, resulting in cellular hypoxia. In addition, COHb shifts the oxyhemoglobin saturation curve to the left, impairing O_2 release at the tissue level.
- CO toxicosis often leads to heart and brain damage, as these organs have a high oxygen demand and thus are greatly affected by the severe hypoxia caused by COHb.
- Delayed neurotoxicity has been reported in humans and animals. This is hypothesized to be due to hypoxic-mediated lipid peroxidation and inflammatory-mediated damage to cells in the brain.
- Direct cytotoxicity can occur due to the inactivation of intracellular respiratory enzymes by CO as it is delivered to the tissues.

SIGNALMENT/HISTORY

- Dogs and cats presenting with CO toxicosis often have a history of being in a fire or in an enclosed space without adequate ventilation.

CLINICAL FEATURES

- Based on a few published reports, both dogs and cats respond to CO toxicosis with similar clinical signs, which parallel the effects of CO toxicosis in humans.
- Most patients will present with some degree of neurologic dysfunction, ranging from decreased mentation to a full comatose state.
- Tachycardia and tachypnea were common findings in a case series of dogs and cats with CO toxicosis. These signs are likely due to tissue hypoxia caused by a large concentration of CO in the blood. Pets may also smell of smoke and may have concurrent evidence of smoke inhalation injury.
- A case series describing CO toxicosis in 4 dogs and 2 cats reported deafness in 5 of the 6 patients, diagnosed 18 days after initial discharge from the hospital. All 5 patients were fully auditory at a 6-week evaluation.

DIFFERENTIAL DIAGNOSIS

- Primary respiratory disease resulting in tachypnea, dyspnea, or hypoxemia
- Primary CNS disease
- Primary metabolic disease (e.g., hepatic encephalopathy)
- Toxicities
  - Neurotoxins (e.g., lead)
  - Drug ingestion/overdose

DIAGNOSTICS

- A minimum database, including CBC, serum chemistry profile, and urinalysis should be performed to monitor for end-organ damage and to help eliminate other potential causes for the neurologic signs.
- A blood COHb level should be performed. Most human hospital stat labs are able to perform this test with a very short turn-around time (within a few hours). COHb levels are measured on a co-oximeter machine.
- It is important to note that hemoglobin saturation analysis will be impaired due to the presence of COHb. Pulse oximetry will overestimate the amount of saturated Hb, as the machine cannot differentiate COHb from HbO_2 (oxyhemoglobin).
- Arterial blood gas analysis will measure the amount of dissolved oxygen in the blood (PaO_2) but will not indicate the amount of usable oxygen as HbO_2. In patients experiencing CO toxicity due to smoke inhalation, measures of PaO_2 levels are more important, as secondary lung injury may occur.

THERAPEUTICS

- Oxygen supplementation is the mainstay of treatment for patients experiencing CO toxicosis. On room air ($FiO_2 = 21\%$), the COHb T½ is 4–6 hours. When administering a FiO_2 of 100% (through intubation), the COHb T½ is decreased to 40–80 minutes.

- While *initial* oxygen supplementation at a FiO_2 of 100% is recommended, this should not be continued beyond 18 hours due to the risks of O_2 toxicity.
- Other supportive care measures include IV fluid therapy to maintain tissue perfusion, monitoring of respiratory rate and effort (especially in cases of smoke inhalation, as secondary lung injury is common), serial evaluation of mentation status, and neurologic support (e.g., anticonvulsants, etc.) if indicated.

 COMMENTS/PROGNOSIS

- If CO toxicosis is suspected, blood COHb levels should be performed as soon as possible. COHb levels in the blood not only verify the diagnosis but can provide prognostic information as well. COHb levels of 20%–26% have been reported in dogs, and all dogs recovered with intensive supportive care. Twenty-four hours after therapy of these dogs, CO levels decreased to 0%–3%.
- Delayed neurotoxicity can occur and is characterized by resolution of neurologic signs, followed by recurrence of some form of neurologic dysfunction weeks later. In most cases, these delayed signs resolve and the patient returns to a normal neurologic state.
- If blood COHb levels are very elevated and therapy is delayed, most patients, human and veterinary, do not survive.
- Oxygen therapy should be instituted as soon as possible in any patient with smoke inhalation injury, or if CO toxicosis is suspected.

See Also

Smoke Inhalation

Abbreviations

CBC   = complete blood count
CNS   = central nervous system
CO   = carbon monoxide
COHb = carboxyhemoglobin
FiO_2 = fraction of inspired oxygen concentration
Hb   = hemoglobin
HbO_2 = oxyhemoglobin
IV   = intravenous
O_2 = oxygen
PaO_2 = partial pressure of oxygen
T½   = half-life

Suggested Reading

Aslan S, Karcioglu O, Bilge F et al. Post-interval syndrome after carbon monoxide poisoning. Vet Human Toxicol 2004; 46(4):183–185.

Berent AC, Todd J, Sergeeff J, Powell, LL. Carbon monoxide toxicity: a case series. JVECC 2005; 15(2):128–135.

Brunssen SH, Morgan DL, Parham FM et al. Carbon monoxide neurotoxicity: transient inhibition of avoidance response and delayed microglia reaction in the absence of neuronal death. Toxicology 2003; 194:51–63.

Author: Lisa L. Powell, DVM, DACVECC
Consulting Editor: Justine A. Lee, DVM, DACVECC

Smoke Inhalation

DEFINITION/OVERVIEW

- Smoke inhalation represents an uncommon form of pulmonary injury, cardio-vascular compromise, and neurologic impairment in veterinary patients, which is likely a reflection of high prehospital admission mortality as opposed to infrequent occurrence.
- For small animals, the most common source of smoke inhalation is from home fires.
- Carbon monoxide (CO), cyanide, direct heat injury, combustion products, and particulate matter that result from burned materials in the fire contribute to the pathophysiology of smoke inhalation.
- Common clinical signs include stupor, coma, and respiratory distress.
- Treatment is aimed at alleviating clinical signs and addressing the toxic effects of combusted materials.
- Therapeutic management includes oxygen supplementation, fluid therapy, pain management, and specific treatment of known inhaled toxins.
- The use of empirical antibiotic and corticosteroid therapy is not indicated unless a secondary bacterial pneumonia is present, as clinical benefits have not been detected.
- There are limited clinical studies documenting the prognosis of veterinary patients treated for smoke inhalation; however, information from these sources indicate a fair to good prognosis when severe skin burns are not present.

ETIOLOGY/PATHOPHYSIOLOGY

Mechanism of Action

- The mechanism of action of smoke inhalation and its relation to pulmonary injury is usually attributed to nonirritant gases (e.g., CO, hydrogen cyanide, CO_2), thermal injury, and smoke toxicosis from released irritant gases and particulate matter.
- For most small animals, the resultant clinical syndrome of smoke inhalation is likely a combination of some, if not all, of these components.

- Carbon monoxide is believed to be the leading cause of death in animals exposed to fires and smoke. Carbon monoxide's generation, mechanism of action, and toxicity is discussed in chapter 103.
- Common sources of cyanide in household fires include the combustion of fabrics like nylon, wool, and silk; photographic film containing nitrocellulose; photocopier paper; polyfluorocarbons; polyvinyl acetate; resins containing melamine and phenolic; polyurethane foam; and plastic.
- Cyanide toxicosis causes histotoxic hypoxia when oxidative phosphorylation is inhibited. When aerobic metabolism is affected, there is impaired oxygen extraction and utilization, conversion to anaerobic metabolism to facilitate cellular respiration, and accumulation of lactic acid.
- Increased inspired CO_2 not only functions as a nonirritating asphyxiant gas, but it also functions to increase respiratory rate, which further increases inhalation of the other components of smoke.
- An increase of environmental CO_2 to 7%–10% causes unconsiousness in humans within several minutes.
- Unless steam or superheated particulate matter is inhaled, thermal injury to the lower airways and pulmonary parenchyma is uncommon, given the effective heat dissipating mechanisms of the upper airway.
- The majority of thermal injury secondary to smoke inhalation is restricted to the oral and nasal cavities and larynx. These effects can be delayed for approximately 24 to 72 hours.
- Chemicals released from burned materials, as well as particulate matter, contribute to the toxicosis of inhaled smoke and the resultant mucosal damage, pulmonary injury, and bronchoconstriction. Much of the anatomic localization of impact depends on the solubility of the chemical, the formation of particulate matter, and early and delayed effects of the chemical.
- Common inhaled irritants within smoke include ammonia, acrolein, hydrogen chloride, and chlorine gas.

Pharmacokinetics/Absorption, Distribution, Metabolism, and Excretion

- The amount of time spent in the fire, the type of materials burned, the amount of heat generated, the amount of oxygen available (which is usually a factor of the materials burned), and the animal's health status all determine the severity of insult secondary to smoke inhalation.
- This information is often not available to the emergency response team responsible for removing the animal from the fire, nor is it available to the clinician treating the patient. Therefore, while knowledge of the burned materials can be helpful to better understand the expected impact and specific treatments, most veterinary victims of smoke inhalation must be treated empirically.
- For specific information about the pharmacokinetics, absorption, metabolism, and excretion of carbon monoxide, please see chapter 103.

- Within the context of smoke inhalation, cyanide toxicosis results from inhalation of combustion products containing cyanide. Cyanide inhalation results in rapid exposure and development of clinical signs within seconds to minutes.
- Most cyanide is converted to thiocyanate, which is formed primarily in the liver and then excreted by the kidneys.
- Carbon dioxide produced in fires is inhaled, which exacerbates the lack of oxygen in the environment. In addition, because of its rapid diffusion across the alveoli, it causes increased pCO_2 within the arterial circulation, and subsequent increased respiratory rate due to response by the brainstem. Hyperventilation is effective to decrease the pCO_2, but it also increases the amount of other toxins within the smoke which are inhaled.
- Irritants can be absorbed by inhalation (most common) or by ingestion if there is deposition of the chemical on the pet's hair coat and ingestion during grooming.
- Since there is limited clinical information about small animals suffering from smoke inhalation, and because of the huge variation of chemicals released from fire, as well as the variability of inhaled chemicals even within a single fire, there is very limited information about the metabolism and excretion of inhaled chemicals in small animals.

Toxicity

- The toxicity of carbon monoxide is discussed in chapter 103.
- There are no proven cases of cyanide toxicosis secondary to smoke inhalation; however, cyanide toxicosis is thought to have a role in the clinical signs seen in a study of dogs and cats presented for smoke inhalation.
- In dog experimental studies, the lethal blood cyanide level was found to be $438 \pm 40\,\mu g/dL$.
- In small animal patients, there are no standard or known toxic doses for the other toxins released from fires.

Systems Affected

- Not all small animal patients with smoke exposure demonstrate all clinical signs, and treatment at the scene of the fire, especially with oxygen, may affect the clinical signs observed by the attending veterinarian.
- Respiratory
  - Oropharyngeal, nasopharyngeal, and laryngeal burns, inflammation, and/or edema
  - Coughing, tachypnea, dyspnea due to the following:
    - Inhibition of mucociliary escalator function
    - Deposition of particulate matter along the lower airways and alveoli

- Bronchospasm, bronchoconstriction, and obstruction of small airways
- Hypoxemia
- Hyper- or hypoventilation
- Pulmonary edema
- ARDS and ALI
- Nervous
  - Cerebral vasodilation
  - Cerebral hypoxia
  - Cerebral edema
  - Direct effect of toxins on the CNS
  - Seizures/stupor/coma
- Cardiovascular
  - Myocardial and tissue hypoxia
  - Carbon monoxide–induced cardiotoxic dysfunction
  - Mitochondrial cytochrome oxidase dysfunction
  - Vasodilation
  - Methemoglobinemia
- Ophthalmic
  - Direct corneal injury from heat, smoke, and particulate matter
  - Local irritation from chemicals and particulate matter
- Skin/exocrine
  - Direct burn and chemical injury, especially to nonhaired skin

 SIGNALMENT/HISTORY

- There are no species, breed, or sex predilections for animals exposed to smoke.
- Studies on smoke exposure in dogs and cats showed an age range of 0.5–11 years in dogs (median = 3.2 years) and an age range of 0.25–11 years (median = 3.35 years) in cats. The relatively young median age is speculated to be due to the fact that younger animals are more likely to survive smoke inhalation and arrive at a veterinary hospital for treatment than are older pets.

Risk Factors

- Those animals that are commonly kept as pets in the home, or housed in barns and stalls, are at the highest risk.
- In clinical studies of dogs and cats with smoke exposure, fires were most common in the colder months, from November to March, when more animals are indoors, windows are closed, and heaters are being used with greater frequency. These studies were performed in Philadelphia, Pennsylvania.
- Animals with underlying disease, such as cardiovascular, respiratory, or musculoskeletal diseases, may be at higher risk of prolonged exposure or death from

smoke inhalation if they are physically unable to get out of the burning structure or if they are unable to be moved by their owners.

Historical Findings

- Signs reported at the scene of the fire include the following:
  - Dyspnea
  - Vocalizing
  - Coughing and gagging
  - Open-mouthed breathing (cats)
  - Loss of consciousness
  - Lethargy
  - Weakness and ataxia
  - Foaming from the mouth
- Smoke smell on the hair coat

Location and Circumstances of Poisoning

- Animals have a history of being exposed to a fire or smoke-filled enclosure. Such information may be obtained from an emergency response team, instead of the pet's owner, especially if the owner was also in need of medical care or not home at the time.

CLINICAL FEATURES

- Respiratory—tachypnea; dyspnea; respiratory distress; short, shallow respirations; open-mouthed breathing (cats); increased bronchovesicular sounds, wheezes, crackles, or moist lung sounds on auscultation; coughing; nasal discharge
- Nervous—lethargy, depression, ataxia, stupor, coma, excitement (cats)
- Cardiovascular—hyperemic mucous membranes, grey/cyanotic mucous membranes, decreased pulse quality, decreased heart sounds on auscultation (cats), gallop rhythm (cats)
- Ophthalmic—blephrospasm, corneal ulceration, third eyelid elevation, conjunctival hyperemia, miotic or mydriatic pupils, epiphora (see fig. 104.1)
- Skin/exocrine—smoke odor to fur, singed hair or burnt skin (especially on the face and footpads), soot on the skin, skin lacerations (see fig. 104.2)
- Gastrointestinal—expectoration, hypersalivation (cats)

DIFFERENTIAL DIAGNOSIS

- Inhalation of other toxins or substances
- Pulmonary parenchymal disease such as pneumonia

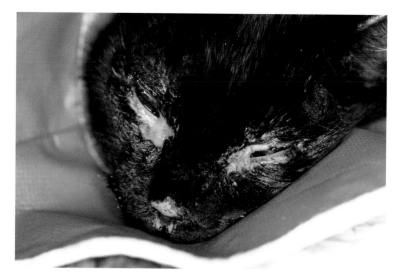

■ Fig. 104.1. Injury in a cat after smoke exposure: The eyelids and nasal planum are burned, and the cat's whiskers have been singed. (Photo courtesy of Dana L. Clarke)

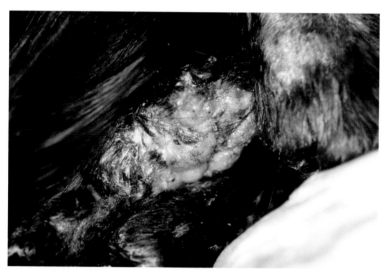

■ Fig. 104.2. The metatarsal and digital pads from the cat in figure 104.1, which have also been burned. (Photo courtesy of Dana L. Clarke)

- Lower airway disease such as asthma or bronchitis
- Upper airway obstruction such as laryngeal paralysis or brachycephalic airway syndrome
- Pleural space disease such as pneumothorax and pleural effusion
- Primary cardiac disease with or without congestive heart failure
- Primary neurologic disease such as seizures or inflammatory CNS disorders

DIAGNOSTICS

- Diagnostics needed to confirm carbon monoxide toxicity are discussed in chapter 103.
- Blood cyanide levels are the gold standard for diagnosing cyanide toxicosis. However, this diagnostic is not widely available and often not on an emergency basis. Severe lactic acidosis in the face of good perfusion suggests cyanide and/or carbon monoxide toxicosis; this can be measured on a handheld lactometer or via blood gas analysis.
- Pulse oximetry is a readily available, noninvasive, rapid diagnostic tool to assess oxygen saturation of hemoglobin. However, when carboxyhemoglobin or MetHb are present, the result obtained from pulse oximetry tends to overestimate the true saturation of hemoglobin with oxygen.
- PCV/TS, BG, and BUN. This should be obtained at presentation and reassessed frequently, especially when therapy such as IV fluids has been initiated. Studies have found that cats and dogs more severely affected by smoke inhalation have a higher PCV and lower BG.
- Blood gas analysis
  - Arterial blood gas analysis provides an accurate assessment of ventilation and oxygenation, even in the presence of carboxyhemoglobin and MetHb. Determination of acid-base derangements can also be made, which is especially important when lactic acidosis is present, as this can be indicative of cyanide toxicosis. If lactate is not routinely measured on the venous blood gas, it should be determined with a lactometer.
  - Venous blood gas analysis can also provide information on ventilation by evaluating the pCO_2 (as long as perfusion is normal), capillary oxygen extraction (caution when the patient is being given supplemental oxygen), and acid-base disturbances.
- Thoracic radiographs are essential, once the patient is stable enough, to assess pulmonary parenchymal changes at presentation and with disease progression. Common radiographic changes seen in dogs and cats with smoke inhalation include bronchial, interstitial, and alveolar patterns, or any combination of these patterns (see figs. 104.3 and 104.4).
- Complete ocular examination is warranted in any patient with a history of smoke exposure, including measurement of tear production, fluorescein staining, and thorough examination of the conjunctiva, scleral, cornea, and eyelids.
- CBC, serum chemistry, and coagulation profile are warranted in any patient that is critically ill secondary to smoke inhalation, receiving large volumes of IV crystalloids or colloids, or for which changes in clinical picture and the above diagnostics require further investigation.
- Endotracheal or transtracheal washes are helpful to confirm smoke inhalation, when carbon particulate matter is retrieved from the wash, and when there is

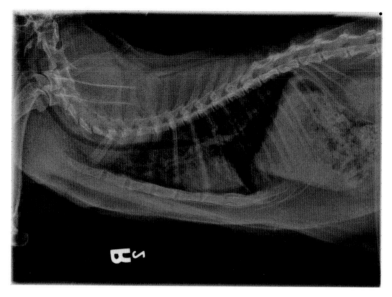

■ **Fig. 104.3.** Right lateral thoracic radiograph taken of a cat exposed to smoke in a house fire. Radiograph shows a generalized bronchointerstitial pattern, with more dense interstitial disease in the left cranial lung lobe.

concern for the presence of pneumonia (e.g., aspiration, complication of severe pulmonary parenchymal injury, ventilator-associated pneumonia).
■ Bronchoscopy, though invasive and not readily available, can help diagnose smoke inhalation, bronchial obstruction, and disease localized to a single lung lobe.

Pathological Findings

■ The gross and histopathologic findings in patients that have died or are euthanized because of the severity of smoke inhalation are a function of the individual inhaled toxins, degree of injury to the respiratory tract and CNS, and extent of burns and ocular injury.
■ On gross examination, there may be burns of varying severity and ocular injury such as corneal edema and ulcers, hyperemia, and foreign material in the conjunctival fornix.
■ Nasopharyngeal, oropharyngeal, and laryngeal burns, inflammation, and edema may be present. Tracheal inflammation, edema, and particulate matter deposition may be present as well. On cut section of the pulmonary parenchyma, there may particulate matter, edema, purulent material consistent with pneumonia, and atelectasis.
■ Other than carbon particulate matter along the airway and within the alveoli, there are no characteristic histopathologic changes associated with smoke inhalation. Instead, the duration of smoke exposure, temperature of the fire, and presence of carbon monoxide, cyanide, and other chemical constituents of smoke will determine the pathology seen microscopically.

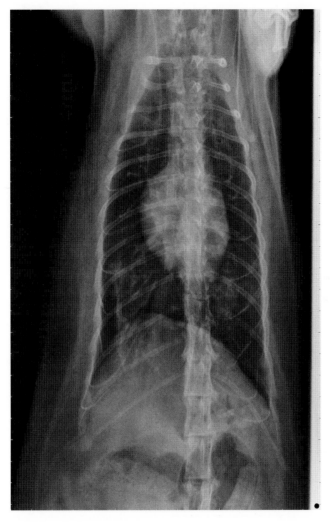

■ **Fig. 104.4.** Ventrodorsal thoracic radiograph of the cat in figure 104.3, which also demonstrates the diffuse bronchointerstitial pulmonary parenchymal changes.

 THERAPEUTICS

- The goals of treating small animal patients presenting for smoke inhalation are provision of supplemental oxygen, administration of toxin-specific antidotes, maintaining patency of the airway (especially the upper airway), preserving hydration, and supportive and nursing care.
- Supplemental oxygen therapy is of the utmost importance for patients presenting for smoke inhalation, especially if there is any concern for carbon monoxide exposure or if the patient is showing neurologic or respiratory signs. Methods

of administering supplemental oxygen include flow-by, mask, nasal oxygen, oxygen cage, and intubation.

■ Treatment of carbon monoxide toxicosis is discussed in Chapter 103, and specific treatment for cyanide is discussed below.

■ Patients should be intensely monitored for signs of progressive upper airway inflammation and obstruction. If upper airway obstruction is present, tracheostomy may be necessary. Should there be signs of respiratory fatigue or failure, severe hypoxemia, or patient distress despite therapy, mechanical ventilation may be indicated.

■ If hypovolemia is present, patients should be treated appropriately with crystalloid and colloid therapy aimed at reversing shock. Once euvolemia is achieved, smoke inhalation patients often require only maintenance fluid therapy, given the concern for pulmonary capillary leak (and secondary pulmonary edema) with aggressive IV fluid therapy, especially in cats.

Appropriate Health Care

■ Patients should be carefully monitored for vomiting, regurgitation, and the inability to protect the airway. Aspiration pneumonia in addition to the pulmonary compromise from smoke inhalation could be fatal.

■ Since smoke inhalation patients, especially those with significant dermal burns, are at increased risk for sepsis, measures to prevent hospital-acquired infections, such as wearing gloves and hand washing, should be adhered to strictly.

Drug(s) and Antidotes of Choice

■ Bronchodilators can be considered in all patients with smoke inhalation and are indicated for those with wheezes heard on auscultation. Inhaled albuterol is readily available, as are xanthine derivatives, such as theophylline and aminophylline (only aminophylline is available for injection), and β-agonists such as terbutaline. Terbutaline can cause tachycardia and CNS excitement, and should be avoided in patients where these effects are a concern.
  • Inhalational therapy (e.g., albuterol) 2–3 puffs q 2–4 hours PRN
  • Terbutaline 0.01 mg/kg IV q 8 hours

■ Cough suppressants should be avoided to promote expectoration of smoke particles within the upper respiratory tract. Likewise, opioids should be avoided as an analgesic due to their suppression of the cough reflex.

■ Antiemetic therapy should be used in the vomiting patient to prevent secondary aspiration pneumonia.
  • Maropitant 1 mg/kg SQ q 24 hours (for up to 5 days)
  • Ondansetron 0.1–0.2 mg/kg IV, SQ q 8–12 hours PRN

■ Sodium thiosulfate (25%) can be used to treat cyanide toxicosis at a dose of 150–500 mg/kg IV as either a bolus or CRI.

Precautions/Interactions

- Corticosteroids are not indicated for patients with smoke inhalation due to increased incidence of bacterial pneumonia without evidence of clinical benefits.
- Empiric antibiotic therapy is not recommended in victims of smoke exposure, due to concerns for bacterial resistance. If bacterial pneumonia is documented via endotracheal or trans-tracheal wash, antibiotic selection should be based on culture and sensitivity testing.
- Sodium nitrate should not be used in smoke inhalation patients to treat cyanide toxicosis, as it can exacerbate decreased oxygen carrying capacity via the formation of methemoglobinemia.

Nursing Care

- Supportive care for patients with smoke inhalation entails maintenance of patient comfort and relief of anxiety, oral and eye care for recumbent patients, and nebulization with saline followed by gentle chest coupage for 15–20 minutes, every 4–6 hours as needed.

Follow-up

- For patients with significant pulmonary changes secondary to smoke inhalation, or for those that develop pneumonia with or without underlying pulmonary parenchymal injury, reexamination and possible follow-up thoracic radiographs should be considered within approximately 1 week from hospital discharge.

Diet

- For patients with any neurologic compromise, vomiting, regurgitation, or those that are sedated, oral food and water should be withheld until the patient is neurologically appropriate and GI signs have resolved.

Activity

- Smoke inhalation patients should have their activity restricted to light exercise only until there is complete resolution of any pulmonary parenchymal disease.

Surgical Considerations

- Surgical tracheostomy could be necessary if there is upper airway obstruction impeding ventilation.
- For patients with significant dermal injuries requiring anesthesia, debridement, and bandaging, sterile ETT and anesthetic tubing should be used; the duration of anesthesia should be limited as much as possible, as should the number of anesthetic events.

COMMENTS

Client Education

- Patients should be carefully monitored for signs of respiratory and neurologic changes, should be rested until pulmonary changes are resolved, and should be isolated from other animals due to concerns for decreased resistance to viral pneumonias.

Patient Monitoring

- Pulse oximetry can be used several times per day to monitor for improvement in oxygenation.
- Arterial or venous blood gas monitoring should be performed at least daily to assess oxygenation (arterial samples only), ventilation, and acid-base balance.
- Thoracic radiography can be used to monitor improvement of pulmonary parenchymal disease. It should also be used if there is an acute decline in the patient's respiratory status to assess for pneumonia. The frequency of follow-up radiography for the smoke exposure patient will depend on the severity of pulmonary changes, interventions such as mechanical ventilation, and the patient's response to therapy.

Possible Complications

- There is very limited information about long-term complications associated with smoke inhalation in veterinary patients. However, patients may have a temporarily increased risk of pulmonary and dermal infections as well as sepsis.
- Depending on the patient's severity of signs at presentation and clinical course, concerns for long-term complications include pulmonary fibrosis, asthma, chronic obstructive pulmonary disease, and neoplasia. These sequelae have not been documented in veterinary patients after smoke inhalation.

Expected Course and Prognosis

- In a retrospective study of 27 dogs with smoke exposure, 4 dogs died and 4 dogs were euthanized. Dogs that were clinically worse by the second day of hospitalization were more likely to die, be euthanized, or have a prolonged course of hospitalization. Less complicated canine smoke exposure patients had improvement in their clinical signs after their first 24 hours of hospitalization.
- Dogs with acute neurologic signs following smoke inhalation were found to have a mortality rate of 46% in another study.
- In a retrospective study of 22 cats with smoke exposure, 2 cats were euthanized because of severe respiratory or neurologic signs, but none died. There were similar findings compared with dogs in terms of clinical course over hospitalization depending on the severity of their signs at presentation.

- A more guarded prognosis is warranted in patients with concurrent significant dermal burns.
- Delayed neurologic signs have been documented in canine patients after initial improvement from acute smoke inhalation injury. In dogs with a history of smoke inhalation and acute neurologic signs at presentation, approximately half of them developed delayed neurologic signs after a period of improvement, and there was a 60% mortality rate in these dogs.

Synonyms

smoke exposure

See Also

Carbon Monoxide

Abbreviations

ALI   = acute lung injury
ARDS = acute respiratory distress syndrome
BG   = blood glucose
BUN   = blood urea nitrogen
CBC   = complete blood count
CO   = carbon monoxide
CO$_2$ = carbon dioxide
CNS   = central nervous system
CRI   = continuous rate infusion
ETT   = endotracheal tube
GI   = gastrointestinal
MetHb = methemoglobin
IV   = intravenous
pCO$_2$ = partial pressure of carbon dioxide
PCV   = packed cell volume
PRN   = *pro re nata* (as needed)
q   = every
RBC   = red blood cell
SQ   = subcutaneous

Suggested Reading

Drobatz KJ. Smoke inhalation. In: King LG. Textbook of Respiratory Disease in Dogs and Cats. St. Louis: Saunders, 2004.
Drobatz KJ, Walker LM, Hendricks JC. Smoke exposure in cats: 22 cases (1986-1997). JAVMA 1999; 215(9):1312–1316.
Drobatz KJ, Walker LM, Hendricks JC. Smoke exposure in dogs: 27 cases (1988-1997). JAVMA 1999; 215(9):1306–1311.

Fitzgerald KT, Flood AA. Smoke inhalation. Clin Tech Small Anim Pract 2006; 21:205–214.
Jasani S, Hughes D. Smoke inhalation. In: Silverstein DC, Hopper K, eds. Small Animal Critical Care Medicine. St. Louis: Saunders, 2009.

Authors: Dana L. Clarke, VMD; Kenneth J. Drobatz, DVM, MSCE, DACVIM, DACVECC
Consulting Editor: Justine A. Lee, DVM, DACVECC

Information Resources for Toxicology

DEFINITION/OVERVIEW

- The tens of thousands of metals, minerals, natural products, and synthetic chemicals used in modern civilization provide numerous opportunities for exposure of small companion animals to dangerous or toxic materials.
- Of the hundreds of drugs and products used in a veterinary practice, many can interact with one another to either increase or mitigate the desired effects.
- Veterinarians receive questions and calls daily about the safety of a variety of products to which pets are exposed.
- Beyond the personal experience and knowledge gained from frequent encounters with the most familiar products, veterinarians need resources to bolster their personal knowledge when less frequently known chemical exposures or questions occur.
- This appendix presents several sources of information that can help veterinarians extend their service to clients by effectively using information resources in toxicology.
- Principle categories of assistance include the following:
  - Persons with in-depth experience relevant to specific toxicants or circumstances. Examples are agronomists, botanists, chemists, limnologists, mycologists, pest control specialists, pharmacists, pharmacologists, pathologists, veterinary extension faculty, wildlife specialists, state and federal regulatory professionals, and many others
  - Textbooks and reference books prepared by knowledgeable experts and provided by reliable publishers
  - Selected peer-reviewed, scientific veterinary journals that routinely accept original reports of toxicology clinical cases or toxicology research
  - Animal poison control centers that maintain a staff of skilled and knowledgeable veterinary specialists for consultation when veterinary toxicology questions arise
  - Government agencies with emphasis on toxicology scientific, regulatory, or educational services
  - Reliable Internet resources for quick and easy access to useful toxicology information on a 24/7 basis

821

VETERINARY AND TOXICOLOGY INFORMATION RESOURCES

- As with all professional service, critical evaluation of resources available is essential to gathering reliable information for toxicology support.
- Sources that are well documented and subject to some form of peer review are usually most reliable.
- If regulatory or legal aspects of toxicology are important, official government sources often provide that aspect of information.
- As with all critical information for patient care, the veterinarian must carefully and critically determine how the information applies to their individual practice needs.

Specialists with In-Depth Expertise Relevant to Veterinary Toxicology

- Examples are agronomists, botanists, chemists, limnologists, mycologists, pest control specialists, pharmacists, pharmacologists, pathologists, veterinary extension faculty, wildlife specialists, state and federal regulatory professionals and many others.
- Knowing about these highly skilled and focused individuals can be invaluable when an infrequently encountered question or exposure demands special knowledge on short notice.
- Prior contact or arrangements with experts that one already knows is often invaluable when a quick and thorough response is required to support a toxicology incident in small animals.

Principal Reference Books and Textbooks

Bonagura JD, Twedt DC, eds. Current Veterinary Therapy XIV. Saunders-Elsevier, 2008.

Bonagura JD, Twedt DC, eds. Kirk's Current Veterinary Therapy: Small Animal Practice XIV. Saunders, 2009. (Note: earlier editions of Current Veterinary Therapy Small Animal Practice contain a range of toxicology topics.)

Burrows GE, Tyrl RJ, eds. Handbook of Toxic Plants of North America. Wiley-Blackwell, 2006.

Campbell A, Chapman MJ, eds. Handbook of Poisoning in Dogs and Cats. Wiley-Blackwell, 2000.

Gfeller RW, Messonnier SP, eds. Handbook of Small Animal Toxicology. Mosby, 2004.

Knight AP, ed. A Guide to Poisonous House and Garden Plants. Teton New Media, 2006.

Morgan RV, ed. Handbook of Small Animal Practice. 5th ed. Saunders, 2008.

Peterson ME, Talcott PA, eds. Small Animal Toxicology, 2nd ed. Saunders, 2006.

Plumlee KH, ed. Clinical Veterinary Toxicology. Mosby-Elsevier, 2004.

Tilley LP, Smith FWK, eds. Blackwell's 5-Minute Veterinary Consult, 4th ed. Wiley-Blackwell, 2008.

Veterinary Clinics of North America Small Animal Practice (Toxicology) 20.2. Saunders, 1990.

Supportive Reference Books and Textbooks

Papich MG, ed. Saunders Handbook of Veterinary Drugs, 2nd ed. Saunders Elsevier, 2007.

Plumb DC, ed. Plumb's Veterinary Drug Handbook, 6th ed. Wiley-Blackwell, 2008.

Plunkett SJ, ed. Emergency Procedures for the Small Animal Veterinarian. Saunders, 2001.

Riviere JE, Papich MG, eds. Veterinary Pharmacology and Therapeutics, 9th ed. Wiley-Blackwell, 2009.

Rozanski EA, Rush JE, eds. Small Animal Emergency and Critical Care Medicine: A Colour Handbook. Manson, 2007.

Selected Veterinary Journals as References in Toxicology

Advances in Veterinary Medicine
American Journal of Veterinary Research
Australian Veterinary Journal
Canadian Journal of Veterinary Research
Journal of the American Animal Hospital Association
Journal of the American Veterinary Medical Association
Journal of Small Animal Practice
Journal of Veterinary Diagnostic Investigation
Journal of Veterinary Emergency and Critical Care
Journal of Veterinary Internal Medicine
Journal of Veterinary Pharmacology and Therapeutics
Research in Veterinary Science
Veterinary Clinics of North America Small Animal Practice
Veterinary Journal
Veterinary Quarterly
Veterinary Record

Animal Poison Control Centers

- ASPCA Animal Poison Control Center
  - http://www.aspca.org/pet-care/poison-control/
  - (888) 426-4435
  - $65 fee
- Pet Poison Helpline (animal poison control hotline)
  - http://www.petpoisonhelpline.com/
  - (800) 213-6680
  - $35 fee

Internet-Based Toxicology Resources

- Agency for Toxic Substances and Disease Registry (ATSDR)
  - http://www.atsdr.cdc.gov/
  - http://www.atsdr.cdc.gov/toxfaq.html
- American Association of Poison Control Centers (AAPCC)
  - http://www.aapcc.org/
  - American Association of Poison Control Centers assists 60 poison centers in the United States on a 24/7 basis.
  - Poison Help hotline at 1-800-222-1222 can be dialed from anywhere in the United States and will be automatically routed to an appropriate center.
  - Certifies poison control center personnel and owns and maintains the National Poison Data System (NPDS).
- Consultant
  - http://www.vet.cornell.edu/consultant/consult.asp
  - Consultant is a diagnostic support system to assist in possible differential diagnoses or causes based on clinical signs entered. When clinical signs are entered, it enables a wide selection of potential differential toxicology diagnoses.
  - Consultant is free of charge, but monetary support is welcome to help defray expenses. It is species specific, provides a brief synopsis of a selected diagnosis/cause, and is supported by 3–6 recent references pertinent to the diagnosis selected.
  - Supported by a database of approximately 500 signs/symptoms, 7,000 diagnoses/causes, and 18,000 literature references, of which 3,000 are Web sources.
- Cornell University Poisonous Plants
  - http://www.ansci.cornell.edu/plants/index.html
  - Maintained by the Animal Science Department at Cornell University as a reference only
  - Includes plant images, pictures of affected animals, and presentations concerning botany, chemistry, toxicology, diagnosis, and prevention of poisoning of animals by plants and other natural flora
  - The images are copyrighted but may be printed, downloaded, or copied, provided it is in an educational setting and proper attribution is provided.
- Drug Compounding—FDA
  - http://www.fda.gov/ora/compliance_ref/cpg/default.htm
- FDA-Approved Animal Drugs
  - FDA Approved Animal Drug Products (Green Book)
  - http://www.fda.gov/animalveterinary/products/approvedanimaldrug products/ucm042847.htm

- Extoxnet (pesticides)
  - http://ace.orst.edu/info/extoxnet/
  - Extension Toxicology Network (EXTOXNET) is maintained by extension services of University of California–Davis, Oregon State University, Michigan State University, Cornell University, and the University of Idaho.
  - Goals of EXTOXNET are to stimulate dialogue on toxicology issues, provide information relevant to extension toxicology, and facilitate exchange of toxicology-related information in electronic form.
- FDA Center for Veterinary Medicine (FDA-CVM)
  - http://www.fda.gov/animalveterinary/default.htm
  - Official Web site for the Center for Veterinary Medicine
  - Provides current information on pet food regulations, labeling, and food safety for pets
  - Monitors and investigates outbreaks of suspected toxicosis related to pet foods
  - Recent examples have included aflatoxins in dogs, melamine/cyanuric acid nephrosis in dogs and cats, and safety of imported pet treats
- InChem
  - www.inchem.org
  - Rapid access to internationally peer-reviewed information on chemicals, including contaminants in the environment and food
  - Primarily human- and environment-oriented
  - Consolidates information from a number of intergovernmental organizations to assist in sound management of chemicals
  - Includes environmental health criteria as well as health and safety guidelines
  - Provides poison information monographs
- International Veterinary Information Service (IVIS)
  - www.ivis.org
  - Free service to veterinarians, veterinary students, and animal health professionals
  - Provides online peer-reviewed references
  - Access to three veterinary toxicology textbooks and the IVIS Drug Database
  - The Drug Database provides rapid access to listings of veterinary drugs by generic name, drug category, biological activity, and manufacturer/distributor.
  - The drug database is under continuing development, and the management advises that some information may be incomplete or contain omissions.
- Merck Veterinary Manual
  - http://www.merckvetmanual.com/mvm/index.jsp
- Medline
  - http://medlineplus.gov/

- Service provide by the National Library of Medicine and National Institutes of Health
- Updated daily and can be bookmarked at the URL www.medlineplus.gov
- Human focused, but can be a good source of information about human drugs encountered by animals
- Also a source of information about human antidotes useful in veterinary medicine
- Public access is allowed, as information is supported by two well-known federal agencies.

- MSDS Search
  - http://www.msdssearch.com/
  - A database service specializing in providing a digital source of MSDS (Material Safety Data Sheets) required by many commercial, business, and manufacturing companies.
  - MSDS sheets contain information about the characteristics and nature of thousands of chemicals to which animals could be exposed.
  - The information is often not assembled consistently in standard references.
  - The MSDS provides a relatively consistent and detailed documentation of composition, use, and potential adverse effects.

- National Institute for Environmental Health Sciences (NIEHS)
  - http://www.niehs.nih.gov/
  - The NIEHS mission is to reduce the burden of human illness and disability by understanding how the environment influences the development and progression of human disease. Some of the NIEHS activities include:
    - Rigorous research in environmental health sciences, and to communicating the results of this research to the public
    - Alphabetical listing of major health topics that are related to or affected by environmental exposures
    - Access to materials and guidance for use by health professionals in educating, diagnosing, and treating patients with conditions and diseases influenced by environmental agents

- Pub Med
  - http://www.ncbi.nlm.nih.gov/pubmed/medline.html
  - Pub Med is a search service of the United States National Library of Medicine.
  - It comprises more than 19 million citations for biomedical articles from Medline and life science journals.
  - Citations include links to full-text articles from Pub Med Central or publisher Web sites.
  - Numerous major scientific and applied veterinary journals can be reliably accessed through Pub Med.

- TOXNET (National Library of Medicine Toxicology Information)
  - http://toxnet.nlm.nih.gov
  - TOXNET is a collection of toxicology and environmental health databases:
    - Hazardous Substances Data Bank (HSDB) is a database of potentially hazardous chemicals (http://toxnet.nlm.nih.gov/cgi-bin/sis/htmlgen?HSDB)).
    - TOXLINE is a database of references to the world's toxicology literature (http://toxnet.nlm.nih.gov/cgi-bin/sis/htmlgen?TOXLINE)).
    - ChemIDplus is a chemical dictionary and structure database (http://chem.sis.nlm.nih.gov/chemidplus/).
- USP Veterinary Drug Information
  - http://www.usp.org/audiences/veterinary/
- Veterinary Information Network
  - www.vin.com
  - A veterinary organization and system of education and databases to help busy veterinary professionals be the best clinicians they can be, providing features to include:
    - Bringing veterinarians together worldwide as colleagues
    - Bringing instant access to vast amounts of up-to-date veterinary information to colleagues
    - Bringing instant access to "breaking news" that affects veterinarians, their patients, and their practice
    - Bringing easy access to colleagues who have specialized knowledge and skills
    - Making continuing education available every day
- Veterinary Toxicology Diplomate
  - http://www.abvt.org/public/index.html

Author: Gary Osweiler, DVM, PhD, DABVT
Consulting Editor: Lynn R. Hovda, DVM, MS, DACVIM

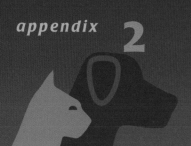
Metallic Toxicants Table

For information on more frequent and serious metallic toxicants for small animals, see individual chapters on iron, lead, and zinc.

Metal & Sources	Toxicity	Clinical Effects	Diagnostics	Therapy/ Prevention
Arsenic (As): Trivalent (+3) and pentavalent (+5) sources are of concern. Natural +5 sources are found in soil, coal, mine tailings, and seafoods (2–22 ppm). Both +3 and +5 valence in pesticides. Other: Pre-2004 treated wood (CCA). Well water ≤21 ppm. Weed and insect killers. Medical: Immiticide (melarsomine) adult heartworm treatment (thiacetarsamide).	Absorbed via GIT, intact skin, inhalation. +3 is 3–10 times more toxic than +5 valence. Storage in liver, kidney, GIT, spleen, skin, hair. Excreted 50% in urine within 48 hours. Lethal dosage range 1–25 mg/kg. More toxic to cats than dogs. Toxicity order is As^{+3}(arsenite) > As^{+5} (arsenate) > trivalent organics. Melarsomine = severe toxicosis at 7.5 mg/kg.	Immediately postabsorption— oral irritation, dysphagia. Acute toxicosis 1–3 hours—GIT pain, vomiting, hematachezia, melena, rice-water stools, hypovolemia from capillary dilation and vascular transudation. Salivation, oral erosion, and ulceration. Subacute—tubular nephrosis, renal failure, azotemia.	Arsenical analysis of: Liver, kidney >10 ppm is toxic. Urine: current exposure = 2–100 ppm. Hair: chronic levels ≥25 ppm. Blood: unreliable for arsenic concentration. *CBC:* Hemoconcentration secondary to dehydration, hemolysis, anemia, ± basophilic stippling, possible pancytopenia, leucopenia, or thrombocytopenia. *Urinalysis:* monitor for whole cells, casts, protein, evidence of hemolysis, hematuria.	No emetics or gastric lavage unless very early and asymptomatic. Charcoal is *not* an effective adsorbent. Intensive care with IV fluids, demulcents, treat for shock, maintain body temp, dialysis for renal failure. Sucralfate, H_2 blockers, antiemetics, antidiarrheas. Monitor renal function. Acute prognosis guarded. Best antidote is succimer (DMSA), a metal chelator. Less toxic, more expensive, more effective than dimercaprol (BAL). *See dosages at end of table.*

(Continued)

Metal & Sources	Toxicity	Clinical Effects	Diagnostics	Therapy/Prevention
Barium (Ba): Rodenticide (obsolete), welding fluxes, depilatories, dyes, glass manufacture, explosive detonators	Acid- or water-soluble barium salts act as strong cardio-suppressants and cause severe hypokalemia by blocking exit channels for K in muscle cells. Barium also stimulates skeletal, smooth, and cardiac muscle. Toxic dose Canine: 50 mg/kg BW.	Acute—vomiting, colic, salivation, diarrhea, ventricular tachycardia/ fibrillation, dyspnea, weakness. Violent peristalsis, arterial hypertension, and arrhythmias. Additional signs may include seizures, tremors, mydriasis.	Hypokalemia, from blocking cellular K+ exit. ECG changes from hypokalemia (ECG: QRS or QTc interval changes). Tissue levels— primarily in bones (replacing Ca^{++}). Soft tissue normal values generally less than 1 ppm. Blood values from acute poisoning expected at 2–10 ppm. Blood gases. ECG: QRS or QTc interval changes.	Emesis and activated charcoal not recommended. Saline diuresis, intravenous K^+ to control hypokalemia and tachycardia is critical. Consider gastric lavage if patient is stabilized and airway protected. Magnesium sulfate (250 mL/kg PO) to form insoluble $BaSO_4$ and reduce absorption. Lidocaine recommended in humans if refractory to potassium.
Cadmium (Cd): Ores, mine tailings, smelters. Also in foods (shellfish), cigarettes, fertilizers, solders, batteries, art pigments, automotive paints, semiconductors, solar cells.	Multisystem effects. Accumulates in kidneys and very slowly excreted— oxidative damage and lysosomal release → renal damage. Competes with Ca and Zn. Dogs tolerate 10 ppm in diet; chronic toxicity occurs at 50 mg/kg.	Acute—dyspnea, vomiting, colic, diarrhea (mucosal damage), weakness, renal failure. Chronic—rhinitis, anorexia, renal tubular dysfunction, sodium retention, osteomalacia/ osteoporosis enlarges joints, testicular damage, potential copper deficiency.	Blood levels ≥100 μg/ dL reflect acute exposure; urine levels represent chronic exposure, but blood or urine values for small animals are poorly defined. Liver accumulates 1–2 ppm and kidney from 3–10 ppm. Diagnosis depends on history of exposure, typical clinical signs, and elevated cadmium in blood, urine, or tissue.	Treat symptomatically and supportive therapy for gastroenteritis and renal insufficiency. Zinc supplementation may reduce accumulation or persistence of Cd residues. $CaNa_2EDTA$ or d-penicillamine. *See dosages at end of table.*

(Continued)

Metal & Sources	Toxicity	Clinical Effects	Diagnostics	Therapy/ Prevention
Copper (Cu): Liver accumulation in dogs enhanced by autosomal recessive trait in Bedlington terrier; also high risk in West Highland, Skye, Dalmatian, Doberman, and Labrador. Sources include coins, wiring, garden sprays, feeds, copper oxide capsules.	Absorbed readily from GIT, stored mainly in liver cell lysosomes, excreted in bile complexed with molybdenum. Excess accumulation causes hepatic cell necrosis. Hereditary copper accumulation is a liver disease. Acute release from liver may cause hemolytic crisis.	Acute exposure to concentrated copper salts— moderate to severe gastroenteritis. Chronic accumulations— hepatic insufficiency, possible encephalophathy, and occasional acute hemolytic crisis with icterus and hemoglobinuria.	Samples for diagnosis: Chemistry panel— elevated LDH, ALT, AST, bilirubin, bile acids. CBC—anemia, hemoglobinaemia, hypoproteinemia. Urine— hemoglobinuria Liver biopsy for histopathology and copper analysis may be diagnostic. Liver normal <400 ppm dry weight. Secondary Cu accumulation 400—800 ppm. Toxicosis >800 ppm.	Treat acute signs of liver disease and anemia symptomatically. If chronic toxicity—chelation of copper storage with d-penicillamine *See dosages at end of table).* Continue therapy with monitoring up to 1 year. Biopsy for liver status again after 1-year therapy.
Chromium (Cr): Occurs in nature in 4 oxidation states. Cr+6 is made and used by industrial processes. Cr+3 is used in leather tanning, pigments, and wood preservation. Few sources are generally available to small animals.	Cats tolerate 100 μg/day or 16 μg/kg/d. Dogs tolerate 50 μg/kg/d. Cr supports glucose tolerance and modulates serum triglycerides and cholesterol.	Reports of poisoning in small animals are rare. Signs in other species include vomiting, profuse diarrhea with mucosal sloughing, and dermatitis.	Cr is widely distributed in mammalian species at very low (ng/g) concentrations. Normal values in rats are 6 ppm (liver) and 8 ppm (kidney). Dosage of 100 mg/kg raises Cr values to 90 and 700 ppm in liver and kidney, respectively. Excreted mainly in urine.	Minimal toxicity is expected after ingestion. Some sources suggest activated charcoal, others do not. Overdose, if it occurs, is treated with general detoxification, fluids, and GIT therapy to manage potential or real gastroenteritis and dermatitis.

(Continued)

Metal & Sources	Toxicity	Clinical Effects	Diagnostics	Therapy/Prevention
Gold: Gold-containing drugs are used primarily to manage rheumatoid arthritis. Forms include gold sodium thioglucose, gold sodium thiomalate, gold thiosulfate.	Rat IM LD_{50} = 35–440 mg/kg. Gold drugs are generally not available in a way that would expose small animals unless by malicious intent or extreme carelessness.	Most data is for parenteral exposure. Signs include ventricular tachycardia, vasodilatation, hypotension, stomatitis, glossitis, ocular inflammation, pneumonitis, toxic encephalopathy, and polyneuropathy.	Urine assay for gold would establish exposure, but diagnostic values are not established. Human therapeutic use produces approximately 1 µg/mL blood levels.	Gold toxicity has been treated in humans with steroids BAL and N-acetylcysteine (NAC). *See dosages at end of table.* Animal treatment regimens are not established.
Lithium (Li): Used in human medicine to treat manic depressive illness. Standard and sustained-release products available. Adult therapy range is 300–1800 mg/day. Tablet strength typically is 300 mg. Lithium batteries low risk: pass through GIT and contain limited lithium.	Rat oral LD_{50} = 525 mg/kg. Feline: Toxic >85 mg/kg. Animals with renal disease, dehydration, sodium depletion, cardiovascular disease, severe debilitation, or receiving diuretics are at higher risk. Crosses the placenta, concentrates in fetus, may be teratogen.	CNS—drowsiness, tremors, weakness, confusion, ataxia, seizures, or coma. GIT—vomiting, diarrhea, nausea, anorexia. Other—blurred vision, PU/PD, T-wave ECG changes. Signs prolonged if sustained-release product ingested.	History: excessive and/or sustained high dosages. Human serum values: Moderate tox = 1.5–2.5 mEq/L Severe tox = 2.5–3 mEq/L Fatal = >3 mEq/L. Recheck serum Li as needed. Follow clinical course with baseline labs, electrolytes, BUN, and creatinine.	Activated charcoal not effective. Decontaminate—gastric lavage if <1 hr postingestion. Whole bowel irrigation if >1 hr postingestion, using PEG @ 25–50 mg/kg followed by 0.5 mg/kg/hr oral infusion until effluent is clear. IV fluids @ 1.5–2x maintenance with 0.9% NaCl to aid renal excretion. Acetazolamide (10 mg/kg q 6 hrs) and aminophylline to enhance renal excretion. Hemodialysis may be option in some cases. *(Continued)*

Metal & Sources	Toxicity	Clinical Effects	Diagnostics	Therapy/ Prevention
Mercury (Hg): Current sources are limited. Ointments, leather preservatives, thermometers, fungicides, barometers, anti-mildew paints, fluorescent bulbs, mercury vapor lamps.	Vapors and organic mercurials absorbed by inhalation and from GIT. Metallic mercury concentrates in GIT and kidney. Organic mercury concentrates in brain. All forms pass the placenta. Cats are highly susceptible.	Organic mercurials cause erythema, conjunctivitis, stomatitis, depression, ataxia, incoordination, proprioceptive deficits, abnormal postures, paresis, and blindness. Hypoproteinemia, proteinuria, and azotemia typical in inorganic Hg poisoning.	Blood (>6.0 ppm) and urine (>1.5 ppm) are good samples for acute to subacute exposure. Hair (>45 ppm) for chronic exposure. Liver (>30 ppm) and kidney (>20 ppm) associated with toxicosis in cats.	Acute inorganic mercury—egg white to inactivate mercury; activated charcoal results variable. Whole bowel irrigation with PEG recommended. Oral sodium thiosulfate (0.5–1.0 g/kg BW) may bind mercury. Antidote: Oral *d*-penicillamine or DMSA may bind Hg. *See dosages at end of table.*
Selenium (Se): Selenium dietary supplements, gun bluing compound, pigments, photocells, photography developing products.	Canine lethal dosage is 1.5–3 mg/ kg both oral and parenteral. Dietary levels of 10–20 ppm are toxic. Selenium causes glutathione depletion, lipid peroxidation, and replaces sulfur in amino acids. May also depress ATP formation.	Acute–vomiting, diarrhea, dyspnea, ataxia, hypovolemia and collapse result from acute exposure. Signs are similar to acute arsenic or iron toxicosis. Chronic—exposure may cause rough, dull hair coat, alopecia, weight loss, and infertility.	Normal blood Se value in dogs is 0.220 ppm. Blood Se >1–2 ppm is presumptive of toxicosis. Kidney and liver values >12 ppm are considered toxic. Chronic exposure is detected with hair analysis.	Life support includes acute therapy for gastroenteritis and shock. Activated charcoal is recommended by some, not by others. Alternatively, gastric lavage with sodium thiosulfate 20% solution may be helpful. Treatment: NAC *See dosages at end of table.* *(Continued)*

Metal & Sources	Toxicity	Clinical Effects	Diagnostics	Therapy/ Prevention
Tin: Food preparation, toothpaste, pigments for ceramics and textiles. Organotins (alkyl tins) used as fungicides, insecticides, wood, leather, textile, preservatives.	Two valence forms (+2 and +4). Prior use of trimethly/ triethyl tin as a fungicide. Organic tins are toxic and well absorbed from GIT, but inorganic forms are highly tolerated.	Organotin target organs are brain, liver, immune system, and skin. Cause skin and eye irritation, colic, diarrhea, hepatotoxicity and neurotoxicity (hyperactivity), seizures, ataxia.	Myelin edema (status spongiosis) and demyelization in CNS. Blood levels >0.3 ppm and liver levels of 0.6 ppm have been associated with organotin toxicosis.	Acute exposures not likely. If occurs, activated charcoal is recommended. BAL for 4 days effective in experimental animals. Sodium thiosulfate may improve response. *See dosages at end of table.* Control fever and hypotension.

Antidotes and dosages: For more details, consult Plumb DC, Plumb's Veterinary Drug Handbook, 6th ed. Wiley-Blackwell, 2008.

- CaNa$_2$EDTA, 100 mg/kg/day SQ in 4 divided doses diluted in D$_5$W. Duration of dosing depends on toxin.
- BAL dogs/cats: 2.5–5 mg/kg IM q 4–12 hours. Multiple days of dosing required (see Plumb's).
- DMSA, metal chelator. Dosage 10 mg/kg PO q 8 hours for 4–15 days depending on metal.
- *d*-penicillamine: 10–15 mg/kg PO q 12 hours. Drug may cause vomiting. Give 1 hour prefeeding.
- NAC: 140 mg/kg PO or IV (5% solution) initially, then 70 mg/kg q 4 hours PO or IV for 3+ treatments.
- Sodium thiosulfate: 40–50 mg/kg IV as 20% solution q 8–12 hours.

Abbreviations

ALT	= alanine aminotransferase
AST	= aspartate aminotransferase
ATP	= adenosine triphosphate
BAL	= British anti-Lewisite (dimercaprol)
BW	= body weight
CaNa$_2$EDTA	= calcium disodium ethylene diamine tetraacetate
CBC	= complete blood count
CCA	= chromated copper arsenate
CNS	= central nervous system
D$_5$W	= dextrose 5% in water
DMSA	= dimercaptosuccinic acid (succimer)
ECG	= electrocardiogram
GIT	= gastrointestinal tract
IM	= intramuscular
IV	= intravenous
K	= potassium

LD_{50}	= median lethal dose
LDH	= Lactate dehydrogenase
NAC	= N-acetylcysteine
PEG	= polyethylene glycol
PO	= *per os* (by mouth)
PU/PD	= polyuria/polydipsia
SQ	= subcutaneous

Author: Gary Osweiler, DVM, PhD, DABVT; Ahna G. Brutlag, DVM

Toxic Plant Tables

Toxic Plants and Their Clinical Signs—Antidotes and Treatment

Plant and characteristics	Clinical signs	Antidotes and treatment
Angel's trumpet (*Brugmansia* spp.; *Datura* spp.) Two genera for same common name. Garden annual with white trumpet-shaped flowers Whole plant toxic: toxicity highest in seeds	Thirst, GI atony, disturbed vision, delirium, hallucinations "Dry as a bone, blind as a bat, red as a beet, mad as a hatter"	Parasympathomimetic drugs (physostigmine)
Autumn crocus (*Colchicum autumnale*) Houseplant Whole plant toxic; toxicity highest in bulbs	Burning sensation in throat and mouth, thirst, nausea, hemorrhagic diarrhea, seizures, cardiac abnormalities	IV fluids, analgesics, anticonvulsants, cardiovascular support
Belladonna lily (*Amaryllis* spp.) potted plant Bulbs are most toxic	Nausea, diarrhea, hypotension, depression	Gastric lavage, charcoal, fluids, and supportive treatment
Bittersweet (*Celastrus* spp.) Weed, vine with red berries Immature fruits are toxic	Gastric irritation, vomiting, diarrhea	Fluids
Bleeding heart (*Dicentra* spp.) Garden, woods, potted plant Roots more toxic than leaves	Vomiting, diarrhea, muscle tremors, convulsions or paralysis	Fluids and seizure control
Castor bean (*Ricinus communis*) Garden shrub or ornamental, grows to 2 m Seeds are 1 cm, dark and light mottled, and highly toxic	Latent period: colic, emesis, severe and hemorrhagic diarrhea, muscle tremors, sudden collapse	Emesis, charcoal, fluids, and electrolytes

(Continued)

835

Plant and characteristics	Clinical signs	Antidotes and treatment
Chinaberry tree (*Melia azedarach*) Ornamental tree in temperate to subtropical areas Berry is most toxic	Salivation, anorexia, vomiting, diarrhea. Followed by weakness, ataxia, seizures	Fluid and electrolyte replacement, anticonvulsants and supportive care
Christmas rose (*Helleborus niger*) House and garden plant Entire plant is toxic	Hypersalivation, vomiting, diarrhea. Cardiac arrhythmias, heart block	Gastric lavage or emesis; activated charcoal or saline cathartics to decontaminate the GI tract
Daphne (*Daphne mezereum*) Landscape shrub Entire plant is toxic	Vesication and edema of the lips and oral cavity, salivation, thirst, abdominal pain, emesis, hemorrhagic diarrhea	Fluid and electrolyte replacement, analgesics
Delphinium or larkspur (*Delphinium* spp.) Outdoor garden, mountains; tall with blue, purple, or pinkish flowers Seeds more toxic than leaves	Trembling, ataxia, weakness, lateral recumbency	GI detoxification; physostigmine to treat muscarinic signs
English holly (*Ilex* spp.) Landscape plant Fruit is toxic	Nausea, vomiting, diarrhea	Fluid and electrolyte replacement
English ivy (*Hedera helix*) Houseplant Fruit and leaves are toxic	Salivation, thirst, emesis, gastroenteritis, diarrhea, dermatitis	Supportive care
Golden chain (*Laburnum anagyroides*) Landscape tree with long chains of yellow flowers Entire plant is toxic	Emesis, depression, weakness, incoordination, mydriasis, tachycardia	GI decontamination with lavage or emesis followed by activated charcoal
Horse chestnut or buckeye (*Aesculus* spp.) Landscape or forest tree; palmate leaves Nuts and twigs most toxic	Gastroenteritis, diarrhea, dehydration, electrolyte imbalance	Fluid and electrolyte replacement, demulcents, and therapy for gastroenteritis

(Continued)

Plant and characteristics	Clinical signs	Antidotes and treatment
Iris or flag (*Iris* spp.) Perennial garden flower Rootstock most toxic	Hypersalivation, vomiting, diarrhea	Fluid and electrolyte replacement
Irish potato (*Solanum tuberosum*) Vegetable garden Vines, green skin, and sprouts are toxic	Vomiting, diarrhea, depression, rapid heart rate, mydriasis, muscle tremors. Signs may vary from atropine-like to cholinesterase inhibition. Use antidotes accordingly and with caution.	GI decontamination. If atropine-like signs predominate, use physostigmine. If salivation and diarrhea are present, use atropine cautiously.
Lantana (*Lantana camara*) Garden and wild in mild temperate to tropical areas: bright orange and yellow, red, purple, or pink flowers Foliage and immature berries are toxic	Weakness, lethargy, vomiting, diarrhea, mydriasis, dyspnea. Advanced signs are cholestasis, bilirubinemia, and photosensitization.	GI decontamination, fluids, and respiratory support. Protect from sunlight and treat for hepatic insufficiency.
Lupine (*Lupinus* spp.) Garden ornamental Seeds more toxic than leaves	Salivation, ataxia, seizures, dyspnea	GI decontamination, anticonvulsants
Mistletoe (*Phoradendron* spp.) Parasitic shrub on other trees Access to pets in homes at holiday time Leaves, stems, and berries are moderately toxic	Vomiting, GI pain, diarrhea	Fluid and electrolyte replacement; demulcents for gastroenteritis
Monkshood (*Aconitum* spp.) Perennial garden ornamental Entire plant is toxic	Salivation, vomiting, diarrhea. Muscle tremors, cardiac irregularities, respiratory depression	GI decontamination, fluid and electrolyte replacement. Manage similar to digitalis glycoside overdose, with caution about potassium administration.
Morning glory (*Ipomoea purpurea* and *Ipomoea tricolor*) Garden annual, potted plant Seeds most toxic; risk increased when seeds are pre-soaked Occasionally used as hallucinogen	Nausea, mydriasis, hallucinations, decreased reflexes, diarrhea, hypotension	Activated charcoal; dark, quiet surroundings; tranquilization as needed

(Continued)

837

Plant and characteristics	Clinical signs	Antidotes and treatment
Mountain laurel (*Kalmia* spp.) Native of eastern and southeastern woods, mountains Leaves and flowers are toxic Honey from nectar also toxic	Oral irritation, salivation, projectile vomiting, diarrhea, weakness, impaired vision, bradycardia, hypotension, AV block	Emetics are contraindicated. Use activated charcoal, fluid replacement, and respiratory support as needed.
Narcissus, daffodil, jonquil (*Narcissus* spp.) Garden ornamental bulb Bulb is most toxic	Nausea, vomiting, hypotension, diarrhea	Gastric lavage, charcoal, fluid replacement, supportive treatment for gastroenteritis
Nettle (*Urtica doica*) Garden weed Hairs on leaves contain toxin that enters skin on contact	Oral irritation and pain, hypersalivation, swelling and edema of nose and periocular areas or other areas of skin contact	Antihistamines and analgesics. Local or systemic anti-inflammatory supportive therapy to treat affected contact areas
Poinsettia (*Euphorbia pulcherrima*) Garden or potted plant, especially at Christmas holidays Sap of stem and leaves is mildly to moderately irritant or toxic	Irritation of mouth: may cause vomiting, diarrhea, and dermatitis	Demulcents and fluids to prevent dehydration
Rosary pea or precatory bean (*Abrus precatorius*) Native of Caribbean islands Seeds (when broken or chewed) are highly toxic Illegal to import into United States	Nausea, vomiting, diarrhea, weakness, tachycardia, possible renal failure, coma, death	Emesis or lavage followed with charcoal, demulcents, fluids, and electrolytes.
Thorn apple or jimsonweed (*Datura stramonium*) Annual weed, some species are ornamental (*Datura metel*) Entire plant is toxic, but seeds are most toxic and available	Thirst, disturbances of vision, delirium, mydriasis, GI atony. "Hot as a pistol, blind as a bat, red as a beet, mad as a hatter"	Parasympathomimetic drug (e.g., physostigmine)
Tobacco (*Nicotiana tabacum*) Garden plant, weed, cigarettes Whole plant is toxic	Rapid onset of salivation, nausea, emesis, tremors, incoordination, and ataxia, followed by collapse and respiratory failure	Assist ventilation and provide vascular support. After respiratory support, decontaminate the GI tract with lavage and activated charcoal.

(Continued)

Plant and characteristics	Clinical signs	Antidotes and treatment
Wisteria (*Wisteria* spp.) Woody vine or shrub with blue to white legume flowers Entire plant is toxic	Nausea, abdominal pain, prolonged vomiting	Antiemetics and fluid replacement therapy
Yellow jessamine (*Gelsemium sempervirens*) Mild temperate to subtropical climates Yellow trumpet-shaped flowers grow on evergreen vines	Weakness, seizures, paralysis, respiratory failure	Symptomatic and supportive therapy of respiration. GI decontamination and fluid replacement therapy

Authors: Gary D. Osweiler, DVM, PhD, DABVT; Lynn R. Hovda, RPH, DVM, MS, DACVIM

Topical Toxins: Common Human OTC Dermatological Preparations

For information on topical preparations with a greater potential for toxicity, including 5-fluoruracil (5-FU), calcipotriene (vitamin D), imidazoline decongestants, nicotine or fentanyl transdermal patches, pyrethrin/pyrethroid insecticides, salicylate (aspirin) creams, and tea tree oil (melaleuca oil), see the individual chapter.

Product Category and Trade Name	Active Ingredients	Toxicity	Clinical Signs	Treatment	Prognosis
Analgesics (camphor): Campho-Phenique Carmex Tiger Balm Arthritis Rub; White; Red Vicks VapoRub	Camphor, up to 11%	Toxicity is not well established in cats/dogs. <1 g of camphor has caused death in children. Mouse LD_{50} (oral) = 1310 mg/kg. Camphor is readily absorbed across the skin.	Onset of signs is 5–20 minutes. Dermal application can cause local irritation. Any ingestion can cause GI distress Large ingestion can cause CNS depression and seizures (humans). Death from respiratory depression/seizures.	No antidote. GI protectants if needed. Benzodiazepines or barbiturates for seizures. Respiratory support. Monitor blood pressure and vitals.	Good with treatment/mild signs. Severe signs without treatment have a poorer prognosis. If no signs by 60 min, toxicosis unlikely.
Antibiotics: Duospore Polysporin Lanabiotic Medi-Quik Neosporin Triple Antibiotic	Bacitracin Neomycin Polymyxin B	Not established. Severe toxicity is not expected from acute ingestion/application.	Self-limiting vomiting and diarrhea (partly from the petroleum-based carrier). Anaphylaxis in cats with ocular administration (very rare).	Supportive GI care. Treat for anaphylaxis with O_2, epinephrine, fluids, diphenhydramine, possible steroids.	Excellent with acute ingestions and appropriate treatment for anaphylaxis if needed.

(Continued)

Product Category and Trade Name	Active Ingredients	Toxicity	Clinical Signs	Treatment	Prognosis
Antifungals: Femstat Lamisil AT Lotrimin AF Monistat Neosporin AF Nizoral A-D Spectazole Vagistat	Butoconazole, 2% Clotrimazole, 1%–2% Econazole, 1% Ketoconazole, 1%–2% Miconazole, 2%–4% Terbinafine, 1% Tioconazole, 1%–6.5% Tolnaftate, 1%	Generally, all OTC antifungal preparations have a wide margin of safety, especially in acute ingestions.	Self-limiting vomiting and diarrhea (partly from the carriers).	Supportive GI care.	Excellent with acute ingestions.
Antihistamines: Benadryl Caladryl Dermamycin Ziradryl	Diphenhydramine (DPH), 1%–2%	Toxicity unlikely with ingestion of topical DPH or significant topical application (poor dermal absorption). Oral: 2–4 mg/kg (therapeutic dose), mild CNS depression and anticholinergic effects. Large oral overdoses may cause severe CNS stimulation.	Following ingestion: Common—vomiting and diarrhea, especially from carriers. Lethargy, dry mouth, urinary retention. Uncommon—CNS stimulation, agitation, and tachycardia from large oral overdoses.	Emesis and activated charcoal (large ingestions only). Sedation and GI support as needed.	Excellent following ingestion of topical preparations.

(Continued)

Product Category and Trade Name	Active Ingredients	Toxicity	Clinical Signs	Treatment	Prognosis
Antiseptics (benzoyl peroxide): Clean & Clear PERSA Gel-10 Clearasil Acne Treatment PanOxyl Acne Face Wash Proactiv Acne Cleanser	Benzoyl peroxide, 2.5%–10%	Minimal systemic absorption may occur from topical administration. Severe toxicity is not expected from small, acute ingestions/applications. Large ingestions may cause tissue irritation. Mouse oral LD_{50} = 5,700 mg/kg	Dermal and ocular irritation, including hyperemia and blistering or ulceration (rare) following topical exposure. GI irritation (vomiting, pain, gas, diarrhea) likely with small ingestions. Erosion/ulceration possible with massive ingestions.	Dermal or ocular decontamination. Dilution or gas decompression if ingested. Supportive GI care and GI protectants.	Good with acute ingestions or topical reactions.
Corticosteroids: Cortaid Penecort Procort Scalpicin	Hydrocortisone, 0.5%–1%	Ingestion, even in massive doses, is unlikely to cause harmful effects. Therapeutic dose = 5 mg/kg PO.	Self-limiting vomiting, diarrhea (partly from carriers) with possible PU/PD.	Supportive GI care. Access to water.	Excellent with acute ingestions.

(Continued)

Product Category and Trade Name	Active Ingredients	Toxicity	Clinical Signs	Treatment	Prognosis
Local anesthetics: Cetacaine Chigger X Plus Goodwinol Solarcaine	Benzocaine, 5%–20% Dibucaine, 1% Lidocaine, 0.5%–2.5% Prilocaine, 2.5%	Oral toxic dose is not established. 1–2 licks are unlikely to cause toxicity. Larger ingestions pose greater risk. Dibucaine is more toxic than lidocaine. Topical lidocaine is systemically absorbed; toxicity unlikely unless used chronically. High first-pass effect makes oral toxicity less likely.	Anesthetization of the pharynx can lead to aspiration. Methemoglobinemia and Heinz bodies can occur with ingestion. Cats are more sensitive and can develop methemoglobinemia or seizures more readily than dogs. Dibucaine can cause seizures, arrhythmias, hypotension, death.	Emesis of questionable efficacy. Charcoal if no risk of aspiration (stomach tube). Treat for methemoglobinemia if present. More aggressive treatment needed for some exposures and species.	Good with appropriate care.

Abbreviations

AC = activated charcoal
CBC = complete blood count
CNS = central nervous system
GI = gastrointestinal
LD_{50} = median lethal dose
OTC = over-the-counter
PO = *per os* (by mouth)
PU/PD = polyuria, polydipsia

Suggested Reading

Welch S. Local anesthetic toxicosis. Vet Med 2000; 95(9);670–673.
Welch S. Oral toxicity of topical preparations. Vet Clin Small Anim Pract 2002; 32:443–453.

Authors: Ahna G. Brutlag, DVM; Catherine Adams, DVM

Index

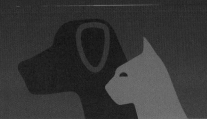

Clinical Toxicology of Agents Toxic to Small Companion Animals

User Note: Clinical toxicology often involves the dual role of treating and advising clients about specific toxicant exposures or potential risks, or the process of reaching a clinical diagnosis when a known or suspected exposure is not available. Often, the patient presents with clinical signs suggestive of a poisoning and key different diagnoses of specific toxicants must be investigated.

Section 1 provides traditional access to information about specific toxicants. This section is beneficial when clients ask specific questions about a product, or when there is a known exposure to a poison.

Section 2 is designed to assist approaching a clinical diagnosis using clinical signs and history reported or observed, but when a confirmed or suspected exposure is not available. Forty-four clinical effects commonly associated with toxicosis are presented with 104 associated toxicants or toxicant groups discussed in this volume. We hope you find this two-part index useful.

Index by Toxicant

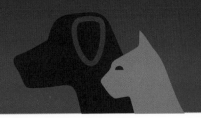

Note: Chapter titles are bolded and chapter paging shows inclusive pages. Page numbers followed by "t" refer to tables; page numbers followed by "f" are figures. Cross references to chapter titles are not bolded.

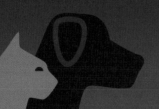

Index by Clinical Signs

- This index provides a quick review of clinical signs or physiological conditions documented for toxicants discussed in this book. This section is intended to assist clinicians with differential diagnoses of specific toxicants.
- Four appendix tables are designated by the letter A (A1, A2, A3, A4) for their respective categories.
- The chapter numbers are preceded by a capital C (e.g., C6).
- Page numbers follow the chapter numbers.
- Users are also encouraged to use a reliable online resource such as the Cornell University Consultant database (www.vet.cornell.edu/consultant/consult.asp) or www.ivis.org as described in Appendix 1.

Clinical Sign(s) or Physiological Abnormality and Selected Relevant Toxicants